CULTURE
&
CLINICAL CARE

CULTURE
&
CLINICAL CARE

EDITED BY
JULIENE G. LIPSON
SUZANNE L. DIBBLE

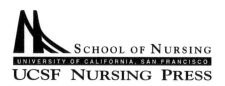

SCHOOL OF NURSING
UNIVERSITY OF CALIFORNIA, SAN FRANCISCO
UCSF NURSING PRESS

Senior publications coordinator: Kathleen McClung
Design/production: Patricia Walsh Design, Monica Lacerda
Editor: Paul Engstrom
Front cover photographer: Jan Watson
Weaver: Susan Hayes

For information, contact:
UCSF Nursing Press
School of Nursing
University of California-San Francisco
521 Parnassus Avenue, Room N-535C
San Francisco, CA 94143-0608 U.S.A.
Phone: (415) 476-4992
Fax: (415) 476-6042
Internet: http://nurseweb.ucsf.edu/www/books.htm

ISBN # 0-943671-22-1

Printed in U.S.A.

TABLE OF CONTENTS

PREFACE

THE INSPIRATION FOR OUR first book, *Culture & Nursing Care: A Pocket Guide*, was *Beyond Boundaries*, a resource manual initiated by Tereza De Paula and developed by the Cultural Diversity Enhancement Committee at the University of California-San Francisco Medical Center in the early 1990s. In 1994, UCSF's Alpha Eta chapter of Sigma Theta Tau created an ad hoc cultural committee that decided to publish a quick, easy-to-use reference for nurses to help them care for patients from diverse cultural/ethnic backgrounds. Several contributors to *Beyond Boundaries* rewrote and expanded their chapters for *Culture & Nursing Care: A Pocket Guide*.

The pocket guide was a success; numerous hospitals, health care agencies, and health science curricula have used it. However, readers encouraged us to include information about European Americans, given that not all clinicians in the U.S. are of European descent. Therefore, the cultural groups in this new edition, *Culture & Clinical Care*, were selected based on their size according to the U.S. Census (each one numbers at least 100,000) and/or on the lack of readily obtainable information elsewhere about a particular group.

Except for African Americans, American Indians/Alaskan Natives, and the European groups, most chapters describe immigrants who came to North America in the second half of the 20th century. The stimuli for this large influx of refugees and immigrants were the 1951 United Nations policy on refugees and the 1965 immigration law that loosened the U.S. quota system so people from all continents could immigrate.

It is very difficult to describe both the common characteristics of cultural/ethnic groups and the diversity within them, and still keep the information brief enough to be easily accessible. Chapters range in scope from cultural groups that are more homogeneous, such as Cambodians, to those that are highly heterogeneous, such as African Americans and immigrants from India. To keep the book to a reasonable length, we have combined tribes or ethnic groups that could probably be described in separate chapters, citing differences among them that are important for health care.

We changed the book title to *Culture & Clinical Care* to be more inclusive of all clinicians and other health care providers, such as chaplains and social workers. It is a practical guide rather than an academic text for college or university coursework, although some might use it for that purpose. *Culture & Clinical Care* certainly is not a cookbook for providing health care to any particular patient in a designated cultural/ethnic group. Rather, its guidelines alert clinicians to issues that may affect health care. If clinicians have doubts or questions, they should ask the patient and family.

We want to thank the following individuals for their contributions to our first book, whose information is included in *Culture & Clinical Care*; contributors to the new edition revised and expanded their previously published chapters. Pamela Minarik, a member of the Sigma Theta Tau cultural committee, helped to conceive—and, as an editor, wrote—the chapter on religion in *Culture & Nursing Care: A Pocket Guide*. Others who contributed to the first book were Linda Boateng (Black/African Americans); Josea Kramer (American Indians); Joyceen S. Boyle (Central Americans); Eden Rivera (Filipinos); Ghislaine Paperwalla (Haitians); Tatiana Reardon (Koreans); Tereza de Paula, Kathleen Laganá, and Leticia Gonzalez-Ramirez (Mexican Americans); Rozina Rajwani (South Asians); and Nenita Nguyan (Vietnamese).

ACKNOWLEDGMENTS

WE WISH TO THANK the chapter authors for their fine work and patient cooperation with our many queries. We also thank Dean Kathleen Dracup for her encouragement and support for beginning this book. In addition, we thank Paul Engstrom, copy editing; Monica Lacerda and Patricia Walsh, design and layout; and Kathleen McClung, senior publications coordinator, for their assistance.

Juliene thanks her husband, Chris Bjorklund, and sons Trevor and Colin for their constant support and patience during the writing and editing process, as they have waited for her to "really" retire.

Sue thanks her partner, Jeanne DeJoseph, PhD, CNM, FAAN, for all of her assistance and support during the construction of this book. She also thanks her mother for providing an environment of cultural interest and respect while she was growing up.

INTRODUCTION

PROVIDING CULTURALLY APPROPRIATE HEALTH CARE

Juliene G. Lipson and Suzanne L. Dibble

DIVERSITY IS PART OF THE FABRIC of American public life. References to diversity, with all its various meanings, permeate the media as well as the popular and academic literature. Sources of diversity must be considered *within* each of the groups that the following chapters describe and, indeed, in any work about the health beliefs and practices of a specific ethnic, racial, or immigrant group.

People have various beliefs about the transitions that accompany health, illness, birth, and death. Most of these beliefs are mediated by culture, age, and length of time in the U.S. "Culture" refers to integrated patterns of human behavior that include the language, thoughts, communications, actions, customs, beliefs, values, and/or institutions of racial, ethnic, religious, and/or social groups. Culture mediates between human beings and chaos, influences what people perceive, and guides their interactions. However, while important, culture is only one of a number of influences on human behavior in the face of illness and other life transitions. One definition of culturally appropriate care includes sensitivity to issues related to race, gender, sexual orientation, social class, and economic situation among factors such as disability (Meleis, Isenberg, Koerner, and Stern, 1995).

Health care providers cannot provide good care without assessing both cultural group patterns and individual variation within a cultural group. Providing appropriate, cross-cultural health care is impossible without partnerships based on trusting, respectful, and responsible relationships between health care providers and patients, their families, and communities.

Yet, as health care providers, we cannot develop good partnerships without knowing what *we* bring to such relationships. It is important that we reflect on our own beliefs about, and approach to, health transitions because openness to other practices begins with self-knowledge. We must acknowledge our own beliefs and biases about specific groups of people that may be inadvertently communicated to patients and families. Awareness of our own verbal and nonverbal communication styles allows us to avoid social gaffes that may offend patients and families. Flexibility in how we communicate enhances our trust-worthiness. We need a sensitive approach to cultural similarities as well as differences, and we need knowledge to inform our practice.

This perspective can be summarized as ASK™ (awareness, sensitivity, and knowledge). Patients are the experts regarding their lives. When we approach a patient and ASK,™ our care can be more appropriate, no matter what group we are working with. The authors anticipate that health care providers will use the information in this book to enhance their ability to ASK.™

LIMITATIONS OF INFORMATION

This guidebook emphasizes information. Its purpose is to sensitize health care providers to cultural variations within each group it describes, to encourage asking questions, and to stimulate learning about how patients identify with and express their cultural background. By itself, information about a specific cultural/ethnic group does *not* make for culturally appropriate care, but neither can good care be provided in the absence of such information. Many health care providers believe that good clinical skills, interpersonal sensitivity, and treating the patient and family members as individuals are sufficient. However, the authors believe that all health care providers need to know something about their patients' sociocultural backgrounds because it is easy to inadvertently insult a patient or family when clinicians act only on what they believe is correct, which is usually based only on their own values and/or education.

Cultural information can lead to insensitive care if it is used in a cookbook manner, as in attempting to apply cultural "facts" indiscriminately to a patient of a particular ethnic group. Such information can lead to stereotyping patients, particularly by providers who lack self-awareness, are ethnocentric, or fail to recognize variability within any cultural group. In *stereotyping*, one makes an assumption about a person based on group membership without learning whether or not the individual in question fits that assumption. It is different from *generalizing*, which begins with an assumption about a group but leads to a quest for further information as to whether the assumption fits the individual. So it is important to learn whether people consider themselves typical of, or different from, others in their cultural group because many factors may influence how individuals express their culture and under what circumstances such expression is important. The authors do not use the term "culturally competent" to describe cross-cultural, health-care interactions. They believe that the term "competence" indicates mastery—an unreachable goal, given the variety and large number of cultural groups. The ASK™ perspective is a more realistic and effective approach to providing cross-cultural health care.

CULTURAL ASSESSMENT

A thorough cultural assessment can take many hours, but health care providers rarely have that luxury. The authors believe that, at a minimum, the following questions (adapted from Lipson and Meleis, 1985) should be asked and the answers to them recorded:

- What is the patient's ethnic affiliation?
- Who are the patient's major support persons and where do they live?
- With whom should we speak about the patient's health or illness?
- What are the patient's primary and secondary languages, and speaking and reading abilities?
- What is the patient's economic situation? Is income adequate to meet the patient's and family's needs?

When patients are immigrants, it is useful to know where they grew up as well as the decade of their arrival in the U.S. because time has an impact on acculturation, communication, health beliefs, and practices. Health care providers must be aware, however, that some patients are reluctant to divulge their birthplace or time of arrival in the U.S. for fear of deportation, even when they have legal documents. If asked, they may not return for care.

SOURCES OF DIVERSITY

Immigrants and refugees. Except for American Indians/Alaskan Natives and Hawaiians, the U.S. has been populated by immigrants from all parts of the world who arrived during different eras. Some groups did not leave their country by choice. For example, Africans were brought to the U.S. as slaves, and many refugees cared more about finding a safe haven than they did about reaching a particular destination. In considering the health and adjustment of immigrants and refugees, it is important for clinicians to take into account why they left their homeland and what drew them to the U.S.

The U.S. Immigration and Naturalization Service defines an *immigrant* as a "nonresident alien admitted for permanent residence." A *refugee* is someone who is admitted outside normal quota restrictions based on a well-founded fear of persecution because of race, religion, nationality, social group, or political opinion. *Asylum-seekers* come to the U.S. and apply for refugee status. An *undocumented person* (the term we prefer to "illegal alien") is an entrant who does not possess documents that would allow him/her to reside legally in the U.S..

Migration within North America also is an important consideration. Some groups have had to relocate; examples are American Indians forced onto reservations and Japanese who were interned during World War II. Migration is stressful even when people choose it. Among those who have experienced a radical change of environment in the U.S. are African Americans, who moved from the rural South to northern cities, and farmworkers, who move frequently from place to place as they follow the crops.

Race/ethnicity. These terms often are erroneously interchanged. *Race* refers to human biological variation, even though there is no scientific basis for discrete biological categories corresponding with social definitions of race. At the DNA level, studies show that humans are 99% alike, regardless of racial differences. Thus, from a genetic standpoint, skin color and other characteristics of appearance are insignificant. On the other hand, race is socially and politically significant because of racism, which Krieger, Rowley, Herman, et al. (1993) define as "an oppressive system of racial relations, justified by ideology, in which one racial group benefits from dominating another and defines itself and others through this domination." Epidemiology links race to higher disease risks, such as those for hypertension and low birth weight among African Americans. However, the social context of racism or poverty, rather than biology, is probably the basis for such differences because they expose people to economic and environmental risks and they influence interpersonal experiences.

Ethnicity refers to a socially, culturally, and politically constructed group that holds in common a set of characteristics not shared by others with whom members of the group come into contact. These characteristics typically include, but are not limited to, a common ancestry, language, and religion; a sense of historical continuity; and interactions with persons in the same group. *Ethnic identity* is a sense of peoplehood, a consciously shared system of beliefs, values, loyalties, and practices that demonstrates identification with a distinctive group. Some people demonstrate their ethnic identity through a symbolic aspect of culture, such as language (e.g., by speaking "Black English") or clothing (e.g., by wearing turbans or head scarves). In any ethnic group, the strength of individuals' ethnic identity varies. Moreover, ethnic identity is not static; the social, political, historical, generational, and interpersonal situation may influence how strongly someone expresses it. For example, since the "war on terrorism" began in the U.S., significant numbers of persons with a Middle Eastern appearance or name have encountered social bias, prejudice, and harassment, and therefore may be less inclined to express their ethnic identity.

Socioeconomic status and social class. Socioeconomic status is related to income, education, and occupation. Within any ethnic/racial group, one must assess socioeconomic status because it may well be a stronger influence on health and access to care than cultural factors are. For example, numerous studies show that poverty is a stronger influence on health and use of health care than ethnicity is. Poverty imposes environmental risks, such as inadequate or no housing, exposure to high levels of lead or industrial toxins, and little access to green open space, and also imposes social risks, such as isolation, gangs, drug traffic, and poor schools. The death rate among U.S. residents with an annual income below the poverty level is several times higher than that among those with a median or higher income (Kaplan, Pamuk, Lynch, Cohen, and Balfour, 1996).

Health care providers must acknowledge that, among immigrants, social-class origin may be a very powerful determinant of how people relate to each other. This influence may or may not decrease in succeeding generations. In addition, acculturated and educated, middle-class immigrants among different ethnic or immigrant groups may have more in common with each other and with persons in the dominant culture than they do with new immigrants or less financially fortunate persons from their home country.

Sexual orientation. Variations in sexual orientation also cross ethnic, racial, and socioeconomic boundaries, so health care providers must consider orientation when assessing a patient in any cultural group. In some areas of the U.S., gay and lesbian subcultures are rich and visible, while in other areas, social stigma keeps gays and lesbians closeted. However, health care providers may inadvertently offend their gay and lesbian patients by assuming they are heterosexual instead of routinely asking, "If you are sexual with others, are they men, women, or both?" Providers may miss important data as well as an opportunity to communicate a nonjudgmental attitude. They must record this information carefully or not at all if the patient has any concerns about how their medical records might be used.

Gender identity. This term means having a subjective, but continuous and persistent, sense of being male or female regardless of one's biological sex. In every cultural group, there are behaviors, attitudes, values, and beliefs deemed appropriate for males and females based on their biological sex. Although gender identity is subjective and internal, others perceive the presentation of self through personality or bodily habitus; at best, they may view such presentation as "different" or, at worst, as "a reason to kill." (See www.lgbthealthchannel.com/transgender for more information.)

Disability. The largest minority in the U.S. comprises disabled persons, 15–20% of whom have a disabling condition that interferes with life activities (Davis, 1997). *Disability* is usually defined as a physical or mental impairment that substantially limits one or more major life activities—i.e., a restriction or inability to perform or accomplish an activity within a "normal range." In contrast, a *handicap* is a social or other kind of disadvantage that accompanies and stems from the disability. For example, less education among disabled persons is a key source of greater poverty and unemployment.

Like sexual orientation and race, cultural perceptions of disability depend on the social context in which someone lives and interacts. The concepts of disability, handicap, and rehabilitation originated in North America and Northern Europe, both of which value autonomy over dependence (Ingstad and Whyte, 1995). In the U.S., disabled persons are entitled to the same rights as others are and their integration into society is expected. The Americans with Disabilities Act of 1990 seeks to make society more accessible in terms of employment, public services and accommodations, and telecommunications. It also prohibits coercion, threat, or retaliation against disabled persons or those attempting to help them assert their rights under the law. In contrast, group-oriented cultures in which interdependence is valued may take it for granted that families help disabled members and that dependence on others does not carry a stigma.

VARIATIONS IN COMMUNICATION

Even when a health care provider and patient speak the same language, different values or beliefs may hamper communication. Nonverbal differences or regional or ethnic dialects can inhibit mutual understanding. Variations in communication include:

Conversational style and pacing. Silence may indicate respect or acknowledgment that the listener has heard the speaker; in cultures in which saying "no" directly is considered rude, silence may mean "no." Style of conversation varies: Answers can be blunt and to the point, indirect, or entail storytelling. The patient may speak loudly or repetitively to convey anger or simply to emphasize something.

Eye contact. Culturally appropriate eye contact may vary from intense to fleeting. Avoiding direct eye contact may be a sign of respect, an effort not to invade someone's privacy, or an appropriate behavior between genders. It is easy to misinterpret cultural differences as negative personality characteristics.

Personal space. Individuals react to others based on their own culture, rarely recognizing that cultural conceptions of personal space differ. For example, someone may be perceived as "aggressive" for standing too close or as "distant" or "cold" for backing off when approached.

Touch. Every culture has norms governing how and when it is appropriate to touch someone else. For example, there may be cultural prohibitions against touching certain parts of the body—perhaps the head or touching the feet before the head. In some cultural/ethnic groups, physical contact among those of the same gender, such as greeting with an embrace or walking hand-in-hand, is more appropriate than among unrelated persons of the opposite gender. In health care, examination of the genitals by someone of the opposite gender may be particularly problematic. Even discussing reproduction might be acutely embarrassing.

Time orientation. Some cultures pace life according to clock time, which they value more highly than personal or subjective time. Others place greater value on interacting with people and completing interpersonal encounters; being "on time" is of secondary importance.

COMMUNICATION AND INTERPRETERS

Language differences pose a barrier to even the most basic cultural assessment. The Office of Minority Health at the U.S. Department of Health and Human Services (2000) has issued standards for culturally and linguistically appropriate care. Standard 4 states: "Health care organizations must offer and provide language assistance services, including bilingual staff and interpreter services, at no cost to each patient/consumer with limited English proficiency at all points of contact, in a timely manner during all hours of operation." Standard 6 states that "family and friends should not be used to provide interpretation services except on request by the patient/consumer."

As numerous chapters in this book illustrate, role conflicts or lack of medical vocabulary often interfere with accurate interpretation. For example, family members often base their messages to both the patient and health care provider on their own perception of the situation and, as interpreters, may withhold vital information out of embarrassment. When communicating serious or terminal illness, it may be culturally acceptable for family members to withhold bad news from the patient to protect him/her. Even bilingual friends, community members, or agency employees may be ineffective as interpreters if they are not trained or the health care provider does not use them appropriately. It is also important to remember that some cultural/ethnic communities are small and an interpreter may know everyone in the community; thus, training in confidentiality issues becomes even more critical.

The following guidelines (adapted from Randall-David, 1989, p. 32) are helpful when working with an interpreter:

- During the interaction, look at, and speak directly to, the patient, not the interpreter.
- Listen to the patient, observing his/her nonverbal communication, such as facial expressions, voice intonations, and body movements, to learn about emotions associated with the topic.
- Be patient. An interpreted interview may take more than twice as long as an ordinary interchange takes because careful interpretation often requires long, explanatory phrases.
- Before the session, meet with the interpreter to explain its purpose.
- Encourage the interpreter to meet with the patient before the session to assess the latter's educational level and attitudes about health and health care. That way, the interpreter can gauge the depth and type of information and explanation that are necessary.
- Speak in short units of speech; do not use long, complicated sentences or paragraphs. If a discussion is complex, do not address more than one topic in a single session.
- Use simple language; avoid technical terms, abbreviations, professional jargon, colloquialisms, abstractions, idioms, slang, and metaphors.
- Encourage the interpreter to use the patient's own words as much as possible rather than paraphrase them in professional jargon. The patient's words provide a better sense of his/her ideas and emotional state.
- Encourage the interpreter to refrain from inserting his/her own ideas or interpretations, and from omitting information.
- Check the patient's understanding and accuracy of the interpretation by asking him/her to repeat the message or instructions in his/her own words with help from the interpreter.

Potential cultural conflicts may arise as a result of the Health Insurance Portability and Accountability Act (HIPAA) of 1996, which seeks to guarantee the security and privacy of health information. A clinician who informs the head of the family about a patient's condition—the most appropriate course in some cultures—is violating HIPAA. One way to circumvent HIPAA and still be culturally appropriate is to have patients complete a form detailing how their personal information should be delivered and to whom.

SUMMARY

There is considerable variation in every cultural group. The intersection of these variations creates experiences unique to individuals, each of whom views experiences through the lens of his/her own personality and resources. The chapters in this book should *not* be used as blueprints for patient characteristics. Rather, their purpose is to alert clinicians to potential factors they should consider in order to provide good care. People, even if ill, are experts regarding their own lives, culture, and experiences. If providers have a genuine desire to learn and ASK™ with respect, people typically help clinicians provide culturally appropriate care.

REFERENCES

Davis, L. (1997). Introduction. In L. Davis (Ed.), *The disability studies reader*, pp. 1–6. New York: Routledge.

Ingstad, B., & Whyte, S. R. (1995). Disability and culture: An overview. In B. Ingstad & S. Whyte (Eds.), *Disability and culture*, pp. 3–32. Berkeley, CA: University of California Press.

Kaplan, G., Pamuk, E., Lynch, J., Cohen, R., & Balfour, J. (1996). Inequality in income and mortality in the U.S.: Analysis of mortality and potential pathways. *British Medical Journal*, 312, 999–1003.

Krieger, N., Rowley, D., Herman, A., Avery, B., & Phillips, M. (1993). Racism, sexism, and social class: Implications for studies of health, disease, and well-being. *American Journal of Preventive Medicine*, 9 (suppl. 6), 82–122.

Lipson, J. G., & Meleis, A. I. (1985). Culturally appropriate care: The case of immigrants. *Topics in Clinical Nursing*, 7, 48–56.

Lipson, J., & Rogers, J. (2000). Cultural aspects of disability. *Journal of Transcultural Nursing*, 11, 212–219.

Meleis, A., Isenberg, M., Koerner, J., & Stern, P. (1995). *Diversity, marginalization, and culturally competent health care: Issues in knowledge development*. Washington, DC: American Academy of Nursing.

Office of Minority Health, U.S. Department of Health and Human Services. (2000). Assuring cultural competence in health care: Recommendations for national standards and an outcomes-focused research agenda. *Federal Register*, 65, 80865–80879. Available at http://www.OMHRC.gov/CLAS

Randall-David, E. (1989). *Strategies for working with culturally diverse communities and clients*. Bethesda, MD: Association for the Care of Children's Health.

ABOUT THE EDITORS

JULIENE G. LIPSON, RN, PHD, FAAN, is a professor emerita in the Department of Community Health Systems and the Department of Anthropology, History, and Social Medicine at the University of California-San Francisco, where she taught international, cross-cultural, and community health nursing. Her ethnographic research has focused on women's birth transitions; on immigrants and refugees from the Middle East, Afghanistan, Bosnia, and the former Soviet Union; and, most recently, on disability and stigmatized, chronic health conditions. She has authored or edited eight books and 78 articles and book chapters.

SUZANNE L. DIBBLE, DNSC, RN, is a professor at the Institute for Health & Aging, Department of Social and Behavioral Sciences at the University of California-San Francisco. She has authored more than 75 articles and given more than 200 presentations nationally and internationally, primarily about living with chronic illness. She has twice received the prestigious Schering Corporation Award for excellence in cancer nursing research from the Oncology Nursing Society.

CULTURE
&
CLINICAL CARE

CHAPTER 1

AFGHANS

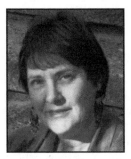 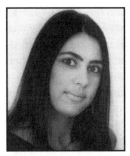

Juliene G. Lipson   Razia Askaryar

CULTURAL/ETHNIC IDENTITY

- **Preferred term(s)**. "Afghan," sometimes "Afghanistani." "Afghani" (the unit of money) used erroneously. Share some religion and nationality, but the heterogeneous population is strongly divided along tribal, political, ethnic, and social-class lines.
- **Census**. The 2000 U.S. Census reports 53,709 persons of Afghan descent, but this significantly underrepresents actual number. Estimates range from 60,000–100,000; some 40,000–50,000 live in the San Francisco Bay Area, about half of whom were born in U.S.
- **History of immigration**. Began to leave Afghanistan after the 1978 communist coup. Was the world's largest refugee population for more than a decade. The country has experienced 25 years of war, including intertribal strife (1989–1996) and Taliban control until 2002. Arrivals in North America in the early 1980s were urban, formerly wealthy, and highly educated. Later arrivals were less-educated, middle-class relatives. Many lived in Pakistan, India, or Europe before coming to U.S., but relatively few came from refugee camps. A small minority are of rural origin, highly traditional, and illiterate in their own languages.

SPIRITUAL/RELIGIOUS ORIENTATION

- **Primary religious/spiritual affiliations**. Most are Muslim, the majority Sunni (84%). Shi'a Muslims make up 15% and others 1%. Muslims believe in one God (Allah) and that Mohammed is God's final messenger.
- **Usual religious/spiritual practices**. Muslims pray directly to God privately or together (*jamaa'a*) at home or in a mosque when an *imam* or *mullah* (spiritual leaders) may lead prayers. Usually, women and men are separated in the

mosque. Expected to act in accordance with God's commands as described in the Koran (*Qur'an*), which includes rules for cleanliness and hygiene, diet, prayer, and moral values. Muslims range from very strict to more relaxed; e.g., they may pray to themselves rather than at specific times.

- **Use of spiritual healing/healers**. Some *mullahs* do religious healing through prayer and by writing Koranic verses on paper; the patient imbibes these verses by drinking water in which the paper has been soaked. Staff should give the patient and family privacy when spiritual healer present. There is no conflict with Western medicine.
- **Holidays**. Muslim holy days include *Eid al-Fitr* (end of Ramadan) and *Eid al-Adha* (end of the annual pilgrimage to Mecca). Observed by going to the mosque, where *mullah* leads families in prayer. A breakfast feast at home follows. Later, there are visits to other family and friends for tea, lunch, or dinner. Secular holidays include Afghan New Year (*Norooz*) (March 21), celebrated with a large picnic and social activities in a park.

COMMUNICATION
ORAL COMMUNICATION

- **Major languages and dialects**. National languages are Dari (50%), a dialect of Persian, and Pashto (35%). There are more than 30 minor languages and many Afghans speak more than one dialect. Young immigrants/refugees, the most well-educated, and the U.S.-born speak English.
- **Greetings**. Address elderly persons with respectful terms such as "Uncle," "Aunt," or "Mother"—e.g., *Bibi* (aunt) Asifa. Strangers not told the legal or familial name of an adult woman. Greetings between nonfamily members may be a simple nod or handshake. Women greet each other with a kiss on each cheek. A man may greet another man with hugs and kisses but greets an unrelated woman with a respectful hand on his chest, without any touching or eye contact.
- **Tone of voice**. Women tend to speak loudly in public to express affection; at home, the mother's voice symbolizes power over children. Men prefer soft tones to demonstrate their control over the situation; a show of aggression means losing control and is disrespectful in public. Pashto speakers may sound argumentative, while Dari speakers may emphasize polite words even when they have strong feelings about an issue.
- **Direct or indirect style of speech**. Tend to speak in stories rather than brief answers. Can be direct when giving medical history, but they avoid personal topics related to genitals, breasts, or sex. Older persons communicate less directly than younger or acculturated people do, but it depends on whom one is speaking with.
- **Use of interpreters**. Clinician should avoid using children or other family members. Ideal interpreter is trained, respected in the community, and of the same gender as, and about the same age as or older than, the patient.

- **Serious or terminal illness**. Family generally hides bad news from the patient. Communicate first to spouse, then eldest child. Clinician can mention cancer but should educate the family about it. Immediate family members want to know about a poor prognosis right away but prefer not to tell extended family members because "they talk." When a patient learns that he/she has a serious illness, the news is communicated selectively—e.g., to the eldest adult daughter.

WRITTEN COMMUNICATION

- **Literacy assessment**. Many are highly educated and bi- or trilingual but may not read or write English well. Most elderly women are illiterate. Clinician should ask directly if and how well the patient reads English before giving forms or instructions. Useful to provide important medical information by audiotape or by giving written information to a close family member who is literate in English.
- **Consents**. Willing to sign English consent forms for tests or procedures even if forms not understood, so a nonfamily member should translate them. Family member or interpreter rarely explains potential side effects on consent form to protect patient from fear.

NONVERBAL COMMUNICATION

- **Eye contact**. Sustained eye contact varies by acculturation and/or generation. Youth do not look elders directly in the eye; they keep their head slightly to the side and down to convey respect. Traditionally, unrelated men and women do not sustain eye contact nor do they make eye contact with someone they perceive to be of higher status; that would be an insult. Do not wink at a person of the opposite gender, as that may be interpreted as flirting. Do not touch a person of opposite gender except to provide care (after asking permission).
- **Personal space**. Varies according to relationship, gender, and acculturation. Space between close friends and family is closer than that in the culture at large. Traditional or older, unrelated men and women maintain a greater distance from each other, often socializing in separate rooms or separate areas of one room.
- **Use and meaning of silence**. In situations where one needs to show respect, silence may mean disagreement or disapproval and is related to generation and age. For example, a younger person remains silent when he/she disagrees with, or is disappointed by, an older person's decision.
- **Gestures**. Men may place their right hand on their heart to show respect. Inappropriate gestures include thumbs up and pointing the finger in conversation, which show disrespect or dismissal. May make a point in discussion by tapping finger on table or holding index finger and thumb together. Very expressive with hands when speaking with anyone; male gestures are broad,

while female gestures are closer to the body. Disrespectful for women to sit with legs apart.

- **Openness in expressing emotions**. Facial expression tends to be flat when a person is upset, depressed, or angry with extended family members, friends, or health care providers. Open expression of emotions is situational and generational; younger persons are more open with siblings, parents, friends, and others.

- **Privacy**. Generally reluctant to share personal and family issues with non-family members, including health care professionals. Women more willing than men to discuss their problems with friends; men do not discuss their personal problems with anyone. Privacy is gender- and age-related: Young women much more open than are men of any age.

- **Touch**. Touching most parts of the body is acceptable when necessary for care. Patients extremely uncomfortable when clinician must touch genital areas or women's breasts. Most cooperate if asked permission and the clinician explains what he/she intends to do and why.

- **Orientation to time**. Depends on the situation. Includes past, present, and future orientation—e.g., the present in social interactions and the future in hard work and commitment to children's education. When guests are present, finishing the interpersonal encounter gracefully and naturally is more important than being on time for an appointment elsewhere. Acculturation encourages stricter use of clock time in business, at school, or for health care appointments.

ACTIVITIES OF DAILY LIVING

- **Modesty**. Clinician gender an issue for older and more traditional people. Women avoid being touched by male clinicians. More-acculturated persons are willing to be cared for by health care providers of the opposite gender but may not be entirely comfortable. In general, people are extremely modest in dress and regarding any topic related to hygiene. Nudity is extremely embarrassing.

- **Skin care**. Afghans are said to be obsessive about cleanliness—they bathe daily. Do not use special soaps or lotions but carefully avoid skin preparations that contain lard or pork products. *Uzoo* is a cleansing ritual done before prayer. It begins with washing the hands three times with soap and water, washing the teeth with one's finger, cleansing inside the nose, washing the whole face (including ears and behind the ears), washing the feet and ankles, and, finally, washing the genital area. While washing, a prayer is said three times.

- **Hair care**. Hair is washed frequently so it stays very clean. Shampoos and conditioners are by individual choice, although people avoid any that contain pork products. Men generally keep their hair very short to avoid appearing feminine.

- **Nail care**. Men keep fingernails very short; for women, length and manicures are by individual choice. Both genders keep toenails short.
- **Toileting**. Washing the genital area is required after toileting and before prayer. After toileting, especially stool, elderly people prefer to wash themselves by pouring water from a pitcher over the genital area instead of using toilet paper, which they think cannot clean them adequately. Patients use a commode/bedpan if necessary, even though they may be embarrassed. Clinician should ensure privacy.
- **Special clothing or amulets**. Clothing is related to age and acculturation, but baring the skin is immodest for both genders. Older women often wear a white head scarf and long pants under their dresses. Traditional or very religious persons dress to show only their face and hands. Women may completely cover their hair with a *hejab* (a head covering that fastens beneath the chin and covers the neck) or partly with a scarf, while men may wear a turban or hat. On a neck chain, both genders may wear a charm inscribed with the name Allah or a small gold box representing the Koran, as protection from illness, death, or other bad fortune. They may not want to remove the charm unless necessary for a medical procedure. Occasionally, one wears *taweez* (Koranic verses written on folded paper) on string around the neck to help cure illness.
- **Self-care**. Expectations regarding self-care vary by age and acculturation. Elders expect help from hospital staff and from children at home with all care of their bodies. Younger and more-acculturated persons prefer to do at least some self-care. Afghans comply with most requests and procedures.

FOOD PRACTICES

- **Usual meal pattern**. Three meals per day and a snack in the late afternoon or when guests arrive. A hot lunch, with rice, and a larger dinner, which may be quite elaborate and lavish when guests are present.
- **Special utensils**. None in U.S. Traditionally, meals eaten only with right hand.
- **Food beliefs and rituals**. Prefer food that is warm or hot in temperature, flavorful but not highly spiced. Some adhere to traditional humoral concepts of "hot" and "cold" foods, keeping them in balance to prevent illness. Examples of hot foods are rice or Afghan curry dishes. Cold foods include yogurt and, as a condiment, chutney made of hot green peppers and finely minced herbs.
- **Usual diet**. Breakfast is typically cheese with mint and *nan* (flat wheat bread like pita) or eggs, milk, and tea. Lunch is rice with another dish; dinner is similar but includes more dishes. Diet is based mainly on rice seasoned with herbs, vegetables, and small amounts of meat or poultry, with fresh fruit, dried fruits, and nuts as snacks. Unhealthy practices include cooking with a large amount of oil, fatty meats, and loss of nutrients in overcooked vegetables. Teens and children are becoming addicted to fast food.

- **Fluids**. Black tea is served after every meal and with snacks, and always offered to guests. Soft drinks often served at lunch or dinner. Adults often drink milk at breakfast.
- **Food taboos and prescriptions**. Taboos include pork, alcohol, shellfish, and tobacco. *Halal*, from the Koran, means substances permitted by Allah—the Supreme Law Giver—for consumption; *haram* are those He absolutely prohibits. Any food of suspected or unknown *haram* status is avoided. A widely used pamphlet assembled by members of the mosques lists generic ingredients and brand names, and categorizes them as *halal*, *haram*, or unknown. It includes foods, cleaning products, pizza restaurants, cosmetics, toothpaste, and medications. Most *haram* ingredients are from animals—e.g., fat, collagen, di- or monoglycerides, enzyme, gelatin, hormones, pepsin, shortening, and phospholipids. To promote health, people eat fresh *halal* foods, balance hot and cold foods, and strictly avoid *haram* foods and drinks.
- **Hospitality**. An extremely important Afghan value. Visitors are treasured and treated lavishly, seated in the most comfortable or desirable seat (facing everyone), served first, and given the choicest pieces of meat. Parents give up their marital bed to family members from out of town and children sleep on the floor.

SYMPTOM MANAGEMENT

- **Pain**. Elderly may see pain as God's punishment or as an expected part of life but pray for it to go away. Many experience emotional distress as pain, most often in the stomach or head. Pain tends to keep people from moving or talking. Clinicians can use a number to gauge pain level, but older persons prefer words, such as "someone is sticking needles in me," "throbbing," or "aching." Women may exaggerate their physical pain, which may be depression. Most want immediate relief through medication. A nonpharmacological method for reducing pain is listening to the Koran on audiocassette or compact disk.
- **Dyspnea**. Women may experience dyspnea in a panic or anxiety attack. Persons with dyspnea tend to report it immediately, fearing they are dying. Most can use a numerical scale for dyspnea, but the elderly might use words such as "my heart is about to stop" or "I have difficulty breathing." They want immediate oxygen and medications. As with pain, prayer and listening to the Koran are useful.
- **Nausea/vomiting**. Elderly persons and women accept vomiting and are not embarrassed by it. They describe nausea and vomiting openly and can use a numerical scale. The elderly may use words such as "my food is coming up" or "I have a stomach ache." After vomiting, they may want to drink a glass of water. They desire medications to decrease nausea and vomiting, and accept rectal or IV medications. Reading or listening to the Koran is a useful nonpharmacological method of control.

- **Constipation/diarrhea**. Diarrhea is very embarrassing, especially for elderly persons. May spontaneously tell a daughter about diarrhea but not report it to a clinician unless asked. A family member saying that "my grandma goes to the bathroom constantly" usually means diarrhea. Constipation is less embarrassing, but the patient still must be asked and will not offer the information otherwise. May describe it as "I can't go to the bathroom." Most accept nutritional controls for diarrhea or constipation if educated about how these would be helpful. Most accept enemas if the need and procedure are explained.
- **Fatigue**. Afghans, especially the elderly, tend to complain that they are always tired, making it difficult to distinguish illness-related fatigue. Fatigue also may be a sign of depression. Most can use numbers to describe their fatigue level, but the elderly also use words such as "I sleep all day." Women are more likely than men to report fatigue. Patients are open to medications and other methods of reducing fatigue if these are explained clearly.
- **Depression**. Many do not know what depression is and seek medical care for physical symptoms. Clinician should be cautious about relaying such a diagnosis, as the patient may think it implies that he/she is crazy or something is very wrong with him/her. Patients are open to antidepressants but less open to nonpharmacological methods, such as exercise or psychotherapy. Suggesting more-frequent reading of the Koran may help older persons. Younger persons are more open to counseling and psychotherapy.
- **Self-care symptom management**. Prefer Western medications for treatment of symptoms but may use herbal/home remedies initially or simultaneously. May be initially uncomfortable with chronic disease management, such as glucose monitoring and insulin injection. But this varies according to how disease management is taught and to the age and education of patient.

BIRTH RITUALS/CARE OF THE NEW MOTHER AND BABY
- **Pregnancy care**. Use regular prenatal care. Childbirth preparation classes were not available in Afghanistan, so older persons find them foreign. Younger adults' use of such classes depends on their knowledge of them and when they came to U.S. Husbands may or may not want to attend.
- **Preferences for children**. Boys preferred to girls because girls marry and move to their husband's family. Sons are ongoing providers for elderly parents; the eldest son may live with them or take them into his home. The ideal family size in Afghanistan is six children. In U.S., because of financial issues, 2–3 children common.
- **Labor practices**. Women in labor go to the hospital and generally cooperate with staff directions about eating, walking, showering, and pain control if the directions are explained. Women want the least pain possible and request medication. A more traditional husband may be very uncomfortable having a male obstetrician touch his wife (the husband might even leave the

hospital), but it depends on the family and acculturation level. Clinician should respect modesty and keep the expectant mother's breasts and genitals covered as much as possible.

- **Role of the laboring woman during birth**. A laboring woman is expected to express her pain and she may shout. Most women are active in the birth process; they push vigorously because they want the pain to end.
- **Role of the father and other family members during birth**. A woman expects her spouse to remain in the labor and delivery rooms at all times. She may also want her mother present. The mother holds her daughter's hand, reassures her, washes her face, and rubs her back. The husband may provide more care if the mother is absent.
- **Vaginal vs. cesarean section**. Prefer vaginal to cesarean birth, which is seen as more dangerous.
- **Breastfeeding**. New mothers breastfeed for at least three months and typically continue until baby begins to eat solid food. Bottle-feeding is rarely combined with breastfeeding, unless the mother must return to work, in which case she pumps breast milk for baby. Many women think that formula does not contain the natural healthy nutrients of breast milk.
- **Birth recuperation**. The woman's mother typically stays with her daughter to help during the first three weeks to a month after birth, especially with the first baby. In the first few days, the postpartum woman is expected to eat a soup that her mother makes from flour, nuts, and water. She also is expected to rest and avoid housework and cooking. Within a week or two after the birth, the immediate family hosts a party so friends can meet baby.
- **Baby care**. Grandmothers are expected to take care of the new baby until the daughter or daughter-in-law is able—for 2–6 months.
- **Problems with baby**. Both parents together should be told as soon as staff perceives a problem. Parents generally prefer that extended family members not be told, to prevent the news from spreading through the community.
- **Male and female circumcision**. Circumcision of male children is required by Islam but is rarely performed on neonates in Afghanistan. Some refugees were unable to circumcise their sons while fleeing or temporarily staying in another country; they may request circumcision for an older boy. In North America, boys are circumcised before they leave the hospital. Girls are never circumcised.

DEVELOPMENTAL AND SEXUAL ISSUES

- **Celebration of menarche or becoming a man**. Traditionally, menarche means a girl has become a woman who can give birth and is available for marriage. When a young woman begins to menstruate, she tells only her mother. Because of embarrassment, menstrual periods are not mentioned in the presence of male family members. Becoming a man is not celebrated.
- **Attitudes about birth control**. Use birth control in Afghanistan and U.S.,

but it is acceptable only in marriage. Single women who are sexually inti-mate use oral contraceptives in secret. Birth control is more common in the younger generation.

- **Attitudes about sexually transmitted infection (STI) control, includ-ing condoms**. Norms regarding sexuality are changing and depend on age and acculturation. Older generation believes there is no risk of acquiring an STI in marriage. Young adults are more knowledgeable about STIs and more likely to protect themselves, such as by using condoms.
- **Attitudes about abortion**. Islam strictly forbids it. If a woman becomes pregnant outside of marriage, she might have an abortion, but she would never tell her parents.
- **Attitudes about unwed sexual experimentation**. Sexual activity is taboo for unmarried women. If the family learns that a young woman has been sexually active, she may be disowned, punished, or, rarely, even killed by a male family member. Men's sexual activity outside of marriage is regarded negatively but may be accepted with resignation. Some accultur-ated young persons have strictly secret sexual relationships.
- **Sexual orientation**. Homosexuality is against Islamic law. A gay or lesbian person hides orientation from family and community. If family finds out, he/she is disowned.
- **Gender identity**. Very strong expectations of women to be ladylike and of men to be highly masculine. Parents may pressure children who do not fit these stereotypes to change. Family may disown a son or daughter whose gender identity is ambiguous or the opposite of his/her birth gender.
- **Attitudes about menopause**. Discussion of sexual or anatomical topics is highly embarrassing, even for acculturated women. Some women do not know about menopause and think they are sick when they first develop symptoms. Menopause generally regarded as a normal life change; some wel-come it as reducing the risk of pregnancy. Some women discuss their symp-toms and treatment choices with sisters and close women friends.

FAMILY RELATIONSHIPS

- **Composition/structure**. Family life is at the core of Afghan culture and psychological well-being. Most Afghans spend free time socializing with family and old friends. Among those older than 30, new friendships may be slow to develop because of distrust of those outside the family circle. Both extended-family and nuclear-family households common. Considerable fam-ily obligations, especially to parents and older siblings, often supersede other responsibilities, including allegiance to spouse, job, and one's own needs. These norms are loosening in the younger generation.
- **Decision-making**. Varies by acculturation level, urban or rural origin, and age. Clinician should ask who makes decisions for the family: father, mother, or both? Family obligations and traditional hierarchy may interfere with

making decisions or compliance. Strong aversion to interference by school or social service agency in family affairs, which Afghans consider to be private.

- **Spokesperson**. In most families, the father makes decisions about matters outside the home, but the mother makes them in the home.
- **Gender issues**. Traditionally, men expect wives to stay home, cook for family and visitors, care for children, clean house, and socialize only with Afghan female friends. More cosmopolitan women enjoy their freedom and the opportunity to be active in the community, but they are expected to maintain lifelong modest behavior. Once her reputation is tarnished, a woman is no longer respected and becomes the target of gossip. In U.S., the man's role as head of the family is damaged when he cannot obtain respected work and when children become the parents' translators and spokespersons. Even acculturated and cosmopolitan men who have been in the U.S. for two decades maintain a tribal consciousness that favors women's submission to husbands/fathers, despite the fact that classical Islam promotes gender equality and mutual spousal respect.
- **Changing roles among generations in U.S.** Enormous generational differences between the elderly, those in their late 30s through 50s, and young adults. Elders are similar to how they were in Afghanistan. The middle generation is caught between Afghan and American cultures. Those who immigrated as children or were born in U.S. are American but uphold Afghan values. Women experience more role conflict than men do, as women acculturate more quickly. Remaining single may be viewed as unnatural. Finding a husband may be difficult because many men older than 30 perceive acculturated women as insufficiently naive or submissive.
- **Caring roles**. The mother takes primary role in caring for an ill person. If that person is elderly, the oldest daughter is the primary caregiver. If there is no daughter, the patient's sister provides care.
- **Expectations of and for children**. Expected to work hard in school and return home for homework; strict parents do not allow after-school activities. Parents are concerned about school influences, especially sex education or their children being served pork. Even while sounding and appearing completely American in speech and activities, children and teens respect Islamic and family values, although some teens rebel until high school. Boys have much more freedom than girls do. Parents perceive independent and assertive children, who resemble their dominant-culture peers, as "having no respect" and not following the cultural value of strict obedience to elder family members, particularly the father. Parents value higher education so greatly that they may allow their college-age children to live on campus. However, such students are expected to come home on weekends.
- **Expectations of and for elders**. When an elderly person enters the room, others stand and/or kiss the back of that person's hand as a sign of respect and acknowledgment of wisdom, which comes with age. A young person

should not contradict an elder, although this is changing and varies among families. Elderly women who had high status in Afghanistan are often depressed because of the loss of family members and culture. Their adult children work full-time and cannot dote on them, and the adult children may expect elderly women to care for the grandchildren. Elders are not expected to live alone; they usually live with the eldest son and may completely depend on his family for support.

- **Expectations of hospital visitors**. Visiting a sick person is very important. Numerous family members and friends gather at the bedside and remain until asked to leave. If an Afghan is crying, one should just sit beside him/her without touching, hugging, or calling further attention to him/her. The patient usually wants a close female family member to stay overnight in the hospital room.

ILLNESS BELIEFS

- **Causes of/attitudes about physical illness**. Illness can have natural causes, such as "germs," dirt, cold or wind, seasonal changes, or not taking proper care of one's body. A traditional humoral belief is that "hot" and "cold" imbalances cause sickness; hot/cold qualities describe food, drinks, medicinal herbs, individual human nature, and specific illnesses. Supernatural causes of illness, which cleanses one's sins, engenders God's mercy, and is to be borne with patience, include God's will; a less common cause is *jinns* (ghosts or spirits). The evil eye is a social cause of illness instigated by another person. Afghans often perceive illness as due to failure to abide by Islamic principles.
- **Causes of/attitudes about mental illness**. Commonly acknowledged that there are many Afghans with psychological problems, mainly stress, depression, and post-traumatic stress disorder. Despite such recognition, families tend to seek psychiatric care only as a last resort because they perceive such care as shaming the family. Fears include gossip, losing face, and that therapist will share personal family information with others.
- **Causes of genetic defects**. Such defects are considered to be the result of God's will. Disabled person perceived as God's child and the genetic problem is His choice. The disabled are usually loved and cared for without bias.
- **Attitudes about disabilities**. Believed to be God's will. Family does not discriminate against a disabled member. Parents or eldest sibling care for him/her.
- **Sick role**. The ill person should rest in bed under the care of spouse or children. Ill women do not wear make-up and are not expected to cook or clean.
- **Home and folk remedies**. Treat mild natural illnesses only with home remedies and by dietary means. Most older women know how to prepare herbal remedies (available in Afghan, Iranian, and Indian food stores) for injuries, colds, and stomach complaints. "Hot" illnesses, such as fever and measles, are treated with a diet emphasizing cold foods and medicines; "cold"

illnesses, such as arthritis and chicken pox, are treated with hot foods and herbs. May consult a *mullah* for supernatural illness or evil eye.

- **Medications**. Normally comply with Western medications, which they like. Want to rid themselves of symptoms quickly. Many use folk remedies, such as herbal teas, while taking Western medications.
- **Acceptance of procedures**. Generally accept surgery, transfusions, and organ transplants. No restrictions regarding the gender, race, or religion of donors. However, Islam forbids donating body parts.
- **Care-seeking**. Prefer biomedical care to folk healers, though some persons consult a spiritual healer if the illness is incurable through biomedical means or they perceive it as having a supernatural cause. May use both biomedical and spiritual healers simultaneously, inviting the spiritual healer into the hospital room when death is near.

HEALTH ISSUES

- **Concept of health**. Most Dari words for health mean "wholeness" or "completeness." Afghans have both natural and supernatural concepts of health.
- **Health promotion and prevention**. Believe that health is maintained by regularly exercising, eating fresh food and a balanced diet, staying warm, and getting enough rest. Generally favor health promotion and prevention but may lack the knowledge, time, or resources for regular practice. Islam forbids alcohol and street drugs; abuse exists but at a relatively low rate.
- **Screening**. Regular examinations and screening for disease were not normal in Afghanistan and are foreign to older persons. Elderly women rarely undergo mammograms or gynecological or clinical breast exams. Childbearing women do, mainly while pregnant, but some are beginning to accept the need for annual exams. Younger persons and acculturated persons are being screened.
- **Common health problems**. Heart disease, stroke, arthritis, and diabetes are acknowledged as community problems. Many diabetics are unaware of it despite clear symptoms. Thalassemia is common. Glucose-6-phosphate dehydrogenase deficiency, which can cause hemolytic crises when eating fava beans, is common among Pashtuns and Uzbeks.

DEATH RITUALS

- **Beliefs and attitudes about death**. Grieve expressively and strongly. Muslims believe that when their time comes, they must go to the other world where God is calling them. This belief makes "letting go" easier for some families. They may view the withdrawal of life support as "playing God" but accept the initiation of life support as a gift of medical technology.
- **Preparation**. When death seems inevitable, clinician should tell the spouse and parents directly and immediately. They need time to notify family members, especially those who are far away so they can be present when patient dies. A family member will bring in a *mullah* when patient is near death.

- **Home vs. hospital**. Prefer death in the hospital so family does not feel responsible. Hospice still a foreign concept.
- **Special needs**. The most important need is to have the entire family and a *mullah* there for the passing and afterward.
- **Care of the body**. The body is washed in a ritual manner only by another Muslim, preferably a *mullah*. The washing may be delayed to await the arrival of family members. Body is wrapped in a white cotton shroud and placed in a coffin. Only close female family members are allowed to see the face of a deceased woman. Only close male family members and friends are allowed to see the face of a deceased man, with the exception of his wife. Islam does not permit embalming.
- **Attitudes about organ donation**. Islam forbids organ donation.
- **Attitudes about autopsy**. Islam forbids autopsy; traditional persons do not believe in it. Family members sometimes allow autopsy when they must clarify the cause of death to resolve arguments among them. If autopsy is critical, clinician should educate the family about the need for it.

SELECTED REFERENCES

Lipson, J., Askaryar, R., & Omidian, P. (2004). Afghans and Afghan Americans. In J. Giger & R. Davidhizar, R. (Eds.), *Transcultural nursing: Assessment and intervention* (4th ed.) (pp. 363–377). St. Louis, MO: Mosby Year Book.

Lipson, J. G., & Omidian, P. (1992). Health issues of Afghan refugees in California. *Western Journal of Medicine*, 157, 271–275.

Lipson, J. G., Omidian, P., & Paul, S. (1995). Afghan Health Education Project: A community survey. *Public Health Nursing*, 12, 143–150.

AUTHORS

Juliene G. Lipson, PhD, FAAN, a nurse-anthropologist, is professor emerita in the School of Nursing and Department of Anthropology, History, and Social Medicine at the University of California-San Francisco, where she taught community health and cross-cultural nursing. She has done research on the health and adjustment of immigrant and refugees to the U.S. from Arab countries, Iran, Afghanistan, Bosnia, and the former Soviet Union. Her recent research is on disability. She is currently conducting an ethnographic study of persons who have multiple chemical sensitivities.

Razia Askaryar, MA, was born in Afghanistan and came to the U.S. at age 5. She is a doctoral candidate in psychology at the California School of Professional Psychology-San Francisco Campus. Her dissertation is "Somatization Underlying Depression in Relation to Acculturation Among Afghan Women in the Bay Area." She used three questionnaires and interviews to capture underlying issues among this population.

CHAPTER 2

AFRICAN AMERICANS

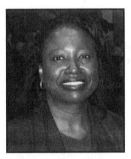
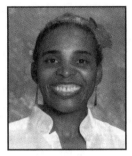

Catherine M. Waters   *Salamah Locks*

CULTURAL/ETHNIC IDENTITY

In this chapter, "African American" refers to the Black or African American population whose origins are any of the Black racial groups of Africa, most of whom did not come to the U.S. voluntarily. Blacks who more recently immigrated from Africa and the West Indies/Caribbean are described in other chapters. African Americans exhibit a diverse range of cultural patterns according to regional, urban, and rural differences; age; education; socioeconomic status; religious beliefs; socialization; and assimilation/acculturation. Many aspects of African American culture are similar to those of the dominant culture because of historical ties.

- **Preferred term(s)**. Preference depends on person's age and socialization. Younger persons tend to prefer "African American"; older persons refer to themselves as "Colored." Some African Americans who are multiracial prefer to self-identify as African American or multiracial, or they would rather not use any racial-group term. Best to ask which term is preferred: Colored, Negro, Black, Afro-American, or African American. Do not assume African American ethnicity based on skin color, as the color range is from the lightest light to the darkest dark.
- **Census**. According to the 2000 U.S. Census, about 34.7 million people, or 12% of the total population, self-identify as African American, of which 55% are younger than 18 years. An additional 1.8 million self-identify with at least one other race. African Americans reside in all regions of the U.S. (55% in the South) and are socioeconomically diverse (22% live in poverty).
- **History of immigration**. The earliest arrivals are believed to have been in 1619, when 20 Black indentured servants were brought to Jamestown, VA.

Some 4 million slaves were brought to the U.S. between the 17th and 19th centuries; none were voluntary immigrants nor can their descendants be considered immigrants. Important historical influences include emancipation, migration from rural areas to cities, and the civil rights movement. Immigrants from Africa and the West Indies/Caribbean share some history with African Americans but perceive it differently.

SPIRITUAL/RELIGIOUS ORIENTATION

- **Primary religious/spiritual affiliations**. As a group, African Americans are religious/spiritual. They have strong church affiliations. Baptist and other Protestant denominations, Catholicism, and Islam are the primary affiliations. Many African Americans believe that God is a union of three divine persons—the Father, Son, and Holy Spirit.
- **Usual religious/spiritual practices**. Church an important African American institution. Typical religious/spiritual practices include attending church on Sunday, praying and singing, reading the Bible daily, and visits from the minister or deacon. Promoting one's health considered essential to good religious/spiritual practice. As a part of such practices, many churches maintain a health ministry.
- **Use of spiritual healing/healers**. May use faith and root healers (herbalists) along with biomedical resources but do not readily divulge these practices to health care providers. Clinicians should assess a person's understanding of illnesses and beliefs about their causes and proper treatments. There is no conflict with biomedicine.
- **Holidays**. Important cultural holidays are Juneteenth, the oldest known celebration of the end of slavery. It was first celebrated on June 19, 1865, after enforcement of President Lincoln's signing of the Emancipation Proclamation nearly two-and-a-half years earlier. Kwanzaa, established in 1966 by Dr. Maulana Karenga, has origins in the age-old African first-harvest celebrations. Kwanzaa, which means "first fruits" in Swahili, is celebrated December 26–January 1 in honor of family, community, and culture. Each day observes the values of unity, self-determination, collective work and cooperative economics, purpose, creativity, and faith. Dr. Martin Luther King Jr.'s birthday is celebrated on the third Monday in January. Religious holy days are observed according to one's religious affiliation.

COMMUNICATION
ORAL COMMUNICATION

- **Major languages and dialects**. English. Some indigenous dialects spoken in the coastal areas of South Carolina, Georgia, northern Florida, and Louisiana—e.g., Gullah, Creole, patois (*patwa*). Vernacular Black English is an expressive dialect that refers to a range of nonstandard varieties of English spoken by African Americans of any educational or social level. May switch between vernacular Black English and standard English depending on circumstances.

- **Greetings**. Unless indicated otherwise, address others—especially elderly African Americans—as "Mr." or "Mrs." or by professional title and last name. Many women greet each other with a hug and/or kiss on the cheek. Some men greet each other with a modified handshake hug. When greeting strangers, a handshake is acceptable; may hug if it is solicited.
- **Tone of voice**. When speaking with each other, conversations often loud and animated, with body movements. These gestures often express affection. Tone of voice can be low- or high-pitched in both positive and negative encounters. Most accurate way to interpret meaning of voice tonality is to ask the person in a direct manner; clinician should not assume he/she knows what the patient means.
- **Direct or indirect style of speech**. Style is direct and frank but depends on age. Older African Americans tend to be less direct than younger people are. At times, conversations can be lengthy and circuitous in the form of story-telling, an essential form of communication. Storytelling was primary source of communication during American slavery, when slaves were prohibited from reading and writing. Because of slaves' illiteracy, stories were the only means of passing down the history of their ancestors. Storytelling continues to be an important form of communication among 21st-century African American elders.
- **Use of interpreters**. Not applicable.
- **Serious or terminal illness**. To convey a serious or terminal illness, family-centered approach ideal. Often, oldest relative selectively reveals poor prognosis or conveys nothing; this may not be universally practiced. Many African American elders are private about their health, especially if it involves a serious or terminal illness. They tend to be skeptical about allowing other family members to accompany them to health visits and be present during their examination for fear that their condition will be revealed. Many elders believe that their illness is between themselves and God. If the family lacks cohesiveness, it seeks the guidance and direction of the family minister or a close family friend, who are important members of African Americans' social networks. These relationships go beyond consanguinity. Discussions of advanced directives and organ donation are suspect, especially when the patient is seriously or terminally ill. Usually one or several persons in the family knows of the person's health-care wishes. Clinician should share patient information with family and friends only as directed by patient.

WRITTEN COMMUNICATION

- **Literacy assessment**. Literacy may vary by generation; level is not easily discernible. Clinician should ask indirectly what level of schooling the patient has completed. Refusal to sign any forms or documents could indicate illiteracy rather than "just being difficult."

- **Consents**. Clinician should involve the family in consent process, avoid using medical jargon, and elicit feedback to check patient's understanding. Verbal consent or a waiver from signed consent may be preferable. The long history of abuse of African Americans as experimental research subjects may dissuade them from readily volunteering for research. Including African American researchers and/or staff and thoroughly explaining the study may ease concerns.

NONVERBAL COMMUNICATION

- **Eye contact**. Sustained eye contact varies by generation. Youth do not look elders directly in the eye. Many elders may make direct eye contact, but it is fleeting. In general, maintaining appropriate eye contact shows respect and can help to establish trust.
- **Personal space**. African Americans are affectionate people who express their affection by touching, hugging, and being close to friends and family. Personal space between close friends and family is closer than in the dominant culture. If clinicians are invited, sharing close personal space is acceptable. A clinician's nonresponse to such an invitation may be viewed with suspicion and can hamper trust and rapport.
- **Use and meaning of silence**. Silence may indicate lack of trust, disagreement, or nonacceptance.
- **Gestures**. Body and hand gestures often used to accentuate a point in conversation. Are a form of expression and do not necessarily indicate disgruntlement or hostility. A hand on the hip, for example, emphasizes a point of view or opinion.
- **Openness in expressing emotions**. African Americans openly express their emotions with each other but may subdue those related to depression until trust and rapport established. In general, both genders mask negative emotions, which makes a diagnosis of depression difficult.
- **Privacy**. Clinicians should respect African Americans' privacy. African Americans generally reluctant to share personal and family issues with non-family members, including health care professionals. Expressing genuine, nonjudgmental interest in African Americans' health is essential in obtaining accurate and complete personal health information. Patient will provide such information if trust and respect established. Women willing to discuss their personal and health problems with friends, but men typically do not. Privacy also age-related: Younger persons tend to be more open than older persons are about their health problems.
- **Touch**. Although African Americans are affectionate people, clinician should always obtain permission, either verbally or nonverbally, before touching. Most accept touch if the clinician explains what he/she intends to do and why.

- **Orientation to time**. Time frame is typically flexible and nonlinear. Life and social issues may take priority over keeping appointments. Primarily present-oriented, but this varies among individuals. Older persons tend to be more punctual and more willing to wait.

ACTIVITIES OF DAILY LIVING

- **Modesty**. Both genders appreciate respectful approaches. Women may prefer a female clinician for both nursing and ob/gyn care. Muslim women prefer to have head, arms, and legs covered at all times, but the degree of expression of this tradition is individually determined by the marital couple.
- **Skin care**. Daily skin care and bathing in the sink, tub, or shower important. African Americans tend to have dry skin; staff should provide moisturizer and lotion. They use soap and other bath products daily. Common skin problems: keloids, pigmentary disorders, pseudofolliculitis (razor bumps and ingrown hairs), and melasma (patchy tan to dark brown discoloration of the face in pregnant and older women).
- **Hair care**. As hair tends to be naturally dry, use hair oils daily. Hair texture ranges from straight to kinky, and length from long to short. Women's and men's hairstyles include braiding, "natural kinky," straightened, permed, or relaxed. Typically, a "pic" or comb with big teeth is needed for longer, thicker hair. Hair is shampooed every 7–10 days but varies among individuals.
- **Nail care**. Manicures and pedicures a matter of individual choice. Decorative fingernails of some length common among women. Both genders typically prefer short toenails. Women's toenails may be painted and the toes adorned with a ring.
- **Toileting**. Staff should provide and ensure privacy regardless of the mode of elimination, be it a restroom, bedpan, urinal, or bedside commode. Hand washing and washing of the genital area after toileting essential. Muslims may observe additional bathing rituals associated with daily prayer times.
- **Special clothing or amulets**. Varies among individuals. Some African Americans use prayer beads and wear crosses and copper or silver bracelets. For both genders, dressing in their "Sunday best" for church services is not complete without a hat of some kind. An individual may make a special effort to select a hat that is special to, or an expression of, him/her. Muslim women may cover their hair.
- **Self-care**. In general, prefer independent self-care. If that is not possible, prefer a family member to help. Appreciate assistance with difficult-to-reach areas of the body.

FOOD PRACTICES

- **Usual meal pattern**. Three meals daily. A traditional, large meal (supper) often eaten in late afternoon, frequently on Sundays after church with friends and family.

- **Special utensils**. None.
- **Food beliefs and rituals**. Family and friends sharing food is a social event for any occasion. One is expected to taste everything. Prefer cooked foods. For religious reasons, may not eat pork. All varieties of leafy greens, such as collards, mustard, kale, and cabbage, often deemed essential for good health. Family greetings often include, "Are you hungry?" or "Have you eaten?" Muslims celebrate the holy month of Ramadan with 30 days of fasting from dawn to sunset; breaking the fast and evening meals may include some traditional Middle Eastern or African dishes. All religious observances in Islam are based on the lunar calendar. Thus, the month of Ramadan rotates gradually through all seasons. Those who celebrate Kwanzaa also may consume traditional foods originally from Africa.
- **Usual diet**. Prefer cooked foods. Usual diet consists of hearty meals with meat, fish, greens, rice, grits, white and sweet potatoes and other starches (e.g., corn and yams), and a variety of homemade desserts. Prefer home-cooked foods to processed and fast foods. Meals typically light during the week and heartier on weekends. Supper served on Sundays after church services often is the large meal of the day, followed by a light dinner in the evening.
- **Fluids**. Prefer coffee and cold drinks with ice, such as ice water, tea, flavored drinks, and sodas.
- **Food taboos and prescriptions**. Food taboos, such as pork and catfish, often related to religious restrictions, including those imposed by Islam and Seventh Day Adventists. Otherwise, generally no prohibitions. Cooked greens important for maintaining bowel function. Other prescriptions: fresh fruits for hydration and constipation, and red and yellow vegetables for adequate blood circulation or anemia.
- **Hospitality**. An important African American value. Visitors welcomed with open arms. Out-of-town family members and friends often stay in host's home, lavish meals are prepared, and other family, friends, and neighbors participate in the visit.

SYMPTOM MANAGEMENT

- **Pain**. Expression of pain is generally open and public but can vary. All forms of pharmacological and some forms of nonpharmacological, alternative, and complementary methods acceptable. May avoid pain medication for fear of addiction but will become agitated if denied pain medication. Numerical, pictorial, and word pain scales helpful for rating discomfort levels. Choice of pain scale should be based on literacy level and patient preferences.
- **Dyspnea**. Often described as "difficulty catching breath." If explained, oxygen and opiates are acceptable means to control dyspnea; however, fear of addiction is strong.
- **Nausea/vomiting**. Prefer nonpharmacological methods, such as ginger ale, soda crackers, and teas, to control nausea and vomiting, which are often

described as "feeling sick to the stomach." Welcome pharmacological agents when symptoms are severe.

- **Constipation/diarrhea**. Open attitude about reporting constipation, often described as "bowels blocked up." Preferred means for restoring bowel functioning is nutrition, such as eating fruits and prunes to provide roughage. Secondary means are laxatives and enemas. Older persons become upset if they do not move their bowels daily.

- **Fatigue**. African Americans will report feeling fatigued or tired, although not readily. May take sleeping pills to foster sleep. Fatigue may be a masked indication of depression.

- **Depression**. Seldom acknowledged. Symptoms typically masked. May be reported as feeling tired. Depression tends to be higher among African American women than men. Tend to accept medications and therapy reluctantly to alleviate symptoms. Often use social support networks to cope with depression.

- **Self-care symptom management**. Prefer Western medications to treat symptoms but may use herbal and home remedies initially or simultaneously. Usually, the mother or wife provides or obtains a remedy from a "knowing person" (herbalist). Self-care management, such as that for diabetes, asthma, blood-pressure monitoring, keeping health appointments, giving injections, and attending health education classes, is important and expected.

BIRTH RITUALS/CARE OF THE NEW MOTHER AND BABY

- **Pregnancy care**. Varies by level of education and health care knowledge. Use regular prenatal care; more than 70% of African Americans initiate such care during the first trimester. Attend childbirth preparation classes. Partners are actively involved in pregnancy care. Some women crave or eat boxed starch as a substitute for eating clay or dirt (geophagy) while pregnant. This craving is possibly related to the woman's diet: There may be an insufficiency of a mineral or substance necessary for proper fetal development. Geophagy, an African ritual that slaves practiced, is believed to contribute to the good health of mother and fetus. African Americans view pregnancy as a normal life process. No special limitations on activities during pregnancy. Many women continue to work and perform other daily routines.

- **Preferences for children**. Generally conservative about marriage, family, and children. No preference for gender. The contemporary, ideal family size is two children; in rural areas, families with many children are often viewed as healthy and blessed.

- **Labor practices**. Expression of labor pain can be open and public. Use of medications varies, but African Americans do not avoid such medications. Women go to the hospital when in labor and generally cooperate with staff directions about eating, walking, showering, and pain control if these are explained. Partners actively involved in the labor process.

- **Role of the laboring woman during birth**. Most women are active participants. Expect all persons present, including themselves, to do their job and may be quite loud and verbally expressive. Emoting fully is acceptable.
- **Role of the father and other family members during birth**. Varies by education level. Traditionally, only females were in attendance, but this tradition has shifted over time. Partners are now active participants.
- **Vaginal vs. cesarean section**. As medically indicated, though prefer vaginal delivery.
- **Breastfeeding**. Varies by level of education and information from female associates. Compared to other ethnic/racial groups, African Americans have the lowest rates of breastfeeding initiation and continuation, especially among low-income and less-educated women. Most are willing to breastfeed if instructed about the benefits and if the father and other close relatives support them.
- **Birth recuperation**. Family members care for mother and baby, depending on socioeconomic level and family resources. No tub bath, shower, or hair washing after birth until cessation of postpartum bleeding. Clinician should offer sponge baths and provide privacy as needed.
- **Baby care**. Mother is expected to care for baby with help as needed from female relatives, such as her mother, aunt, grandmother, and sister.
- **Problems with baby**. Women rely on older female relatives, such as their mother, grandmother, and aunt, to provide reassurance and advice about baby problems. Physician should inform parents immediately and directly if baby has a health problem, even if one is only suspected.
- **Male and female circumcision**. Many follow the biomedical tradition of newborn male circumcision before leaving the hospital. Females never circumcised.

DEVELOPMENTAL AND SEXUAL ISSUES
- **Celebration of menarche or becoming a man**. Neither is celebrated.
- **Attitudes about birth control**. All forms of birth control acceptable. Many African Americans believe that using contraception is a moral right of choice for women. Contraceptive use varies and is associated with education, religious beliefs, socioeconomic status, and marital status. African American couples tend to prefer female sterilization, condoms, and the pill as primary contraceptive techniques.
- **Attitudes about sexually transmitted infection (STI) control, including condoms**. Both genders accept condom use to minimize risk of unintended pregnancy and STI. Women are more likely than men to insist that men use condoms, an attitude that varies by education, socioeconomic status, and religious beliefs.
- **Attitudes about abortion**. Abortion does occur but is uncommon (children viewed as gifts from God) and varies according to religious beliefs, edu-

cation, and socioeconomic status. Many women hide or deny unplanned pregnancy until second trimester, at which time abortion is not an option.

- **Attitudes about unwed sexual experimentation**. Such experimentation is discouraged. Depending on religious affiliation, an unwed woman who becomes pregnant may be required to receive counseling from her pastor or be counseled by elder women in the church. She also may be required to attend church services openly during pregnancy. Level of family education greatly influences degree of adolescent promiscuity. Many young women hide or deny pregnancy. Abortion of unplanned pregnancies is unusual.
- **Sexual orientation**. Homosexuality is typically stigmatized and may be an embarrassment to the family and community. However, the homosexual family member is not disowned. A lesbian or gay person is discreet about his/her sexual orientation. Increasing age, more education, being female, having a higher income, and being urban associated with positive attitudes about sexual minorities. Most African Americans likely to support laws prohibiting antigay discrimination.
- **Gender identity**. Have traditional beliefs about gender identity and roles, although these beliefs vary. In general, women are expected to be feminine and men are expected to be masculine. Family and community may disown one whose gender identity is ambiguous or opposite to his/her birth gender.
- **Attitudes about menopause**. Women have positive attitudes about aging and menopause, viewing it as a normal life change. Usually do not take hormone replacement therapy; many use home remedies, such as garlic, to minimize symptoms such as hot flashes or night sweats. Depression may accompany menopause. Some women discuss their symptoms and treatment choices with female relatives and friends.

FAMILY RELATIONSHIPS

- **Composition/structure**. Family structure is often nuclear, extended, and matriarchal, and may include fictive kin—e.g., a godmother or "my sister." Family life is the core of African American culture and psychological well-being. Most spend their leisure time socializing with family, friends, and neighbors. Homosexuality as a family structure viewed as aberrant, but families are becoming more tolerant. Allegiance to family and friends, who often make up a wide and diverse social network, overrides other responsibilities.
- **Decision-making**. In nuclear family, father typically has the final decision-making role inside the household; outside, egalitarian decision-making occurs. The mother often makes health care decisions for family.
- **Spokesperson**. The father or eldest family member speaks for family, although family has likely discussed the topic about which he/she speaks.
- **Gender issues**. Typically vary by generation. Older African Americans may have traditional views about separate male and female roles. Younger persons are usually egalitarian: Both men and women cook, clean house,

participate in child care and child-rearing, and work inside and outside of the home. Women viewed as equal and autonomous.

- **Changing roles among generations in U.S.** There are generational differences in practically every aspect of African American life. Older African Americans tend to be conservative and traditional. Younger African Americans tend to be liberal and not to conform with traditional values. More African American women than men are unmarried and educated at the college level. Many women would like to get married and have a family, but finding a husband is difficult for various social and historical reasons. Women tend not to date persons of a different race, whereas men tend to do so. Family members often shun interracial dating, especially by women. This trend is changing gradually.
- **Caring roles**. Wife or eldest sister often assumes family-caretaker role, but this depends on family structure. Sons, especially in the absence of female relatives, often care for ailing parents.
- **Expectations of and for children**. Early walking and toileting encouraged. Children are expected to help with household chores and to attend and complete school. Developing talents in sports and music are encouraged as a way to establish a socioeconomic base. Discipline and appropriate behavior are always emphasized. Children may attend private schools but are not boarded out. Child education is a central value of the African American culture. Both male and female children are expected to expand their learning through advanced degrees.
- **Expectations of and for elders**. Elders are a source of wisdom and demand respect. They are revered and often involved in caring for and raising grandchildren. Many elders live with their children or the children live with them to maintain the elder's independence. Institutionalization of elders for any reason is avoided and unacceptable, although this view is changing and varies among families.
- **Expectations of hospital visitors**. Visitors welcome; they frequently bring food, flowers, and/or a card. Family members may sleep at the bedside. Numerous family members, friends, and clergy gather at the bedside and remain until asked to leave, particularly on Sunday afternoon after church. Visiting a sick person is expected of family, friends, and clergy.

ILLNESS BELIEFS

- **Causes of/attitudes about physical illness**. Typically view health as being in harmony with nature and illness as a state of disharmony. Believe physical illness is a result of natural causes, improper diet and eating habits, exposure to cold air/wind, and unnatural or supernatural causes. May view illness as God's punishment for improper behavior or not living according to His will, or as the work of the devil. Those who are superstitious or believe in witchcraft or voodoo think illness occurs when someone casts a spell.

African Americans tend to have a fatalistic attitude about physical illness.

- **Causes of/attitudes about mental illness**. View health and illness as inseparable from mind, body, and spirit. Thus, mental illness often is related to spiritual imbalance. Although mental illness is no longer stigmatized or considered aberrant (when someone is thought to be possessed by demons), many African Americans still mask it. However, they encourage seeking help from family, friends, clergy, or a mental health professional.
- **Causes of genetic defects**. Consider defects to be the result of God's will. This belief varies by level of education. Family members and friends provide love and care in a nonjudgmental manner.
- **Attitudes about disabilities**. Believe that physical and developmental disabilities are a result of God's will, which should not be questioned. This attitude varies by level of education. Family members and friends love and care for the disabled person in a nonjudgmental manner, usually at home. Seek appropriate services, such as adult day care and respite care, to cope with the disability. Institutionalization usually a last resort.
- **Sick role**. Acknowledge that one cannot work and perform usual roles while sick. Expect attention from family and relatives but maintain independence.
- **Home and folk remedies**. Include teas, herbs, warm medicated compresses on the chest for colds, and cotton balls in the nostrils to protect against cold wind. May seek advice or prescriptions from folk healers who are stable, respected, and powerful resources, particularly for ailments whose origin is believed to be the result of a "fix," "hex," or "spell" (used interchangeably to mean a negative influence/presence by an external force or person). Those in rural areas may practice magic or voodoo to remove spells.
- **Medications**. Accept all forms of biomedical and alternative pharmacological methods and typically adhere to them as prescribed. Adherence is based on the belief that medication will improve one's health and feeling of well-being, and on trust in the health care professional who prescribes the medication. Medication-sharing uncommon but may occur.
- **Acceptance of procedures**. Historically skeptical about procedures but will accept surgery, transfusions, organ transplants, and other medically necessary procedures if these are explained and there are no religious restrictions. Generally do not consider organ transplantation, except for members of immediate family. Desired norm is to die as an intact person.
- **Care-seeking**. Use both folk and biomedical systems. Highly respect biomedicine and use it for serious illnesses. Often, African Americans seek care when they perceive a problem or when they think care is helpful and accessible.

HEALTH ISSUES

- **Concept of health**. View health as harmony among mind, body, and spirit, including a feeling of well-being, fulfillment of role expectations, and freedom from pain.

- **Health promotion and prevention**. Proper diet, stress management, and exercise in fresh air are prescriptions for maintaining health if they do not interfere with family obligations. Open to, and accepting of, culturally relevant and appropriate healthy-lifestyle information that fits in context of their everyday lives. Health-promotion and illness-prevention practices vary by education and socioeconomic level.
- **Screening**. Regularly participate in screening and routine exams. These health practices vary by gender and by socioeconomic and education levels. Men tend to participate less in screening, so clinicians should obtain a health history. Persons with more education, socioeconomic resources, and steady employment and adequate health benefits are more likely to participate in screening and routine exams if they have sufficient access to care.
- **Common health problems**. African Americans tend to be affected disproportionately by the top 10 leading causes of death in U.S. Typically have a higher body mass index, are more sedentary, smoke cigarettes, receive less prenatal care, have more low-birth-weight babies, have higher infant-mortality and homicide rates, report more stress, and have more morbidity and mortality from heart disease, hypertension, stroke, cancer, type 2 diabetes, and HIV/AIDS. Also a high incidence of lactose intolerance and periodontal disease. Sickle cell anemia the most common genetically inherited condition.

DEATH RITUALS

- **Beliefs and attitudes about death**. Consider death inevitable, a natural part of living. One dies when God is ready for him/her. African Americans may grieve expressively and strongly, but this varies. Have a paradoxical view about religion's influence and end-of-life care: Although death is God's will, life support typically should not be withdrawn; it is an extension of God's gift and omnipotence.
- **Preparation**. Clinician should report impending death to eldest family member, spouse, or parents. Notification should be immediate and direct when death is inevitable. Time is needed to notify family members, especially those far away, so they can be present when patient dies.
- **Home vs. hospital**. Prefer death at home, although this varies among families. Dying elders are frequently cared for at home until death is imminent, then brought to the hospital. Some African Americans believe that death at home brings bad luck.
- **Special needs**. None related to the death ritual. This varies among families and according to religious practice (e.g., prayer or having a cleric present).
- **Care of the body**. Family members usually want professionals to cleanse and prepare the body unless a religious ritual is requested. African Americans show great respect for the deceased and avoid cremation.
- **Attitudes about organ donation**. Generally a taboo. Often view organ donation as desecration of the body. Some believe that it hastens one's

death. May make exceptions for donations between family members.

- **Attitudes about autopsy**. When the need for autopsy is explained, most families understand and are accepting. Physician must discuss these issues with family members before death occurs.

SELECTED REFERENCES

Alexander, G. R., Kogan, M. D., & Nabukera, S. (2002). Racial differences in prenatal care use in the United States: Are disparities decreasing? *American Journal of Public Health, 92*, 1970–1975.

Harrison, A. O. (1997). Contraception: Practices and attitudes in the black community. In H. P. McAdoo (Ed.), *Black families* (pp. 301–319). Thousand Oaks, CA: Sage.

Karenga, M. (1998). *Kwanzaa: A celebration of family, community, and culture*. Los Angeles: University of Sankore Press.

Lewis, G. B. (2003). Black-white differences in attitudes toward homosexuality and gay rights. *Public Opinion Quarterly, 67*, 59–78.

Thomas, S. B. (2000). The Black organ and tissue donor shortage: A review of the literature. *African American Research Perspectives*, Fall, 11–23.

Waters, C. M. (1999). Professional nursing support for culturally diverse family members of critically ill adults. *Research in Nursing & Health, 22*, 107–117.

Waters, C. M. (2001). Understanding and supporting African-Americans' perspectives of end-of-life care planning and decision-making. *Qualitative Health Research, 11*, 385–398.

Waters, C. M., Times, R., Morton, A. R., Crear, M., & Wey, M. (2001). Perception of health status and participation in present and future health-promotion behaviors in African American women. *Journal of Prevention & Intervention in the Community, 22*, 81–96.

AUTHORS

Catherine M. Waters, RN, PhD, is an associate professor in the University of California-San Francisco School of Nursing, Department of Community Health Systems. She teaches courses related to program planning, advanced practice in community and public health, and cultural concepts in health. Her research focuses on lifestyle education and behavioral changes as mechanisms for disease-risk reduction, using culturally focused, community-based interventions in at-risk and underrepresented populations, especially African Americans.

Salamah Locks, RN, MS, CS, is a clinical nurse III in a cardiology, cardiothoracic/vascular surgery, and telemetry unit at the University of California Medical Center-San Francisco. She is a doctoral student in the UCSF School of Nursing with research interests in elder health care and longevity in African American males. Salamah's greatest inspiration, her mother, was raised by her slave-born paternal grandmother.

CHAPTER 3

AMERICAN INDIANS/ ALASKAN NATIVES

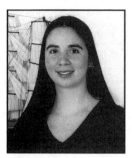
Janelle Palacios

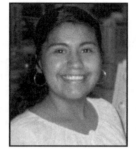
Rose Butterfly

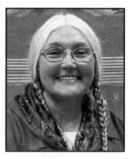
C. June Strickland

The American Indian/Alaskan Native (AI/AN) population is highly diverse. Retention of traditional customs and the level of acculturation are vastly different. There are more than 550 federally recognized tribes, bands, and nations and an additional 200 tribes that are not federally recognized. Tribes from different regions, such as those in the Southeast and Northwest, vary immensely in terms of cultural practices, language, and life situations. Tribes within regions, such as the Yakama Nation and the Quinault, differ as do people within tribes. Clinicians should recognize that reservation-dwelling AI/AN may not be of that particular reservation tribe and may feel isolated from their own tribal culture and distant family. Even an indigenous individual may not fit tribal enrollment requirements and therefore not have access to health care through Indian Health Services. Reservation lifestyle differs from urban living, creating different experiences.

CULTURAL/ETHNIC IDENTITY

- **Preferred term(s)**. Varies. Clinician should take care to ask each individual. Often use tribal names (e.g., Chippewa, Hopi, Seneca, Colville) when referring to themselves. Tribal affiliation names such as Navajo and Nez Perce are not the real names; people may prefer Dine to Navajo and Nimi'ipuu to Nez Perce. The designation of all tribes as "American Indians" or "Alaskan Natives" sometimes preferred rather than "Indians," "Native Americans," or "Eskimos."
- **Census**. According to the 2000 U.S. Census, there are nearly 4.1 million AI/AN, accounting for 1.5% of the total U.S. population. In this group,

0.9% reported they were solely of AI/AN heritage and 0.6% reported AI/AN heritage in combination with other ethnicities. Forty-three percent of all AI/AN live in the western U.S. The largest numbers are in California, Oklahoma, Arizona, and Texas, with 25% in California and Oklahoma. The largest AI populations by number of tribes are Cherokee, Navajo, Latin American Indian, and Choctaw. The largest AN populations are Eskimo, Tlingit-Haida, Alaskan Athabascan, and Aleut.

- **History of migration**. AI/AN people had original rights to all U.S. land and slowly lost their rights through colonialism and government expansion policies. Under these policies, only federally recognized tribes were granted smaller designated areas of land called reservations. The General Allotment Act of 1887 further divided the reservations, giving each tribal member a small parcel of land if the member signed a contract and pledged to follow U.S. law. Allegedly surplus reservation land (often of higher quality) was sold to non-natives, which created a checkerboard of ownership within reservations. The act also sought to "civilize" people by establishing a legal system that encouraged Christian education. The Congressional Termination and Relocation Act of 1954 cancelled recognition of some tribes and subsidized the relocation of AI/AN from rural to urban settings. This often left entire families stranded without promised financial and social-service support. Today, most AI/AN live in urban areas, but many families return to reservations to visit relatives and contribute to tribal activities.

SPIRITUAL/RELIGIOUS ORIENTATION

- **Primary religious/spiritual affiliations**. Religious and/or spiritual affiliation is by individual choice. Due to past colonization and Christian conversion, many AI/AN have some Christian ties, although they also may hold traditional beliefs. Some of them respect and combine different religious practices, such that an individual can be both highly acculturated and very traditional. Clinicians should not make assumptions. It is important and acceptable for clinicians to ask if spiritual beliefs/religion should be incorporated into biomedical health care.
- **Usual religious/spiritual practices**. May use sweet grass, cedar, sage, or tobacco smoke along with prayers, blessings, cleansing, and healing. Also view dancing, singing, and drumming as routes of spiritual connectedness, health, and healing. May sit for long hours in a steamy place and sweat. If a patient discloses that he/she practices sweats and if dehydration is a medical issue, it may be appropriate to negotiate the length of sweating time. Some patients choose not to disclose traditional practices.
- **Use of spiritual healing/healers**. Varies among individuals. Some may be suspicious of biomedicine but use it in conjunction with healers to promote fully integrated healing and to realign the body into harmony with life. Clinician should discuss with the healer how staff can help—e.g., by providing

privacy for a ceremony. If sacred objects such as feathers, a medicine bag, or bundles are present, do not remove or handle them. If need be, ask the patient or family to move items. If surgery is indicated, a sacred object may accompany the patient; place it in a plastic bag and attach it to his/her chart.

- **Holidays**. Vary by tribe/religion and individual choice. Holidays can also be social gatherings to celebrate seasonal changes—e.g., winter to spring; the harvest of certain crops, roots, or berries; and the beginning of fishing or hunting season. Many celebrated holidays were introduced and taught in school.

COMMUNICATION
ORAL COMMUNICATION

- **Major languages and dialects**. More than 100 indigenous languages. English usually spoken. Metaphors, anecdotes, and storytelling may convey meaning in a given context. Clinicians should listen closely and not interrupt the speaker. To facilitate conversation, can ask questions after a monologue has ended. Careful listening may answer further questions. Inappropriate to ask, "Do you have an Indian name?" or "Can you say something in Indian?" Appropriate to ask, "Which tribe are you from?" or "Who are your people?"
- **Greetings**. Strangers should always introduce themselves to the patient and/or family. A light handshake is culturally appropriate and respectful; a hard grip or pumping handshake is not. Take care when addressing patients. Appropriate to use their first name, but inappropriate to refer to someone as "chief," "squaw," or "medicine man." During provider introductions and visits, validate what the patient has done correctly in terms of his/her health care before suggesting changes.
- **Tone of voice**. Patient may be soft-spoken with clinician. Clinician should be clear, direct, and calm when expressing urgent instructions. Loudness may suggest aggressive, rude behavior. Humor may foster a comfortable, positive environment and rapport.
- **Direct or indirect style of speech**. Indirect style of speech common, with stories communicating key points. Clinician should listen carefully to speaker for subtle indications of desires. Pauses are sometimes a part of conversation and should not be misinterpreted as the end of discussion.
- **Use of interpreters**. Clinician should enlist a mature person and ask about preference for same gender. Older AI/AN, such as Dine (Navajo), may speak Dine, English, Spanish, or a combination. Be clear and distinguish between fact and probability, as grammar may alter translation from English to another language. Listening carefully to a story and responses is respectful, facilitates rapport, and provides context for answers. Excessive questions may suggest to patient/family that clinician is being invasive and/or not listening.
- **Serious or terminal illness**. Propose and facilitate a family meeting to discuss a patient's condition and course of treatment, especially regarding sen-

sitive topics such as do-not-resuscitate codes. Hospice may be desired and, depending on the individual, culturally appropriate.

WRITTEN COMMUNICATION

- **Literacy assessment**. Compared to other ethnic minorities, fewer American Indian youth graduate from high school. Boarding-school experiences in the 19th and 20th centuries had a negative effect on the AI/AN language, culture, and perception of education. Often modeled on military schools, boarding schools taught AI/AN to read, write, and speak English; to be individualistic; to adopt Christian values and religion; and to be good citizens. Sometimes their education was reinforced by brutality that included physical and psychosocial harm, withholding food, and taking children unwillingly from families. If a patient's ability to read and write English is questionable, oral health education of him/her and family—including demonstrating ideas and concepts—is warranted. Appropriate for clinician to ask if he/she may read and explain procedures.
- **Consents**. Due to historical abuse of signed documents, some patients are wary of signing consents. Clinician should explain the procedure and ask patient if he/she needs to consult with family members or others first. Indicate if it is OK for patient to wait for such consultation. Full discussion of procedures with everyone who should be involved, and gaining group consensus, may increase an individual's willingness to sign consents. In emergency situations when family members are unavailable to give consent, the prudent choice is to limit medical procedures to the least invasive. Be sure to talk with patient and family afterward. Double check to find out if patient or family needs to have the care plan or procedure clarified.

NONVERBAL COMMUNICATION

- **Eye contact**. Avoidance of direct eye contact should not be interpreted as inattentiveness or evasiveness. In fact, it may reflect a patient's or family member's respect for clinicians. Providers should behave naturally and forego mannerisms, such as avoiding eye contact, that might make the interaction uncomfortable or awkward.
- **Personal space**. AI/AN greatly appreciate adequate personal space in the health care setting, especially during a healing ritual or when they need time with family or friends. It is prudent to maintain a respectful distance (a few feet) when meeting someone for the first time.
- **Use and meaning of silence**. AI/AN cultures observe silence in a variety of circumstances. Context of a situation influences the meaning of silence. If the clinician does not understand a period of silence, he/she should openly ask patient and family what it means. This shows that the clinician is listening to and respects them.
- **Gestures**. Nodding the head, pursing the lips, or pointing the chin may indi-

cate acknowledgment. A rude and disrespectful gesture is the stereotypical greeting "How," with the arm extended and palm facing the visitor. Nodding the head in someone's direction may be an acceptable informal greeting.

- **Openness in expressing emotions**. Sharing emotions physically and verbally varies among tribes and individuals. Is generally reserved for close kin and friends.

- **Privacy**. There may be resistance or an unwillingness to disclose information, out of respect for the patient or family members. They may expect the clinician to discuss a medical condition, test results, and prognosis with the extended family. Ask patient about what is appropriate.

- **Touch**. Sensitivity to modesty is appreciated during physical examination. Explain why an examination is necessary and why touching may be helpful.

- **Orientation to time**. Focus is on the present, described as "Indian time," rather than on the future, but this is flexible. It often conflicts with rigidly scheduled appointments. Pauses may be a natural part of conversation. Pressuring someone to respond or act is considered rude and disrespectful, especially among elders. Patients feel more comfortable sitting down with a clinician and getting to know him/her. Some AI/AN may not grasp the notion of future illness, so the relevance of preventive health care may escape them.

ACTIVITIES OF DAILY LIVING

- **Modesty**. Flexible, depending on the individual and tribe. Nakedness appropriate when body exposure is necessary, although clinician should offer a gown or drape. Same-gender clinician important for certain examinations— e.g., Pap smear or prostate exam.

- **Skin care**. Best to ask the patient.

- **Hair care**. Care and treatment of hair may be associated with health or mourning practices. Some Pacific Northwest women prefer that no one except a close family member touch their hair. Clinician should always ask before touching. If cutting or shaving is necessary, ask the patient or family if they would prefer a health provider or family member to do this. If that cannot be arranged, ask the patient or family how hair should be disposed of, as some tribes require hair to be stored by the family or an individual, or to be disposed of ceremoniously. A traditional hairstyle may require an appropriate person to fix it. Ask the patient. The hair of very ill patients, including infants, may be washed and dressed ceremoniously.

- **Nail care**. Some tribes may collect nail parings. Ask the patient or family if parings should be disposed of or collected.

- **Toileting**. Patient may use nonprescription aids, such as teas or special foods, for diarrhea or constipation. Respect for privacy and modesty is appreciated. Best to ask if a bedpan or commode is preferable.

- **Special clothing or amulets**. If the patient wears a medicine bag or has special items such as feathers or herb bundles nearby, clinician should make every effort not to remove them. Allow the patient or family to move items to another visible place. If a procedure necessitates removal of a special item but the patient asks to keep it, place the item in a plastic bag and attach it to his/her chart.

- **Self-care**. Self-care is expected, for the most part. Help is generally offered to elders and disabled persons, but they may not take advantage of it. In a hospital or clinic setting, clinician should state the location of, and provide information about, amenities such as the library, magazines, TV, radio, cafeteria, vending machines, meal schedule, and how to get extra food or fluids if needed. Tell visitors about parking, the visitation policy, staying overnight, and adjunct areas—e.g., the playroom, pool, and private family conference rooms.

FOOD PRACTICES

- **Usual meal pattern**. Three meals daily have become the norm, but this varies with social and other activities. Sharing food often reflects hospitality and respect; patients may want to share hospital food with visitors or eat food that visitors bring.
- **Special utensils**. None.
- **Food beliefs and rituals**. Food may be blessed or specially prepared for ceremonies. For example, wakes or funerals may include feasts at which "fry bread" or other high-fat foods are served. Despite the negative aspects of AI/AN diet, the social and cultural rituals associated with food have positive benefits.
- **Usual diet**. Traditional diets were low in fat. But due to a lack of natural resources and the historical removal of people from their native lands, the availability of low-fat foods may be limited. Today's typical diets—consisting of high-fat, salty, and sugary foods that are filling—may be related to their low cost and accessibility. Some urban and rural families receive government-subsidized staples and food from the Women Infants and Children (WIC) Supplemental Nutrition Program. When assessing AI/AN who have diabetes, clinicians should be aware that potential diet choices—especially fresh produce—may be limited by low income and dependence on commodity foods.
- **Fluids**. Clinicians should encourage fluid intake between meals. Some patients prefer herbal teas. If so, teas brought in by visitors might contain substances that, given patients' particular medications, may be contraindicated. Consuming water with every meal may be desirable.
- **Food taboos and prescriptions**. Many view water as a sacred, life-sustaining source, a way of connecting with the earth. May request water with each meal and/or before or after invasive procedures. Some southwestern tribes believe that corn, beans, and squash promote health. Foods to avoid vary among tribes and individuals.

- **Hospitality**. For AI/AN, food- and gift-giving often is fundamental. Hospitalized patients may want to share food with visitors or accept food or gifts from them. Clinician should keep in mind that kinship boundaries are extended in AI/AN culture; visitors who are not the patient's blood relatives may feel entitled to the same food or parking rights that the patient or his/her family has.

SYMPTOM MANAGEMENT

- **Pain**. Undertreated in this population, often due to stereotypes of AI/AN as substance abusers or as people who can stoically manage pain. Patient may be unwilling to express pain, so the clinician must frequently ask about it. Use of number scale understood. Patient may explain pain in general terms—e.g., "not feeling good" or "something not feeling right." If pain is not treated, patient may express pain to a family member or friend who may relay the message to the health care provider.
- **Dyspnea**. Lungs are associated with freedom, so tightness of breath may be construed as a hindrance. Wide use of oxygen to alleviate symptoms, especially among elders.
- **Nausea/vomiting**. Patient may express embarrassment. Clinician should offer basins and access to water, soap, and towels. Appropriate to ask patient how this is normally handled.
- **Constipation/diarrhea**. Patient may express embarrassment. Clinician should ask how he/she usually tolerates or alleviates the problem. Constipated patients may want to walk around or they might ask a family member or friend to prepare special food. Ask if patient is taking additional therapy. Appropriate to ask the patient how this is normally handled.
- **Fatigue**. Physical as well as psychosocial issues may result in fatigue. Clinician should consider external sources of fatigue, such as poverty, living conditions, and/or family dynamics that lead to elevated stress/anxiety. Patient may use prescription drugs or adjunct therapy. Ask how he/she handles fatigue.
- **Depression**. Highly prevalent. Standard screening tools have inadequately captured the extent of the problem and may mask depression or magnify preexisting depression. Feeling "out of harmony" or "heavy," or somatizing psychological problems (e.g., sensing a dull ache), may indicate depression. AI/AN have the highest rate of teen suicide in U.S. This could be related to socioeconomic status, education, limited opportunities, and intergenerational pain resulting from memories of colonization or stories told and retold in families about sexual and physical abuse at boarding schools in earlier times.
- **Self-care symptom management**. Depending on how traditional and acculturated one is, AI/AN may use traditional medicine first or in conjunction with biomedicine. Biomedicine might be the first choice for certain diseases, such as diabetes, in more-educated AI/AN communities. Smudg-

ing—cleansing oneself with herbal smoke from burnt sage, cedar, tobacco, or sweet grass—may augment self-healing at home or in the hospital. If this creates problems, clinician should give the patient and/or visitors an alternative place to smudge. In some cultures, extended family members help care for patient. Individuals living in rural or urban areas may not have any familial or tribal support.

BIRTH RITUALS/CARE OF THE NEW MOTHER AND BABY

- **Pregnancy care**. AI/AN women have the lowest prenatal care rates of all population groups in U.S., which may reflect cultural (e.g., concept of time) and social (e.g., access to transportation) differences. If a woman continually misses prenatal care appointments and schedules them late in pregnancy, clinicians should ask how they can accommodate future visits. Teen pregnancy rate among AI/AN is higher than U.S. average and early pregnancy may be more culturally acceptable; therefore, clinician should treat young mothers respectfully. Some pregnant women may abstain from negative experiences such as attending funerals or seeing dead animals. In some tribes, it is appropriate for a pregnant woman to "sweat" as a way of ensuring her health and that of the baby.
- **Preferences for children**. Traditional stories typically taught that both genders contribute equally to the tribe. Children often are highly valued and recognized as the protectors of cultural legacy.
- **Labor practices**. Vary among tribes. AI/AN expect female attendants from among family or friends. Analgesics may be used minimally for a normal delivery.
- **Role of the laboring woman during birth**. While stoicism may be encouraged, clinician should not assume patient does not need support. Should always offer support, encouragement, and analgesics according to the birth plan. Some families may want the placenta returned. Ask if they do and who should receive it.
- **Role of the father and other family members during birth**. Varies among cultures. Father may be absent during birth but present at other times—e.g., to hold or name the baby after delivery. Clinician should not assume that father's absence during birth means the infant lacks a father figure.
- **Vaginal vs. cesarean section**. Vaginal birth strongly preferred. Clinician should ask patient (or a family member if patient is unable to answer) if she wants an episiotomy. Due to a history of imposed sterilization, women may fear cesarean birth. If cesarean section is necessary, properly educate mother about the procedure and assess her understanding of it. She may fear that she will not be able to deliver more children without difficulties or become pregnant again after a cesarean.
- **Breastfeeding**. Breastfeeding and bottle-feeding acceptable. Clinician

should explain advantages and disadvantages of each. If bottle-feeding preferred, discuss proper technique, formula type, and when to use whole milk.

- **Birth recuperation**. Exercise versus bed rest varies according to tribal tradition, acculturation, and economic resources. Women may want family present while resting after delivery instead of being isolated.

- **Baby care**. In addition to birth parents, it is normal and culturally acceptable for grandparents, uncles, aunts, and cousins to provide or supplement baby or child care. Clinician may have to delicately negotiate care of the infant or child with the caregivers and parents. Some families bind infants into cradleboards (comparable to slings), which provide a swaddled, protective environment.

- **Problems with baby**. Clinician must inform the baby's caretaker—a parent, grandparent, aunt, or uncle—of any problems. Some AI/AN families may congregate to make decisions. If the infant is not expected to live, family may wish to remain with baby and pray or perform a ritual until his/her death. American Indian babies often are born with Mongolian spots—darkly pigmented areas on the lower back—that should not be mistaken as a sign of abuse.

- **Male and female circumcision**. Male circumcision may be performed for hygienic reasons.

DEVELOPMENTAL AND SEXUAL ISSUES

- **Celebration of menarche or becoming a man**. Celebrating rites of passage varies among tribes, traditions, and individuals. Some tribes honor a girl's first menstrual period and new role in the community with a special ceremony. For example, she may be entrusted with more responsibility related to ceremonies, such as root-digging. In some tribes, hunting may be the rite of passage for boys, in recognition of their contributions to community and family.

- **Attitudes about birth control**. Couples make their own decisions. Generally use intrauterine devices, birth control pills, condoms, and tubal ligation. In the 1970s, systematic sterilizations were performed mainly on reservation-dwelling women of childbearing age. As a result, AI/AN women may distrust health care providers who endorse birth control. Some southwestern tribes may have taboos that forbid women from talking about sexual matters with males—including clinicians—who are not their partners. Clinicians must approach birth control topics cautiously, giving the patient adequate time and respectful distance when answering questions.

- **Attitudes about sexually transmitted infection (STI) control, including condoms**. STI education may be limited to what the public schools teach. Some AI/AN believe that because they know their partner, there is no need to worry about STIs and, later, present with advanced disease. It is appropriate for clinicians to educate patients and discreetly discuss condom use with them.

- **Attitudes about abortion**. Individuals make their own decisions. Some want an abortion. Providers must be aware that abortions often are culturally incompatible with AI/AN values and should monitor the woman who chooses abortion for potential depression and suicide. Unplanned or unwanted pregnancies may be carried to term. After delivery, infant may be placed with a caregiver, often a member of the extended family.
- **Attitudes about unwed sexual experimentation**. Sexual experimentation generally viewed as a fact of life, but family attitudes within tribes vary. Teen pregnancies are higher among AI/AN (58.3 per 1,000 live births in 2002) than the U.S. national average (42.9 per 1,000 live births).
- **Sexual orientation**. Acceptance of nonheterosexual practices varies among tribes, families, and individuals. Many tribes have traditional stories alluding to variations in sexual orientation, and some have always long accepted homosexual and bisexual orientations—e.g., Berdache or Two Spirited People.
- **Gender identity**. Acceptance has varied historically. Some tribes have recognized genders other than female and male. Some cultures have accepted role reversal and, today, may not pressure individuals to identify with one gender. Contemporary views depend on the tribe and individual.
- **Attitudes about menopause**. Generally regarded as a normal part of life. AI/AN do not view physiological signs of menopause as disruptive to overall health, although some women may seek symptom relief via traditional herbal remedies/practices or biomedicine.

FAMILY RELATIONSHIPS

- **Composition/structure**. Cultures vary in kinship structure. Extent of acculturation to the dominant culture throughout history should be considered. In matrilineal/matrilocal clans, the family lives near the wife's family, and land, house, and other possessions are passed down through females. In patrilineal/patrilocal clans, the family lives near the husband's family and possessions are passed down through males. Kinship roles are extensive; they often include friends as family members who may be identified in specific terms or referred to as cousin, brother, or sister.
- **Decision-making**. Varies among tribes, kinship structures, and families. Sometimes decisions are made by individuals, sometimes by group consensus. Providers should facilitate decision-making by providing private space and time for family discussion.
- **Spokesperson**. Age and gender of the spokesperson may vary individually and among tribes. Be aware that a child or a family friend may be the appropriate spokesperson. Ask who should receive information.
- **Gender issues**. Vary among cultures, locations, and demographics. In matrilineal clans, women and/or their brothers may make important decisions, while men protect the family's and community's well-being. Each gen-

der may have specific roles. In addition, some roles are limited to particular situations or times. For example, respect dictates that women refrain from drumming and performing or attending ceremonies while menstruating.

- **Changing roles among generations in U.S.** Today, many tribal communities emphasize the connection between education and culture. As younger generations become more educated, an increasing number of AI/AN return home to help their families, community, and tribe deal with issues central to their cultural legacies.

- **Caring roles.** When a family member is ill, women (daughters, aunts, grandmothers) may be caregivers. So might friends, depending on situation. Caregiving varies among kinship structures. Often, grandparents help care for young children, who are expected to help care for elder grandparents. It is culturally acceptable to be raised by members of the extended family— aunts, uncles, or cousins. Sometimes a grandmother may be called "Mother."

- **Expectations of and for children.** Children are generally expected to respect elders, take pride in Indian culture, and develop natural talents. Cultivating independence also is valued; one fosters this by fulfilling responsibilities to family, community, and tribe.

- **Expectations of and for elders.** Status of elders is characterized by their health or physical decline, the counseling or teaching they provide to the younger generation, or having grandchildren. Elders highly value caring for themselves, although in times of need, families usually take the initiative to care for them. In skilled nursing facilities on reservations, male residents tend to outnumber female residents 2-to-1.

- **Expectations of hospital visitors.** Vary among tribes, although central focus is on promoting the patient's well-being—e.g., through prayer, song, dance, and smudging. Providers should be aware of the need for space, time, and privacy. Transportation to and from the hospital may be difficult, which may affect the length of visits. Family members may prefer to remain at the bedside if they stay overnight.

ILLNESS BELIEFS

- **Causes of/attitudes about physical illness.** Some AI/AN relate physical illness to violation of taboos or being out of harmony, although beliefs vary depending on culture, assimilation, and individual beliefs.

- **Causes of/attitudes about mental illness.** Some cultures believe that such causes include violation of taboos, loss of harmony with the environment, or ghosts. Clinician should consider both the individual's and the tribe's degree of acculturation in assessing how mental illness is perceived. Traditional persons may avoid psychotherapy or medication. Inquire if the patient is willing to try different therapies.

- **Causes of genetic defects.** Beliefs vary by tribal culture and acculturation. Some tribes believe that taboos broken by parents cause genetic defects, others believe that the parents were too closely related. Various tribes believe that a child with a genetic defect bears all of the tribe's pain, guilt, and burden, and therefore is highly valued and respected.

- **Attitudes about disabilities**. Depend on the context and individual experiences with disabilities. If a sole provider becomes disabled, he/she may have negative feelings about the disability. Sometimes disability is deemed to have occurred for an unknown reason. Providers should cautiously discuss disability in terms of its meaning and degree of function. Disabled persons generally are socially integrated into the community.

- **Sick role**. In order to get well, AI/AN typically focus on health and wellness of the body, mind, and spirit rather than on sickness, and on activity rather than rest.

- **Home and folk remedies**. Herbs and roots for common maladies, such as cough, diarrhea, constipation, or headache, especially if they are prescribed by a healer or knowledgeable person. When prescribing medication, changing a patient's diet, or preparing for a medical procedure, clinician should ask if patient uses any home remedies.

- **Medications**. Clinician should ask patients if they use traditional medicine, recognizing that some are not comfortable disclosing such information. Also should ask if they partake in any strenuous activity related to ceremonies (e.g., dancing or sweating), as that has implications regarding hydration and prescription drugs. Some persons are skeptical about medications; they think medications will be habit-forming or cause lifelong illnesses if taken over a lengthy period. Providers should explain why taking a particular drug—e.g., an antibiotic—is important and how to do so appropriately.

- **Acceptance of procedures**. Varies among individuals. Full discussion of procedures will educate the patient and greatly enhance provider-patient relationship. Some may refuse to accept donated organs or be reluctant to give up body parts (limbs, blood, gall stones) because of personal beliefs.

- **Care-seeking**. Because AI/AN focus on the present, they may not consider the future consequences of current habits—e.g., how a high-sugar diet and inactivity may lead to diabetes. Thus, they may not seek care until symptoms are advanced. Some may visit a recognized healer before contacting a physician.

HEALTH ISSUES

- **Concept of health**. Oriented toward holistic health and wellness. Aligning mind, body, and spirit with personal beliefs about nature/God/the universe enhances an individual's harmony.

- **Health promotion and prevention**. Some tribes hold ceremonies—dancing, singing, drumming, sweating—to promote health. Clinician should inquire about such activities and how long the patient participates in them, as some rituals last up to 24 hours or longer and may be contraindicated by his/her medical condition. Be sensitive, realizing that some people may not willingly discuss traditional behavior.

- **Screening**. Clinician should explain its importance to the patient and family but also recognize that lack of resources and/or fear of appearing inferior may be barriers to health screening. Special concerns that necessitate screening include diabetes, suicidal risk, prenatal care, mammograms, cervical cancer, and dental problems.
- **Common health problems**. AI/AN populations have the highest rates of depression, suicide, and diabetes of any ethnic minority in U.S. and are the most likely to lack prenatal care. Smoking and alcoholism are more prevalent among AI/AN than among Americans in general. Some of these problems are related to low socioeconomic status, poverty, limited education, high unemployment, and intergenerational pain (cultural heaviness) as a result of historical injustices and disenfranchisement.

DEATH RITUALS

- **Beliefs and attitudes about death**. Some AI/AN take care to honor the body, regarding it as the spirit's home. Some believe that upon death, the spirit reunites with the Creator. Others believe in reincarnation. Still others believe in a Christian-oriented philosophy (going to heaven). Depending on the cause of death, reactions range from acceptance to denial. For example, if a person dies while sleeping, an explanation is that a deceased loved one visited and took him/her. Dealing with death as a result of a car crash or homicide may be more difficult, but AI/AN often believe that the deceased rests in peace with other relatives and friends who have died.
- **Preparation**. Family members must be told if a patient is not expected to live so arrangements can be made and loved ones can gather.
- **Home vs. hospital**. Depends on the culture and family. Some families may prefer that the patient be in a hospital and, as would occur in a more natural setting, undergo minimal procedures.
- **Special needs**. Privacy is appreciated, especially if the family wants someone who is a recognized healer to facilitate the patient's spiritual health. To promote healing, smudging (burning special herbs) or singing might take place. If so, the provider may help find an appropriate place for this practice.
- **Care of the body**. Preparation depends on the tribe and family. Special persons may step forward to take care of the body. Providers can ask how these persons might help care for the body. They can ask family members if the health-care-setting protocol is adequate or if the hospital protocol is inappropriate. Some may request that the body be cleansed by a special person before it is moved.
- **Attitudes about organ donation**. Not usually practiced. Body parts are deemed integral to the deceased, in accordance with cultural beliefs. However, if interest is expressed, clinician should explain the procedure.

- **Attitudes about autopsy**. State laws and cultural beliefs may clash. Autopsies conducted for the appropriate reason (e.g., litigation) are generally acceptable, although it is important for clinician to ask if the entire body should be returned to the family and to discuss legal or jurisdictional mandates. Providers must be sensitive to special religious proscriptions regarding the time period within which the body must be buried.

SELECTED REFERENCES

Adams, D. W. (1997). *Education for extinction: American Indians and the boarding school experience, 1875–1928*. Lawrence, KS: University Press of Kansas.

Dick, R. W., Manson, S. M., & Beals, J. (1993). Alcohol use among American Indian adolescents: Patterns and correlates of students drinking in a boarding school. *Journal of Studies on Alcohol, 54*, 172–177.

Klebe, E., & Judge, K. (1993). *Health services for American Indians and Alaska Natives* (CRS Report to Congress, 93-975 EPW). Washington, DC: Library of Congress.

Manson, S. M. (1995). Culture and major depression: Current challenges in the diagnosis of mood disorders. *Psychiatric Clinics of North America, 18*, 487–501.

Norton, I. M., & Manson, S. M. (1996). Research in American Indian and Alaska Native communities: Navigating the cultural universe of values and process. *Journal of Consulting and Clinical Psychology, 64*, 856–860.

Rhoades, E. R., Reyes, L. L., & Buzzard, G. D. (1987). The organization of health services for Indian people. *Public Health Reports, 102*, 352–356.

Rudy, R. H., & Brown, J. A. (1988). *Indians of the Pacific Northwest*. Norman, OK: University of Oklahoma Press.

Strickland, C. J. (Winter 1996–97). Suicide among American Indian, Alaskan Native, and Canadian Aboriginal youth: Advancing the research agenda. *International Journal of Mental Health, 25*, 11–32.

Utter, J. (1993). *American Indians: Answers to today's questions*. Lake Ann, MI: National Woodlands Publishing.

AUTHORS

Janelle Palacios, RN, BSN, is Salish/Kootenai and grew up on the Flathead Reservation in Montana. She graduated from the University of Washington School of Nursing in 2003 and currently attends the University of California-San Francisco, where she is pursuing a master's degree in nurse-midwifery and a PhD. After completing her education, she plans to offer her skills to native communities.

Rose Butterfly is an enrolled Blackfeet member and descendent of the Colville and Yakama tribes. She grew up in Nespelem, WA, on the Colville Reservation. She will graduate from the University of Washington with a BS degree focusing on health care for American Indians and with a minor in American Indian studies.

C. June Strickland, PhD, RN, is an Echota Cherokee and graduate faculty member at the University of Washington. She is committed to developing culturally appropriate research instruments, examining the cultural appropriateness of research methods (such as focus groups), and exploring the appropriateness and fit of mainstream theories and strategies in Indian communities. Her current research focuses on health-related behavior change (prevention) among American Indians in the Pacific Northwest.

ACKNOWLEDGMENTS

To our family members, friends, and colleagues, thank you for sharing your insight and helping us write this section. To our native communities, thank you for your support. We extend a special thanks to Polly Olsen and Walt Hollow at the University of Washington.

CHAPTER 4

ARABS

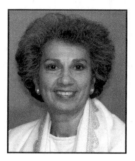

Afaf Ibrahim Meleis

CULTURAL/ETHNIC IDENTITY

Most speak Arabic and are Muslim, but there is great variation based on country of origin (there are 21 Arab nations), social class, education, urban or rural origin, and time in U.S. (e.g., third and fourth generations usually are assimilated).

- **Preferred term(s)**. May identify themselves by regional origin, such as Arab Americans or Middle Eastern Americans; by country of origin, such as Egyptian Americans or Palestinians; by city of origin, such as Ramallah; or by ethnic minority group, such as Armenians or Assyrians. Clinician should ask what the patient prefers to be called.

- **Census**. The 2000 U.S. Census cites nearly 1.24 million people of Arab ancestry, of whom the largest groups are Lebanese and "Arab/Arabic." However, they are likely undercounted, as many list themselves as "White." Other estimates range from 3 million to nearly 5 million. Largest Arab-American communities in Michigan (Detroit), California, and New Jersey.

- **History of immigration**. Began arriving in early 1800s. First serious wave came between 1887–1913, including many single, uneducated men from what was then called Greater Syria seeking better jobs and a higher standard of living. The second wave (1940–1970) was driven by political events and wars; many were refugees. Creation of State of Israel in 1948 markedly increased Arab immigration, especially of Muslims. The third wave (1970–2000) also was driven by wars and deteriorating economic and political circumstances. These immigrants were more often highly educated and professionals. Since 1990, immigrants to U.S. have been selected by lottery. Mostly well-educated but work in small businesses and transportation (e.g., driving taxis) due to limited employment opportunities.

SPIRITUAL/RELIGIOUS ORIENTATION

- **Primary religious/spiritual affiliations**. Early immigrants were Christians, including Protestants and Greek Orthodox. Recent immigrants are Muslims and almost exclusively of the Sunni branch, although many from Iraq are Shi'ite. Differences in branch of Islam are not reflected in health and illness practices.
- **Usual religious/spiritual practices**. Christians attend church and pray. Those who worship Islam believe in God (Allah) and His messenger, Prophet Mohammed; fasting during the month of Ramadan; giving alms to the poor; making pilgrimages to Mecca; and praying five times a day (usually in silence) and washing before prayers. Some attend communal prayer on Friday afternoon, a holiday/day of rest in all Muslim countries.
- **Use of spiritual healing/healers**. Christians may request a Middle Eastern minister. Muslims do not expect a Muslim religious leader (*imam*) to visit; *imams* only summoned after death. Families may want to pray for patient in silence or want another room for privacy.
- **Holidays**. All celebrate New Year's Eve. At the end of the month of Ramadan, the date of which is determined by lunar calendar, Muslims celebrate four days of *Eid al-Fitr*, or "Small Eid." Also important is *Eid al-Adha*, or "Big Eid" (Feast of Sacrifice), a holy time that commemorates the story of Ibrahim and his son Ismail, and the lamb as a sacrifice. Those who can make a pilgrimage to Mecca leave during this time. Many Muslims celebrate the birthday of the Prophet Mohammed; the date rotates in the Christian calendar. All holidays also observed in the U.S. Christians celebrate Catholic and Orthodox holidays, such as Christmas on December 25 or January 7 (Orthodox on Julian calendar), Easter, and others.

COMMUNICATION

ORAL COMMUNICATION

- **Major languages and dialects**. Arabic. Variations in dialects, words, and meanings in different Arab countries (e.g., Egyptian-Arabic). Most understand each other, but there are exceptions, such as Yemenis, who speak a local version of Arabic not widely understood. Though all Muslims read the same Koran written in Arabic, not all speak Arabic. Some ethnic minorities also speak their own language (e.g., Armenian). Arabic spoken at home among nearly 600,000 people in U.S. Arab professionals and business people usually speak English fluently.
- **Greetings**. Use title and first name. Adults or elderly may prefer to be called mother (*Om*) or father (*Abu*) followed by the first name of the eldest son (e.g., *Om* Waheed, or "mother of Waheed"). Clinician should ask family how friends or distant relatives address a person. Family members greet each other by handshake and kisses on both cheeks. Clinician can approach by shaking hands and acknowledging country of origin or something personal

about the patient or family. Smiling and direct eye contact, even if patient avoids them, are helpful.

- **Tone of voice**. Loud voice means message is important. Patients and/or family members usually express anger in high, intense voice. Arabs tend to repeat same information several times if they think others do not understand them or for emphasis.
- **Direct or indirect style of speech**. Very polite. With strangers, may express agreement that does not reflect true feelings. They avoid outward show of disagreement and may respond in ways they think others want them to respond. Head-nodding and smiles do not always mean comprehension. Clinician should ask person to repeat information to assess his/her understanding. Narrative style rather than short answers preferred in describing illness experience and symptoms. Clinicians should take time to discuss illness using a personal approach and soft tone of voice.
- **Use of interpreters**. After assessing patient's English ability, clinician should inform him/her that an interpreter is available. Arabic is a very flowery language with elaborate metaphors. Use same-sex interpreters whenever possible. Use only a same-sex family member for translating sensitive topics regarding sex, elimination, marital problems, reproduction, or highly sensitive diseases—cancer, HIV/AIDS, tuberculosis, venereal diseases. Sometimes family members edit messages to protect patient. The more sensitive an issue, the less likely families are to discuss it.
- **Serious or terminal illness**. Clinician should avoid blunt presentation of diagnosis and prognosis. A careful, caring, indirect style is preferable when presenting grave news. Family members buffer sick persons from knowing the whole truth. Confide first in family spokesperson and consult on best way to approach patient with news. Family prefers to disclose information to patient but may request presence of a health professional. If a family member provides the information in Arabic, there is no guarantee that the seriousness of the situation will be conveyed. Accommodate family needs for gradual and prolonged disclosure of information.

WRITTEN COMMUNICATION

- **Literacy assessment**. Some who claim to speak English fluently or moderately well in fact have difficulty understanding health professionals or following directions. May be too proud to admit they do not understand. Clinician should first ask patient about his/her comfort with spoken and written English, then speak slowly in simple terms and ask for validation. Insulting to assume a lack of language skills among those who are educated or have been living in U.S. for a long time. Assume fluency until information indicates otherwise.
- **Consents**. Written consent forms may be problematic; verbal consent based on trust more acceptable. Dislike hearing all possible complications before a

medical procedure; think it is bad luck to dwell on potential complications. Clinician should explain need for written consent, emphasize positive consequences, and humanize the process. For example, when asked for advice, clinicians should indicate what they would do for member of their own family.

NONVERBAL COMMUNICATION

- **Eye contact**. More sustained eye contact conveys more trust. Modesty may affect eye contact with opposite sex. Traditional women may avoid eye contact with men and persons they do not know. Health professionals should always make direct eye contact.
- **Personal space**. Families expect very little personal space. With someone of same gender, closeness (10–12 inches) expected and encouraged. When comfortable with clinicians, prefer close proximity as a way to build trusting relationship.
- **Use and meaning of silence**. Silence may indicate respect for authority but may not mean agreement. It could mean patient does not understand an instruction and therefore is embarrassed.
- **Gestures**. Expressive use of hands in conversation. Older or more traditional immigrants may use *salaam* gesture—touching heart with right hand, then forehead and gesturing forward. Those from Saudi Arabia may signal "yes" by turning their head side to side and "no" by tipping head backward and clicking tongue. For emphasis, may point and shake a finger at others, which may be offensive to non-Arabs. Patient may interpret an open palm facing him/her as warding off the evil eye. Showing bottom of foot is in bad taste and pointing it toward others is disrespectful. Right hand used for eating, left for bodily hygiene.
- **Openness in expressing emotions**. Expressive, warm, other-oriented, shy, and modest. Facial and bodily expressions indicative of inner emotions, more exaggerated than those of European Americans. Show feelings more openly through nonverbal cues and by the voice they use while speaking with family members. More vocal and use more gestures. Flat affect in presence of strangers may prevent others from gauging their inner feelings. Traditional women may be reserved and unexpressive, withholding some emotions until they trust the other person and feel accepted.
- **Privacy**. Value privacy and modesty, particularly in presence of strangers. Respect for professionals enables disclosure and loss of privacy, especially after trust is established. Clinician should segregate genders when a procedure calls for undressing. Disclosure is enhanced by matching gender of clinician and patient.
- **Touch**. Comfortable touching those of own gender only. Touch enhances trust, acceptance, and communication. When patient touches area of body about which he/she has a complaint, it helps pinpoint the problem and improves diagnosis. If clinician also touches the area of complaint, it con-

firms understanding and reassures the patient about clinician's ability to make a better diagnosis.

- **Orientation to time**. More past- and present-oriented than future-oriented. Tend to have two time conceptions: "on time" for official business and more spontaneous and flexible time for social and informal gatherings. Human interaction more valued than adhering to a clock or schedule. If importance of being on time emphasized, will comply. Prevention education (future orientation) may be influenced by God's control over events rather than individual efforts. When patient and family say, *"Inshallah"* (God willing), they believe there are higher powers that facilitate or impede, although the patient will take responsibility for care.

ACTIVITIES OF DAILY LIVING

- **Modesty**. Great modesty expected of men and women. Most women need a long gown and robe. Men's modesty is intensified in presence of women. Clinician should drape patient appropriately and carefully, particularly if patient is of opposite gender. Patient may be attended by a female chaperone from family. Unwed young women do not undergo pelvic exams because of concern about potential loss of virginity.
- **Skin care**. Varies by country of origin and level of biculturalism. Some prefer daily shower. Some reluctant to use foreign bathrooms and need careful orientation and support. Some may refuse showers postnatally or during menstruation, believing they are harmful. Others may not want to shower because they believe it will undermine their recovery. Some women may wish to use make-up in the hospital.
- **Hair care**. Prefer to wash hair weekly. Concerned they may catch cold from washing hair, that washing it will interfere with recovery, or about management of hair after washing (e.g., women who cover their hair require hair care by another woman and, after care, immediate covering of hair).
- **Nail care**. No special routines.
- **Toileting**. Toilet paper not sufficiently purifying. Most prefer to wash after every urination and bowel movement; clinician should provide small pitcher. May insist on using a bidet to wash after urination and bowel movement. May be willing to use urinal or commode if their privacy is respected.
- **Special clothing or amulets**. Depends on country of origin. Many women consider head scarves important or essential. Some patients want a Koran or Bible (*Ingeel*) next to bed or under pillow. Parents may want to pin a blue stone, bead, or hand with five fingers on children's clothing to ward off the evil eye. Even highly educated, nontraditional Arabs may believe in the evil eye and keep special amulets during illness.
- **Self-care**. Believe in complete rest and abdication of all responsibilities during illness. Expect family and hospital personnel to care for them. Clinician can enhance self-care by carefully orienting patient to all hospital routines.

May avoid postoperative activities, such as coughing or ambulation, for fear of pain. Patient and family believe that energy should be reserved for healing, not expended on self-care. Clinician should clearly and constantly explain to patient the rationale for self-care, such as exercise and hydration, in his/her recovery.

FOOD PRACTICES

- **Usual meal pattern**. Three meals per day, largest usually preferred at about 2 p.m. New immigrants need to be oriented about meal routines in U.S. and the hospital.
- **Special utensils**. Per the dominant culture. Prefer to eat with right hand.
- **Food beliefs and rituals**. Offering food is associated with nurturing, acceptance, and trust. Someone who shares tea, coffee, and chocolates is reaching out. Eating important for recovery, especially hot soup. May avoid mixing milk and fish, sweet and sour, or hot and cold in meals as unhealthy. In observance of Ramadan, Muslims fast (which includes not drinking fluids) from sunrise to sunset, breaking the fast at sunset and eating another meal before sunrise (usually at 2–4 a.m.). Children, pregnant women, and ill persons are exempt, but some insist on fasting.
- **Usual diet**. Vegetables simmered with tomato sauces, chicken, lamb, beef, or fish. Rice and legumes common. Bread often served with every meal, like fruit and desserts. Prefer own food cooked from scratch rather than prepackaged food.
- **Fluids**. Water and juices, such as orange juice. Do not serve ice in drinks. Like strong black tea with or without milk, and sugar with beverages. Islam prohibits alcohol, but some Christians and nonpracticing Muslims drink. Though excessive drinking is uncommon, clinician should not rule it out.
- **Food taboos and prescriptions**. Most Muslims avoid pork products and food cooked in alcohol. Christians may eat pork and ham. No cold beverages in the morning, no iced beverages when sick. Do not offer hot and cold food simultaneously. Do not eat raw fish or meat prepared rare or medium-rare; prefer well-done meat or poultry to avoid eating "blood." Drink mint tea for abdominal discomfort. Chicken and chicken soups help in recovery. Clinician should ask the kitchen about the availability of Middle Eastern foods; include all-wheat pita bread or Syrian bread. Receiving and accepting offers of tea, coffee, or sweets demonstrates acceptance and trust.
- **Hospitality**. Food plays a central role in the family and relationships with friends, and at gatherings. Are proud of their hospitality and value generosity and sharing. Accepting their hospitality akin to accepting their culture. Sharing food breaks the ice, enhances relationships. Clinician should accept offer of a cup of tea or a sweet; guests may initially refuse, then eat when host insists.

SYMPTOM MANAGEMENT

- **Pain** (*waga* or *allam*). Very expressive about pain, particularly in presence of family members with whom they feel comfortable. Focus is on present pain experience. Pain feared and causes panic when it occurs, and should be avoided at all costs. Some may have low pain threshold. Better able to cope with pain if they understand source and prognosis. Higher tolerance for painful procedures when understand the benefits. Express pain metaphorically, using symbols such as fire, iron, knives, and rocks, so clinician should learn meaning of symbols. Some respond to numerical pain scale, others cannot; less able to assign number to other symptoms. Response on pain scale may not reflect reality of pain—e.g., even minor pain may be a "10." Believe injections more effective than pills. Some perceive intravenous fluids as indication of severity of situation; clinician should explain meaning. Some able to manage self-medicating; clinician should provide detailed information about advantages and disadvantages, and be prepared to offer advice. Helpful nonpharmacological methods for all symptoms include reading Koran or Bible.

- **Dyspnea** (*deekat nafas*). Panic accompanies feeling of not being able to breathe. Tend to hyperventilate. Need careful coaching about meaning of oxygenation associated with severity and urgency of situation. May be unable to translate dyspnea discomfort into numbers. Prefer medications to control dyspnea, believing they are best method. Clinician needs to rehearse oxygenation, including timing and length of use.

- **Nausea/vomiting**. *Nefsi ghama aleya* means nausea, but some may not translate it as such. Many embarrassed when they vomit. Most do not differentiate between nausea and vomiting; they say, "I will vomit," but not "I am nauseated." Consider vomiting serious because of loss of nutrients. Need assurance that vomiting is not as devastating as it seems. Clinician should coach patients on ways to prevent nausea and vomiting. Tend to trust that medications help, though not as much as other noninvasive strategies.

- **Constipation/diarrhea** (*imsaak/ishaal*). Expect routine bowel movement and become very distressed if it does not occur at particular time. May not volunteer information due to modesty but will be uncomfortable and distressed. Clinician should ask about bowel movements, then teach that the routine and time are not significant. Constipation prevalent due to low fluid intake (except tea), lack of mobility, and low roughage in American diet, which substitutes sweets and proteins for roughage and fruits. Some use laxatives for regularity; clinician should ask about such use. Accept medication for diarrhea. Education can help them understand relationship between nutrition and bowel movements.

- **Fatigue** (*taab, taaban, andy doukha, habtaan*). "Tired," "fatigued," "dizzy," "cannot open my eyes," and "my blood pressure is low" are all expressions of fatigue. Clinician should encourage an afternoon nap and ask family members to allow patient to rest. Give family "permission" to be away from patient so everyone can rest. Encourage hydration and teach relationship between diet and energy. Preference is for pharmacological intervention, which should be accompanied by careful coaching and monitoring of other lifestyle patterns and medications.

- **Depression** (*metdiagh, tabaan nafsian, makboud*). Will not acknowledge depression because emotional well-being believed to be a family matter. Depressive symptoms never reported—viewed as a personality defect. Because of stigma, depression should never be referred to as mental illness. Clinician should explain that depression is an illness, not a personality weakness, and that it is treatable like other illnesses. Encourage patient to discuss and give permission to feel depressed. Fatigue, sadness, restlessness, oversleeping, and flat affect all are expressions of depression. Often manifested by anger and hostility that are diffused and/or directed at others. Careful assessment of lifestyle, sleep patterns, level of satisfaction, eating habits, family relationships, disappointments, and perception of achievements may reveal depression. Losses, isolation, and mainstream society's bias against Arab countries predispose patient to depression. Neither accept nonpharmacological treatments nor believe they are useful.

- **Self-care symptom management**. Prefer biomedicine for treating symptoms but may use home remedies simultaneously. Clinician's expectations of self-care may connote lack of caring. They expect to be cared for by family or caregivers. Responsive to education for long-term self-care (e.g., diabetic self-care, monitoring blood pressure, wound treatment). Higher adherence congruent with extent of training and periodic monitoring by clinicians. Adhere less to regimens requiring lifestyle changes. Family members should be included in training and monitoring.

BIRTH RITUALS/CARE OF THE NEW MOTHER AND BABY

- **Pregnancy care**. Some delay prenatal care until late in pregnancy because they believe that a normal pregnancy does not warrant medical attention or because of expense. Much attention given to pregnant women, who are encouraged to rest, do minimal work, and eat well. Pregnant women should be given anything they crave. Preparation for birth or baby not culturally practiced, as people respond to birth in a very present-oriented manner— i.e., they will deal with the birth when it happens. Clinicians should encourage women to start prenatal care, be active, and eat a balanced diet. Women need assurance that they can maintain normal routine. Clinicians should strongly and repeatedly suggest that they enroll in childbirth preparation classes, and should support and help facilitate enrollment. Prenatal and postnatal classes should be presented as a prescription for couples.

- **Preferences for children**. Birth of a boy greeted with more rejoicing than birth of a girl. If family is "blessed" with one or more boys, it may welcome

a girl's birth. Fear of Western influence on girls' upbringing enhances preference for boys. Larger families valued to make up for loss of extended family
through immigration, but immigrants prefer smaller families. Serious family
planning usually begins after third child.

- **Labor practices**. Women believe many myths about labor pains, which
  they greatly fear. Very expressive during labor—make loud noises, moan,
  groan; some scream. Female family members expected to be present and
  available. Prefer medications to control pain. Husbands need support, as
  they feel overwhelmed and powerless.
- **Role of the laboring woman during birth**. Active participation in labor
  is a foreign concept to most Arab American women. Tend to tense their
  muscles and wait for delivery to take place. Clinician should hold woman's
  hand, fan her, dry her perspiration, talk with her, remind her of her other
  labor experiences and that this labor will soon end.
- **Role of the father and other family members during birth**. Father not
  expected to participate in labor or delivery. Mother, sister, or mother in-law
  expected to be present and provide support.
- **Vaginal vs. cesarean section**. Vaginal delivery preferred. Cesarean greatly
  feared.
- **Breastfeeding**. Modernization often means giving up breastfeeding. Clinician should help mother make decisions and explain the advantages of
  breastfeeding. Will need help with first baby. May not offer breast for first
  few days because colostrum believed to be harmful to baby. May not request
  assistance for fear of imposing on staff, so clinicians need to offer assistance.
  Monitoring and tangible support will enhance adherence to breastfeeding.
- **Birth recuperation**. New mother expected to be on complete bed rest after
  delivery. Her mother or sister is expected to take charge of household and
  family. New mother should eat enriching proteins, such as chicken, and
  drink rich fluids made with milk and other ingredients. Tea used to cleanse
  body, lentil soup to increase breast milk. It may take the new mother considerable time to bathe or shower for fear of hurting incision and/or episiotomy or of introducing infection into uterus. Washing breasts may "thin"
  the milk. Clinician should explain the disadvantages of not washing. Very
  difficult for first-time mother without extended family; needs more understanding, support, networking.
- **Baby care**. Father may whisper call to prayer in newborn's ear. Some wrap
  umbilical area to prevent cold from entering body. They expect nurses to
  care for baby in hospital and extended family members to help with baby
  care during first few weeks at home. Absence of extended family postpartum
  may be distressing for new immigrants.
- **Problems with baby**. News should be conveyed to both mother and father,
  interjecting caring and hope. Better to give information in phases to help
  them process it and cope. Then clinician may include aunts or grandparents

in further discussion of baby, as they will be caring for it.

- **Male and female circumcision**. Male circumcision expected and required of Muslims. Some prefer it when a son is about 6 years old, others prefer it in hospital. Female circumcision never discussed at birth. If subject comes up, usually arises when a daughter is school age or adolescent. Not based on religious beliefs but passed on culturally. Arab Americans usually do not attempt to have daughters circumcised. Some have been circumcised in their home country.

DEVELOPMENTAL AND SEXUAL ISSUES

- **Celebration of menarche or becoming a man**. In some families, mothers may congratulate daughters when they experience their first menstrual episode. Becoming a man is not acknowledged in most families.
- **Attitudes about birth control**. Acceptable only for married couples and most often after first or second child is born. Birth control pills or diaphragms are methods of choice. Tubal ligation accepted option after third child is born. Resist use of condoms, and vasectomy is a rare choice, but these should always be suggested and/or encouraged as viable options. Clinician should discuss advantages of vasectomy. Discuss options early in childbearing years with married couple and educate regarding all options. First- and second-generation single women use birth control without disclosing it to family. If disclosed, use must be presented as a prescription for hormonal purposes.
- **Attitudes about sexually transmitted infection (STI) control, including condoms**. STIs feared and never anticipated as an infection among immigrants from Middle East. Wives, husbands, and extended family members should never be included in discussions about STIs. Clinician should discuss them in great detail, provide opportunities for follow-up questions, and use professional interpreters rather than family members. Also should use caution in relating condom use to STIs because of stigma.
- **Attitudes about abortion**. While abortion at one time was the method of choice for planning family size, the rise of Islamic fundamentalism and religiousness in the Middle East, and of Christianity in the West, have influenced attitudes. Becoming the least-practiced option. If indicated for married couples, topic should be handled with great care and discussed in context of religious norms.
- **Attitudes about unwed sexual experimentation**. Premarital sex strictly forbidden for single women and tolerated, though discouraged, for men. When practiced by young people, not disclosed. Must be kept strictly confidential between patient and clinician.
- **Sexual orientation**. Homosexuality is never acknowledged or tolerated. Culture and religion discourage any open expression of homosexual orientation. Families feel stigmatized by homosexuality of anyone in immediate or extended family. Gays and lesbians remain closeted, though there have been some recent efforts to raise awareness in U.S.

- **Gender identity**. Gender is congruent with sex. Families do not accept cross-gender traits and responses. There is pressure on girls to be feminine and on boys who exhibit any feminine mannerisms to change and conform to masculine behavior. Any gender ambiguity is stigmatized and unacceptable. If ambiguous, clinician should ask questions and provide support and options for discussing it. Look for cues and be sensitive to issues of security or disclosure.
- **Attitudes about menopause**. General lack of knowledge about, or awareness of, the process and experience. Menopause considered part of growing old—inevitable but not welcomed. Arabic term is *sin el yass*, or, literally translated, "age of despair." There is growing awareness among educated immigrants that menopause can be discussed, that it is accompanied by some discomfort and symptoms. Women generally do not easily associate their symptoms with menopause. Prefer hormonal therapy and medication to control symptoms.

FAMILY RELATIONSHIPS

- **Composition/structure**. Family is central in Arab society and culture. It takes precedence over the desires of individual members. Relatively few persons remain single or live alone. Family includes nuclear and extended family; a household may encompass uncles, aunts, nephews, nieces, and grandparents. Families are traditionally patriarchal, with males and elders receiving the most respect and having the most power; women and children are subservient. Little tolerance for alternative family structures—e.g., gay and lesbian couples. Changes in, and deviations from, the traditional structure may be a source of tension even in bicultural families.
- **Decision-making**. In traditional families, the eldest male makes decisions. Among generation born and raised in U.S., make their own individual or nuclear-family decisions, but parents and siblings still very involved in diagnostic and treatment decisions. Extended-family members also participate in decision-making. Adherence to treatment better when families make informed decisions.
- **Spokesperson**. Father, eldest son, or elderly uncle usually the family spokesperson. If there is a grandmother, many families defer to her counsel. Physicians are expected to make decisions regarding patient care.
- **Gender issues**. Men are typically breadwinners and family protectors. Women are responsible for care of children and house. Women may be very powerful in the family but do not show it in public. In health care, men in the immediate family are responsible for logistics of patient transportation, financial arrangements, and funeral plans.
- **Changing roles among generations in U.S.** Immigrant family roles vary depending on extent to which American values and beliefs have been integrated into the family's repertoire of choices and responses. Roles also vary

according to English language proficiency and to type and context of employment. Children of immigrants tend to adopt American norms and behaviors. They serve as interpreters, thus becoming more central in the family's decision-making. Elderly parents may depend on their adult children or grandchildren. The newly adapted family structure may be stressful for all parties, as the lines of authority become more ambiguous. The next generation's relationships are more egalitarian and the empowerment of women is more noticeable.

- **Caring roles**. Mothers, grandmothers, sisters, sisters-in-law, or daughters assume caring functions, such as meeting the daily needs of patients in or out of the hospital.
- **Expectations of and for children**. Children considered sacred. Families sacrifice money, time, and country of origin to raise children who are well provided for and well-educated. Child-rearing based more on negative than positive reinforcement. To Westerners, there appears to be total permissiveness in some cases—e.g., roaming in clinics, loud voices, and demanding behaviors. But in other cases, such as academic achievement, girls' modesty and chastity, respect for adults, the prohibition against talking back, and friendships approved by parents, there are very strict expectations. Parents more strict with girls than boys. Children expected to be obedient to all adults. Arab children may morbidly fear injections and invasive procedures, as some parents threaten their kids with these as negative reinforcement in daily life.
- **Expectations of and for elders**. Elders respected—and they expect to be respected. Sons especially responsible for supporting elderly parents. Women gain more power in family as they age, particularly if they have children. Elderly parents are to be accommodated in their son's or daughter's home and cared for by sons, daughters, and daughters-in-law. They need to be educated and helped when moving to a skilled-nursing or assisted-living facility. Children expected to be available at the bedside to care for and support the elderly at all times.
- **Expectations of hospital visitors**. Family vigilance and the demands family members place on medical staff regarding a patient demonstrate concern for him/her. Expectations to visit and to be visited are high for immigrants and Arab Americans. Visitors are expected to support grieving or rejoicing families. Entire families visit sick person and his/her family. Visitors may be treated as family or as acquaintances. Those considered family may be expected to help care for the patient.

ILLNESS BELIEFS

- **Causes of/attitudes about physical illness**. Naturalistic and social causes of illness include bad luck, stress in family, loss of person or objects, "germs," winds and drafts, imbalance in hot/cold and dry/moist, and sudden fears.

Among children, deprivations of love by family members may be considered a cause. Supernatural causes include the evil eye, God's punishment for sins, and the curse of the devil (*shaitaan*). The elderly and religious may endure illness and suffering in the belief that these are Allah's will, that Allah also may cure them.

- **Causes of/attitudes about mental illness**. Caused by sudden fears, pretending to be ill to manipulate family, wrath of God or God's will, or devil's curse. Causes are individually, not family, focused. Mental illness might also be caused by loss of country, family, and friends. Mental distress often expressed psychosomatically in terms of vague bodily symptoms. Mental illness highly stigmatized; it brings shame on family and could affect whether a child is marriageable. Mental health care or hospitalization sought only in advanced stages of illness and only after all family and community resources have been exhausted.

- **Causes of genetic defects**. Wrath of God, God's will, or a test of endurance. Religious beliefs call for acceptance, but social expectations oblige isolation from distant family and friends. Disclosure an issue; prefer to conceal genetically defective family members. May refuse genetic counseling, believing it defies God's will. Tend to care for children with genetic defects at home; shun institutionalized care.

- **Attitudes about disabilities**. A stigma to be camouflaged, kept a family secret, and shielded from public view. Within the extended family, disabled persons are treated with sympathy and overindulgent care that may interfere with development and healthy self-care.

- **Sick role**. The ill are treated well. Expected to be passive in any decisions regarding them or others. Patients expect to be pampered. Family members may insist that patient refrain from ambulation, and may take over preventive and other usual self-care, believing energy must be preserved for healing. Mentally ill persons are believed to be able to control their illness. They may be treated less well by family.

- **Home and folk remedies**. Amulets, sweating, reciting verses from Koran or Bible, prayers, well-balanced diet. Folk remedies include herbal teas, camphor ointment, and hot chicken soup. Herbs for a common cold, intestinal disturbances, and menstrual cramps; herbal poultices for stiff muscles and abdominal pain. Often, Epsom salts and castor oil for constipation, and castor oil for minor burns. Yogurt with garlic and dried mint flakes for diarrhea. May use cupping or moxibustion, particularly Saudis and Yemenis.

- **Medications**. Western medications are treatment of choice, but consultations with health care professionals in country of origin may yield additional medications to take concurrently with prescribed drugs. Usually a high level of adherence to biomedicine, but must see benefit. Will comply if given clear instructions about when to terminate medication. Medications often exchanged between family members. Clinician should ask specifically about other providers and medications other than those prescribed in U.S. Folk remedies usually not a threat.

- **Acceptance of procedures**. High acceptance of procedures that are expected to cure, such as blood transfusions, surgery, and organ transplants. However, low acceptance of complications, which are deemed a result of negligence or lack of expertise. Donation of blood may be reserved for loved ones. Clinician should explain procedures clearly and slowly, with a family member supporting the patient, and de-emphasize potential pain and complications.
- **Care-seeking**. Western biomedicine respected and sought early for symptoms, immediately for pain if resources such as money, transportation, or babysitting permit. Preventive health care not well understood nor a priority. May delay care for natural conditions, such as pregnancy, or if condition is stigmatized. Prefer care from health professionals who provide personal attention.

HEALTH ISSUES

- **Concept of health**. A gift of God manifested in being able to eat well, meet social obligations, be in a good mood, have strength, and not experience stressors or pain. Being overweight associated with health and strength.
- **Health promotion and prevention**. Based on traditional humoral theory, Arabs and Arab-Americans believe in promoting health by avoiding hot/cold and dry/moist shifts, avoiding wind and drafts, staying warm, being well-fed, and resting well. May not accept clinician's suggestions about diet change and exercise.
- **Screening**. Arabs respect the health care system and providers. Accept recommended screening if they trust a provider's intentions and expertise, and if they understand the rationale for screening and how it will help them get better. Otherwise, because of their focus on the present or lack of health insurance, less likely to initiate preventive health care/yearly screening and regular follow-ups. Some women (especially those who are single, due to the high value of virginity) avoid mammograms and Pap smears out of modesty or fear that tests may reveal a stigmatized condition like cancer.
- **Common health problems**. Common genetic conditions include sickle cell anemia, thalassemia, glucose-6-dehydrogenase deficiency, and other disorders as a result of consanguineous marriages. Coronary heart disease, hypertension, and diabetes relatively common and likely increased by smoking, obesity, high-cholesterol diet, and sedentary lifestyle.

DEATH RITUALS

- **Beliefs and attitudes about death**. Death is expected and inevitable, accepted as God's will. But believe death should be delayed or prevented by biomedical interventions. After death, peoples' behaviors and actions on earth are judged by a score card of good and bad deeds. Death is feared and never discussed. All care should be in context of hope for life.

- **Preparation**. Arabs do not openly anticipate or grieve for a dying person before death. Clinician should inform designated head of family privately of impending or actual death of a patient and allow him to decide how to inform rest of family. Family will find it difficult to decide on do-not-resuscitate orders. It may lose trust in health care system if this option is offered.
- **Home vs. hospital**. Critically or terminally ill patient prefers to die in hospital with family surrounding him/her. Hope that Western medicine may delay death prompts family's preference for patient to die in hospital.
- **Special needs**. Prepare private room for family members to meet and grieve together. In some families, young women are barred from being with the dying or dead patient. Clinician should respect wishes of family. Arab Christians may request visit by minister or priest. Let family initiate visit, but provide support. Muslims do not need an *imam* present before or during death process; he reads the Koran after death. Family's grief is open, loud, and uncontrollable.
- **Care of the body**. Christians usually have body embalmed; religious funeral follows. Muslims turn body toward Mecca. It is washed three times by same-gender Muslim and all orifices are sealed with cotton to retain soul of the deceased. Body is then wrapped in layers of white cotton fabric and taken to the mosque for final prayers of the dead. Muslims believe in immediate burial in the ground without embalming. Coffin used in U.S.
- **Attitudes about organ donation**. May not allow organ donation due to respect for burying the body whole and the deceased meeting the Creator with integrity. Asking about organ donation before death may be extremely insensitive. It depends on length of time patient has been in U.S. and degree to which he/she has adopted new values.
- **Attitudes about autopsy**. Autopsy problematic. Clinician should broach this topic with care, allowing family the option of refusing. Rationale for autopsy should be presented in terms of benefit and outcome for family.

SELECTED REFERENCES

Meleis, A. I. (1981). The Arab American in the health care system. *American Journal of Nursing*, 81, 1180–1183.

Meleis, A. I. (2002). Egyptians. In P. St. Hill, J. Lipson, & A. Meleis (Eds.), *Caring for women cross-culturally: A portable guide*, pp. 123–141. Philadelphia: F. A. Davis.

Meleis, A. I., & Hattar-Pollara, M. (1994). Arab Middle Eastern American women: Stereotyped, invisible but powerful. In D. Adams (Ed.), *Women of color: A cultural diversity health perspective*, pp. 133–163. Newbury Park, CA: Sage Publications.

Meleis, A. I., & Jonsen, A. (1983). Ethical crises and cultural differences. *Western Journal of Medicine*, 138, 889–893.

AUTHOR

Afaf Ibrahim Meleis, RN, PhD, FAAN, is a professor and the Margaret Bond Simon dean of nursing in the School of Nursing at the University of Pennsylvania. A nurse and medical sociologist educated in Egypt and the U.S., she immigrated to the U.S. in 1962 and formerly held professorships at the University of California-Los Angeles and University of California-San Francisco. Her research on the experiences of immigrants in the health care system and on the work and health of women in Colombia, Brazil, Mexico, Kuwait, Egypt, and the U.S. has been widely published, as has her work in theoretical nursing.

CHAPTER 5

BRAZILIANS

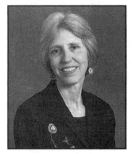 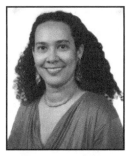

DeAnne K.
Hilfinger Messias

Tereza Cristina
Macedo de Paula

CULTURAL/ETHNIC IDENTITY

Numerous cultures, populations, invasions, and immigrations contributed to modern Brazilian culture and ethnic identity. The mix included more than 200 indigenous tribes, French and Dutch traders, black African slaves, and Italian, German, Japanese, Syrian, and Lebanese settlements. Ethnic intermarriage was/is widespread, resulting in rich cross-fertilization and Brazilianization of cultures and traditions in art, architecture, music, styles of social interaction, and cuisine, which is regionally diverse. Concepts of class and social status, including economic and educational levels, are very strongly embedded in Brazilian society. Social identity is based on these concepts and on skin color from blended ethnicity or backgrounds—e.g., *moreno* (medium brown mixture), *mulato* (African and European), *caboclo* (indigenous and European), and *pardo* (mixed).

- **Preferred term(s)**. Brazilian. Distinct from other populations in Latin America in culture, language, ethnicity, and history. Immigrants to U.S. resent being identified as Hispanics. However, the U.S. Census Bureau description of "Hispanic" includes people from South America, which encompasses Brazil. Brazil's ethnic, cultural, and linguistic individuality can be traced to the 1494 Treaty of Tordesillas between Spain and Portugal that divided their empires in South America. Portugal claimed the eastern coast and, after exploration and settlement, vast areas of the interior, all of which became one country, Brazil. Spanish colonization in the region resulted in many separate nations.
- **Census**. According to the 1997 Second Census of Brazilians Overseas, compiled by Brazil's Foreign Ministry, there are 1.5 million Brazilian expatriates

globally. The vast majority live in the U.S. Because immigration has been relatively recent, most adults are foreign-born.

- **History of immigration**. Before 1980, Brazilians' presence in the U.S. was virtually unrecognized. Since the mid-1980s, the number of documented and undocumented Brazilians has increased significantly, although official statistics do not accurately reflect undocumented immigration. Large concentrations of immigrants are in Massachusetts, Pennsylvania, New York, New Jersey, Florida, Texas, and California. They left Brazil because of economic instability, chronic hyperinflation, underemployment, low wages, and a relatively high cost of living. Many are of middle-class or lower-middle-class origin and well-educated but often are employed in low-status service jobs they typically would not have held in Brazil. Large numbers come as tourists or students. Some seek specialized medical care in the U.S. if they can afford it.

SPIRITUAL/RELIGIOUS ORIENTATION

- **Primary religious/spiritual affiliations**. Vast majority are Roman Catholic, but many do not practice Catholicism. Evangelical and Protestant churches are growing rapidly, particularly in low-income communities. There are also spiritists and Kardecists who follow the doctrines of the French psychic researcher Allan Kardec. Brazil's constitution guarantees religious freedom. There are Mormons, Jews, Muslims, and Buddhists in Brazil. An indigenous religion is *Umbanda*, a blend of African and Amerindian spiritism and folk Catholicism. A significant minority of Brazilians are devotees of *candomblé*, which Yoruba slaves originally brought from Western Africa to Brazil. At that time, practicing *candomblé* was forbidden, so slaves matched their animistic deities with Catholic figureheads in order to continue their traditional worship. For example, Oxala, a male god of procreation and harvest, was identified with Jesus; Iemanja, the goddess of the sea, was associated with Our Lady of the Immaculate Conception.
- **Usual religious/spiritual practices**. Catholic folk practices focus on saints, promises, and pilgrimages. Regular church attendance not necessarily an indication of religiosity. Syncretism (blending beliefs and practices from different religions) is common. Catholics may also take part in an Iemanja ceremony on New Year's Eve and spiritists may attend mass sometimes. Strong belief in miracles and miracle cures, many of which the devout attribute to saints. Spirit mediumship and spiritual healing are part of popular Catholic practices and various spiritist religions.
- **Use of spiritual healing/healers**. Brazilians have strong traditions of religious/spiritual healing. Catholic priests are called in emergencies and for the sacrament of the sick. Spiritists practice laying on of hands (*passes*). Folk healers (*benzedeiras, curandeiras*) often give blessings and prayers along with herbal remedies. Practicing spiritists are in U.S. urban areas with large Brazil-

ian enclaves, such as New York. *Benzedeiras* and *curandeiras* are less common in U.S.

- **Holidays**. Religious holidays include Carnival Monday, a Brazilian national holiday the Monday before Lent; Shrove Tuesday, a Brazilian national holiday the day before Ash Wednesday (called Mardi Gras or Fat Tuesday in U.S.); Ash Wednesday, the first day of Lent, 46 days before Easter; Good Friday (traditional to have fish with the main meal on the Friday before Easter); Easter Sunday; Our Lady of Aparecida (*Nossa Senhora Aparecida*) (October 12), patron saint of Brazil; All Souls' Day (November 2), when family members make cemetery visits to honor the dead; and Christmas (December 25), when Santa Claus (*Papai Noel*) must wear shorts. In the Middle Ages, celebration of Jesus Christ's birthday replaced pagan festivals celebrating the winter solstice (summer in Brazil). Secular holidays include New Year's Eve (December 31), when women traditionally wear a new white dress to a party, and New Year's Day (January 1); Tiradentes Day (April 21), which commemorates the execution of Joaquim José da Silva Xavier, a hero in the 1789 revolt against the Portuguese; Labor Day (May 1); Independence Day (September 7), which celebrates the declaration of independence from Portugal by Dom Pedro in 1822; and Republic Day (November 15), the anniversary of the Proclamation of 1889, which removed Emperor Dom Pedro and established Brazil as a republic.

COMMUNICATION
ORAL COMMUNICATION

- **Major languages and dialects**. Portuguese is the official, prevailing language. Some regional variations in pronunciation and slang words but no regional dialects. English and French main second languages of educated Brazilians. More than 100 indigenous languages; the most prevalent are Tupí, Guarani, Gê, Arawak, and Carib. The Portuguese borrowed many African and Indian words, particularly from Tupí, the common language among indigenous tribes in coastal areas. Many settlements and physical features still have Indian names.

- **Greetings**. Except in business situations, Brazilians greet everyone with a hug. If the newcomer is a family member, friend, or acquaintance, a kiss on each cheek is included. A kiss on the lips often exchanged between family members. In business situations, women may hug, but men usually do not unless their relationship is long-term. Handshakes are appropriate when strangers are introduced or in formal situations, both for greetings and good-byes; often prolonged and may be accompanied by, or replaced with, an embrace (*abraço*). If two men are well-acquainted, a slap on the shoulder or stomach, or a sustained pat on the back, may accompany the handshake and last into the conversation. Women may shake hands upon meeting, but typically they greet with a kiss, usually twice on alternate cheeks. They may kiss the air while brushing cheeks, beginning on the left. Greetings with kisses are now common between men and women, but the man kisses only one of the woman's cheeks. When entering or leaving a group, a newcomer ensures that he/she personally greets or says good-bye to each individual. In greetings and leave-takings, personal comments are exchanged regarding clothing, hairstyle, weight gain or loss, the other's general appearance, or home. Saying good-bye can take a very long time, sometimes almost an hour. Persons of lower social class may use the title *doutor/doutora* (doctor) when addressing someone of higher status; it is an expression of social deference and not necessarily related to educational degrees or profession. Brazilians are more likely to refer to business colleagues by first name—e.g., "*Senhor* Angelo" or "*Senhora* Clarice." Priests, physicians, professors, and other professionals usually go by their title and first name—e.g., "*Padre* Jurandir."

- **Tone of voice**. Brazilians tend to speak more loudly than dominant-culture Americans do and to "step" on each other's words. They respond quickly and their words literally tumble over one another in lively discussions. As discussion becomes more interesting, voices become louder and interruptions more frequent. Interruptions are not considered rude.

- **Direct or indirect style of speech**. Brazilians provide many details when offering information. Always very courteous. Will stop the conversation to summarize it for those who cannot keep up. Comfortable with verbal confrontation, although confrontation does not usually take place between a younger and older person. In unpleasant or potentially awkward situations, an indirect approach is considered a gracious way of sparing another's feelings and awkwardness. Considered impolite to say "no" directly to a health care provider; clinician should not assume patient has necessarily concurred.

- **Use of interpreters**. Clinician should not use Spanish speakers as interpreters; key words will not be understood. Family or friends can translate, but their knowledge or understanding of medical terminology may be limited.

- **Serious or terminal illness**. Family members should be consulted before patient is informed, as some families do not want patient to know or want diagnosis/prognosis presented to him/her in an indirect manner.

WRITTEN COMMUNICATION

- **Literacy assessment**. About 86% of Brazilians are literate, the result of a literacy campaign that began in Brazil in 1971. Literacy varies regionally and among rural and urban areas (e.g., 27% illiteracy in the Northeast, which has a high proportion of rural poor). Literacy in Portuguese has a direct influence on English fluency. Brazilians vary in fluency or knowledge of English; some recent immigrants have very limited comprehension and speaking ability even if they read and write Portuguese. Most Brazilians do not speak Spanish, as few study it, but some immigrants learn Spanish through contact with Hispanic populations.

- **Consents**. Written consent uncommon in Brazil. Medical language of consent forms and explanation of possible complications and risks may cause concern, confusion, or fear. Patients and family members may be reluctant to question medical professionals about treatment options or to request second opinion.

NONVERBAL COMMUNICATION

- **Eye contact**. Similar to that in dominant American culture, although more persistent and with some distinctions. For example, in settings in which most people stare straight ahead, as in an elevator, Brazilians look around at each other. Exception to direct eye contact is when speaking to someone of a different age or status. Younger or lower-class persons may show respect by avoiding direct eye contact with health professionals.
- **Personal space**. Quite close. If others back away from a Brazilian because personal distance is too close, they will probably hurt that person's feelings. Brazilians stand very close while speaking and do not apologize for bumping or brushing against another person. Rarely wait in line in public places, as in the public market; whoever pushes to the front is next. The dominant-culture habit of constantly apologizing in crowded situations seems very odd to Brazilians.
- **Use and meaning of silence**. Associated primarily with solemn occasions. Rare in everyday life.
- **Gestures**. Attentive to body language, gestures, and body movement, perhaps more than to the spoken message. Using hand gestures and signs common in everyday conversation and among specific groups, such as bus drivers. To beckon someone, Brazilians stretch out their hand, with palm down, and make sweeping movements with the fingers. The "OK" sign ("O" made with thumb and forefinger) is an obscene gesture. Appropriate sign for "all is well" is a "thumbs up." To emphasize a statement, may snap fingers while whipping hand down and out. To express appreciation, may pinch earlobe between thumb and forefinger. To dramatize further, may reach behind head and grasp opposite earlobe.
- **Openness in expressing emotions**. Generally quite comfortable with disclosing emotions; open about feelings and sharing common frustrations of daily living. Immigrants probably less open with health care providers due to barriers such as language and social class.
- **Privacy**. Home and family are private matters, but little privacy exists among family members. Being alone is often equated with being sad.
- **Touch**. Touch and body contact common in communication; occur more frequently among peers and family members of the same sex. Touch equated with friendship and concern rather than intimacy. Women touch more than men do; often walk down street with arms around each other, arms linked, or holding hands. May touch or tug at each other's clothing or jewelry while

talking. Men and women might pat the other's shoulder or arm as reassurance. A man may put an arm around another's shoulders, pat or poke his back or tummy, or squeeze his shoulder, sometimes in greeting, sometimes to emphasize a point, and sometimes as a gesture of goodwill and friendship. A Brazilian who thinks the other person's attention is wandering may touch that person's chin to redirect his/her gaze.

- **Orientation to time**. More flexible than northern European Americans regarding arrivals and departures. Tend to arrive a few minutes—sometimes hours—late for a social event. People expect tardiness and adjust their plans accordingly. For example, hosts invite dinner-party guests to arrive about two hours before the meal will be served; guests may arrive at any time during that period. May stay very late at an enjoyable party, even if it does not begin until 10 p.m. Lunch breaks are longer than an hour and frequently used for doing errands. People take unexpected holidays. Lateness in business less acceptable; tend to arrive at business meetings on time and to attend to business rather than socialize, even over lunch. Take time obligations seriously, as in honoring a promise to do or deliver something by a certain time or date. But if deadline is not met, tolerance rather than annoyance more common. Time may be subordinate to personal and social relationships. For example, meetings may start when certain persons arrive rather than at an appointed hour.

ACTIVITIES OF DAILY LIVING

- **Modesty**. Women may prefer a female caregiver. Young girls and older women tend to be more modest. In health care situations, women may be more modest than they would be in other situations (e.g., at the beach), particularly in presence of male health care providers. Clinicians should appropriately cover female patients during physical examinations.
- **Skin care**. Hygiene is very important; shower or bathe in bed daily. Brazilians expect hospital to provide hygienic care.
- **Hair care**. Value physical appearance. Men frequently comb hair. Both genders shampoo daily. If patient is bedridden, clinician should offer to shampoo his/her hair. Brazilians may cut hair according to a phase of the moon.
- **Nail care**. Women keep all nails well-manicured. Going to beauty parlor for manicure is a social activity. Men generally keep nails short and clean.
- **Toileting**. Soap and water peri-wash after bowel movement or urination a common custom. If patient is bedridden, clinician should offer a daily peri-wash (*higiene íntima*). Women hand wash their intimate apparel daily.
- **Special clothing or amulets**. Commonly use crucifix, rosaries, religious medallions, and *figas*—amulets in the figure of a clenched fist with thumb clasped between forefinger and middle fingers, to ward off evil. Special colored ribbons tied around wrists or ankles as part of petition to the Virgin Mary are not removed until they fall off. Spiritists and followers of *Umbanda* may prefer white clothing.

- **Self-care**. If patient is ambulatory, will perform most self-care; family member may assist. If family not available, clinician should offer nursing help.

FOOD PRACTICES

- **Usual meal pattern**. Traditionally, breakfast is smallest meal. Main meal at noon and lighter meal in evening. Sandwiches considered a snack, not a meal.
- **Special utensils**. None.
- **Food beliefs and rituals**. Bathe before meals, as bathing afterward is believed to interfere with digestion. Vitamin supplements are believed to enhance appetite.
- **Usual diet**. Breakfast usually consists of coffee with hot milk, French bread, and butter. Rice and beans are daily staples. Main meal consists of rice, beans, meat, and a vegetable or salad. Evening meal may be similar to lunch or be a light meal—e.g., soup or hot milk and coffee with bread or cake. Food usually well-seasoned; prefer food to be seasoned during preparation and not salted at table.
- **Fluids**. No ice in water or drinks. Soft drinks often consumed at meals. Coffee and tea not consumed with meals; drink strong black coffee with sugar (*cafezinho*) after meals and in mid-morning or mid-afternoon.
- **Food taboos and prescriptions**. Certain foods or food combinations are thought to be potentially harmful or to make one ill (*faz mal*). When someone has a cold, sore throat, or respiratory ailment, avoids cold drinks or foods (e.g., ice cream, popsicles). Do not consume milk or milk products at same time as fruits such as watermelon, mango, pineapple, or lemon. Often eat fish on Fridays. Catholics avoid meat, especially on Fridays, during Lent. Soups, such as chicken and rice soup (*canja*), appropriate for ill person. Bland diets and avoidance of fatty and spicy foods prescribed for cases of "liver dysfunction" (*mal do fígado*).
- **Hospitality**. Brazilians are warm and friendly. Commonly invite someone to share a meal or other festivity soon after establishing an acquaintance. Quite acceptable to arrive unannounced at the home of a family member or close friend.

SYMPTOM MANAGEMENT

Brazilians cannot easily use numerical scales for symptoms; qualitative descriptors more likely.

- **Pain** (*dor*). Generally low threshold for pain. Men thought to be less tolerant of pain than women are. Usually use words to describe location and intensity. Moaning, crying, or screaming may accompany pain. Often prefer intramuscular and IV injections to other forms of medication. Many do not consider over-the-counter analgesics (e.g., aspirin, acetaminophen) to be effective. Immigrants may avoid or delay visiting a doctor in U.S. if they think clinician will "only prescribe Tylenol." Rely on medications from Brazil.

- **Dyspnea** (*falta de ar*—lack of air). Attributed to both emotional and physical causes. Generally accept oxygen, although its use may suggest increase in gravity of illness.
- **Nausea/vomiting** (*nausea/vômito*). May be concerned about characteristics of vomitus (e.g., presence of blood). Usually refuse food if nauseated. Generally attribute GI disturbances to "liver" problems (*doença de fígido*). Clinicians should inquire about liver function and self-medication for liver problems.
- **Constipation/diarrhea** (*prisão de ventre/diarréia*). Alterations in bowel function, especially diarrhea, often attributed to food ingestion or intestinal parasites. Homemade oral rehydration solution (*soro caseiro*), medicinal teas, or rice water indicated for diarrhea. Enemas (*lavagem intestinal*) used only in severe or complicated cases. In Brazil, the relatively high-fiber diet and higher incidence of intestinal parasites probably contribute to a low prevalence of, and societal concern about, constipation. Immigrants may have more constipation due to dietary changes.
- **Fatigue** (*cansaço*—tiredness). Associated with both physical and emotional exhaustion. Management includes bed rest, tonics (*fortificantes*), and increased nutritional intake.
- **Depression** (*depressão*—depression; *tristeza*—sadness; *desgosto*—sorrow). May be reluctant to acknowledge depression or seek help from a mental health professional due to social stigma. Reluctance to take psychotropic medications may be related to fear of addiction. For immigrants, longing for home and family (*saudades*) may be related to depression.
- **Self-care symptom management**. Use home remedies or treatments but expect medications to be prescribed. Varies in cases of chronic illness. Some seek alternative treatments or approaches; others comply with prescribed medications and procedures.

BIRTH RITUALS/CARE OF THE NEW MOTHER AND BABY

- **Pregnancy care**. Family and society give special attention to pregnant women. Family tries to satisfy woman's specific desires or cravings (*desejos*). Pregnant woman expected to eat larger quantities—enough to "feed two." May solicit ultrasound examination, regardless of medical necessity, to learn baby's sex. Prenatal care the norm; immigrants desire it, but insurance may be a barrier. Middle- or upper-class immigrant women may take childbirth preparation classes. Lower-class immigrants less likely to take such classes, but they use prenatal care if it is accessible and affordable.
- **Preferences for children**. Although male children are highly valued, Brazilians do not disregard or neglect girls. Common to want children of both sexes. Voluntary childlessness is uncommon. Large families were previously the norm, but with rapidly declining fertility rates, current rate is about 2.5 children per woman. Immigrant women avoid having many children due to lack of family support in U.S.

- **Labor practices**. Receptiveness to, and acceptability of, walking, shower-ing, or family labor coaching depend on immigrant woman's exposure to U.S. models of family-coached childbirth and previous birth experiences in Brazil. Women often particularly fearful of pain during childbirth. Clinicians should offer options for pain relief and anesthesia.
- **Role of the laboring woman during birth**. Women often become less active. Some react to pain by screaming.
- **Role of the father and other family members during birth**. Male part-ner generally not present during labor or delivery. His presence often dis-couraged due to belief that he may become faint or "not be able to take it." Presence of female family member depends on exposure to childbirth prepa-ration classes and family presence in U.S.
- **Vaginal vs. cesarean section**. Woman may choose cesarean section for fear of difficult birth, for convenience, or due to belief that vaginal birth follow-ing C-section is not possible or advisable. Rate of C-sections in many private Brazilian hospitals ranges from 50–85%. May desire an episiotomy to restore tight vaginal opening to afford male partner sexual pleasure.
- **Breastfeeding**. A social norm. But the belief that breast milk is "weak" or insufficient in quantity and fears of milk "drying up" are common deterrents to successful breastfeeding. Average breastfeeding duration in Brazil is eight months; women usually breastfeed exclusively for first 4–6 months. Labor law allows two half-hour rest periods during working hours to breastfeed infant in first four months. Brazil has largest stocks of "human milk" in the world. Women open to storing their own milk. May use manual expression more frequently than electric pumps.
- **Birth recuperation**. Traditionally, new mother expected to rest at home, assisted by her mother, sister, or other family member. Expected to avoid stren-uous physical activity and outside social engagements for 40 days after birth.
- **Baby care**. During first 40 days, baby generally not taken out in public except for visits to doctor. When in public, infant often completely covered. Baby girls often have ears pierced soon after birth.
- **Problems with baby**. Both parents should be informed, preferably by a physician. If mother is single, inform her in the presence of family member or friend. Parents may appear to face infant death with stoic resignation.
- **Male and female circumcision**. Neither practiced routinely.

DEVELOPMENTAL AND SEXUAL ISSUES

- **Celebration of menarche or becoming a man**. No particular social or cultural rituals or celebrations related to menarche itself. Female family members are the usual source of information, although public-health sex education is becoming more prevalent. Traditionally, it was socially sanc-tioned for boys to be sexually initiated by domestic workers or prostitutes, but that is not typical now. Rite of passage for both girls and boys is 15th birthday celebration (*quinze anos*); more commonly celebrated by girls. In middle- and upper-class families, an important rite of passage to adulthood is the highly competitive university entrance exam (*vestibular*), a more difficult version of the Scholastic Aptitude Test in U.S.

- **Attitudes about birth control.** Fertility and childbearing highly valued; childlessness uncommon. But fertility rates have rapidly decreased over the last several decades. Despite the Catholic Church's official position, most married or partnered women use contraception, most frequently tubal ligation and oral contraceptives. Tubal ligation frequently performed in conjunction with C-section and often is the primary indication for it. Requires consent of the male partner of married women older than 25 who have at least two living children. Such consent not required for other forms of contraception. Men rarely participate in women's choice of contraceptive method.

- **Attitudes about sexually transmitted infection (STI) control, including condoms.** Early in the HIV/AIDS pandemic, Brazil had very high incidence rates. Public health campaigns promoted condom use to prevent HIV/AIDS and other STIs. Men use condoms. Government distribution of antiretroviral therapies has resulted in a dramatic reversal of projections of HIV/AIDS morbidity and mortality within the last few years. Although women still represent a minority of those living with HIV/AIDS, it is spreading rapidly among teenage girls. IV drug use plays a significant role in HIV transmission in Brazil. Traditional stigmas regarding STIs in general are becoming less prevalent due to public-health media campaigns and changing social norms.

- **Attitudes about abortion.** Abortion is illegal in Brazil, punishable by a jail sentence for a woman who induces or consents to an abortion and for the person who performs it. Although legal abortions are extremely rare, both professionals and lay persons perform clandestine, illegal abortions. Personal feelings about abortion vary and may include guilt or shame, particularly among religious women. Due to its illegality, women rarely have opportunities to discuss their feelings about abortion with health care providers and therefore may not be very comfortable discussing it in U.S.

- **Attitudes about unwed sexual experimentation.** Although not formally sanctioned, sexual activity among teenage girls and boys is acknowledged and the rate of teenage pregnancies is on the rise. Initiation of sexual activity occurs earlier among boys (at around age 14) than girls (at an average age of 15–16).

- **Sexual orientation.** Acceptance of gay, lesbian, and bisexual orientations varies widely. Large metropolitan areas have openly gay and transsexual communities. Public health campaigns to prevent HIV/AIDS have stimulated more open, public discourse. In smaller towns and rural areas, gays and lesbians are included in regular family activities or relationships. However, some individuals may not formally disclose their homosexuality to the family, which, in turn, never explicitly acknowledges what is common knowledge. Some gay and lesbian persons emigrate to U.S. partly out of a desire to join a more open gay or lesbian community.

- **Gender identity**. Ambiguous or opposite gender identity not discussed openly. More acceptance or tolerance of transsexuals and persons with ambiguous gender identity in Brazil's large urban areas than in smaller communities or rural areas.
- **Attitudes about menopause**. Generally viewed as a natural part of aging and as a reprieve from the worry of unwanted pregnancy. Herbal or homeopathic remedies may be first choice of treatment for symptoms such as headache, hot flashes, or nervousness. Long-term use of hormone replacement therapies not widespread.

FAMILY RELATIONSHIPS

- **Composition/structure**. Close family network usually includes parents, children, grandparents, aunts, uncles, cousins, and their respective spouses and siblings. Also may include godparents (*padrinhos*). Family is center of social activities and a resource for mutual economic and social aid. Brazilians have a strong sense of family loyalty and of duty to help relatives. They often prefer to seek help from family rather than professionals or social agencies. Being separated from their traditional family support system is often a great source of stress and sadness for immigrants.
- **Decision-making**. Within the nuclear family, decisions made by parents or spouse. In the extended family, those with more education and/or economic means usually play the role of family counselor or adviser and provide material support in times of need.
- **Spokesperson**. Parent or spouse.
- **Gender issues**. Traditional families patriarchal. The male, as head of the family (*chefe da família*), is expected to meet family's material and economic needs. The female, as head of house (*dona da casa*), is responsible for managing the home, even if she has a job. Different standards for boys and girls. Families are more tolerant of boys' than of girls' freedom to have many experiences, such as coming home late from parties.
- **Changing roles among generations in U.S.** Emphasis is on *machismo*. Gender roles vary by social class and education. Middle and upper classes are traditionally patriarchal, lower-income households are more matriarchal. Immigration and employment challenge the traditional expectation regarding gender. For example, in more egalitarian cases, men do some housework. Middle-class women immigrants may do more housework than they did in Brazil, where it was delegated to paid domestic workers. Intergenerational tension, particularly between adolescents and immigrant parents, is typical.
- **Caring roles**. Women are principal caregivers. Also, women—particularly

older women—are main source of knowledge and expertise regarding home remedies and treatments.

- **Expectations of and for children**. Parental treatment of, and expectations for, sons and daughters differ. Girls generally are expected to be docile, submissive, calm, and interested in school. Boys are considered to be more competitive. Boys also have more freedom than girls do and are not held to the same discipline standards. Adult children often remain in parents' home until marriage; some remain after marriage.

- **Expectations of and for elders**. Elders usually remain in home. Social contacts revolve around family. Adult children are expected to provide both economic security and social companionship for parents in old age. Family members are the primary caregivers. Home care preferred over institutionalization or nursing home. Those with economic means employ home health aides.

- **Expectations of hospital visitors**. The patient, especially if he/she has a private room, expects a companion (*acompanhante*) at all times. Family members or close friends may rotate through that role 24 hours a day. Patient expects frequent visits by friends and family for social and emotional support.

ILLNESS BELIEFS

- **Causes of/attitudes about physical illness**. May be attributed to divine intervention or fate. Acute illnesses often attributed to activity, change in temperature, food ingestion, or strong emotion before onset. A common belief is that infants and young children can become ill if exposed to bursts of fresh air or wind (*pegar vento*). May attribute some childhood illnesses to a spiritual origin, such as the evil eye (*mau olhado*) or a spell (*feitiço, quebranto*), or to jealousy or revenge (*inveja*).

- **Causes of/attitudes about mental illness**. Attribute folk syndromes known as *nervos, ataque de nervos,* and *susto* to suppression of strong negative emotions, such as anger, fear, envy, worry, sadness, or grief. Stigma attached to institutionalization for mental problems.

- **Causes of genetic defects**. A common fatalistic explanation is God's will (*vontade de Deus/Deus quis*). May also be attributed to events during pregnancy (e.g., accidents, emotional shocks), to defective sperm, or to excessive alcohol use. Some parents accept child's genetic or congenital defects; others harbor strong feelings of guilt or shame.

- **Attitudes about disabilities**. Family members may view disabilities as divine punishment or a "cross to bear." Tend to confine disabled person to home, fearing possible public humiliation. In Brazil, some public and private institutions provide support and rehabilitation. Disabled children usually do not attend regular classes at school. Brazilian parents not accustomed to "mainstreaming" disabled persons, as is common in U.S.

- **Sick role**. Not expected to make decisions about their own health issues. Families, when present, handle decisions and details regarding patient care.

Patient likely to be totally passive and to prefer complete care by others. When someone is hospitalized, family members rotate shifts to maintain a constant presence.

- **Home and folk remedies**. Use a variety of herbal baths and teas as household remedies, sometimes along with special prayers and blessings. A mainstay of Brazilian folk medicine is drinking herbal and medicinal teas, especially for gastric symptoms such as indigestion, heartburn, and diarrhea. Medicinal teas include lemon grass (*cidreira, capim santo*) and orange rind (*casca de laranja*) for indigestion, guava flower (*flor de goiaba*) for diarrhea, and garlic (*alho*) and ginger (*gengibre*) for colds.
- **Medications**. Biomedicine well-accepted, but so are herbal and home remedies; often take both simultaneously. Some persons helped by a folk remedy or pharmaceutical treatment suggest or recommend it to others. Family members and friends often share medications, including prescription drugs. Self-medication with antibiotics and other drugs available over-the-counter in Brazil is common, often before seeking health care from professionals. Immigrants frequently bring supplies of drugs with them or have them sent from Brazil, aware that such drugs require a prescription in U.S.
- **Acceptance of procedures**. Tend to accept surgery, blood transfusions, and organ transplants. Patient and family may monitor duration and quantity of IV infusions as an indication of severity or prognosis of patient's condition.
- **Care-seeking**. Often concurrently use a variety of treatments, such as homeopathy, acupuncture, medicinal herbs, and spiritual healing, along with biomedical care. May delay biomedical care based on insurance, cost, or transportation, or "put health on hold" until they can return to Brazil.

HEALTH ISSUES

- **Concept of health**. Usually considered to be an absence of pain, suffering, or disease, and sometimes a divine blessing. Weight gain in children and adults viewed as a sign of health.
- **Health promotion and prevention**. Seek medical care primarily for treatment of existing illness rather than to promote health or prevent disease. If physician prescribes a specific diet or exercise regime, patient may accept it or at least try to comply with the "doctor's order." May be less open to health education by nurses. Vast majority of Brazilians accept vaccinations, but immigrants are unaccustomed to paying for them.
- **Screening**. May not actively seek screening for conditions when there are no apparent symptoms. Reluctance to undergo screening may be rooted in fear of uncovering a disease or not wanting to face bad news.
- **Common health problems**. In young children, acute respiratory infections. In adults, leading causes of death are cardiovascular disease (e.g., heart disease, stroke), followed by malignant neoplasms and trauma such as acci-

dents and violence. Communicable diseases include respiratory diseases, intestinal parasites, tuberculosis, STIs and HIV/AIDS, Hansen's disease (leprosy), malaria, hepatitis, and Chagas disease (caused by the protozoan parasite *Trypanosoma cruzi*, which enters the body through broken skin).

DEATH RITUALS

- **Beliefs and attitudes about death**. Unexpected death may be perceived as God's will. Hold Catholic/Christian beliefs about life after death.
- **Preparation**. Clinician should inform family members as soon as death is certain and offer to call priest or chaplain. Family members may feel need to say final good-byes to begin grieving. Delayed funeral services must be explained to new immigrants; in Brazil, health department mandates burial within 24 hours of death.
- **Home vs. hospital**. In cases of acute illness, usually prefer hospital. In chronic or terminal cases, may prefer home. Might be reluctant to accept terms of hospice care (e.g., no therapeutic measures) because they do not want to give up hope.
- **Special needs**. Family may want to arrange for extended visitation to be with the body before it goes to morgue. Clinician may need to explain American hospital and mortuary procedures to recent immigrants.
- **Care of the body**. Final good-byes may involve kissing and caressing the body. No specific rituals, but family chooses clothing for the deceased. In Brazil, there is no embalming and the body is prepared at the hospital. Family and friends maintain constant vigil by open casket until burial. Some want the body sent to Brazil for burial.
- **Attitudes about organ donation**. Donation uncommon. Immigrants may not be amenable because of fear, distrust, or desire to send body to Brazil for burial.
- **Attitudes about autopsy**. Autopsy not routine or common. If medically indicated, clinician should provide information and support to help family make a decision.

SELECTED REFERENCES

Hess, D. J., & DaMatta, R. A. (Eds.). (1995). *The Brazilian puzzle. Culture on the borderlands of the Western world.* New York: Columbia University Press.

Levine, R. M. (1997). *Brazilian legacies.* New York: M. E. Sharpe.

Levine, R. M., & Crocitti, J. J. (Eds.). (1999). *The Brazilian reader: History, culture, politics.* Durham, NC: Duke University Press.

Margolis, M. L. (1995). Brazilians and the 1990 United States census: Immigrants, ethnicity, and the undercount. *Human Organization, 54,* 52–59.

Margolis, M. L. (1994). *Little Brazil: An ethnography of Brazilian immigrants in New York City.* Princeton, NJ: Princeton University Press.

Messias, D. K. H. (2002). Transnational health resources, practices, and perspectives: Brazilian immigrant women's narratives. *Journal of Immigrant Health*, 4, 183–200.

Rebhun, L. A. (1994). Swallowing frogs: Anger and illness in Northeast Brazil. *Medical Anthropology Quarterly*, 8, 360–382.

AUTHORS

DeAnne K. Hilfinger Messias, RN, MS, PhD, is associate professor in nursing and women's studies at the University of South Carolina-Columbia. She lived in Brazil for more than 20 years, participating in nursing education programs and directing a rural primary health care program on the Amazon River. Her research has focused on women's work, health, and migration, particularly among Brazilian immigrants in the U.S.

Tereza Cristina Macedo de Paula, RN, BSN, MSN, is assistant patient care manager at the Adult Medical Surgical Intensive Care Unit at the University of California Medical Center in San Francisco. She immigrated from Brazil in 1982 and established residence in San Francisco in 1987. Her field of interest is educating nursing staffs about culturally diverse patient and family responses to hospitalization.

CHAPTER 6

CAMBODIANS (KHMER)

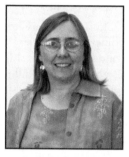 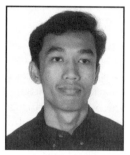

Judith C. Kulig *Sanom Prak*

CULTURAL/ETHNIC IDENTITY

- **Preferred term(s)**. Cambodian or Kampuchean. Prefer to be called Khmer. Sino-Khmer refers to Chinese-Cambodians.
- **Census**. According to the 2000 U.S. Census, there are nearly 172,000 Khmers in the U.S. Census figures are widely considered to undercount actual population; many Khmer did not report culture of origin because of fear/distrust of government, misinformation, language and cultural barriers, and high mobility, and because they were not accustomed to completing the form. The largest populations have settled in Long Beach, CA, and Lowell, MA.
- **History of immigration**. Before 1970, only a few hundred Khmer resided in U.S. In 1975, well-educated professionals affiliated with American government were evacuated directly to U.S. due to impending civil war. Some spoke English or French. Many were young and single or married with small children. Between 1975–79, large numbers of mostly urban Cambodians escaped to Thai refugee camps and, after brief stays, were resettled in U.S. and Canada. In the brutal civil war, cities were evacuated, schools and factories were closed, the population was herded into group farms and forced labor, intellectuals and skilled workers were killed, and 1.5–2 million died as a result of execution, starvation, illness, or hard labor. After 1980, those who were resettled from refugee camps included more rural families and individuals (often widows and orphans), including elderly and extended-family members who had varying health needs and problems. Large percentage did not know English, lacked skills necessary for life in U.S., and were in poorer physical condition than those who arrived earlier. Since 1985, most arrivals have been immigrants sponsored by family members who are American citizens.

SPIRITUAL/RELIGIOUS ORIENTATION

- **Primary religious/spiritual affiliations**. Predominantly Theravada Buddhist but some have converted to Christianity. Syncretism—blending Buddhism, animism, and sometimes Christianity into native beliefs and practices, even though the precepts of each differ—is characteristic of Khmers. Evangelical Christian churches and the Church of Jesus Christ of Latter Day Saints (Mormons) are active in most Khmer communities. Khmer are comfortable with attending both Christian and Buddhist worship services.
- **Usual religious/spiritual practices**. Numerous Buddhist celebrations throughout the year. Elders attend temple service weekly. Most homes have an altar on which food offerings and incense are offered daily. Monks and religious laypersons (*aacha*) use holy water. *Aacha* always male and perform marriage as well as healing ceremonies. Inappropriate for women to touch a monk. *Yiey chii* are Buddhist nuns (often postmenopausal) who may live in the temple (*wat*) all year or on specific days each month that correlate with phases of the moon signifying Buddha's birth. At each meal, including weddings, a dish of food set out for ancestral spirits.
- **Use of spiritual healing/healers**. Khmer are slow to seek care from biomedical practitioners and often hold traditional healing ceremonies in someone's home. *Kruu Khmer* are healers who specialize in dealing with certain illnesses. They may visit patients but do not disclose to health professionals who they are. *Thump* are evil *kruu Khmer* who cast spells.
- **Holidays**. Major ones include Cambodian New Year, or *Chaul Chhnam* (April 13–15); *Phchum Ben* (in September), a feast of the ancestors similar to Thanksgiving; *Bon Om Touk* (November 7–9), a water festival; and *Bon Kathen* (in October), a celebration to provide for monks. Religious and other holidays incorporate religious activities with a festive party. These holidays also are celebrated in U.S.

COMMUNICATION

ORAL COMMUNICATION

- **Major languages and dialects**. Khmer is the major dialect and also name of the people. Some speak Chinese and Vietnamese. Earlier refugees spoke French as well. Khmer tribal dialects exist, but few people speak them. Written language based on Sanskrit from India. Most youth speak English predominantly; elderly Cambodians remain more comfortable speaking Khmer and need translators. Literature and handouts should be in both languages.
- **Greetings**. *Sompeah*—gesture of both palms brought together with fingers pointed upward. Height of *sompeah* indicates status of person being greeted. More acculturated *Khmer* greet with handshakes. Terms such as *Om* (great aunt or uncle), *Pu* (uncle), *Ming* (aunt), and *Bang* (older sibling) used when talking with friends. Otherwise, *Look* (Sir, Mr.) or *Look Srey* (Mrs.) used for persons of higher status.

- **Tone of voice**. Respect essential, demonstrated by speaking softly and being polite. Speaking in loud tone with excessive gestures considered rude, especially for women. Effusive, loud, or over-familiar behavior toward Khmer (including children), and showing anger or confrontation, deemed inappropriate.
- **Direct or indirect style of speech**. Khmer avoid speaking bluntly, not wanting to hurt others' feelings. Instead, they speak carefully and indirectly. May couch requests or questions in seemingly vague terms. Unusual for elderly, in particular, directly to say "no" to a question or request. Impolite to disagree; thus, Khmer may say "yes" but not do as expected. They often agree with health care provider to avoid loss of face. Smile should not be interpreted as happiness or agreement. May laugh in situations in which, to Westerners, laughter is inappropriate. This is not a sign of rudeness or rebuke but instead may reflect nervousness.
- **Use of interpreters**. Trust friends and family members as interpreters. Include family members when discussing health condition. Sensitive issues, such as sexuality, should include interpreter of same gender. Helpful to use interpreter who is respected because of his/her personal or professional health care experience.
- **Serious or terminal illness**. Most families prefer that discussion of end-of-life issues be with family members rather than patient. Family often attempts to "protect" patient from knowledge of a poor prognosis. Clinician should allow family to speak with patient in its own way and time, and offer to answer questions or clarify concerns.

WRITTEN COMMUNICATION
- **Literacy assessment**. Khmer speak slowly without jargon or idioms. Many elderly cannot read or write their own language. Younger Khmer have lost the ability to read and write their language and are more fluent in English. Asking the patient is the best way to assess his/her literacy in Khmer and English.
- **Consents**. Middle-age and older Khmer may be uncomfortable with written consents, due to Khmer Rouge war in which signed life histories were required from persons later executed. Clinician should ensure accurate translation and patients' understanding of consents for health-related procedures. Younger Khmer are more familiar with providing consent and understand forms more easily than elders do. For research, clinician should use only verbal consent.

NONVERBAL COMMUNICATION
- **Eye contact**. Direct eye contact acceptable, but polite women lower their eyes or avoid direct eye contact to some extent. Avoiding eye contact generally deemed a sign of respect and is not associated with age, gender, or status differences.

- **Personal space**. Shy but affectionate with one another and have a smaller personal space than dominant culture does. This also applies to their relationships with non-Khmer and to health care providers with whom they have a trusting relationship.
- **Use and meaning of silence**. Welcome silence. It is more appropriate than meaningless chatter.
- **Gestures**. Lower head when walking in front of elders. To beckon someone, Khmer extend the hand, palm down, and pull fingers in toward themselves. If palm faces up, it is equivalent to beckoning someone as if he/she were an animal.
- **Openness in expressing emotions**. Khmer reluctant to complain or express negative feelings, such as anger, toward one another or toward other persons, such as health care providers. Crying is controlled, quiet sobbing is acceptable. Communication barriers may prevent expressing emotions through verbal means.
- **Privacy**. Respect authority figures. Willing to discuss some issues but hesitant to discuss sexuality, mental health symptoms, and alternative healing practices. Clinicians should acknowledge importance of saving face and limiting confrontation.
- **Touch**. Inappropriate to touch person's head without permission because some Khmer believe that the soul is in the head. Backslapping considered improper for the well-bred. Public displays of affection and public contact between members of opposite sex are inappropriate, but holding hands with someone of the same sex is a sign of friendship.
- **Orientation to time**. Flexible. May arrive early for appointments, but tardiness also should be expected. Strong orientation to the past (remembering ancestors), but there is also a focus on the present because actions today determine the future. *Samsara* refers to continual birth and death, an important concept. Buddhists believe in rebirth and karma.

ACTIVITIES OF DAILY LIVING

- **Modesty**. Very modest. Uncomfortable exposing body. More comfortable with clinician of same gender, but both men and women are comfortable with male physicians.
- **Skin care**. Shower or bathe daily. Infants and children (up to age 2) "washed down" after each diaper change. Young women take considerable time caring for their skin. Make-up extremely important.
- **Hair care**. Wash hair daily. Young persons use many hair products. Young women have long hair; after marriage (particularly after first child is born), they cut it.
- **Nail care**. Men keep nail of right little finger longer than other fingernails for good luck. Women meticulous about nail care.
- **Toileting**. Older Khmer more accustomed to squatting on toilet. May be

uncomfortable with bedpan or urinal due to inexperience with such devices.

- **Special clothing or amulets**. Young unmarried women who are menstruating wear a protective string and cloth bag around their waist to prevent "love magic"—having a love spell cast on them. For protection, adults and children may wear string around waist or chain around neck with amulet containing Buddha or inscriptions in the Pali dialect. May wear *katha* (amulets or what appears to be a piece of string). Some children wear a bracelet made of string to scare away evil spirits. Clinician should not remove these without permission. Tattoos, usually on men, are a more traditional means of protection against harm or illness.
- **Self-care**. Family members help provide care and bring food to an ill family member. Patient performs hygiene and other self-care activities, such as ambulating.

FOOD PRACTICES

- **Usual meal pattern**. Rice a staple, eaten at all three meals. Largest meal of the day is at noon, but since their relocation to U.S. and due to employment obligations, all family members normally gather for supper. Each has a bowl and takes food from communal bowls.
- **Special utensils**. Fork, spoon, and chopsticks.
- **Food beliefs and rituals**. Believe "hot"/"cold" properties are inherent in food and should be balanced. Rice considered neutral, chicken hot, vegetables cold. Combinations of ingredients also determine hot/cold properties. For example, adding coconut cools food. Some traditional foods, including pickled vegetables, fermented soybean curd, and soy sauce, are high in sodium. Rarely consume dairy products. Fat intake generally low.
- **Usual diet**. Breakfast often is chicken soup or noodle dish. Other meals include rice or noodles with fish paste and vegetables. More elaborate meals also prepared, such as pancakes (similar to crepes) with pork, bean sprouts, and fish sauce. Younger Khmer like Western foods.
- **Fluids**. Many Khmer are lactose intolerant. Like soy drinks and specially brewed coffee. Do not use ice. Prefer warm tea or water.
- **Food taboos and prescriptions**. "Hot"/"cold" balance in diet to enhance health.
- **Hospitality**. Very hospitable. Offers of food and drink should be accepted, as should an offer of the only chair in a room.

SYMPTOM MANAGEMENT

Clinician must ask very directly and specifically about each symptom a Khmer patient—especially an older one—may be experiencing. General or passing questions are meaningless. Khmer prefer traditional practices before they seek pharmacological treatment.

- **Pain** (*chhoeur*). Often endure pain and other symptoms stoically. Prefer intramuscular or subcutaneous injection. May use acupressure or home remedies for pain management. Understand numerical pain scales.

- **Dyspnea** (*pibak dok dong hoem*). Become anxious if cannot breathe. Some Khmer have died from sudden, unexpected nocturnal death syndrome, characterized by an inability to breathe plus cardiac symptoms. They describe dyspnea as no air to breathe or shortness of breath. Will use inhaler and oral medications.
- **Nausea/vomiting** (*choeung khmort/khmort*). Interpret nausea/vomiting as a balance problem in gastrointestinal system and are likely to restrict particular foods. Clinician should ask patient if he/she felt in balance at the time of nausea/vomiting.
- **Constipation/diarrhea** (*tuol leak mouk/reak ach*). Modesty prevents open discussion of altered bowel habits, but Khmer usually respond if clinician asks directly. Enemas must be explained carefully. Folk remedies for constipation include soap or gallbladder of a boa or other snake mixed with beeswax and inserted into anus. For diarrhea, most Khmer drink herbal tea.
- **Fatigue** (*oess kamlang*). Believed to be related to other symptoms or problems.
- **Depression** (*chom ngee oess sangkhim*). Uncomfortable discussing mental symptoms. Explain depression as sadness. Khmer believe that Western medicine is "too strong" for their bodies; may reduce drug dosage or not take pills. Older Khmer women attribute memory loss and post-traumatic stress disorder to brutalities of Khmer Rouge War.
- **Self-care symptom management**. Use alternative healers and healing practices, and home remedies. Often go to Western and Vietnamese or Cambodian physicians simultaneously to receive adequate care. Usually seek help from medical system after symptoms appear rather than practice preventive self-care.

BIRTH RITUALS/CARE OF THE NEW MOTHER AND BABY

- **Pregnancy care**. Elderly women give prenatal advice about diet and activities. Khmer are uncomfortable with prenatal classes, a Western approach. Pregnant women follow specific activity restrictions (e.g., not standing in doorways, as baby will be stuck in birth canal, and not stepping over others while pregnant). Pregnant women are active. They pay close attention to diet during pregnancy, especially if the pregnant woman's mother or mother-in-law is present. Avoid some foods, but special foods with coconut are sanctioned. Diet includes high-protein foods, such as eggs, meat, and bean curd. Mother takes herbal medicines in last trimester for healthy baby and these also are prepared for postpartum use. Sexual intercourse not permitted during last trimester. Believe that *vernix caseosa* is sperm.
- **Preferences for children**. Historically, large rural families were the norm, but urban families commonly controlled the number of pregnancies and births. After the war years, it became important to bear children in refugee

camps. In U.S., Khmer limit number of children because of economics; typical family size is 2–3 children. No preference for gender of child.

- **Labor practices**. Walking during labor acceptable. Husband may choose not to be with wife. Her mother or midwife (*chomp*) may assist.
- **Role of the laboring woman during birth**. Expected to be stoic but participates by actively pushing. Pain relief should be offered.
- **Role of the father and other family members during birth**. Depends on situation. Some laboring women do not want husband present but accept their mothers, who provide emotional support and offer encouragement.
- **Vaginal vs. cesarean section**. Prefer vaginal delivery but accept C-section when necessary.
- **Breastfeeding**. Breastfeeding delayed a few days because colostrum believed to be inappropriate for baby. Bottle-feeding implies higher status. Mother is modest when exposing breasts; reluctant to ask questions—e.g., about positioning. Routinely holds baby down and away. Breastfeeding may occur for the first few months and may be combined with bottle-feeding. Many mothers work, so they may curtail breastfeeding.
- **Birth recuperation**. New mother should rest for first few weeks. Mother or mother-in-law very involved in care of baby and new mother. New mother wears heavy clothing, including scarf and close-fitting hat to prevent heat loss. Eats special foods to restore heat lost during birth, and drinks warm tea and water. Usually sleeps on heated bed for several days. For three months, takes regular herbal saunas in which she sits on a stool under a blanket, next to a pan of hot water containing a mixture of herbal roots and leaves that have been boiled. This is believed to help her regain heat, prepregnancy skin tone, and appearance. "Cold" foods, such as vegetables, are restricted; "hot" foods, such as chicken, are acceptable. Takes herbal medicine 3–4 times daily to restore body heat. Peri-care and cleanliness important, but she avoids full body shower for first few weeks. Family members and friends of both genders come to see baby and mother. Baby shower held a few weeks after birth; entire families attend.
- **Baby care**. New mother's mother or mother-in-law very involved in baby care for first few weeks to help ensure new mother is rested. Father also involved; in some families, he takes a more active role in care of child. Cuddling uncommon. Babies (and adults) not kissed but rather sniffed to show affection. Complimenting and praising a baby or child may bring him/her bad luck.
- **Problems with baby**. Clinician should discuss problem with father and family, then with new mother. Accurate translation essential. Couple may blame problem on their own incorrect behavior (e.g., violating activity restrictions during pregnancy). Limited understanding of genetics.
- **Male and female circumcision**. Neither practiced.

DEVELOPMENTAL AND SEXUAL ISSUES

- **Celebration of menarche or becoming a man**. Historically, when young women experienced menarche, a celebration was held in their honor, more commonly among urban, wealthier Khmer. But this tradition has not carried over to U.S. No special recognition of young men who reach adulthood.
- **Attitudes about birth control**. Exposed to birth control in Thai refugee camps. Have adopted a variety of birth control methods in U.S. In the past, it was unacceptable for unmarried women to use birth control, but such rules are relaxing.
- **Attitudes about sexually transmitted infection (STI) control, including condoms**. Limited knowledge about STIs. Do not like condoms, which often are associated with having sex with prostitutes.
- **Attitudes about abortion**. When Cambodians first settled in U.S., they often used abortion to control the number of births. But abortions have declined due to Buddhist beliefs suggesting that such behavior will negatively impact a woman's karma.
- **Attitudes about unwed sexual experimentation**. Young girls are expected not to engage in unwed sexual behaviors. Community closely observes couples' behavior. To prevent loss of face, families attempt to avoid rumors about inappropriate behaviors.
- **Sexual orientation**. Do not acknowledge homosexual behavior. Lesbians and gay men do not openly express such behavior.
- **Gender identity**. Clear gender roles; men and women expected to behave accordingly. Cambodian society and individual families may have difficulty accepting deviations from appropriate behavior and appearance. Pressure to conform is in the form of verbal comments and rejection of choices a person makes.
- **Attitudes about menopause**. Accepted as part of life. Elderly women expected to have more leisure time after menopause because child-rearing is completed. However, they may be asked to care for grandchildren, due to limited family resources.

FAMILY RELATIONSHIPS

- **Composition/structure**. Family-oriented. Maintain the tradition of raising large families if financially able to do so. Extended families living together or in close proximity are the cultural ideal, but nuclear families are common. Due to loss of many family members in war, Khmer practice fictive kinship (i.e., nonbiological relatives are considered to be kin).
- **Decision-making**. Elders key in decision-making. Wives "convince" their husbands to make certain decisions.
- **Spokesperson**. Father, eldest son, or eldest daughter.
- **Gender issues**. Men are head of the household, and are expected to work and support the family financially. Increasing numbers of households are

headed by widowed, divorced, or separated women. Traditional roles common, including those regarding child care and housework, but some women work in a trade at home—e.g., as jewelry sellers. Men help with domestic chores and child-rearing. Women expected to be caregivers.

- **Changing roles among generations in U.S.** Younger family members in U.S. are becoming decision-makers because of language differences and education. Very important that younger family members and clinicians show respect for older family members. More women are working outside of the home in a variety of positions. Independence among women has become more socially acceptable, but families may experience problems if changes occur too abruptly.

- **Caring roles**. Adults, especially women, care for ill family members at home until their health is restored. Elderly often take care of children.

- **Expectations of and for children**. Polite, quiet, obedient children are the norm. Khmer use vocal sounds to discipline children. Girls' behavior more restricted; family is dishonored if a girl loses her virginity before marriage. Children expected to care for parents. Also expected to complete postsecondary education.

- **Expectations of and for elders**. Elders highly respected. Others use special words to address them. They help with child care but otherwise visit or play cards with other elders. Children expected to care for parents. Elders usually live with their adult children; do not like to live in senior or convalescent homes. An organized group of senior Khmer in U.S. assists financially in providing appropriate funeral services.

- **Expectations of hospital visitors**. Expect many family members and friends to visit. Important that patient not be alone. Visitors like to sleep at bedside with patient.

ILLNESS BELIEFS

- **Causes of/attitudes about physical illness**. May attribute illness to natural or supernatural causes. Natural causes include imbalance in "hot"/"cold" or other forces. For example, Khmer believe that "wind" (*kchall*) influences blood circulation, causing illness. A person's past experiences can cause illness. For example, many Khmer have back or limb problems due to time spent in Khmer Rouge labor camps. Supernatural causes of illness include spells cast by *thump* (evil *kruu*). Believe that some illnesses result from sins of past life. Some believe that illness is punishment for faults.

- **Causes of/attitudes about mental illness**. Blamed on Khmer Rouge brutalities. Many Khmer experience post-traumatic stress disorder. Many believe that evil spirits or ancestors cause mental illness. Mentally ill family members are tolerated and cared for with kindness and compassion. Most seek *kruu Khmer* or *aacha* for healing first and/or use both Eastern and Western therapies simultaneously.

- **Causes of genetic defects**. Do not understand genetics. Blame past sins or parents' indiscretions during pregnancy. Clinician must explain defects carefully.
- **Attitudes about disabilities**. Immediate family accepts and cares for, and the community watches over, disabled persons.
- **Sick role**. Passive when ill. Expect health care providers or family members to care for them. Extra attention given to the ill.
- **Home and folk remedies**. Uncomfortable discussing alternative remedies. Herbal medicines common. Chinese and Indian influence evident in types of herbal medicine used. Some use Tiger Balm® or medicated strips of adhesive tape on painful area. Tiger Balm® also inhaled to clear air passages blocked by cold or allergy. "Coining" (*koo'* [rub] *kchall* [wind]) is a treatment for fever, upper respiratory infection, nausea, weak heart, and malaise; it releases heat. A coin is dipped in a mentholated medicine and rubbed in one direction (away from the center of the body) in a symmetrical pattern on the chest, back, and/or extremities. In "cupping," a penny supporting a small candle is placed on the forehead, a candle is lit, and an inverted glass jar placed on top. Suction produces dark circle on forehead. This treatment (e.g., for headache) is believed to suck out pain. Pinching on forehead and neck (*jup* [pinch] *kchall*) treats headache and malaise. Moxibustion (*oyt pleung*) treats gastrointestinal and other disorders. Pain treatments are supplemented by acupressure: Family member puts pressure on arm or leg energy points for 5–15 minutes to release bad air and restore flow of good air.
- **Medications**. Many folk remedies used in Cambodia, some in U.S. But appropriate practitioners and materials are not always available. Use herbal medicines and biomedical drugs concurrently. There are some compliance issues regarding Western medications, due to lack of basic understanding of physiology. The common Khmer orientation to symptoms rather than cause of illness may result in discontinuation of biomedical treatment as soon as symptoms are resolved.
- **Acceptance of procedures**. Uncomfortable with giving blood or blood specimens, due to a belief that it results in heat loss. Clinician should carefully explain procedures such as transfusions. Khmer may not accept organ transplants. They fear surgery; clinician should take time to explain the benefits and risks carefully.
- **Care-seeking**. Often try traditional measures at home before seeking health care elsewhere; may use such treatments simultaneously with Western medicine. Traditional healing practices provide psychological comfort.

HEALTH ISSUES

- **Concept of health**. Good health a result of equilibrium. One must strive for health. It must be individually maintained, but family and community members can influence health. For example, if a young couple has premarital sex, ancestral spirits (*meba*) can make family members ill.

- **Health promotion and prevention**. Most Khmer are oriented more to illness than prevention. Nutrition important, physical activity is not. Clinician should provide health education in the patient's language and in a culturally appropriate manner (e.g., by explaining diabetic diet using Cambodian food).
- **Screening**. Most Khmer do not value early detection or disease screening. Modesty can be an issue regarding some diagnostic tests, such as Pap smears and colonoscopies. Clinician may screen after carefully explaining a procedure to patient and family.
- **Common health problems**. Nutritional deficits, hepatitis B, tuberculosis, parasites (roundworm, hookworm), malaria, HIV/AIDS, Hansen's disease, post-traumatic stress disorder.

DEATH RITUALS

- **Beliefs and attitudes about death**. Buddhists believe that a person will return in another life based on his/her current experiences and karma. The moral precept of karma is that misfortune or accomplishment in this or a past life impacts the next life. One can earn merits by doing good deeds and be reborn into a higher state; immoral acts may result in a lower state. Thus, people may return as humans or animals, depending on how they live. Equanimity in the face of death is highly valued; one should go into death calmly and mindfully.
- **Preparation**. Clinician should inform parents or older children of impending death. Should encourage them to call other family members, monks, and a religious layperson (*aacha*) to provide support at the time of death, and to prepare for funeral and subsequent grieving period.
- **Home vs. hospital**. Chronically ill patients prefer to die at home, as it enables significantly greater cultural/community support and family care. Are comfortable with acutely ill person dying in hospital. If a person dies at home with hospice, body may be kept at home for up to 24 hours. This allows for ceremonies and visitation that are very helpful to the family.
- **Special needs**. Monks and *aacha* must be called to recite prayers. Family members also should be present. Family faces death in quiet, passive manner. May burn incense.
- **Care of the body**. Family, monks, and *aacha* may want to wash body. It is shrouded in white cloth, with hands (holding candles and incense) placed in a prayerful position. Some families place a coin in mouth of the deceased. Prayers by monk on night of the death also important. Clinician should explain to family about releasing body to funeral home. Sorrow phase is limited because the soul of the dead will not rest if sorrow prolonged.
- **Attitudes about organ donation**. Unlikely to allow donation. Due to belief in rebirth and possible better reincarnation, want body to remain intact. Body cremated.

- **Attitudes about autopsy**. Unlikely to agree to autopsy. If essential, careful explanation necessary.

SELECTED REFERENCES

Frye, B. (1991). Cultural themes in health-care decision making among Cambodian refugee women. *Journal of Community Health Nursing*, 8, 33–44.

Kulig, J. (1995). Cambodian refugees' family planning knowledge and use. *Journal of Advanced Nursing*, 22, 150–157.

Rasbridge, L., & Kemp, C. (2003). Cambodian refugees & health care in the inner-city. Retrieved March 15, 2004, from http://www3.baylor.edu/~Charles_Kemp/cambodian_health.html

Rasbridge, L., & Kulig, J. (1995). Infant feeding among Cambodian refugees. *American Journal of Maternal Child Nursing*, 20, 213–218.

Sargent, C., Marcucci, J., & Elliston, E. (1983). Tiger bones, fire, and wine: Maternity care in a Kampuchean refugee community. *Medical Anthropology*, 7, 67–80.

AUTHORS

Judith C. Kulig, RN, DNSc, is a professor in the School of Health Sciences at the University of Lethbridge in Alberta, Canada. She teaches nursing courses in which she incorporates the importance of cultural issues related to nursing practice. She maintains a research program that focuses on rural health issues, including working with unique populations.

Sanom Prak, BS, was born in Phnom Penh, Cambodia, in 1970. He survived the Khmer Rouge regime but lost his father and two siblings. After living in many refugee camps in Thailand and the Philippines, he came to the U.S. in 1984. He is a graduate of San Francisco State University and currently works as a registered nurse at California Pacific Medical Center in San Francisco and at Children's Hospital in Oakland.

CHAPTER 7

CENTRAL AMERICANS
(GUATEMALANS, NICARAGUANS, AND SALVADORANS)

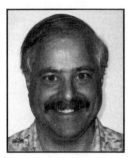
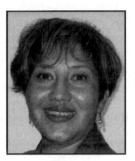
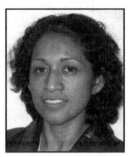

Paul J.
Kunkel

Damaris R.
Aragón

Mirna M. Meoño
de Kunkel

CULTURAL/ETHNIC IDENTITY

- **Preferred term(s)**. After Central America gained independence from Spain in 1821, it gradually split up, with individual countries establishing their own sovereignty. Most Central Americans prefer to be identified with their specific country. Terms such as Guatemalan, Nicaraguan, or Salvadoran are appropriate. However, the dominant cultures in this region retain many broad similarities.

- **Census**. U.S. Census Bureau does not distinguish Central Americans from other Latino groups, so it is difficult to determine actual numbers. Census surveys in 2002 indicate that there are 37.4 million Latinos (excluding Puerto Ricans) living in U.S., of whom 5.3 million (14.3%) are from Central *and* South America. Of foreign-born people in U.S., 36.4% come from Mexico *and* Central America. In fiscal years 1992–2002, 100,344 immigrants arrived from Guatemala, 110,644 from Nicaragua, and 232,483 from El Salvador. These totals are unreliable, given that many undocumented immigrants refuse to participate in a census.

- **History of immigration**. Central Americans have come to U.S. for many years, primarily for economic reasons. In the late 1970s and 1980s, Guatemala, Nicaragua, and El Salvador experienced considerable political violence that had profound effects on all citizens. Consequently, many fled their country of origin to escape devastating circumstances. Although some qualified for political asylum, legal status of most in U.S. often has been precarious.

SPIRITUAL/RELIGIOUS ORIENTATION

- **Primary religious/spiritual affiliations**. Traditionally Catholic, although many have converted to Evangelical religions, whose membership has steadily increased. Mayan Indians may adhere to beliefs associated with a combination of 16th-century Catholicism and traditional Mayan religion.
- **Usual religious/spiritual practices**. Catholics recite the rosary and use the services of priests for confession, communion, or the sacrament of the sick. Evangelicals may attend revivals, prayer meetings, and actively proselytize. Central Americans of Mayan heritage often consult the ancient Mayan calendar to determine appropriate times of year for various religious practices. Their spiritual events frequently mix centuries-old indigenous rituals with newer Catholic rites.
- **Use of spiritual healing/healers**. May summon a priest or physician. May seek advice of traditional healers (*curanderos[as]*). Consider it very therapeutic for a minister or layperson to lay hands on afflicted individual, combining this with prayer.
- **Holidays**. All Central American countries celebrate September 15 as Independence Day. Observe Easter, Christmas, and many minor Catholic feast days. May 10 always reserved for special honors as Mother's Day, no matter which day of the week it falls on.

COMMUNICATION
ORAL COMMUNICATION

- **Major languages and dialects**. Spanish is the national language of all Central American countries. Guatemala has a large Mayan population; slightly more than half of all residents are indigenous Maya. There are 21 Mayan dialects in use today. Some rural Mayan villagers do not speak Spanish. Guatemala has a Black Carib (*Garífuna*) culture with its own language. El Salvador and Nicaragua have Amerindian populations with distinct languages and dialects. There is a small English-speaking region on Nicaragua's Atlantic coast.
- **Greetings**. Central Americans are friendly, outgoing, and gracious. Middle- and upper-class women commonly greet each other by brushing cheeks while kissing the air. Use titles such as *Don* and *Doña* in greeting very familiar persons. Clinician should address new male/female patient as *Señor/-Señora*. Shaking hands appropriate. Long-term patients may greet their health care provider with a hug (*abrazo*).
- **Tone of voice**. Spanish is a rich language, full of intonations and meanings that might be difficult for a novice. Important to closely observe body language while listening to someone speak. Loud, boisterous voices are acceptable and even expected among family and friends.
- **Direct or indirect style of speech**. Central Americans are somewhat formal; for "you," tend to use formal Spanish (*usted*) rather than the informal

version (*tú*). To avoid personal conflicts, they are rarely blunt or direct when discussing important life issues. Commonly tell a prolonged, indirect story to describe a problem.

- **Use of interpreters**. If possible, clinician should allow time for interpreter and patient/family to become acquainted. Should also be sensitive to issues such as gender and age, especially if family member is the interpreter. Preferably, a child should never interpret for a parent, especially when discussing personal or medical issues. When addressing sexual issues, ideally the interpreter is of same gender as patient.

- **Serious or terminal illness**. Clinician should consult with father or eldest son before disclosing serious illness to patient. Disclosing a prognosis may not be valued in Latin cultures; family members may choose not to tell patient that he/she is terminally ill. Clinician should solicit family members' preference.

WRITTEN COMMUNICATION

- **Literacy assessment**. Most Central Americans speak and understand Spanish, except for Mayan Indians from rural and isolated areas of Guatemala, although most Mayans speak some Spanish. Ability to read and write Spanish may be limited. Many Mayan Indians have not had an opportunity to attend school and thus may not be able to read or write proficiently. May value traditional mother/homemaker role of women more than school attendance. If patient has some proficiency with English, important for clinician to speak very slowly and use simple terms and phrases. Most first-generation immigrants have at least rudimentary reading and writing skills in Spanish. They also are eager to attend English as a Second Language (ESL) classes. When giving out patient education materials, important to assess English or Spanish literacy. Acceptable to ask patients direct questions about how long they attended school in their native country and if they have attended any ESL classes. Level of education is a reliable indicator of ability to understand these materials. Usually, members of the second and later generations easily master English.

- **Consents**. Clinician should explain procedures very carefully. Legal concepts and procedures in Central American countries are different from those in U.S. Informed consent and patients' rights are unfamiliar concepts to those entering the American health care system for first time. Feel comfortable signing a consent form only after establishing a relationship with health care provider.

NONVERBAL COMMUNICATION

- **Eye contact**. Persons of same gender maintain a steady gaze when interacting; men and women tend to glance at each other more briefly. Quite common for patients to look down and avoid direct eye contact with clinician, but those who are more highly educated tend to make more direct eye contact.

- **Personal space**. Family members probably maintain the closest proximity, about 18 inches. Strangers keep a few inches farther apart. Central Americans do not have same need for personal space as most North Americans do. Understand clinician's need to work close to them—e.g., when conducting a physical exam.
- **Use and meaning of silence**. Depending on situation, silence can signal respect, acceptance, disappointment, or displeasure.
- **Gestures**. Routinely use nonverbal gestures to convey silent messages. These messages may be secretive and targeted to a particular person without alerting others. For example, people sometimes "point" to someone or something with their lips. An obscene and very rude gesture (a phallic symbol) is pushing the thumb between the index and middle fingers, then making a fist.
- **Openness in expressing emotions**. Only among family and close friends, not in presence of strangers. Indigenous people are stoic.
- **Privacy**. Central American women, especially Mayans, may be very shy around strangers, such as physicians and nurses. Isolation from extended-family members during hospitalization may create stress and feelings of vulnerability because it interferes with traditional support systems. Allow family members to be present. No topics are considered taboo in discussions with health care provider as long as good rapport has been established, which demonstrates respect.
- **Touch**. In Latin cultures, touching someone of same gender common—e.g., patting each other's arms and back or walking arm in arm. Before male clinician begins a physical examination of female, should carefully explain to her parents or her spouse/partner why he must perform exam and steps he will take. No body parts are off limits as long as rapport has been established, procedures are explained in advance, and patient is treated with respect.
- **Orientation to time**. Traditionally, Latin American cultures have a different temporal view. Place less importance on punctuality than North Americans do. Coming from societies in which fatalism is pervasive, they emphasize just living from day to day. Have more of a social focus, with little concern for exact time of day. Lunch can be leisurely with little thought about a later appointment. Promptness and concern about schedules not important. Central Americans are bewildered by health professionals' impatience or annoyance when patients are late for appointments. Regarding education for risk prevention, may be difficult to get patients to acknowledge long-term consequences of their behavior, as they do not easily understand or accept such concepts.

ACTIVITIES OF DAILY LIVING

- **Modesty**. Very modest, particularly women. Clinician should offer hospital gowns and robes. Screens and reassurance during procedures are important. Modesty includes covering legs. Indigenous women comfortable breastfeeding babies in public. Many Latin women prefer a female physician if available. Men generally prefer a male medical provider.

- **Skin care**. Clinician should offer an opportunity to bathe or shower daily. Some patients who recently arrived in U.S. may prefer not to bathe or shower that frequently.
- **Hair care**. Indigenous women may conform to traditional values and not cut their hair but rather braid it. May cover head with traditional scarf or head covering. Long hair not washed daily.
- **Nail care**. Women from higher socioeconomic levels may seek regular manicures and use nail polish. Because of traditional values, work roles, or religious teachings, other women do not wear nail polish. Not uncommon to find dirt under the nails of manual laborers.
- **Toileting**. Privacy important to both genders when hospitalized. A patient hospitalized for first time may need to be oriented to use of bedpan, urinal, and other hospital procedures. Usually cooperative in dependent situations.
- **Special clothing or amulets**. Crosses, rosary beads, or figures of saints may be important. Female children may be protected from evil eye (*mal de ojo*) by wearing red earrings because red is a "strong" color offering protection. Male babies may wear red knitted caps. Both genders may wear a little red bag (*bolsita*) of herbs around the neck to protect them from harm. Clinician should check with parents before removing any red item on baby.
- **Self-care**. Generally expect a nurse to care for hospitalized patient. If the nurse expects a patient to participate in care, specific instructions necessary. Family members of same gender happy to help with personal hygiene.

FOOD PRACTICES

- **Usual meal pattern**. Three meals daily. Lunch is the major meal, perhaps followed by a traditional nap (*siesta*). Evening meal usually smaller and served later in evening. In traditional Mayan culture, man eats and wife serves him; she eats separately.
- **Special utensils**. Indigenous people are accustomed to eating without utensils, using corn tortillas as an all-purpose, edible tool. Otherwise, no special utensils.
- **Food beliefs and rituals**. Many Central Americans believe that mind/body well-being is related to strong/weak or "hot"/"cold" influences. An ill person is said to be too hot, too cold, chilled, or weakened by a variety of causes. Hot/cold qualities also ascribed to foods and liquids but are unrelated to temperature. If someone has a "hot" illness, "cold" foods eaten to restore balance. Some Central Americans believe that if the time for a meal has passed and they have not eaten, appetite diminishes and it is best to wait until the next meal rather than eat between meals.
- **Usual diet**. Coffee and tortillas or bread for breakfast. Soups, meat, rice (or beans), and vegetables for main meal at noon. Rice, beans, and *tortillas* are

staples. Traditional foods are spicy. Many enjoy *tamales*, a traditional food. A hot sauce condiment is always offered at meals.

- **Fluids**. Central Americans do not serve ice in water or drinks; generally serve water and juices at room temperature. Many believe that mind/body well-being is related to strong/weak or "hot"/"cold" influences. Chamomile (*manzanilla*) and mint (*hierba buena*) teas are served hot. Many enjoy very sweet coffee or chocolate. Cold beer served in hot weather.

- **Food taboos and prescriptions**. Avoid drinking or eating "cold" food during "hot" activities, such as ironing. Some persons believe that cold food, such as ice cream, or iced beverages cause stomach pain. Often avoid raw fruits and vegetables because these are thought to cause illnesses. Women may avoid certain foods (milk, avocados, and eggs) during menses because they believe that such foods give the blood an offensive smell. Frequently use herbal teas and other traditional folk remedies when ill.

- **Hospitality**. Central Americans are very social and love to share food, drink, and stories with visitors. Often they prepare special dishes from their native country. Guests are honored with a special meal.

SYMPTOM MANAGEMENT

- **Pain** (*dolor*). View pain as a necessary part of life, something to be endured. Also may consider pain to be a consequence of "earthly misconduct" or "imbalance" of nature. Expressing pain (moaning or crying) acceptable. Numerical scale to determine patient's pain perception works very well. Often use heat packs to reduce pain. Do not typically use ice to treat pain because ice not readily available in Central America. Clinician can offer pain medication.

- **Dyspnea** (*corto de respiración*). Anxious when dyspneic. View the use of oxygen or other "high-tech" interventions as signs of increasing gravity of illness. Very commonly apply Vicks VapoRub™ to help improve breathing.

- **Nausea/vomiting** (*náusea/vómito*). Vomiting uncomfortable and embarrassing in presence of others. May take over-the-counter medications such as Alka Seltzer™. At home, patients may take laxative to "purge" stomach. Highly prefer an IV (*suero*) for fluid replenishment or medications, which they consider to be the most potent form of intervention aside from hospitalization.

- **Constipation/diarrhea** (*estreñimiento/diarrea*). May attribute these conditions to eating spoiled or bad food. Patient may be reluctant to disclose symptoms to a nurse of opposite gender. Patients accept enemas with reluctance and embarrassment. Accept suggestions regarding adequate fluid intake and special diets.

- **Fatigue** (*cansancio*). Attribute fatigue to a lack of vitamins and proper food or may associate it with preoccupation or worry. Men may be reluctant to report fatigue because of masculinity issues related to strength. Central Americans from peasant (*campesino*) backgrounds associate fatigue with overwork rather than illness. Intramuscular injections of vitamin B and iron are common remedies, but they prefer IVs (*sueros*). Prevailing belief is that the more invasive the treatment, the better it is for the patient.

- **Depression** (*depresión*). Believe that a tangible event, such as death of a family member, or illness causes it. Most often associate depression with family problems or being away from family. Commonly somaticized. Those who have experienced catastrophic life events related to political violence or war may suffer post-traumatic stress disorder. Family support, hot soup, stress-reducing activities such as exercise, and prayer groups all are considered to be helpful ways to control depression. Central Americans use medications only as a last resort. Those who are not first-generation may accept psychotherapy.
- **Self-care symptom management**. Frequently use over-the-counter medications. In Central America, prescription drugs are readily available at pharmacies without a prescription, so many people self-medicate. Unfortunately, this can lead to poor compliance with medication regimes, such as taking an antibiotic for a viral infection or only taking half the prescribed amount of an antibiotic. Because many Central Americans are very poor, may not seek early or preventive care. Clinician should talk with patient about the effects on the entire family if he/she does not follow a care regime.

BIRTH RITUALS/CARE OF THE NEW MOTHER AND BABY

- **Pregnancy care**. Latin cultures value mothers and babies. Pregnant women receive much attention and are encouraged to eat well and rest often. In rural areas, midwives often attend pregnant women; in urban centers, physicians typically care for them. Culturally specific beliefs include avoiding cool air and not eating "hot" foods. Strong emotional states are to be avoided. Some women believe that strong moonlight or an eclipse will cause birth defects.
- **Preferences for children**. Desire at least one son as an heir. Traditionally, youngest girl or last child is the designated caregiver for aging parents.
- **Labor practices**. Women may vocalize expressions of pain and discomfort. Often a pregnant woman's mother wants to be with her during delivery. Customary for several women to attend to the mother. Often, pregnant women walk to promote contractions. Squatting and getting on hands and knees are common birthing positions. A shower after delivery is very common.
- **Role of the laboring woman during birth**. Mother may scream and become emotional. Other women who are present offer encouragement and advice.
- **Role of the father and other family members during birth**. Father usually has a passive but sympathetic role. He is expected to be with his wife, to observe how she suffers, in bringing their child into the world.
- **Vaginal vs. cesarean section**. Prefer vaginal delivery. View cesarean section as a serious event, possibly detrimental to mother's health.

- **Breastfeeding**. Varies by social class. Mothers with higher income may pre-fer to bottle-feed. Most poor women breastfeed and cannot afford to buy for-mula. Adequate supply of clean water to prepare formula not available in many areas of Central America, so breastfeeding may be the only option. Working mothers may bottle- and breastfeed concurrently or may choose only bottle-feeding. Breastfeeding occurs in public. Breastfeeding mother may avoid "strong" foods—e.g., avocados, onions, beans, spices—for fear they will change the taste of the milk, such that baby may not want to nurse.
- **Birth recuperation**. Some mothers may follow the practice of *la cuarentena*, a 40-day recovery period after delivery that includes dietary and rest pre-scriptions. New mothers must avoid "cold" foods or drinks, and drafts of cold air. The mother is believed to be in a "cold" state and therefore should eat or drink "hot" substances and keep herself physically warm. "Cold" foods or drinks also will make the mother's milk "cold," causing infant to become ill. New mothers should avoid strong emotional states. Postpartum woman is considered to be in a weak state and must take special precautions during this period. Certain foods, such as chicken soup, bananas, and meat, are thought to strengthen the mother. Traditional remedy for bleeding is sitz baths with Bidens pilosa (*chilca*). Often drink *chilca* tea to boost milk production. If a baby is thought to be colicky, from day one he/she may be given herbal tea, such as mint (*hierba buena*), or, if the condition is believed to be more seri-ous, an herbal tea brewed from anise (*pericón*).
- **Baby care**. Mother is primary caregiver; often, an unmarried female relative helps. The affluent hire a young woman (*muchacha*) to serve as a nanny, but they always prefer a family member.
- **Problems with baby**. Clinician should talk to mother with father present and, for example, say, "I'm worried that…" and "I think you should…." Aunts and grandmothers provide advice about infant care. Central Ameri-cans adhere to prescriptions regarding "hot"/"cold" qualities. Babies often dressed too warmly by U.S. standards.
- **Male and female circumcision**. Male circumcision not traditionally per-formed. Occasionally, some parents wish to emulate U.S. patterns of new-born care, so they may request male circumcision. Female circumcision never performed.

DEVELOPMENTAL AND SEXUAL ISSUES

- **Celebration of menarche or becoming a man**. Great sense of pride when a young woman starts menstruating. She is now considered to be a woman. *Quinceañera fiestas* are elaborate religious debutante parties for girls cele-brating their 15th birthday. For a young man in puberty, the onset of overt masculine signs (facial and pubic hair) is a rite of passage.
- **Attitudes about birth control**. Birth control not restricted to married cou-ples. Youth tend to be more informed than their parents are about family plan-

ning options and tend to use them more. Some indigenous groups have charged that government-sponsored, birth-control programs in Central America are thinly disguised plans for genocide and have refused to participate. In U.S., they remain suspicious of government family-planning programs.

- **Attitudes about sexually transmitted infection (STI) control, including condoms**. Most still naively think they can determine whether or not a potential sexual partner has an STI just by how he/she looks or dresses, which leads to more unprotected sex. Most men are quite reluctant to use condoms. Among married couples, STI is a sign of infidelity. Shameful for a woman to admit to a physician that she has an STI. Most often, people delay treatment for an STI out of fear or ignorance.
- **Attitudes about abortion**. Strong sentiments against abortion due to prevalent Catholic and Evangelical beliefs.
- **Attitudes about unwed sexual experimentation**. Acceptable, without birth control. The widespread conviction that one should "live for today" tends to promote this attitude.
- **Sexual orientation**. Mothers often more accepting of sexual minority family members than are other members of the family. Fathers tolerate this variance. Most often, families do not acknowledge gay or lesbian sexual orientation outside the home. Central American society still has many negative perceptions of sexual minorities.
- **Gender identity**. Transsexuals and persons with ambiguous gender identity are accepted only within a limited circle of family and friends.
- **Attitudes about menopause**. Many women view "the change" (*el cambio*) as the end of their ability to be sexual. Women accept menopause as a normal life stage and discuss it with peers and friends. If symptoms bother them, those who are familiar with traditional medicine often use herbal remedies. For hot flashes, scrapings from an avocado seed are made into a broth. To alleviate intermittent bleeding, shavings from a coconut husk are boiled to make a liquid for consumption.

FAMILY RELATIONSHIPS

- **Composition/structure**. Extended families common, often consisting of three or more generations. They can include cousins and even close friends. Relationships among family members and among persons from same geographical area are close and enduring.
- **Decision-making**. Father or eldest son is primary decision-maker.
- **Spokesperson**. Father or eldest son.
- **Gender issues**. Men and women have traditionally defined roles. Men are generally breadwinners and protectors. Women are typically confined to the home and family. Women who chose a career in their home country were limited primarily to office work, teaching, or nursing. In U.S., they consider many more options.

- **Changing roles among generations in U.S.** Many foreign-born parents worry about their children becoming Americanized. Much to the chagrin of adults, children accept the values of dominant-culture youth and can work and gain more independence than adults ever dreamed possible. Parents are grateful for the extra income their children bring home. However, they fear that the second generation (born in U.S.) will lose the native cultural values and language. The change in roles is dramatic, especially in inner cities. Second-generation persons are better educated and have higher expectations than their parents do. There are few changes in family roles, although women achieve higher levels of education. Each successive generation adopts more values of the dominant U.S. culture.

- **Caring roles**. Women care for the sick. Sometimes men perform aspects of this role. Men may be very caring and attentive to their sick mother, to the detriment of their own marriage.

- **Expectations of and for children**. By U.S. standards, children may be pampered. Parents tend to be very lenient. Value boys' education more than girls'.

- **Expectations of and for elders**. Great respect for elders in all Central American societies. Families are expected to care for elders. Reluctant to place elderly in a nursing home even if family can afford it. Nursing homes are almost nonexistent in Central America.

- **Expectations of hospital visitors**. Because Central Americans are very family-oriented, many may visit a hospitalized family member. Clinician should orient visitors to the unit and encourage family to participate in patient's care.

ILLNESS BELIEFS

- **Causes of/attitudes about physical illness**. Ill health results from imbalance, thus the concern about "hot"/"cold" and strong/weak. Also believe that strong emotions, such as anger, fright, and sadness, cause or aggravate physical illness. Other perceived causes include the evil eye (*mal de ojo*), a witch's curse, or a ghost, and "bad wind" or "forces" that may enter the body directly. At times, the prevailing attitude is "I'm just getting old."

- **Causes of/attitudes about mental illness**. Very private issue. May attribute abnormal behavior, especially depression, to a significant life event (e.g., death of husband or birth of child). Intense emotions, such as anger, grief, or surprise, may lead to sadness, anxiety, or nervousness. "Nerves" (*nervios*) is a common state of anxiety or worry. May attribute mental illness to the supernatural. Strong stigma associated with mental illness; it taints the family's reputation, which is then deemed to have "bad blood." Counseling is a foreign idea. Take medications only as a last resort.

- **Causes of genetic defects**. May attribute defects to the mother's behavior during pregnancy (e.g., not resting or eating properly, strenuous activities, or failing to avoid moonlight, especially during an eclipse). May view birth defects as God's will. Family loyalty is very strong, so family cares for the child at home and rarely institutionalizes him/her. There is a growing awareness of the full spectrum of available health care resources.

- **Attitudes about disabilities**. Family fully accepts a disabled member and cares for him/her at home. "Such is life" (*asi es la vida*) is a common response to disability.
- **Sick role**. A sick person often assumes a passive role and family members provide care. Patient is urged to eat nutritious food, avoid cold air, and get adequate rest for recovery.
- **Home and folk remedies**. Resurgence of interest in medicinal plants and herbs. Commonly drink herbal teas, such as chamomile (*manzanilla*) and mint (*hierba buena*). Believe that lemons and eggs have special healing and protective powers. Great reliance on over-the-counter (OTC) medications. Frequently combine biomedical drugs with home remedies and OTC medications. Clinicians must be especially thorough in this regard when they take patient histories. As rapport grows, patient discloses more information.
- **Medications**. Central Americans are accustomed to obtaining whatever remedy they want from a pharmacy without a prescription. Seek pills first. Consider intramuscular injections to be even better, but believe that IV medications are the best and most potent.
- **Acceptance of procedures**. Clinician should explain procedures clearly. Some Central Americans may be reluctant to donate blood, believing it would make them weak. Accept transplants, although fear of general anesthesia is quite common.
- **Care-seeking**. Seek care from physicians but may delay doing so because of cost. Most prefer to see health professionals—especially physicians—who speak Spanish. Many also seek concurrent care from traditional healers such as *curanderos* if available. *Curanderos* make recommendations about herbal treatments. Many Central Americans who go to pharmacies in U.S. to obtain medications or injections become frustrated when they cannot get what they want without a prescription.

HEALTH ISSUES

- **Concept of health**. Good health related to "hot"/"cold" and strong/weak. Associate good health with ability to perform functional roles. By nature, men considered to be stronger than women.
- **Health promotion and prevention**. Fresh air, eating well, regular exercise, rest, and adequate sleep considered essential. Also important are thinking positive thoughts and not getting angry, upset, or hassled. Lemons and pure water promote health. Laxatives for children "keep them cleaned out." Government-sponsored immunization campaigns have led to a growing appreciation for disease prevention. Families open to health care providers' suggestions about changing their health habits.

- **Screening**. Respect medical authority, so screening for various procedures should not be a problem. Readily disclose medical diagnoses to family. Sexually inactive women tend to avoid Pap smears and breast exams. Rectal exams not a priority. Most immigrants do not have access to affordable health insurance.

- **Common health problems**. Hypertension, associated with a high dietary salt intake. Many suffer the ill effects of alcoholism exacerbated by social isolation. Intestinal parasites endemic in rural areas, where diarrhea contributes to a high infant mortality rate. Elevated cholesterol levels common due to high consumption of red meat.

DEATH RITUALS

- **Beliefs and attitudes about death**. If young person dies, believed to be a greater loss because of the unfulfilled life. Consider prolonged death a relief as long as the person is kept comfortable such that any pain is tolerable. This enables more relatives to say their good-byes.

- **Preparation**. The eldest male in family should be informed of impending death. Catholic patients and families may want to call a priest to administer the sacrament of the sick.

- **Home vs. hospital**. If possible, most Central Americans prefer to die at home surrounded by family members. Especially welcome hospice services.

- **Special needs**. Clinician should ensure an atmosphere of privacy and quiet for sacrament of the sick; if patient can swallow, glass of water helps him/her swallow the small, wafer-like host. Candles appreciated if patient is not receiving oxygen.

- **Care of the body**. Traditionally, family members prepare body for burial. Clinician should ask if they want to prepare body for the mortuary. Central Americans consider death a spiritual event, so family members need time to say good-bye to deceased. Cremation uncommon.

- **Attitudes about organ donation**. Acceptable if body is treated with respect and deference, and if body is made to appear as close to life-like as possible, the way the family remembers him/her. Ideal for deceased to appear to be asleep and peaceful. Will delay organ harvesting if relatives come from far away to view body.

- **Attitudes about autopsy**. Body should be treated with respect. All family members may be involved in the decision. Mayan families may not be comfortable with autopsy because of their beliefs about the afterlife. Many Central Americans do not approve of autopsy because the deceased has "already suffered enough."

SELECTED REFERENCES

Ailinger, R., Molloy, S., Zamora, L., & Benavides, C. (2004). Herbal remedies in a Nicaraguan barrio. *Journal of Transcultural Nursing, 15,* 278–282.

Andrews, M. M., & Boyle, J. S. (Eds.) (1995). *Transcultural concepts in nursing care* (2nd ed.). Philadelphia: J. B. Lippincott.

DeStefano, A. M. (2001). *Latino folk medicine: Healing herbal remedies from ancient traditions*. New York: Ballantine Books.

Glittenberg, J. (1994). *To the mountain and back: The mysteries of Guatemalan highland family life*. Prospect Heights, IL: Waveland Press.

Huber, B. R., & Sandstrom, A. R. (Eds.). (2001). *Mesoamerican healers*. Austin, TX: University of Texas Press.

McGoldrick, M., Giordano, J., & Pearce, J. K. (Eds.). (1996). *Ethnicity and family therapy* (2nd ed.). New York: Guilford Press.

Morrison, M. (1993). *Central America*. Austin, TX: Steck-Vaughn.

Villarruel, A. M., & Ortiz de Montellano, B. (1992). Culture and pain: A Mesoamerican perspective. *Advances in Nursing Science*, 15, 21–32.

AUTHORS

Paul J. Kunkel, RN, MS, CS, worked in a rural clinic in Guatemala from 1984–86. He earned a master's degree in international and cross-cultural nursing from the University of California-San Francisco. He now works primarily with Latino immigrant farmworkers as a public health nurse for the Chelan-Douglas Health District in East Wenatchee, WA.

Damaris R. Aragón, RN, came to the U.S. from Nicaragua in 1978 to avoid political unrest. She earned an associate degree in nursing from Wenatchee Valley College. She is a medical-surgical and psychiatric nurse in Wenatchee, WA.

Mirna M. Meoño de Kunkel, M.Ed, was a teacher in Guatemala before she emigrated to the U.S. in 1988. She earned a master's degree in education from Lesley University in Cambridge, MA. She now teaches a migrant, bilingual, second-grade class at Lewis and Clark Elementary School in Wenatchee, WA.

CHAPTER 8

CHINESE

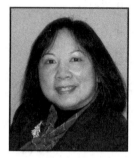

Pauline Chin

CULTURAL/ETHNIC IDENTITY

- **Preferred term(s)**. Chinese, Chinese American. Generation and acculturation influence communication, beliefs, values, family style, etc. For example, early immigrants (40–60 years ago) are strongest believers in Chinese folk medicine; newer immigrants (within last 20 years) combine both Chinese folk and Western biomedical practices; and first- and second-generation Chinese Americans mostly oriented to Western biomedicine.
- **Census**. According to U.S. Census figures for 2002, nearly 2.7 million Chinese, not including Taiwanese. In 2000, 1.5 million Chinese in U.S. were foreign-born. Most live on the East and West coasts.
- **History of immigration**. From 1840–82, Chinese laborers came to U.S. for jobs; many worked on railroads. The 1882 Chinese Exclusion Act suspended immigration of Chinese to America. The National Origins Quota Act of 1924 limited Chinese immigrants to 105 per year, but the act was abolished in 1965. By 1970, U.S. Chinese population had increased by 84%.

SPIRITUAL/RELIGIOUS ORIENTATION

- **Primary religious/spiritual affiliations**. Four major traditional religions/philosophies in China: Confucianism, Buddhism, Taoism, and ancestor worship. In addition to these, many Chinese Americans practice Christianity. Confucianism has played an important role in forming Chinese character and behavior. Its primary philosophy is achieving harmony, the most important social value. Family plays central role and comes before the individual. Buddhist teachings emphasize "face" (dignity). An individual's wrongdoing causes immediate family to lose face. Taoism is an ancient Chinese philosophical tradition whose origins extend back to 3000 B.C. Its central principle is that all life is part of an inseparable whole, an interconnected organic unit that arises from a deep, mysterious, and essentially unexplainable source.

- **Usual religious/spiritual practices**. Depend on religious/spiritual beliefs. Chinese Americans pray alone or in a shrine or church. Common for Chinese families to honor their ancestors, especially during major holidays, such as Chinese New Year. Many Chinese maintain "ancestor tables" or shrines in their homes where pictures of loved ones are displayed and food is left for special events (birthdays or holidays). Incense-burning and eating special foods usually occur on special occasions. May display good-luck symbols, such as statues of Chinese deities, in homes.

- **Use of spiritual healing/healers**. Some use herbalists and acupuncturists in conjunction with Western medicine or before seeking medical help. Rarely, Chinese Americans seek a traditional Chinese healer, such as an acupuncturist, to rid psychiatric patients of evil spirits.

- **Holidays**. Chinese New Year is the most important one. Date varies because it is based on the lunar calendar. Goal is to bring good luck and prosperity to the new year. For example, visitors bring cookies/sweets and oranges to wish their host good luck. People clean their houses and pay their debts before the new year to make a fresh start. For good luck and good health, married persons give money in red envelopes to unmarried persons (mostly children).

COMMUNICATION
ORAL COMMUNICATION

- **Major languages and dialects**. Cantonese and Mandarin most common. Mandarin is national language. Variety of dialects not mutually understood, but all use the same written characters.

- **Greetings**. Chinese are often shy, especially in an unfamiliar environment; socializing and friendly greetings helpful. Clinician should address older patients using "Mr.," "Mrs.," or title and last name. Name order in home country is last name, then first name. Older persons may consider use of first name disrespectful. Shaking hands appropriate, but some just nod head or make a slight bow.

- **Tone of voice**. Chinese language is very expressive and often sounds loud to non-Chinese. Often, this loudness carries over to the English language and, unintentionally, may seem abrupt.

- **Direct or indirect style of speech**. Usually indirect in communicating. To avoid confrontation and loss of face, Chinese Americans rarely say "no" directly. Out of respect, patients may not ask questions but rather nod politely at everything that is said. Clinicians should assess their understanding by asking clear questions.

- **Use of interpreters**. Family members usually available for interpreting, but it is better to have professionals translate information about complicated medical procedures. Clinician should ensure that trained interpreter is fluent in the patient's/family's dialect and avoid male interpreters for older female patients, due to modesty.

- **Serious or terminal illness**. Some families may prefer to be present for information concerning serious or terminal illness. Clinician should ensure involvement of head of household—usually eldest male member of the family. Check with family to find out if head of household should be informed first and/or be present when breaking bad news to patient. Family members may prefer that patient not be told about terminal illness or may prefer to tell patient themselves.

WRITTEN COMMUNICATION

- **Literacy assessment**. Ability to speak or read varies among individuals. Those educated in U.S. are literate in English but may not be able to read and write in Chinese. Newer immigrants usually can read and speak English, but it depends on their education and background. Elderly Chinese (especially women) may be unable to read or write Chinese. Clinician should ask questions to ascertain their understanding but avoid questions that require only a "yes" or "no" answer.
- **Consents**. Clinician should involve eldest male in the family when explaining consent, especially if patient is a young female. Chinese patients usually willing to sign consent forms for procedures that are medically necessary, but they are reluctant to participate in research because of mistrust.

NONVERBAL COMMUNICATION

- **Eye contact**. Usually avoid direct eye with authority figures as sign of respect, and especially with older-generation Chinese. Direct eye contact more common among family members and close friends. It also is more common between persons of the same gender; may be viewed as flirtatious between persons of the opposite gender.
- **Personal space**. Prefer a respectful distance, usually 4–5 feet. Some prefer to sit side by side rather than face each other.
- **Use and meaning of silence**. Can mean lack of understanding or disagreement. May be a sign of respect.
- **Gestures**. Chinese do not use many hand gestures while talking.
- **Openness in expressing emotions**. With family and close friends, use facial expressions and body to show emotion. Otherwise, consider emotions to be private; rarely share them with strangers. Asking questions, especially of authority figures, may be disrespectful.
- **Privacy**. Very important. To "save face," may not want to disclose personal information to health care providers but often do once trust is established or if patient is acculturated. Clinician should involve close family members when necessary.
- **Touch**. Relatively uncommon; more common among family members and

close friends. May view touching someone's head, particularly that of an older person, as disrespectful. Clinician should explain need to touch for health care purposes, which is acceptable. Men and women do not touch affectionately in public.

- **Orientation to time**. Traditional Chinese societies do not value being on time; focus instead on completing present activities. Clinician must reinforce importance of being on time for medical appointments.

ACTIVITIES OF DAILY LIVING

- **Modesty**. Extremely modest, especially women. Clinician should avoid assigning male health care providers to female patients.
- **Skin care**. Good hygiene important. No special needs. Allow family to assist with bathing.
- **Hair care**. Patients may not want to wash hair while sick.
- **Nail care**. No special needs.
- **Toileting**. Privacy important. Prefer to use toilet instead of bedpan or urinal. Older women may prefer to wash afterward rather than using just toilet paper.
- **Special clothing or amulets**. May wear articles (e.g., jade or rope around waist) to ensure good health and good luck. Clinician should avoid removing articles; if removal necessary, encourage family members to take them home for safe-keeping.
- **Self-care**. Most patients prefer to handle daily self-care, but some older men may expect family members or staff to care for them.

FOOD PRACTICES

- **Usual meal pattern**. Three meals a day. Largest is dinner.
- **Special utensils**. Chopsticks, if available.
- **Food beliefs and rituals**. Consider food important for maintaining body's balance of "cold" (*yin*) and "hot" (*yang*). Believe that *yin-yang* imbalance causes illness. Also use food to treat illness and disease. Patients may refuse certain foods due to beliefs about illness and which foods should be used to treat it. If patient is hospitalized, clinician should obtain dietary consult from nutritionist when appropriate to determine food preferences and diet restrictions. Also should encourage families to bring food from home if possible.
- **Usual diet**. Rice and noodles are important staples. Usually do not eat lots of meat; patients may prefer well-done beef. Frequently mix vegetables with meat to maintain *yin-yang* balance. Prefer cooked vegetables, not raw.
- **Fluids**. Drink lots of hot liquids, especially tea, when sick. Prefer hot beverages, believing that cold water shocks the system. Clinician should ask patient before putting ice in drinks or water pitcher.
- **Food taboos and prescriptions**. Food thought to be "cold" (*yin*) or "hot" (*yang*) depending on the energy it is believed to yield when metabolized. *Yin*

foods include fruits, vegetables, cold liquids, and beer. *Yang* foods include meat, eggs, hot soup and liquids, and oily and fried foods. Treat illness caused by *yang* excesses with *yin* foods (avoid *yang* foods) and vice versa. Family members may bring in special foods for treatment purposes. Clinician should consult dietary specialist to ensure compliance with diet. Some Chinese also use herbal preparations and special soups to treat illness. Can be difficult to determine the content of these special preparations.

- **Hospitality**. Offering food to others is a polite gesture, especially when fulfilling obligations or returning favors. Hosts usually offer food/beverages to guests visiting them at home. Respectful to accept offers of food. Guests usually offered the "best" chair, etc., while visiting.

SYMPTOM MANAGEMENT

- **Pain**. Patient may not complain of pain, so clinician should be aware of nonverbal cues. Some patients believe that being stoic is expected; may not want to "bother" the nurse to ask for pain medication. Clinician should offer medication instead of waiting for patient to request it. Some patients use acupressure or acupuncture to treat pain or illness. Clinicians can use numeric pain scale when patient acknowledges pain.
- **Dyspnea**. Too much *yin* or a stressful event can cause it. Patients readily accept oxygen. Some treat it by eating hot soup/broth and wearing warm clothes.
- **Nausea/vomiting**. Caused by too much *yin*. Patient may not keep emesis; may clean up so as not to "bother" nurse. Treat with hot soup/broth.
- **Constipation/diarrhea**. Both caused by too much *yang*. Patient may not keep stool so as not to "bother" nurse. Some patients treat constipation/diarrhea with fruits, vegetables, and other *yin* foods. Accept other dietary suggestions.
- **Fatigue**. Caused by too much *yin*. Treat fatigue with hot soup/broth. Ginseng a common remedy.
- **Depression**. Somewhat common, especially among new immigrants because of financial pressures and the challenge of learning an unfamiliar language and culture. Chinese view any mental health problem, including depression, as shameful; do not readily discuss it. Some describe physical symptoms, such as sleeplessness, when in fact the underlying cause is emotional. If Chinese acknowledge depression, they accept medication and counseling.
- **Self-care symptom management**. Most Chinese treat minor symptoms with food remedies. However, may ignore major illnesses, such as cancer or heart disease, until an advanced stage. Some patients seek Western biomedicine for treatment. If an illness is chronic, more willing to do self-care (e.g., eat a diet appropriate for diabetics or inject insulin).

BIRTH RITUALS/CARE OF THE NEW MOTHER AND BABY

- **Pregnancy care**. Use regular prenatal care and take childbirth preparation classes if acculturated or if they are second-generation Chinese. Hold traditional beliefs about the effect that certain activities of pregnant mother will have on baby. For example, going to the zoo will cause baby to look like one of the animals; listening to beautiful music and thinking good thoughts will foster a happy, healthy baby. Chinese emphasize good nutrition and discourage vigorous activity. Consider pregnancy a "cold" condition, so *yin* foods should be avoided. Eating watermelon during pregnancy, for example, will cause baby to have asthma.
- **Preferences for children**. Traditionally prefer a son to carry on family name, but this preference weaker or nonexistent in U.S. In China, couples strongly encouraged to have only one child. Most of the children put up for adoption are girls.
- **Labor practices**. No special practices. Readily follow clinician's instructions.
- **Role of the laboring woman during birth**. Although Chinese are stoic, it is acceptable for Chinese women to express pain by moaning and making other noises during childbirth. Clinician should offer pain medications because patients may not request medications for fear that the baby might be harmed.
- **Role of the father and other family members during birth**. Usually female family members present during birth. Father and other male members do not normally attend or coach during birth, but those who are acculturated or second-generation Chinese are more active in this regard.
- **Vaginal vs. cesarean section**. Prefer vaginal delivery but accept cesarean if medically necessary.
- **Breastfeeding**. Usually preferred to bottle-feeding, unless mother works, in which case bottle-feeding is more common. While breastfeeding, mother is expected to ingest "hot" (*yang*) foods to strengthen baby's health. Duration of breastfeeding depends on the individual and whether she works.
- **Birth recuperation**. During first 30 days postpartum, mother's pores are believed to remain open and cold air can enter the body, which may cause illness. Based on this belief, a new mother may be forbidden to go outdoors, shower, or bathe. Diet will be rich in *yang* foods, such as meat, eggs, and liver, and mother may avoid *yin* foods. Many consume specially prepared soups and broths containing pigs' feet and chicken. Common for either grandmother to help new mother with cooking, cleaning, and baby care.
- **Baby care**. New baby is center of attention in Chinese families. Mother is expected to care for baby. Ideally, she should take extended time off from work, but grandparents commonly help with care if mother works.
- **Problems with baby**. Take priority in the family and are treated with utmost importance. Health care decisions must involve head of household in traditional families.

- **Male and female circumcision**. Male circumcision quite common. No special ritual. Usually performed at hospital or in doctor's office. Female circumcision not practiced.

DEVELOPMENTAL AND SEXUAL ISSUES

- **Celebration of menarche or becoming a man**. No formal recognition of puberty or transition to adulthood for either gender.
- **Attitudes about birth control**. Chinese are very modest and traditionally unwilling to discuss anything sexual. Thus, usually do not discuss birth control. It may be used, but responsibility typically rests with the woman. Religious beliefs may influence choice of methods.
- **Attitudes about sexually transmitted infection (STI) control, including condoms**. As sex is not openly discussed, there may be limited knowledge about STIs, including HIV/AIDS. Men may refuse to wear condoms and may not believe they need them.
- **Attitudes about abortion**. No preference for abortion vs. adoption. Abortion is common in China when birth control fails; not shameful or hidden. But abortion is not a routine birth control measure. In U.S., it is by individual choice. Religion may influence attitude.
- **Attitudes about unwed sexual experimentation**. Females expected not to have sex before marriage. Those who do may use birth control secretly because pregnancy would disgrace the family.
- **Sexual orientation**. Family does not usually acknowledge gay and lesbian sexual orientation and relationships. They are concealed from the community and shame the family.
- **Gender identity**. Ambiguous or opposite-gender identity usually not discussed outside of the family. Masculine girls and feminine boys face pressure to change.
- **Attitudes about menopause**. Viewed as a normal event. Compared to European American women, Chinese women may have fewer symptoms, due to lower-fat diet and more regular exercise. Treat symptoms with herbal preparations from herbalists.

FAMILY RELATIONSHIPS

- **Composition/structure**. Traditional Chinese values place family and society above the individual. Extended families common. Two or three generations often live in same household. Wife expected to become part of husband's family.
- **Decision-making**. Patriarchal society. Eldest male makes most decisions. Females usually make decisions about the house and family.
- **Spokesperson**. Usually eldest male in household.
- **Gender issues**. Males usually more highly respected and valued than females. Male expected to be the breadwinner and earn money for the fam-

ily. Mothers often expected to stay home and raise the children if another family member is not available to babysit.

- **Changing roles among generations in U.S.** The longer that Chinese are in U.S., the more their family roles resemble those in dominant culture. In acculturated and second- and third-generation families, women usually work and have more-equal relationships with their spouses.
- **Caring roles**. Caring for sick person usually the responsibility of a female in household—mother, wife, daughter, daughter-in-law. Family members generally care for children rather than putting them in day care.
- **Expectations of and for children**. Chinese families highly value children, who are expected to respect elders, obey parents, and behave well. Also value education highly. Children who do not do well in school bring shame on family. Adult children commonly live with parents until marriage. Second-, third-, and fourth-generation children more closely resemble their peers in dominant culture, except for high academic expectations. Emphasis on filial piety: Children must meet parental expectations and fulfill obligations, such as caring for elderly parents.
- **Expectations of and for elders**. Elders highly respected and honored. In extended families, grandparents often responsible for care of grandchildren. Some elderly widows live alone. Adult children obligated to care for elderly parents when they cannot care for themselves, but it is becoming more common to place them in assisted-living facility or nursing home when adult children work.
- **Expectations of hospital visitors**. Common for many family members and friends to visit patient. Considered polite for visitors to bring food or gifts.

ILLNESS BELIEFS

- **Causes of/attitudes about physical illness**. Imbalance of *yin* and *yang* in body causes most physical illnesses.
- **Causes of/attitudes about mental illness**. Thought to be caused by a lack of emotional harmony. In some cases, Chinese believe that evil spirits or bodily imbalance is the cause. Mental wellness occurs when psychological and physiological functions are integrated. Mental illness highly stigmatized, not usually discussed outside the family because of shame. May try to care for mentally ill family member at home until he/she becomes very ill and care is too difficult; then they accept medication and/or hospitalization.
- **Causes of genetic defects**. Usually blamed on mother—something she did or ate, generally. Defects also may be a consequence of bad luck or not honoring ancestors.
- **Attitudes about disabilities**. No special attitudes. Disabled family member usually receives care at home if possible. May not be taken out in public because of shame. Willing to undergo rehabilitation or receive other necessary services.

- **Sick role**. Family expected to care for patient, who takes passive role during his/her illness, including leaving health care decisions to others.
- **Home and folk remedies**. Ginseng root a common home remedy for a number of ailments, including anemia, colic, depression, indigestion, impotence, and rheumatism. Other Chinese remedies are deer antlers for strengthening bones and treating impotence, turtle shells to stimulate weak kidneys and remove gallstones, and snake flesh for healthy eyes and clear vision. May self-medicate with herbs purchased from a traditional Chinese pharmacy or take those prescribed by acupuncturist.
- **Medications**. May take allopathic medications concurrently with herbs, which might interact (e.g., ginseng and antihypertensives). May avoid telling traditional healer or biomedical practitioner about the other and about medications. Some save leftover prescription drugs or borrow them from/loan them to family members or friends. Some do not comply well, stopping medications when symptoms become less severe. Acculturated and second- and third-generation Chinese usually follow the regimen their biomedical practitioner prescribes.
- **Acceptance of procedures**. Some fear having their blood drawn, believing it will weaken the body and thus reduce vital energy. Many Chinese avoid surgery because the body must be kept intact so the soul will have a place to live when it visits earth in the future. Some educated/acculturated persons may accept organ donations and transplants when essential.
- **Care-seeking**. May first adjust diet for minor ailments or use home remedies for ailments such as colds and skin diseases. Most Chinese seek care from biomedical physicians for more serious diseases, such as cancer. Solicit advice from relatives and friends in deciding whether to seek professional care. Traditional practitioners of Chinese medicine prescribe herbs and acupuncture based on a diagnosis involving *yin-yang* and energy balance.

HEALTH ISSUES

- **Concept of health**. Good health is a balance of *yin-yang* influences—not only in the body but in the whole environment. Important to maintain harmony of body, mind, and spirit.
- **Health promotion and prevention**. Preventing illness and promoting good health accomplished by exercise and eating a diet that balances *yin* and *yang* foods. May use traditional methods of health promotion, such as *t'ai chi* or *qi gong*, to balance body and mind. Also important to maintain harmony with family and friends. Accept immunizations.
- **Screening**. May refuse diagnostic tests they consider to be invasive or dangerous—e.g., amniocentesis or glucose tolerance test. Older or less-acculturated Chinese may under-use cancer screening, such as Pap smears, mammograms, or colonoscopies. Clinician should encourage family involvement and participation, and respect privacy.

- **Common health problems**. Skin conditions such as eczema and psoriasis common, as is tuberculosis among newer immigrants. Cancer the leading cause of death among those 25–64 years old; other major causes are heart disease, stroke, cancer, and chronic respiratory conditions. Diabetes and kidney disease also common. Smoking in men is a risk factor. Higher suicide rates than in White population, especially among adolescents.

DEATH RITUALS

- **Beliefs and attitudes about death**. Death part of the life cycle. Many Chinese believe in the afterlife. Others fear death and avoid discussing it. Common to honor ancestors by leaving food at grave site or by displaying a portrait in the home, especially during special holidays. Honoring ancestors allows their spirits to rest and brings good fortune and good luck.
- **Preparation**. Terminally ill patients may be fatalistic and not want to talk about death. Family may prefer that patient not be told he/she is dying or may prefer to tell patient themselves. Traditional families may prefer that the head of household be told first that patient is dying. When death is imminent, Chinese families like to be present and may hold a vigil at the bedside.
- **Home vs. hospital**. Many believe that people should go to the hospital to die because dying at home will bring bad luck. Others believe that the spirit might get lost if death occurs in the hospital. Accept hospice care, especially when comfort care is the goal.
- **Special needs**. Family members may bring special amulets and clothing from home to place on the body. May request that a window be opened to free the spirit after death.
- **Care of the body**. Some families prefer to bathe deceased after death.
- **Attitudes about organ donation**. Believe that body should be kept intact; otherwise, the spirit may not have a place to go when it visits earth. Organ donation uncommon.
- **Attitudes about autopsy**. May not allow autopsy, as body should be kept intact. Accept autopsy if medically or legally necessary.

SELECTED REFERENCES

Feng, C. (2002). Merging Chinese traditional medicine into the American health system. *Journal of Young Investigators*, 6, 6–12.

Lee, E. (Ed.) (1997). *Working with Asian patients: A guide for clinicians*. New York: Guilford.

Mo, B. (1992). Modesty, sexuality, and breast health in Chinese-American women. *Western Journal of Medicine*, 157, 260–264.

Tom, L.A. (2004). Health and health care for Chinese-American elders. Retrieved June 20, 2004, from http://www.stanford.edu/group/ethnoger/chinese.html

AUTHOR

Pauline Chin, RN, MS, is a nurse educator at the University of California Medical Center in San Francisco and a member of the UCSF Diversity Committee. She is a second-generation Chinese American who has done numerous presentations on health care practices and beliefs of Chinese patients.

CHAPTER 9

COLOMBIANS

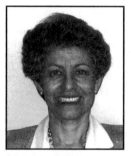

Pilar Bernal de Pheils

CULTURAL/ETHNIC IDENTITY

- **Preferred term(s)**. Colombian (*Colombiano[a]*).
- **Census**. About 2 million in U.S.: 1 million in New York City area, 500,000 in Florida, 100,000 in the Los Angeles area, and the remainder in Boston, Chicago, Atlanta, and Houston areas. Of the total, 490,000 are foreign-born.
- **History of immigration**. Colombians have been coming steadily to U.S. since the 1950s. Represent all levels of education and socioeconomic status; most have at least a high school education. In the last 15 years, many more have come because of conflict in Colombia—guerilla warfare and the war on illegal drugs.

SPIRITUAL/RELIGIOUS ORIENTATION

- **Primary religious/spiritual affiliations**. Catholic (more than 90%).
- **Usual religious/spiritual practices**. Even though patient and his/her family describe themselves as Catholic, may not go to church; if they do, attend mass weekly, either on Saturday, Sunday, or, if very religious, every day. Hospitalized patient's family may bring picture of the Virgin or cross with Christ; if allowed, they place candles around the picture to help with prayer. May do the same at home for a sick person. Religious family members (usually mother/grandmother) may recite prayers or rosary if patient very ill. Clinician should call priest to visit patient for confession, communion, or to receive sacrament of the sick.
- **Use of spiritual healing/healers**. If patient is extremely ill, presence of priest very important. Clinician should facilitate patient-priest privacy. Colombians may seek a traditional healer (*curandero*) or a healer who uses special herb mixtures, prayers, or massage (*sobandero*) if there is no access to

biomedical care or, less likely, in combination with biomedical care. In U.S., *curandero* will not visit hospitalized patient because, in Colombia, biomedical providers do not accept them.

- **Holidays**. Twelve religious holidays celebrated in Colombia, but the most common among immigrants is Christmas Eve (December 24), when there is caroling and dancing. Some immigrants also may celebrate Holy Friday before Easter; in Colombia, Holy Friday and the Thursday before are very important religious holidays. Six national holidays (*fiestas nacionales*) celebrate important historical days in Colombia. The two most relevant secular holidays in U.S. are Independence Day (July 20) and New Year's Day (January 1).

COMMUNICATION
ORAL COMMUNICATION

- **Major languages and dialects**. Spanish is national language. Natives of San Andres and Providencia islands speak a dialect called Papiamento, a mixture of English, French, and Spanish. Very small proportion of population are Indians who maintain their own dialects. Most Colombians in U.S. speak Spanish and English. Most who immigrate are well-educated; they learned English in Colombia or learn it after their arrival in U.S.
- **Greetings**. Out of respect, Colombians address a middle-age or elderly person as "Mrs." (*Señora*), "Mr." (*Señor*), or "Miss" (*Señorita*) followed by the person's last name. Single women are carefully addressed as "Miss." In Spanish, the formal form of "you" is *usted*. Men shake hands with men and women. Women clasp each other's wrists instead of shaking hands. Greetings between friends or relatives are hand-to-hand between men or cheek-to-cheek between women and between women and men.
- **Tone of voice**. May raise voice with family members or friends. May get agitated or emotional when nervous or frightened. Clinicians should make requests politely and avoid talking loudly.
- **Direct or indirect style of speech**. Very respectful of authority figures, particularly physicians. Colombians may nod when a clinician asks them to do something, even though they may not accept it or may not intend to follow through. Clinician should avoid being blunt when giving information/advice, as patient may interpret this as disrespectful. Colombians may take awhile to make their point; like to tell stories, so answers to direct questions may be long and at the end of a story. Introductory greetings and warm-up with superficial conversation may be necessary before patient feels sufficiently at ease to confide a problem. Best if clinician takes time to explain problems in a simple way.
- **Use of interpreters**. May use family members as interpreters. Patient needs professional interpreter if family member is not an adult. When sensitive issues (such as sexual history) must be discussed, clinician should choose a close family member of same gender if possible.
- **Serious or terminal illness**. Clinician should consult with a close family

member about how to communicate bad news. Family may choose to disclose news to patient or may ask clinician to do it (and want to be present). Family members may choose not to disclose seriousness of illness to patient, particularly in the case of a child or sick elderly parent.

WRITTEN COMMUNICATION

- **Literacy assessment**. Literacy level varies depending on socioeconomic background. Colombians of high socioeconomic status—especially young to middle-age adults—may speak, read, and write English well. To assess literacy, clinician should ask patient directly and respectfully, "Can you read?" Also should offer information in Spanish if available; clinicians can assume that most immigrants read Spanish.
- **Consents**. Written consent forms not customary in Colombia. Clinician must begin consent process by explaining that most procedures in U.S. require written and signed form from patient. Should explain this slowly, obtain frequent feedback from patient, and allow questions. Patient may be embarrassed to ask questions.

NONVERBAL COMMUNICATION

- **Eye contact**. May avoid direct eye contact with authority figures (e.g., doctors and nurses) or in awkward situations. May not sustain direct eye contact with an older family member (*persona mayor*), such as a parent or grandparent, or with friends in an embarrassing situation. However, in normal communication, they sustain eye contact with family members and friends.
- **Personal space**. Closer than the Northern European American norm. Frequently share personal space with family members or close friends. With health care providers or strangers, social space is no more than 3 feet.
- **Use and meaning of silence**. May mean failure to understand what has been said and embarrassment about asking or disagreeing.
- **Gestures**. Frowning means disapproval, a common gesture parents use in communicating with children. Colombians avoid placing feet on furniture or yawning in public without covering mouth. Tapping underside of elbow with fingers of other hand suggests someone is cheap. Frequently move hands while talking.
- **Openness in expressing emotions**. Very open. Often loudly express all emotions to family, friends, health care providers, even strangers.
- **Privacy**. If clinician is warm and approachable, patient may open up and confide any problem, personal or not. Communication, particularly regarding sexuality problems, may be better if provider and patient are of same gender.
- **Touch**. Colombians typically are very affectionate and friendly. Appropriate to touch someone when he/she is confronting hardship (e.g., while relaying bad news). Clinician may hold patient's hand or put hand on his/her shoulder.

- **Orientation to time**. Unaccustomed to long-term planning; most plans are short-term. Always expect a social event to start later than the announced time; frequently, ending time of event is not provided. May be a few minutes late for appointments. Clinician should emphasize importance of keeping appointments and canceling ahead if necessary.

ACTIVITIES OF DAILY LIVING

- **Modesty**. Very modest, particularly if clinician is of opposite gender. Clinician should offer gown, robe, and hospital pants to both women and men, and take care not to expose patient's body unnecessarily. Men uncomfortable when female clinician needs to examine, or intervene in area of, private parts.
- **Skin care**. Customary to shower daily. Patient may choose not to shower if feeling weak/feverish or if it is medically contraindicated. Men shave daily, and most women shave their legs and axillae daily. May not routinely wash hands before meals.
- **Hair care**. Do not customarily wash hair daily, especially women with long hair, which is commonplace. Men prefer short hair. No special practices regarding shampoos or conditioners.
- **Nail care**. Women prefer long nails and use nail file instead of scissors. Men cut their nails very short with scissors; prefer to do it themselves if not very sick. Parents cut children's nails short.
- **Toileting**. Done privately. If bedpan or urinal necessary, clinician should protect patient's privacy.
- **Special clothing or amulets**. Amulets common (predominantly Roman Catholic) and include medallions (*escapularios*), rosary beads, and religious figures and pictures. Clinician should not remove these unnecessarily. Girls often have pierced ears and gold earrings. Both genders wear gold bracelets and chain necklaces.
- **Self-care**. Hospitalized patients do not expect to provide any self-care; rather, with exception of eating, they expect to be cared for, including hygiene. A child may expect to be fed, but adults feed themselves unless very ill. Patients perform self-care—e.g., bathing, ambulation, deep breathing, or special physical exercises—if asked to do so for health reasons.

FOOD PRACTICES

- **Usual meal pattern**. Three meals a day. Lunch larger than dinner. For farmworkers (*campesinos*), largest meal may be breakfast. Many Colombians in U.S. have their major meal at night because families cannot meet midday due to work or school schedules.
- **Special utensils**. None.
- **Food beliefs and rituals**. Influenced by Catholicism. For example, most Colombians eat fish on Friday during Lent.
- **Usual diet**. Varies by region in Colombia. Rural people hold more strongly to

traditional diets than those in urban areas do. Coffee or chocolate and bread are part of breakfast. Rice and potatoes a staple at lunch and, for some, also at dinner. Soup common for lunch. Fresh fruit juice frequently accompanies meals. Vegetables scarce in diet (e.g., salad may contain only tomato, lettuce, and carrot). May snack between meals. Sandwiches do not replace meals.

- **Fluids**. Prefer hot drinks first thing in the morning and commonly at breakfast. At other times of day, prefer to drink fresh fruit juices diluted with water, although commonly drink sodas if available.
- **Food taboos and prescriptions**. Colombians avoid cold or iced drinks when sick, particularly if they have a cold, respiratory infection, or fever. But they use ice externally to relieve pain. Women avoid acidic foods during menstruation. Commonly drink a hot infusion of diluted, unrefined sugarcane paste (*agua de panela*), possibly with lime, when they have cold symptoms. Frequently drink hot herbal tea—chamomile, mint, flax seed, thyme, or rosemary—as home remedies.
- **Hospitality**. Serve food at every social occasion. Alcohol common at social gatherings, typically beer and *aguardiente* (similar to tequila), which has 30–32% alcohol and is derived from sugar cane.

SYMPTOM MANAGEMENT

Most immigrants understand, and are comfortable with, numerical scales for reporting symptom level.

- **Pain** (*dolor*). Occasionally report *inflamado(a)*, indicating abdominal pain. Women in pain may be more expressive than men are; tend to cry easily. Men expected to be stoic and do not demonstrate pain easily. Colombians prefer oral or IV routes to intramuscular or rectal. May not take pain medication as directed due to fear of becoming addicted. Use heat/ice to control pain, massage to control muscular pain.
- **Dyspnea**. Express "being without air" or "unable to breathe" as *quedarse sin aire* or *no poder respirar*. Patient/relatives may be very anxious. Expect and accept oxygen when this occurs; may accept other medications if need for them is explained. Nonpharmacological approaches, such as prayer or relaxation techniques, acceptable.
- **Nausea/vomiting** (*náusea/vómito*). Interpret as a sign of illness. Feel embarrassed after vomiting but report it to care provider. Accept medications to control symptoms. Patient may smell alcohol to reduce the desire to vomit. Drink chamomile tea for stomach pain.
- **Constipation/diarrhea**. Constipation in Spanish is *estreñimiento* or *estar dura del estómago*. Expect daily bowel movement and become concerned if none occurs. May use over-the-counter laxatives such as milk of magnesia. Patients mention constipation or report it when asked; accept enemas if necessary. Report loose stools in any form as diarrhea. Usually stop drinking milk if diarrhea occurs. Accept dietary recommendations for symptom management.

- **Fatigue** (*cansado[a]*). May believe that anemia causes fatigue. Accept medications but may fear addiction if sleeping pills necessary. Take naps to relieve fatigue.
- **Depression** (*presión*). Recognize depression. Depressed persons say, "I am sad" (*triste*) but do not talk about depression openly. May drink "tranquilizer" teas, valerian root tea. Clinician should be cautious when asking about high blood pressure ("*¿Sufre de la presión?*" or "*¿Tiene la presión alta?*") because patient may interpret this as asking if he/she suffers from stress/depression. Accept medication and counseling.
- **Self-care symptom management**. Do not expect to care for themselves. Patients may not take action until very sick. Colombians usually expect a family member to care for them. Family pampers patient with attention and services to the point of interfering with appropriate care—e.g., by discouraging early ambulation and self-care activities, such as eating and bathing. In cases of chronic illness, if clinician clearly explains importance and need for self-care, family members comply with his/her recommendations.

BIRTH RITUALS/CARE OF THE NEW MOTHER AND BABY

- **Pregnancy care**. Use prenatal care if patient/family can afford it, but immigrants from rural areas may not, regardless of their financial circumstances. Pregnant women are protected from hard work. Family members encourage them to rest and eat a substantial amount of food and protein-rich food. If childbirth preparation classes available, couples in Colombia and U.S. attend.
- **Preferences for children**. May value boys more than girls, especially the first child, but this is more common among Colombians of rural origin. A son is important for carrying on the family name. Also desire girls, particularly if mother has had only boys. Big families (5–8 children on average) more common in older generation. Young persons and immigrants tend to have smaller families.
- **Labor practices**. Do not eat during labor for fear of vomiting; only sip fluid. Most prefer to lie down but may walk and/or shower early in labor. Relatives generally not present during labor and delivery but welcome the option in U.S. Analgesia welcome but not expected in lower socioeconomic groups; it is not routinely offered to poor women in Colombian hospitals.
- **Role of the laboring woman during birth**. Passive. Follows instructions. Expression of pain varies; frequently very noisy and, less frequently, she suffers in silence.
- **Role of the father and other family members during birth**. Family members not expected to be present at delivery, but younger fathers may welcome the opportunity if they attended childbirth preparation classes. If family members present, mother of laboring woman plays major role in supporting daughter.
- **Vaginal vs. cesarean section**. Cesarean section may be sign of upper-class

status. Mother often requests it when she is experiencing much pain.

- **Breastfeeding**. Expected, particularly among low- to middle-income Colombians. Although breastfeeding has increased at all socioeconomic levels, duration varies from weeks or months (if the mother must work outside home) up to a year. Few continue beyond a year. Longer duration expected if mother is from a rural area.
- **Birth recuperation**. Mother and sister care for new mother and baby; father also may participate. Not allowed to do strenuous physical activities. Some from rural areas do not leave house until 40 days postpartum. Some postpartum women put cotton in their ears to avoid "air entering their system." Mother's diet rich in protein; lots of chicken in first month. Most women shower on second day postpartum. Female relative may provide perineal care.
- **Baby care**. New mother and her mother take care of baby. If baby's maternal grandmother does not live with the family, common for her to move in with family for several weeks or even months to help care for baby, particularly if she lives in Colombia and has the economic means to travel to U.S.
- **Problems with baby**. Clinician should first approach the father or, in his absence, a close relative (her mother if present) to suggest best way to present information to new mother. An authority figure, such as a physician, should present it.
- **Male and female circumcision**. Male circumcision varies. Traditionally performed at birth if parents choose it. Religion does not influence the decision. Female circumcision never practiced.

DEVELOPMENTAL AND SEXUAL ISSUES

- **Celebration of menarche or becoming a man**. Menarche symbolizes becoming an adolescent but is not celebrated. For girls, the 15th birthday (*quinceañera*) is a very important celebration of becoming an adult. Depending on economic means and acculturation, the celebration may range from a tea to a large, debutante-style party with a band. In the past, to celebrate becoming a man, the father or a close relative took boy to a prostitute to initiate him in sex—an isolated practice now. More commonly, the first sexual relationship (an implicit transition to manhood) is with a friend.
- **Attitudes about birth control**. Contraception acceptable for married couples. Catholicism frequently does not influence use. Acceptance for unmarried couples varies. Condoms are the preferred method, particularly in the younger generation. Couples of rural origin and/or with less education, particularly the husband, tend not to adhere to or accept contraception.
- **Attitudes about sexually transmitted infection (STI) control, including condoms**. Stigma attached to having syphilis or gonorrhea. Chlamydia testing relatively unavailable in Colombia, so this infection is not well known. Male partner often rejects condom use if the couple has a stable rela-

tionship and children. Younger couples and those not in a stable relationship more likely to accept condoms. People may be aware of HIV/AIDS, but commitment to the relationship influences condom use.

- **Attitudes about abortion**. Abortions are illegal in Colombia, but health professionals and laypersons increasingly perform them; prosecution is rare. Society mostly accepts abortion, which may be performed in cases of unplanned pregnancy. But acceptance varies according to religious beliefs; Catholicism considers it a sin. More culturally acceptable among families of urban origin.
- **Attitudes about unwed sexual experimentation**. In last few decades, there has been less condemnation of sexual intercourse before marriage and more acceptance of children born out of marriage. That is less true among persons from rural or isolated regions.
- **Sexual orientation**. Being gay or lesbian not acceptable and carries stigma. Patient/family keeps this information secret. Close family members and close friends may be supportive.
- **Gender identity**. Ambiguous gender identity or identity opposite that of birth gender is not accepted and is stigmatized. Parents pressure feminine boys and masculine girls to change their behavior.
- **Attitudes about menopause**. Accepted as a fact of life. Many women just ignore symptoms unless symptoms are very bothersome, in which case they consult a physician. Use few if any specific herbal remedies for peri-menopausal symptoms; middle- and upper-income women with access to herbal or soy-based remedies from natural-food stores use them more often. Medicine for menopausal symptoms and other health problems growing in popularity, but expense limits it to middle- and upper-income persons.

FAMILY RELATIONSHIPS

- **Composition/structure**. Nuclear or single-mother families most common. In Colombia's family-oriented culture, members of extended family—partic-ularly those in older generation—are very influential.
- **Decision-making**. Father or eldest sibling makes decisions with input from wife, mother, and other siblings. Extended family may be influential in decisions.
- **Spokesperson**. Wife and husband speak for each other. Father or eldest sib-ling presents family's decision. Children often influential in elderly parents' decisions.
- **Gender issues**. Men responsible for most decisions, financial support of family, and handling matters outside the home. Women responsible for household and child care; are caregivers for any family member regardless of gender. In recent years, due to economic pressures, common for both parents to work outside the home.
- **Changing roles among generations in U.S.** No major changes in family

roles. As in Colombia, immigrant women are taking a more active role in the workforce than they have in the past.

- **Caring roles**. Expect mother, sister, or close relative to care for children and sick family members.

- **Expectations of and for children**. Highly protected and very dependent on parents. Adolescents expected to live with parents until they marry, unless study or work necessitates living elsewhere. Parents' opinions heavily influence children's future plans. Parents emphasize punishment rather than positive rewards by frightening children. Mothers often threaten children by saying they will have to get an injection if they do not behave well in a hospital or clinic. Both genders are taught to be quiet, obedient, respectful, and shy, and to avoid confrontations with parents and older persons. Older adolescents more independent.

- **Expectations of and for elders**. Treated respectfully. Elders expect family members to care for them when ill. If economically dependent, they expect to live with one of the children, usually a daughter. Often babysit to enable their children and spouses to work. Institutionalization of elder family members is considered to be abandonment; occurs only as a last resort, when they are very sick and no adult family members are available to stay with them at home.

- **Expectations of hospital visitors**. Colombians highly value a companion during hospitalization, primarily a close relative, friend, or someone they trust and who can care for them if a family member or close friend is not available. Patient expects many relatives and friends to visit. Acceptable for clinician to ask respectfully that the family limit the number of visitors. Family member is expected to spend night with the hospitalized adult, either on a sofa or other bed if available. Parent always stays overnight with an ill child. Visitors may become noisy, particularly if patient is not very ill, or tearful if patient is very ill.

ILLNESS BELIEFS

- **Causes of/attitudes about physical illness**. May attribute severe illness to God's design or purpose. Some may associate illness with bad behavior or punishment—e.g., if sick person has drinking problem. May blame respiratory infections on cold weather or getting wet, particularly the cold of the night (*sereño*). Blame gastrointestinal problems, particularly diarrhea, on parasites (often amoebas) but also on poorly cooked food or, in small children, on spoiled milk. One folk belief is that someone who grinds their teeth at night may have parasites.

- **Causes of/attitudes about mental illness**. May attribute mental illness to an overwhelming situation. Believe that mental illness in women results from love deceptions. Mental illness stigmatizes family. Accept psychotherapy as well as medications and hospitalization, if available, for severe mental illness.

- **Causes of genetic defects**. May attribute them to parents, particularly the mother, having done something wrong before or during pregnancy. Family members accept loved ones who have genetic defects. Prefer to care for them at home.
- **Attitudes about disabilities**. Persons with very little education may attribute them to supernatural causes. Family members usually care for persons with disabilities, who typically are confined to the home. Disabled persons stigmatized if there is an obvious physical deformity.
- **Sick role**. Sick person expects to be cared for while ill, usually by a female family member. Patient assumes a passive role and lets family make decisions regarding care.
- **Home and folk remedies**. Often drink herbal teas—chamomile, mint/spearmint, flax seed, or rosemary—for many ailments before seeking medical care, particularly for respiratory and gastrointestinal problems. Frequently use Vicks VapoRub™ on chest for respiratory illness. For a cold, drink very hot, unrefined sugar-cane paste (*agua de panela*) to "sweat out the cold." Patient may be unwilling to disclose use of herbal remedies if he/she does not trust clinician; concerned about being scolded for practicing/accepting folk medicine.
- **Medications**. In Colombia, most medications available without a prescription. Pharmacies often a primary source of health care. People typically medicate themselves, share medications, or use prescriptions that friends give to them. Immigrants may self-medicate with medicines from Colombia. Clinician should always ask patients if they are taking any medication a friend or relative has given them or that has been sent from Colombia, and about herbal teas or other remedies.
- **Acceptance of procedures**. Typically accept procedures if these are explained clearly and slowly. May accept blood donation or transfusion, surgery, or organ transplant if the procedure is deemed necessary.
- **Care-seeking**. Expect and prefer Western biomedicine if herbal remedies do not work or illness becomes severe. May concurrently use a native healer (*curandero[a]*), particularly if patient is from lower socioeconomic class.

HEALTH ISSUES

- **Concept of health**. Good health is freedom from symptoms and illness, ability to fulfill usual roles, ability to sleep well, feeling good, and happiness.
- **Health promotion and prevention**. Relate prevention to temperature, especially cold. For example, if the body is hot from weather or activities, one avoids exposure to cold by not opening refrigerator or going barefoot. Postpartum women put cotton in their ears to prevent cold air from entering the body; also completely cover baby with blanket to avoid exposure to air currents. Vaccination of children widespread in Colombia, particularly in urban areas, so families expect immunizations in U.S. Eating well important

for maintaining health. However, few eat adequate vegetables. Eat sufficient fruits and grains if available, particularly beans (*frijoles*), though not refried beans. Personal cleanliness and keeping the house clean are very important. Exercise becoming more prevalent in younger generations.

- **Screening**. Screening in Colombia for many diseases unavailable because of limited access to health care, due to economics and lack of health insurance in urban areas and to lack of professional providers in rural areas. Pap smear is most common screen among all women, especially when they request family planning. Well-child checks at time of vaccinations are common in Colombia.

- **Common health problems**. Most prevalent ones mirror those in U.S. and in other developed countries generally (e.g., heart disease, stroke, and hypertension). Other health problems are characteristic of less-developed countries (e.g., child deaths from severe gastrointestinal and respiratory infections, especially among recent immigrants). Cervical cancer is third-highest cause of morbidity in women older than 15 years. Because of serious sociopolitical problems in Colombia, homicide is highest cause of mortality among those 15–45 years old. Mental illness has become quite prevalent because of direct or indirect exposure to violence in Colombia; may be reflected in immigrants who arrived within the last 5–10 years.

DEATH RITUALS

- **Beliefs and attitudes about death**. Catholics believe that one should be at peace and without sin at time of death. Most Colombians accept death as God's intention (*designio de Dios*).

- **Preparation**. When patient is dying, clinician should inform head of family (parent or eldest child), preferably away from his/her room, so family can be summoned. Patient may be surrounded by all family members, except small children. Commonly say Catholic prayer at patient's bedside. Patient may want to receive sacrament of the sick from a priest. Family members discuss difficult decisions.

- **Home vs. hospital**. If illness acute, may choose hospital. If disease terminal after chronic illness, may prefer to die at home. Families may need to be introduced to the concept of hospice, as it is not well-known in Colombia. Accept hospice as long as they understand it does not mean abandoning their terminally ill relative.

- **Special needs**. May keep a religious figure or picture of the Virgin, Christ, or saint with lighted candles. Family members may cry uncontrollably and loudly; women may be hysterical.

- **Care of the body**. All family members may want to see body before it goes to morgue. Other than cleaning and dressing body, family does not prepare it in any special way because, in Colombia, the deceased generally is buried within 24–36 hours after death. Cremation becoming more customary. Relatives may need to be warned that in U.S., the body is rarely buried before three days after death.

■ **Attitudes about organ donation**. May be acceptable for clinician to request organ donation. Should ask closest family member, who may consult, and decide with, family. Clinician should characterize organ donation as an act of goodness, a way to benefit others.

■ **Attitudes about autopsy**. Acceptable if viewed as necessary to clarify cause of death. After patient dies, clinician should ask closest family member before he/she leaves hospital.

SELECTED REFERENCES

Bernal de Pheils, P., & Jaramillo, D. (2003). Colombians. In P. St. Hill, J. Lipson, & A. Meleis (Eds.), *Caring for women cross-culturally* (pp. 108–122). Philadelphia: F. A. Davis.

Bernal de Pheils, P., & Meleis, A. I. (1995). Self-care actions of Colombian *por dia* domestic workers: On prevention and care. *Women and Health, 22,* 77–95.

Gomez, L. A., Tovar, H. C., & Agudelo, C. A. (2003). Use of health services and epidemiological profiles as parameters for adjusting the Compulsory Health Plan in Colombia. *Rev Salud Publica (Bogota), 5,* 246–262.

AUTHOR

Pilar Bernal de Pheils, RN, MS, is a clinical professor in the School of Nursing at the University of California-San Francisco, where she teaches in the graduate nurse practitioner program. She also maintains a practice in several primary care clinics as a family nurse practitioner. Bernal de Pheils was educated and worked in Colombia as a nurse for 15 years before she came to live in the U.S. She travels frequently to Colombia and keeps in regular contact with nurse colleagues and the health care system there.

CHAPTER 10

CUBANS

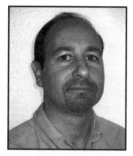

Larry Varela

CULTURAL/ETHNIC IDENTITY

- **Preferred term(s).** Cuban, for either native-born or American-born. Cubans are very proud of their heritage and many do not choose to identify themselves as American. The preferred term for those born in U.S. is Cuban American.
- **Census.** The 2000 U.S. Census estimates 1.2 million Cubans, of whom 60% are foreign-born. Seventy-five percent of Cubans live in southern U.S.; of those, 67% are in Florida.
- **History of immigration.** From 1895–1905, Cubans moved to Tampa and Miami, FL, to work in tobacco industry. Established small, tight communities. In the 1940s and 1950s, with increased trade and commerce between U.S. and Cuba during World War II, there was an influx of workers for war industry. Largest number of immigrants arrived between 1959–79 after the overthrow of Cuban government and the rise of communism under Fidel Castro; most were middle and upper class. Settled and built strong communities in Miami, Tampa, and New York. Were able to sustain much of their culture and language. In 1980, 120,000 Cubans immigrated via the Mariel Boat Lift. Among them were many criminals because Castro emptied the jails. Having lived under communism for about 20 years, this group was socially different from previous immigrants. Cubans continued to immigrate legally and illegally to U.S. in large numbers after 1981. About 30,000 "rafters" landed in 1994. Since then, U.S. policy has been to stop Cubans at sea and send them back; if they reach land, allowed to stay. Since the fall of communism in the former Soviet Union and the rise of tourism in Cuba, the obvious economic disparities between Cuba and other nations have stimulated emigration.

SPIRITUAL/RELIGIOUS ORIENTATION

- **Primary religious/spiritual affiliations**. Mostly Catholic, but many other Christian denominations now represented, such as Jehovah's Witnesses and Baptists. Some in Cuba and U.S. practice Santeria, a 300-year-old Afro-Cuban religion. It includes worship of African gods (*orishas*) associated with specific Catholic saints. When biomedicine and the church fail to heal, some seek help from Santero priests. Healing practices include magic, removing spells, spirit possession, and communication with *orishas* through animal sacrifices. An angry or vengeful person can cause illness in someone else by casting a spell, which must be broken before the patient can heal. Most ceremonies take place in the home, away from public settings. Those who lived in Cuba during Castro's regime experienced a more secular state with fewer ties to the church.
- **Usual religious/spiritual practices**. Praying and reciting the rosary common. Worship of several important saints popular. Attending church for confession and communion important to many. Santeria ceremonies in the home include sacrificing animals or performing blessings to remove spells.
- **Use of spiritual healing/healers**. May call a priest to minister to very ill person in hospital or to administer rites of sick or last rites. Traditional healers who practice Santeria rarely become involved with health care team.
- **Holidays**. Catholic holidays very important, especially Easter and Christmas. Depending on acculturation, secular holidays such as July 4th are reasons for taking the day off and gathering with family and friends.

COMMUNICATION
ORAL COMMUNICATION

- **Major languages and dialects**. Castilian Spanish (common Spanish). Cubans speak quickly and shorten words by dropping letters. Also have incorporated many English words into spoken Spanish that other Spanish speakers do not use. For example, *lonchar* comes from the English verb "to lunch." In Castilian Spanish, the word is *almorzar*.
- **Greetings**. Formal upon introduction, then a more familiar tone. Informal greetings loud, with friendly hug or kiss on cheek. Address each other by first name or other familiar terms. Handshake common among men. Cubans show more respect for elderly persons. Family members and close friends greet by embracing and kissing on cheek.
- **Tone of voice**. Speak loudly in normal conversation. To outsiders, sounds hostile and aggressive.
- **Direct or indirect style of speech**. Most interactions with strangers tend to be polite. Commands or requests are direct, often forceful. Cubans love to talk and hold multiple conversations simultaneously. Tell personal stories to bring drama to most conversations.
- **Use of interpreters**. Prefer the most educated or acculturated family mem-

ber, except to interpret sensitive information—e.g., regarding sexual matters. In that case, clinician should use only an older member of immediate family and match the gender of patient and interpreter.

- **Serious or terminal illness**. Clinician should discuss poor prognosis only with older members of immediate family. Should discuss HIV/AIDS diagnosis only with patient and only through interpretation by a Spanish-speaking health care provider. Acculturated Cubans want to be informed of terminal illness. Typically, less-acculturated persons first inform their spouse, eldest child, or person directing care, then the immediate family, as appropriate. Clinician should allow family members to inform patient, but often they do not, believing that such knowledge will affect patient's will to live and thus diminish his/her fight for life. Cubans often exclude pregnant women, children, and ill family members from such discussion or knowledge. Do-not-resuscitate orders usually unacceptable; Cubans strongly feel that all interventions should be tried. Agreeing to such orders shows that one has given up hope and is allowing patient to die; concerned that others will view this as an uncaring attitude, abandonment, or even abetting or hoping for death.

WRITTEN COMMUNICATION

- **Literacy assessment**. Highly literate in Spanish. Cubans who arrived in U.S. at a young age and those who are American-born often fluent in both English and Spanish. Command of English among older persons who have been in U.S. for many years depends on their acculturation, need to speak English, and location of residence, with great variation in reading and writing proficiency. New arrivals often speak little or no English. Clinician should ask which language the patient feels more comfortable communicating in and whether he/she can read English.
- **Consents**. Clinician should use interpreter when necessary. Often, family wants to consult with the most educated, respected, or eldest family member before giving consent. Usually do not want to be informed of hazards or possible side effects; may want such information withheld from patient out of concern it will cause stress. Cubans do not typically like to participate in research for fear of not obtaining the best treatment. Most comfortable signing a written consent.

NONVERBAL COMMUNICATION

- **Eye contact**. Direct eye contact expected during conversation. Looking away shows lack of respect or dishonesty.
- **Personal space**. Close contact and touching acceptable, as they show affection among family and friends. Personal space with stranger varies depending on one's comfort with that person, but it is considerably closer than what most northern European Americans prefer.
- **Use and meaning of silence**. Usually means awkwardness or uncertainty.

- **Gestures**. Often use hand gestures to add emphasis or drama while speaking.
- **Openness in expressing emotions**. Typically outgoing and confrontational. They have no problem expressing their emotions and often become almost melodramatic. More open with family and friends. May be more guarded with strangers yet express emotions just a few feet away.
- **Privacy**. Extremely important. Only family members appointed by patient or the person directing care should be included in discussions. May withhold sensitive or personal information—e.g., about sexually transmitted infection, abortion, domestic abuse, or alcoholism—from health care workers due to social implications. Family often prefers that information be withheld from patients. Clinician should discuss an issue with family members before informing patient. Withholding information may be per patients' request; may instruct family not to tell them how sick they are or if they are terminally ill.
- **Touch**. Shows affection among family and friends. Hugging acceptable, including between males. Patient or family may hug or kiss a health care provider in gratitude. Touching sexual areas viewed as inappropriate.
- **Orientation to time**. Usually adhere to mainstream business time. Individuals' orientation to social time varies, but some may arrive an hour or two later than scheduled. Time orientation also varies according to situation, acculturation, and socioeconomic status. For example, the more important or formal an appointment, the more likely one is to arrive on time. Cubans who are more acculturated and those of higher socioeconomic status are more likely to adhere to clock time. Elderly Cubans or newer arrivals may focus on past and their possible return to Cuba. Present orientation reflected by their emphasis on current issues and needs rather than on, for example, how their current health behavior may affect future risks. Others focus on the future, as demonstrated by hard work and education.

ACTIVITIES OF DAILY LIVING

- **Modesty**. Both genders very modest. Clinician should provide adequate covering. Women prefer female clinicians but accept males.
- **Skin care**. Prefer to wash daily.
- **Hair care**. Normally wash hair daily but less frequently when ill. Believe that wet hair may cause chills or cold draft that will exacerbate illness. Some women do not wash hair during menses.
- **Nail care**. Important to women even while ill. Women usually wear nails long. Men keep nails short and clean.
- **Toileting**. Regularity a priority for many. Prefer to use bathroom because of lack of cleanliness, awkwardness, and lack of privacy associated with bedpans. Women, in particular, prefer bathroom—it enables good peri-care, often with soap and water.
- **Special clothing or amulets**. Attach religious medallions, rosary beads, or a cross to bed or clothing, so health care workers should take care when dis-

carding sheets or gown. Some Cubans wear amulets, necklaces, or bracelets to protect themselves from evil.

- **Self-care**. Patient's role well-defined: totally submissive in all care activities. If allowed to, female family members provide all care, including bathing, toileting, and feeding; do the same at home. Patients do not accept concept of hastening recovery through self-care. Cooperate with requests to ambulate or breathe deeply. Generally comply with requests in hospital, with help from female family members, but may refuse to do self-care at home.

FOOD PRACTICES

- **Usual meal pattern**. Three meals a day. For the elderly and new arrivals, lunch still is main meal.
- **Special utensils**. None.
- **Food beliefs and rituals**. Important to consume fresh food, soups, and broths when ill. Often believe that eating too much when ill is not good. May omit some foods during illness, believing they are too difficult to digest.
- **Usual diet**. Rice and beans common with lunch and dinner. Most foods fried. Meat important with all meals. Eat small variety of vegetables. Eat sweets frequently. Typical diet is high in calories, simple carbohydrates, and saturated fat, and lacks leafy green vegetables.
- **Fluids**. Cold fluids, juices, and coffee.
- **Food taboos and prescriptions**. Some dictated by religion (e.g., not eating meat during Lent). Cultural practices include eating fish on Fridays, not drinking beer when eating bananas, and not drinking water when eating fish. Home remedies include tea brewed from locally grown herbs (for GI upset) and papaya (for hypertension).
- **Hospitality**. Treat guests very well. Even offer to prepare a whole meal. Food a vital part of hospitality and very important in entertaining. Guests often bring food or drinks as gift.

SYMPTOM MANAGEMENT

Understand numerical scales for all symptoms.

- **Pain** (*dolor*). Culturally acceptable to express pain. Men may seem hypersensitive, women more tolerant. May fear addiction to narcotics. Prefer not to take medication or to stop as quickly as possible. View injections as more effective or stronger than tablets. Underutilize nonpharmacological methods for pain control.
- **Dyspnea** (*corto de aire*, or "short of breath"). May express fear and anxiety by becoming very verbal or crying, by a great show of emotions. Readily accept oxygen. Useful for clinician to suggest nonpharmacological control methods.
- **Nausea/vomiting** (*náusea/vómito*). Often attribute nausea/vomiting to stress or nervousness that affects stomach. View it as marker for increasing illness. Report vomiting quickly. Readily accept rectal administration of medicine.

- **Constipation/diarrhea** (*estreñimiento/diarrea*). May attribute constipation to poor eating habits, and diarrhea to anxiety, illness, or eating something disagreeable. Regularity a priority for many. Lengthy discussion about bowels not uncommon. Accept enemas, suppositories, or nutritional controls.
- **Fatigue** (*fatiga*). Cubans do not customarily nap in the afternoon. Report fatigue. Nonpharmacological treatments probably more acceptable than medical treatments.
- **Depression** (*depresión*). Often ignore or deny it. May attribute depression to "nerves," extreme stress, or anxiety. View depression as mental illness, which shames the family. Probably will not accept either medical or nonpharmacological treatments.
- **Self-care symptom management**. Expect family members (usually women) to direct—and, when possible, take responsibility for—symptom management. Patient does self-care, including for chronic illness, if no help available or he/she has an independent personality.

BIRTH RITUALS/CARE OF THE NEW MOTHER AND BABY

- **Pregnancy care**. Expect prenatal care, if affordable. Rest encouraged. No strenuous activities. Pregnant women expected to avoid loud noises and looking at people with deformities. Diet of fresh foods and low salt encouraged. More-acculturated couples take childbirth preparation classes.
- **Preferences for children**. Prefer boys, but girls have important role in care of family. Prefer small families—1–2 children.
- **Labor practices**. Pregnant woman's mother present during entire labor and delivery. Although the father often is discouraged from participating, his involvement is more common among the more-acculturated. Prefer physicians and hospitals for delivery.
- **Role of the laboring woman during birth**. Assumes a more passive role than her mother does, who will try to direct all activity. Loud expressions of pain common.
- **Role of the father and other family members during birth**. Pregnant woman's mother takes commanding role. Father's participation depends on acculturation level and childbirth education trends. More-traditional Cuban men not involved at all.
- **Vaginal vs. cesarean section**. Prefer safest procedure for the mother.
- **Breastfeeding**. Becoming more popular again among Cubans, after a period of bottle-feeding popularity. Mix breast- and bottle-feeding if mother works. Duration of breastfeeding varies as in dominant culture.
- **Birth recuperation**. Traditionally, new mother and infant not allowed to leave home for 41 days, during which time she rests and devotes her energy to caring for baby. Her mother and sisters help care for new mother and baby. New mother sheltered from bad news and any stress that could harm her or child. She is encouraged to eat more to foster milk production.

- **Baby care**. Commonly is the full responsibility of the birth mother or other women in the family. Grandmothers often are very involved. May place amulet or bracelet on baby to protect it from the evil eye.
- **Problems with baby**. Clinician should inform baby's father and then the woman's mother; should not give information directly to new mother because family may fear she will become hysterical and possibly have a breakdown. Family then decides when to inform her.
- **Male and female circumcision**. Neither practiced routinely in Cuba. Male circumcision commonly practiced in U.S.

DEVELOPMENTAL AND SEXUAL ISSUES

- **Celebration of menarche or becoming a man**. Girls who are Catholic view menstruation as dirty, something not to be discussed. Cubans celebrate girls' 15th birthday to mark their maturation, often with a large formal party similar to the debutante ball for American girls. Fifteenth birthday is when more-traditional girls are allowed to begin wearing make-up and dating boys. No equivalent celebration for Cuban boys nor any real acknowledgment of transition to manhood.
- **Attitudes about birth control**. Contraceptives common, except among more religious persons. Castro blocked the Catholic Church's prohibition on contraceptive use. Most Cubans understand the benefits of smaller families.
- **Attitudes about sexually transmitted infection (STI) control, including condoms**. Promiscuity common among Cuban men. STI control is practiced but not the norm. Cuban men do not like to use condoms. Knowledge of HIV widespread, even among new arrivals in U.S. Practicing safe sex varies, but, in general, Cuban men still practice unsafe sex even though they are concerned about HIV/AIDS. One reason for such behavior is masculinity: Men take charge and put their own needs first, viewing condoms as protection for women, the receptive party. Another reason is homophobia: Gay men often remain closeted and have clandestine, anonymous sex.
- **Attitudes about abortion**. Pre-Castro Cubans do not accept it well. More acceptable among recent immigrants because of declining influence of Catholic Church in Cuba since 1959. Single pregnant women more likely to get abortion.
- **Attitudes about unwed sexual experimentation**. Most Cubans highly value women's chastity before marriage. More-acculturated and recent immigrant women are more open to premarital sex. Men are expected to have premarital sex; they boast about their conquests.
- **Sexual orientation**. Cubans do not readily tolerate any orientation other than traditional heterosexuality. Under the Castro regime, persons accused of homosexuality are imprisoned. Homosexuality uncommon; occurs secretly and families rarely talk about it. Men often consider themselves to be heterosexual if they dominate during sexual encounters with other men. Gay or

lesbian Cubans may have heterosexual relationships to conceal their true sexuality.

- **Gender identity**. Do not tolerate ambiguous gender identity. Families and society harass effeminate men, masculine women, and cross-dressers.
- **Attitudes about menopause**. Likely accepted as part of life, but Cuban-born women rarely discuss it among themselves.

FAMILY RELATIONSHIPS

- **Composition/structure**. Cubans are family-oriented. Extended family important. Often three generations in a household. Reconstituted families (the type created when two, one-parent families join together) still uncommon but becoming more common among new immigrants and more-acculturated persons.
- **Decision-making**. Family usually consults the most educated, most respected, or eldest member, usually a male. He/she and closest family members then make decisions. Cubans usually follow a physician's recommendation because they consider doctors important and highly respect their education.
- **Spokesperson**. Father, eldest son, or daughter, or the most educated family member.
- **Gender issues**. Men traditionally expected to make decisions outside the home and to protect family. Often quick to show anger and aggressive behavior. Women traditionally expected to be closely involved in family care and concerns, even if they work outside the home. Women usually play a submissive, supportive role.
- **Changing roles among generations in U.S.** Most Cubans who arrived before or right after 1959 are more conservative and religious. Each subsequent generation has become more acculturated but continues to hold old beliefs and perform old practices. Those who have come to U.S. since 1980 were raised in a socialist secular system that permitted more modern thinking in some regards (e.g., less negativity about abortion and divorce). New women immigrants typically are more flexible and able to obtain work to help support the family, which increases their power in the family and fosters more equitable gender roles.
- **Caring roles**. Wife, daughter, or mother responsible for caring for sick family members. Patient becomes totally submissive; men, in particular, fall into a helpless, dependent role. Family's assistance may be so pervasive that it hinders recovery.
- **Expectations of and for children**. Boys are taught to be aggressive, competitive, and controlling, and to protect family interests. Girls are taught to be submissive, supportive, and caring. Physical punishment of children common. Respect for elders important. Male children exceptionally protective of mothers. Strong emphasis on, and respect for, education.
- **Expectations of and for elders**. Expect to be cared for and depend on their

adult children. Given great respect. Help care for younger generations. Traditionally, family cares for them at home until death. Placing elderly in nursing homes becoming more common as economics and acculturation influence family structure and life. Extended-family members often assist when possible.

- **Expectations of hospital visitors**. Close ties with family and friends very important in Cuban culture. Visiting the sick is a clear sign of respect and caring. Showing personal and physical affection keeps connections solid. A family member almost always stays overnight with patient. Visitors bring food to share.

ILLNESS BELIEFS

- **Causes of/attitudes about physical illness**. Cubans understand modern germ theory, but they also accept other causes. For example, they often believe that nerves or extreme nervousness causes illness or makes it worse. Supernatural causes include God's will, the evil eye, evil spells, magic, and African gods (*orishas*) who are not appeased. The evil eye is cast by a jealous or envious person with ill intent. Magic includes casting an evil spell so someone becomes sick. Healing spells usually undo evil spells.
- **Causes of/attitudes about mental illness**. Thought to be hereditary or caused by extreme stress. A mentally ill person socially marks a family; the stigma may discourage someone from marrying into that family out of fear the illness will be passed along to offspring. Mental illness often hidden from public view or not acknowledged. If possible, the mentally ill receive care— in most cases, loving care—at home.
- **Causes of genetic defects**. Attributed to heredity or mother's extreme stress or trauma during pregnancy. While pregnant, looking at a child with a defect may cause baby to have same defect. If possible, family member with genetic defect receives care at home.
- **Attitudes about disabilities**. View disabled persons as unfortunate and perhaps deserving of the disability. Often blamed on family or personal misconduct or behavior. Frequently conceal and do not mention disabled persons, who usually receive care at home if possible.
- **Sick role**. Expect a sick person to be totally submissive, helpless, and dependent. Ill person may be passive in terms of decision-making.
- **Home and folk remedies**. Drink a variety of herbal teas to treat minor conditions at home. May not report such treatments.
- **Medications**. Readily use biomedical drugs. Compliance varies. Often self-treat as necessary. Sharing medications with others acceptable and common. High prevalence and acceptance of nontraditional treatments and medication, such as Chinese medicine and over-the-counter herbal remedies, which Cubans often use concurrently with medications. Patient may disclose nontraditional approaches if he/she is comfortable with clinician.
- **Acceptance of procedures**. Most Cubans accept surgery, transplants, and

transfusions. Physician recommendations usually sufficient for acceptance.
- **Care-seeking**. Seek biomedical care if home and herbal remedies do not work or if illness apparently is severe. Pray and seek religious assistance concurrently with medical care. May use Santeria as last resort.

HEALTH ISSUES
- **Concept of health**. Good health is mind, body, and spirit in balance. Any influence that can cause imbalance, such as stress or supernatural forces (e.g., the evil eye), can cause illness. Traditional Cubans think overweight and rosy-cheeked persons are healthy, that skinny persons are poor or sickly. This reflects socioeconomics and the wasting that accompanies illnesses such as tuberculosis. More-acculturated Cubans accept fitness and staying trim as healthy concepts but, like others in the dominant culture, struggle with obesity.
- **Health promotion and prevention**. Avoiding stress, bad news, or extremes—e.g., too much heat, cold, or exercise—important for maintaining good health. Health promotion and prevention becoming more acceptable among Cubans. In Cuba, extensive vaccination and antenatal care programs have resulted in significant decreases in morbidity and mortality under Castro. However, poor dietary habits continue to cause health problems. Exercise uncommon among older persons. Protect themselves from evil eye or spells with amulets or through religious observance.
- **Screening**. Many undergo routine physical exams and make good use of preventive services. With education, screening very acceptable to most.
- **Common health problems**. Cardiac and cerebrovascular diseases, diabetes, malignant neoplasms, and diabetes. Smoking and obesity are risk factors.

DEATH RITUALS
- **Beliefs and attitudes about death**. Generally fear death despite often strong spiritual beliefs. Most view death as unnatural. As Christians do, most believe in life after death.
- **Preparation**. Acculturated Cubans usually want to be informed about terminal illness. For less-acculturated patients, clinician should first inform the person directing care and the male head of family (if none, then closest relative). Should not inform patient that he/she is dying unless family requests it. Suggest to family that it contact affiliated church. Cubans will notify entire family, who are expected to remain with patient until the end, including all night.
- **Home vs. hospital**. Prefer hospital for medical treatment and pain management. Family wants all measures taken to prolong patient's life or to make him/her comfortable. View inpatient medical care as more important than dying at home.
- **Special needs**. Family insists on being with patient at all times, including

overnight. Every family member and friend expected to visit. Clinician should allow visits but maintain firm control of visitor traffic, reinforcing the need for patient to rest. Public expressions of emotion, such as crying and screaming, are common before and after death.

- **Care of the body**. No special requirements.
- **Attitudes about organ donation**. Donations uncommon.
- **Attitudes about autopsy**. Autopsy not common or desired.

SELECTED REFERENCES

Dossick, J. (1992). *Cuba, Cubans, and Cuban Americans, 1902–1991: A bibliography*. Coral Gables, FL: University of Miami North-South Center.

Hispanics in the U.S. (1980). In C. E. Cortes (Ed.), *Cuban exiles in the U.S.* New York: Arno Press.

Purnell, L. D. (2003). People of Cuban heritage. In L. D. Purnell & B. J. Paulanka (Eds.), *Transcultural health care: A culturally competent approach* (2nd ed.), (pp. 122–137). Philadelphia: F. A. Davis.

U.S. Department of Commerce, Economics and Statistics Administration, U.S. Census Bureau. (2001). The Hispanic population: Census 2000 brief. Washington, DC: U.S. Government Printing Office.

AUTHOR

Larry Varela, RN, MS, was born in New York City to Cuban parents and raised in Miami. He earned a bachelor's degree in nursing at the University of Florida and a master's degree in cross-cultural and community health nursing at the University of California-San Francisco. His work experience includes eight years of intensive care, a year in Sudan as a program manager with the International Rescue Committee, and 10 years of home health/hospice care, mainly for the homeless, mentally ill, substance-abusing, and HIV/AIDS populations. He currently is director of hospice services at Kaiser Hospital in Martinez, CA.

CHAPTER 11

DOMINICANS

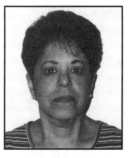 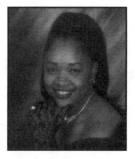

Neddie Valentin Serra   *Jeanette Martinez*

CULTURAL/ETHNIC IDENTITY

- **Preferred term(s)**. Dominican (*Dominicano[a]*). A transnational population with continuous family, social, financial, and political commitments to the homeland. Perceive themselves as temporarily living in U.S. and hope to return someday to "my country" (*mi pais*). Do not want to be referred to as Dominican Americans.
- **Census**. According to the 2000 U.S. Census, nearly 765,000 Dominicans live in U.S., but other survey centers report more than 1 million. Discrepancies likely a result of confusing Census wording (some Hispanics did not identify their national origin) and the undocumented immigrants residing in U.S. The New York metropolitan area has the largest number of Dominican immigrants, due to family connections and chain migration.
- **History of immigration**. The Dominican Republic occupies the eastern two-thirds of the Caribbean island of Hispaniola and shares a border with Haiti. U.S. involvement during political upheavals fostered close economic, sociocultural, and political connections between it and the Dominican Republic. Dictator Rafael Trujillo limited emigration between the 1930s and 1960s. After his assassination, emigration to U.S. increased markedly in the context of unrelenting political unrest and economic problems. Since the late 1960s and after U.S. immigration reform in 1965 that eliminated the quota system, the Dominican Republic has been among the top 10 exporters of emigrants to U.S. In contrast to the elite who left in previous years because of political unrest, economic issues have stimulated emigration in the 1980s and 1990s, including that of many skilled professionals and less-skilled laborers.

SPIRITUAL/RELIGIOUS ORIENTATION

- **Primary religious/spiritual affiliations**. Majority (95%) belong to Catholic Church. African heritage introduced other deities and practices. Dominicans have a religious legacy that merges Christianity, spiritism (*espiritismo*, or promoting spiritual wellness through moral behavior), Santeria (merging Catholic saints and African gods), witches (*brujos*), and healers (*curanderos*).
- **Usual religious/spiritual practices**. Although Catholicism is the official religion and strongly influences people, only about 10% of Dominicans actively participate in church activities. Not unusual for them to have small shrines or altars in corners or closets of their homes containing a variety of saints and images of the Virgin Mary surrounded by flowers and lighted candles. Some Dominicans make a religious promise (*la promesa*) or obligation to God or a saint (usually Saint Alta Gracia)—e.g., to attend church three times a week if God intervenes in a health or crisis situation. Typical practices of Santeria include worshipping African gods (*orishas*) that are associated with specific Catholic saints. In *espiritismo*, believers consult an *espiritista*, a medium who communicates with the spirit world, to receive messages about how to purify the soul through moral behavior.
- **Use of spiritual healing/healers**. Many Dominicans strongly believe in the connection between the spiritual dimension and illness. *Que sea lo que Dios quiera* (what God wills will be) reaffirms the family's belief that God is in control of the illness situation and individuals have limited ability to change fate other than by sacrifice and prayer. In dealing with illness, they often seek support from indigenous healers, who are first called to the home before visiting the patient in the hospital, and also pray and perform other religious rites. Some seek help from Santero priests—who practice healing through magic, removing spells, spirit possession, and communicating with *orishas* through animal sacrifices—or *espiritistas*, especially in cases of mental illness. Clinicians must understand how these beliefs affect decision-making and health care practices, and carefully assess religious and folk interventions to determine how to incorporate them into treatment.
- **Holidays**. Generally very festive, with music and dance, which are at the center of Dominican culture. Religious holidays include *El Dia de Los Reyes* (Three Kings Day) (January 6); *Dia de Virgin Alta Gracia* (patron saint of Dominicans) (January 21); and *Semana Santa* (Holy Week), which begins on Good Friday and extends through Easter Sunday. Secular holidays include the birthday of Pablo Duarte (January 26), who freed the Dominican people; Independence Day (February 27), the day of the revolt that established Dominican independence; Dominican Restoration Day (August 16), which celebrates independence from Spain; and Constitution Day (November 6). Except for Independence Day, most secular holidays are not celebrated in U.S.

COMMUNICATION
ORAL COMMUNICATION

- **Major languages and dialects**. *Castellano* (Castilian) Spanish, from early colonization. English taught in schools. Many Dominicans know some English before they arrive in U.S.
- **Greetings**. Dominicans emphasize politeness and respect in all social encounters. Address older women by last name and *Señora* or *Doña*, men by last name and *Señor* or *Don*. Use formal "you" (*usted*). Upon entering a group, it is polite to address all members, usually with a social kiss on each cheek. Handshake is acceptable to both genders if two persons do not know each other.
- **Tone of voice**. Dominicans tend to be very emotional; tone of voice can be loud and dramatic. Varies according to a person's social, economic, and educational background. For example, persons from rural areas may be loud and demonstrative, while the tone and patterns of speech among persons who are more educated or of higher socioeconomic status may resemble those of dominant culture.
- **Direct or indirect style of speech**. Careful not to offend others in conversation, although tend to be very frank. If they do not agree with someone, will say so. If speaking Spanish, may respond at length, but if answering in English, answers are brief and to the point.
- **Use of interpreters**. Many use a family member as interpreter, especially if they are newly arrived in U.S. or uncomfortable about English pronunciation. Female patients prefer female interpreters, particularly if the topic is sexual. Men prefer male interpreters regarding sexual issues; may not be truthful with female clinician due to embarrassment or fear of being perceived as less than potent.
- **Serious or terminal illness**. Dominicans do not discuss serious or terminal illness with ill person. Family members closest to patient (e.g., wife and older children if husband is ill) should be informed. Often, family members withhold information from sick person. Families respond differently to serious illness depending on social status, financial and family resources, and educational background. If patient is informed first, a man diagnosed with a serious problem then informs the older women, the eldest male child, or another dominant male figure in the family; a woman must first inform the dominant male figure and then her mother and mother-in-law. Dominicans expect health care providers to be sensitive and compassionate.

WRITTEN COMMUNICATION

- **Literacy assessment**. Literacy related to length of time in U.S. and social status in Dominican Republic. An estimated 82% of Dominicans older than 15 years can read and write in Spanish if they were educated in homeland. Those of higher socioeconomic status likely to be literate in English but may lack confidence in speaking, fearing embarrassment. Older, less-educated persons have difficulty with written materials in Spanish, especially materials containing technical or medical terms; less likely to be comfortable with any use of English. Many immigrants in U.S. dropped out of high school and may have limited literacy in Spanish, but more than 90% of second- or third-generation Dominicans have completed at least high school.

- **Consents**. Best to establish a relationship with patient before requesting consent. May be suspicious of written consent unless a trusted individual explains it. Consent forms should be available in Spanish. If not, family member or trusted health care provider should translate. All options must be clearly presented and family should be included in discussion of the rationale for written or verbal consents. Dominicans usually unwilling to participate in research studies—fear being used as "guinea pigs" and not having any protection if something goes wrong.

NONVERBAL COMMUNICATION

- **Eye contact**. Prefer direct eye contact, similar to dominant culture.
- **Personal space**. Tend to place less emphasis on personal space than do most Northern European Americans; expect, and are comfortable with, close proximity to family members while standing or sitting. Most children share bedrooms with siblings if space is limited, even girls and boys until the time of puberty. Infants and young children share sleeping space with parents. Cautious about closeness with opposite gender; do not want it to be interpreted as a sexual advance.
- **Use and meaning of silence**. Can mean that listener is not interested in, or does not want to acknowledge, what the speaker is saying.
- **Gestures**. Very expressive and emotional in conversation, liberally using their hands and body language. Inappropriate gestures similar to those in dominant U.S. culture.
- **Openness in expressing emotions**. Freely express anger, joy, and other emotions to family and friends. Many facial expressions and hand gestures accompany speech. However, Dominicans view strangers very cautiously— may not express feelings to them.
- **Privacy**. Share private information with health care providers if it pertains to their health. Very reticent about sharing sexual information with anyone. Sexuality rarely discussed in families, even when family members are very close.
- **Touch**. Reflects familiarity. Acceptable for women to touch one another on the arms or shoulders. Friendly pinch on the cheek OK (especially with children). Social kiss or handshake permissible between men and women. Other male-to-female touch unacceptable, especially touching a woman's breasts or thighs; denotes disrespect unless specific permission has been granted. Clinician should ask permission to touch patient.
- **Orientation to time**. Dominicans live in the here and now. Value social

interaction more than time. Feelings of others considered more important than strict adherence to a schedule. They may be late for appointments if engaged with guests or friends.

ACTIVITIES OF DAILY LIVING

- **Modesty**. Women, especially those who are older or married, expected to dress and behave conservatively. Immodestly dressed women perceived as having loose sexual morals and are not respected. Men modest in intimate care and personal needs. Dress and behavior among second- and third-generation Dominicans resemble those in dominant culture, but parents and grandparents still uphold modesty as the standard of behavior. Improper for males to care for females, especially if the care is physical. Female patients may refuse to have males help with bathing and toileting. Males prefer male assistance.
- **Skin care**. Very important. Use numerous natural products—e.g., oils, egg masks (egg white on skin), oatmeal water and milk paste, plain yogurt—to protect skin. Leave such products on skin until dry, then rinse them off. Bathe daily. Beliefs about hot/cold may discourage feverish patients from bathing for fear of additional health problems, as getting cold increases humoral imbalance. Young children with a fever are usually wrapped in blankets to protect them from drafts or cool air.
- **Hair care**. Many natural products available, including oils. Local shops catering to Dominican clientele sell some products; family members or friends import others from Dominican Republic. Among these are a combination of almond oil, bear oil (*asceite de oso*), coconut oil (*asceite de coco*), and bee oil (*asceite de aveha*). Also use pureed carrots mixed with avocado to smother hair for 10–15 minutes before shampooing.
- **Nail care**. Varies as in dominant culture.
- **Toileting**. Because of modesty, clinician should ensure privacy if bedpan or commode necessary. Dominicans prefer to wash rather than use only toilet paper; also want perineal care.
- **Special clothing or amulets**. Dominican culture a blend of Spanish, Taino Indian, and African slave influences that include healing and protective practices. Persons who have made *la promesa* often wear all-white clothing with a colored sash to represent their religious obligation. May adorn themselves with various charms, amulets, and healing pouches. Common for babies to be protected against the evil eye by a black onyx charm in the form of a hand (*asabache*) attached to infant's wrist. Wear necklaces with gold charms representing Catholic saints and place statues of saints at the bedside of ill persons. May attach pouches containing various herbal mixtures to clothing for protection or healing. If special amulets or medals must be removed, patient/family complies. Clinician should give the item to a family member for safe-keeping.

- **Self-care**. Individuals perform self-care. If unable, family members provide care.

FOOD PRACTICES

- **Usual meal pattern**. Three meals a day, the biggest at noon. Breakfast often consists of white farmer's cheese (*queso blanco*), eggs, and salami, all fried. Serve green plantains, sometimes mashed, in place of bread. Typical dinner consists of the same simple foods—eggs, salami, plantains, or homemade soup. Expect all family members to be present at meal time and share news of the day, especially positive news. Activities center around those at the table; distractions such as television or radio perceived as rude and are unacceptable.
- **Special utensils**. None.
- **Food beliefs and rituals**. Many believe in the "hot"/"cold" theory of disease: One should treat cold illnesses with hot medications or hot foods (e.g., chicken soup and hot tea) and avoid cold foods (e.g., orange juice). During holiday seasons such as Christmas, many celebrate by eating roasted pig with rice, peas, and salad. During other religious holidays (e.g., Holy Week), many abstain from eating meat products or they fast—i.e., forego enjoyable food as a demonstration of faith to God or the saints.
- **Usual diet**. Varies by socioeconomic status. Most common dishes are rice, beans, meat, and salad. Traditional foods include spices, yams, plantains, and other vegetables grown in Dominican Republic. Relished foods include deep-fried chicken with peppery seasonings (*chicharron de pollo*), avocados, boiled green plantains mashed with oil and sauteed onion (*mangú*), fried meat pies (*empanadas* or *pastellios*), and stew (*sancocho*) containing various meats. A popular traditional dessert is *habichuelas con dulce* made with sweet beans, coconut milk, evaporated and regular milk, sugar, and butter.
- **Fluids**. Most drink espresso coffee at all meals; sometimes hot chocolate also served. Wealthier persons may serve tea with a snack, but persons of lower socioeconomic status view tea as something to consume when ill.
- **Food taboos and prescriptions**. No food taboos. Many believe that herbal teas are useful for treating a variety of ailments. Some drink juices or the vitamin-fortified brand drinks Malta Morena™ or Forty Mart™. These drinks are sold in small, inner-city markets (*bodegas*) that cater to Dominicans.
- **Hospitality**. Receive guests with great hospitality, warm smiles, handshakes, and hugs. Always offer meals; prepare food even if it is not meal time. Guests expected to eat and drink with family. Treat elders with respect. Family members usually give up their bedrooms for overnight guests.

SYMPTOM MANAGEMENT

- **Pain** (*dolor*). Unacceptable for individuals to appear weak. Men, in particular, seldom admit to pain or discomfort and are expected to tolerate such inconvenience; they may not seek health care until symptoms are disabling.

Due to fear of addiction, may not accept narcotics and the explanation that treatment is necessary. Nonpharmacological methods for controlling pain acceptable. Commonly use herbal remedies. Understand numerical pain scale.

- **Dyspnea** (*falta de respiro*). If a person thinks something is seriously wrong, he/she will go to physician and accept treatment, including oxygen. Sometimes family members pour cold water over his/her head. Family may take the person outside for fresh air to see if this improves the breathing problem.

- **Nausea/vomiting** (*náusea/vómito*). No special meaning. Folk remedies usually the first treatment option—e.g., chamomile tea (*manzanilla*) for stomach upset, anise for gas, or linden leaves (*tilo*) for children who have gas or difficulty sleeping. Avoid rectal suppositories (consider them an invasion of privacy) and do not see need for this intervention. More readily accept IV agents.

- **Constipation/diarrhea** (*constipación/diarrea*). Folk remedies—e.g., chamomile tea for diarrhea—are usually the first treatment option. Not embarrassed to report symptoms, but are embarrassed about treatment and avoid it at all costs. For example, they do not accept enemas or suppositories, especially if administered by a care provider of the opposite gender. Nutritional controls acceptable.

- **Fatigue** (*fatiga*). Attribute fatigue to poor nutrition. Afflicted person needs strengthening with extra vitamins; is encouraged to eat red meat and organ meats, such as liver, and to consume special fortified drinks. Older persons may suggest that the individual drink beer for more strength.

- **Depression** (*depresión*). Mental illness is stigmatized. View it as punishment for moral infractions. Some families fear embarrassment and social isolation if outsiders learn of a depressed person, as they may consider depression a mental illness. Depending on degree of depression, family may choose to care for the individual at home using herbs, teas, and homeopathic remedies. May also use prayer, fasting, or obligation/sacrifice (*la promesa*), such as attending church more often. Dominicans often suspicious of outside resources and programs. Length of time in U.S., education, and economic status influence their acceptance of medication and mental health services.

- **Self-care symptom management**. Most are passive recipients of care rather than active in self-care. Even in cases of chronic illness, many cede control to elder family member, spouse, and/or older children.

BIRTH RITUALS/CARE OF THE NEW MOTHER AND BABY

- **Pregnancy care**. Generally seek prenatal care as soon as the woman suspects she is pregnant, if couple is financially able. Only very wealthy or upper-class women attend childbirth preparation classes. According to hot/cold theory, pregnant women should not expose themselves to night air (*sereño*), as cold night air will harm the fetus. Exposure to terrible news or traumatic events also can negatively influence the fetus.

- **Preferences for children**. Most families expect married couples to procreate, often early in the union. Welcome a child of either sex, but most males anticipate male heirs as a sign of virility. Large families common. Second- and third-generation Dominicans in U.S. may have expectations similar to those in dominant culture. Lack of economic resources and difficulties living in U.S. also may limit family size.

- **Labor practices**. Laboring mother is encouraged to stay active—to walk, shower, and prepare for the hospital as in dominant culture.
- **Role of the laboring woman during birth**. Often extremely vocal and emotional; may scream and call on God or family to help her. Wants pain medication.
- **Role of the father and other family members during birth**. Male partner is usually supportive but does not play an active role during labor, preferring to wait outside or observe. Woman's mother and mother-in-law present if at all possible. Other female household members also may be present to coach and support the laboring woman.
- **Vaginal vs. cesarean section**. Expect a vaginal delivery. Elder family members may perceive the need for a C-section as weakness of birthing mother, as an inability to deliver child on her own. Cesarean birth also limits mother's immediate postpartum ability to care for infant.
- **Breastfeeding**. Strongly encouraged for all infants. Mothers who have been in U.S. longer may use a combination of breastfeeding and bottle-feeding. Weaning often left up to the child; not unusual for a toddler or preschooler to still breastfeed.
- **Birth recuperation**. For 40 days after delivery (*la cuarentena*), new mother's mother or mother in-law usually cares for the family while she remains in bed and limits activity. She only needs to breastfeed the baby and heal. Immediately postpartum, she is fed warm soups and stews, oatmeal, dried and salted fish, vitamins, and plenty of fluids so she can regain her strength and well-being. Older female household members may limit new mother's bathing and hair washing during *la cuarentena*. Baby's father is expected to remain supportive and loving, but sexual activity between him and mother not allowed.
- **Baby care**. Mother expected to be fully involved emotionally with baby after delivery (e.g., by holding and cuddling it). But during *la cuarentena*, grandmother or another female household member physically cares for infant. If family has been in U.S. for awhile, father may actively participate in caring for infant.
- **Problems with baby**. Clinician should notify elder family member and father/husband first. Head of family decides if it is OK to tell others, including members of extended family. The eldest person, mother and mother-in-law, or husband informs the new mother. Do not tell outsiders about problems with baby. Make medical decisions within the family; new parents consult with members of immediate family.

- **Male and female circumcision**. Male infants not usually circumcised. Female infants never circumcised.

DEVELOPMENTAL AND SEXUAL ISSUES

- **Celebration of menarche or becoming a man**. Like other Hispanic cultures, Dominicans celebrate 15th birthday (*quinceañera*) as a coming-out for girls. Boys encouraged to be sexually active early on as a declaration of manhood. Traditionally, not uncommon for fathers to take boys to a prostitute for initiation; this practice may or may not occur in U.S.
- **Attitudes about birth control**. Acceptable for married couples to practice natural controls, such as withdrawal or rhythm method. Catholic Church prohibits other forms of birth control.
- **Attitudes about sexually transmitted infection (STI) control, including condoms**. Most men prefer not to use condoms because they feel it limits their sexual experience. STIs a concern because of *machismo*: Men do not think condoms are manly and women usually do not initiate or insist on their use. Dominicans very afraid of HIV/AIDS but too embarrassed to talk about it or any STI. Most parents do not discuss these issues even with adult children.
- **Attitudes about abortion**. Catholic Church prohibits abortion. However, folk healers or older females familiar with herbal remedies that may induce abortion may perform it in secret.
- **Attitudes about unwed sexual experimentation**. Young men expected to have several sexual encounters before marriage. Unmarried women discouraged from having sex. Responsibility of entire family to ensure virginity until marriage; otherwise, a daughter may be unmarriageable. Attitudes among more-acculturated persons similar to those of dominant culture.
- **Sexual orientation**. Dominicans do not perceive homosexuality as a problem because it "does not exist" in their culture. Gays and lesbians most likely remain silent regarding their orientation. Sexuality generally not discussed, even among close family members. Because men pride themselves on sexual prowess, revealing an orientation that the community considers abhorrent exposes them to risk of isolation or possible violence.
- **Gender identity**. Unacceptable to have an ambiguous gender identity or one that is opposite of birth gender. Dominicans may perceive such identities as punishment of parents for having done something bad or evil, or as a curse someone has placed on them. Do not accept transsexuals. Feminine boys and masculine girls are pressured to change; if they do not, family denies the opposite gender identity and behaves as if it is nonexistent.
- **Attitudes about menopause**. Should be suffered as a normal consequence of aging. Women do not initiate discussion of menopause with clinicians, do not reveal problems associated with menopause, and do not seek treatment for symptoms, nor do they discuss sexuality issues. Not likely to be receptive to hormone therapy, especially if they think it is related to birth control.

Men may perceive partner's menopause as a loss of femininity and a reason to seek younger women for sexual pleasure.

FAMILY RELATIONSHIPS

- **Composition/structure**. *La familia* or *los parentes* are nuclear and extended families. They are Dominicans' most fundamental and powerful social unit, characterized by strong emotional, moral, and social bonds supported by trust and affection. Informally adopting someone into the family is referred to as *compadrazgo*, which denotes strong emotional ties. *Compadrazgo* also refers to those chosen to witness or accept responsibility at times of crises or during religious rites, such as baptism and marriage. These relationships between the *ahijado* (child) and his *madrina* and *padrino* (godparents) and with *compadres* and *comadres* (co-parents) persist at all levels of society, including among Dominicans who have immigrated to U.S. There are three forms of marital union: a formal religious church ceremony (*matrimonio por la iglesia*), recognized by the Catholic Church; a civil ceremony (*matrimonio por la ley*), which is state-sanctioned; and a union between consenting individuals (*unión libre*). *Matrimonio por la iglesia* is an irrevocable tie not to be taken lightly; more common in U.S. and usually related to achieving higher socioeconomic status. Some men who can afford it maintain other households and father more than one family. This arrangement never discussed (even though wives may be aware of it) and is less common in U.S. because of high cost of raising a family.
- **Decision-making**. Traditionally, dominant male figure is head of the household; sometimes he is officially called *jefe de la familia*. Female-headed households in U.S. are prevalent; in those cases, *la jefe* (female family leader) makes family decisions.
- **Spokesperson**. Head of the family is usually the spokesperson. Those who know more English or are more educated cannot assume the role of spokesperson but do consult with the head of household/elder and serve as interpreter.
- **Gender issues**. Significant role differences between genders, with clearly established expectations for and behaviors of each, especially along class lines. *Machismo* describes the patriarchal system of male dominance. All Dominicans expect at least the appearance of a male-dominated household. At least in public, men make all major family decisions and have authority to use their power if they so choose. In reality, women have subtle ways to greatly influence family decisions. Women mostly responsible for function of family unit—e.g., for preparing meals, caring for children, and entertaining guests. They also nurture children and are their source of love and affection, in contrast to authoritarian fathers.
- **Changing roles among generations in U.S.** Related to reason they immigrated, when they immigrated, and economic factors. For example, early immigrants came for political reasons, whereas later ones were motivated by

dreams of economic prosperity. Early immigrants established economic stability and typically have maintained traditional male-female roles. Since the 1950s and 1960s, Dominicans have not prospered; recent immigrants are among the most impoverished in New York City. In most families, both parents must work outside the home. Traditional gender roles persist, but most families blend roles to meet the needs of a working dyad. Most Dominican households headed by females (which make up about 40% of households with children younger than 18 years) have economic problems.

- **Caring roles**. Although women usually care for ill family members and themselves, considered improper for a family member of one gender to help a family member of the opposite gender with physical needs. An older son or another male family member, if available, cares for male patient.

- **Expectations of and for children**. Families consider it very important to provide food, love, and protection for their children. Sons and daughters live at home until marriage. Some dependence on parents continues even after marriage. For example, married children always seek family advice and support before they make major decisions. Sharp dichotomy in sex roles begins early in life. Girls protected against any public display of nudity, even exposure of genitalia when their diapers are changed. But public nudity of boys socially acceptable until about age 6, and handling genitals is tolerated. Girls are elaborately and carefully groomed and femininity is expressed as early as age 1 in the form of frilly dresses, gold earrings, charm bracelets, and chains. They are carefully chaperoned until marriage. Boys, in contrast, have a great deal of freedom. A young woman who is not a virgin may be unmarriageable and is expected to remain in parents' home. Dominicans expect children to go to school but do not pressure them to seek higher education. Although all household members are expected to contribute financially, children in school are not expected to contribute until able.

- **Expectations of and for elders**. Expected to live with family. Newlyweds usually move close to their elders to help provide for them and, when necessary, take parents into their home. Dominicans rarely use skilled nursing facilities and home care by unrelated home health assistants. Daughters care for mothers, sons for fathers. However, sons take care of mothers if a female family member is not available; daughters care for fathers under similar circumstances.

- **Expectations of hospital visitors**. Family members usually remain at bedside day and night. At least one family member must stay with patient if possible. All family members and close friends expected to visit. At times, the group will be large. Family members warmly receive visitors, as they provide support and comfort for patient and family.

ILLNESS BELIEFS

- **Causes of/attitudes about physical illness**. Often viewed as punishment, a lesson to be learned, or God's will for the family. May first seek God's healing through prayer and miraculous intervention. Making a religious sacrifice or promise (*la promesa*) may also help family cope with the illness. Family may display complete assurance that a miracle will soon occur. Believe that a "hot"/"cold" imbalance can cause illness. Recommend a hot remedy if a cold disease or illness develops, and a cold remedy (including food items) if a hot disease develops. Some disagreement about which illnesses are cold and which are hot; cold and hot foods may differ among individuals. A common cold condition is menstruation. Two common hot conditions are pregnancy and constipation. Dominicans sometimes attribute illness to a curse placed by, or a spell cast by, another person out of jealousy or revenge.

- **Causes of/attitudes about mental illness**. View mental illness as a disgrace. It is punishment for moral infractions or the consequence of a curse or spell. Family prefers to care for mentally ill person at home if possible. Accept medications and psychotherapy.
- **Causes of genetic defects**. God's punishment. Most children with genetic disorders are cared for at home without help from outside resources. View institutionalization and hospitalization unfavorably; these options may make the family feel incapable of caring for its own.
- **Attitudes about disabilities**. View some disabilities as punishment for a sin committed against God. Keep disabled family member at home; do not take him/her to public places. Sometimes consider such a person an embarrassment to family.
- **Sick role**. Expect sick individuals to be passive and allow family members to care for them.
- **Home and folk remedies**. Wide use of herbal teas for minor ailments, especially chamomile tea for stomach or bowel problems. Some Dominicans use homeopathic remedies purchased at neighborhood markets (*bodegas*) or small stores (*botanicas*) that sell many herbs, ointments, and the like. Those who believe in "hot"/"cold" theory of disease may treat cold illnesses with hot foods (and avoid cold foods), and treat hot illnesses with cold foods. If asked, they divulge such remedies, but they must have confidence in the clinician and know they will not be reprimanded or ridiculed.
- **Medications**. Accept Western medications. Compliance varies. Often combine folk remedies with Western medications.
- **Acceptance of procedures**. Before any procedure, both family and patient must be informed about what will take place. Accept transfusions and, if necessary, surgery. Do not readily accept organ transplants.
- **Care-seeking**. Try home remedies first but use biomedical and folk healers concurrently if their condition does not improve.

HEALTH ISSUES
- **Concept of health**. Attribute health to God's will, and illness to God's pun-

ishment or a spell/curse put on the family by an enemy or someone who is envious of one's wealth, beauty, or happiness.

- **Health promotion and prevention**. Many see little value in prevention, as God makes the final decision about who will be healthy. View the typical Dominican diet as healthy. Do not value exercise as a means to better health. Women with a little extra weight are sexy; very thin women are sickly. Have confidence in health care providers and understand prevention. Will modify behavior if it does not interfere with family relationships—e.g., by creating conflict between husband and wife over dietary restrictions.
- **Screening**. Irregular contact with health care providers for routine screenings and preventive care. Children get regular vaccinations. Women avoid some potentially embarrassing screening procedures, such as rectal exams and self-examination of breasts, because many avoid touching themselves. However, they accept mammography.
- **Common health problems**. High blood pressure, cardiovascular disorders, obesity, diabetes, mental illness, substance abuse, nutritional disorders, teen pregnancy, HIV/AIDS, and other sexually transmitted infections. Domestic violence and/or child abuse are high-risk health concerns. Some health conditions, such as poor nutrition, substandard housing, poor sanitation, environmental hazards, and overcrowding, are associated with poverty. There is stress or depression among women who head a household and are dealing with parenting, changing roles, and racial and gender barriers in U.S.

DEATH RITUALS

- **Beliefs and attitudes about death**. View death as normal but do not believe people should die. For Dominicans, death is very traumatic and painful even if someone is diagnosed with a terminal or fatal illness. Believe that if the dying person has gone to church and is a "good person," he/she will go to heaven; a bad person will go to hell. Death of a young person or child, or death from trauma, means the individual was not ready to go; special masses and prayers necessary so the spirit can go to heaven.
- **Preparation**. Inform first the immediate and extended families of an impending death, then close friends or persons outside the family. Usually do not inform the dying patient. Religious and Catholic families call a priest.
- **Home vs. hospital**. Prefer death at home, with patient surrounded by loved ones. Welcome hospice, but family wants to be directly involved in care.
- **Special needs**. If patient dies in hospital, most family members come to the bedside. Often burn candles near the body. Death necessitates that all family reunite at the wake or funeral; most will travel to the Dominican Republic if the funeral is there. All family and friends expected to provide emotional, financial, and physical support to grieving family members. After burial, Dominicans hold a religious ceremony (*los nueve dias*, the nine days) in the home, hosted by family members who cook meals, provide hospitality,

and lead the service in prayer and supplication for the deceased. Immediate family members refrain from celebrating festive occasions or attending parties for one year, especially if the deceased was a parent or spouse.

- **Care of the body**. In U.S., body taken to mortuary for preparation. Family purchases new, special clothing for body to be buried in—a black suit for a man, often a beautiful white dress for a woman.
- **Attitudes about organ donation**. Do not believe in organ donation; body should remain intact for burial. If a family member needs an organ, someone else will donate it if he/she is able to.
- **Attitudes about autopsy**. Do not believe in value of autopsy; resist it. If autopsy necessary, clinician should ask wife, mother, spouse, or whoever was closest to the deceased.

SELECTED REFERENCES

Foner, N. (Ed.). (2001). *New immigrants in New York* (Rev. ed.). New York: Columbia University Press.

Haeussler-Flore, D. (2002). *An introduction to the culture of the Dominican Republic for rehabilitation service providers (part II)*. Buffalo, NY: Center for International Rehabilitation Research Information and Exchange. Retrieved March 20, 2004, from http://www.cirrie.buffalo.edu/domrep.html

Hendricks, G. (1974). *The Dominican diaspora: From Dominican Republic to New York City—villagers in transition*. New York: Teachers College Press.

Lòpez-De Fede, A. (2002). *An introduction to the culture of the Dominican Republic for rehabilitation service providers (part I)*. Buffalo, NY: Center for International Rehabilitation Research Information and Exchange. Retrieved March 20, 2004, from http://www.cirrie.buffalo.edu/domrep.html

AUTHORS

Neddie Valentin Serra, EdD, RNC, was born in the U.S. and raised in New York City. She is a first-generation Hispanic whose parents emigrated to the U.S. from Puerto Rico in the late 1940s. Inspired by her mother to seek a nursing career, she was the first in her family to earn undergraduate and graduate degrees. She is currently an associate professor and chairperson of the Bloomfield College Division of Nursing in Bloomfield, NJ.

Jeanette Martinez was born and raised in the Dominican Republic. She emigrated to the U.S. with her family in 1997. She completed her basic education in the Dominican Republic and then graduated from high school in Paterson, NJ, where she currently resides with her parents and a brother. Martinez is the mother of a 2-year-old. She is pursuing a degree in cosmetology and hopes to graduate in 2005.

CHAPTER 12

EAST INDIANS

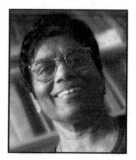

Rachel Zachariah

CULTURAL/ETHNIC IDENTITY

East Indian refers to inhabitants of the Indian subcontinent and anyone of East Indian ancestry around the world; not all can identify their roots. In U.S., East Indians have a heterogeneous language and culture. This chapter focuses on the largest religious groups: Hindus, Christians, and Sikhs. For information on Muslims, refer to the chapter on Pakistanis.

- **Preferred term(s)**. East Indian, South Asian, Asian Indian, and Indo-American. Sometimes identified by religious affiliation, such as Sikhs, Hindus, and Muslims. Also may identify themselves by their mother tongue (see major languages and dialects).

- **Census**. The 2000 U.S. Census counted more than 1.6 million East Indians, the fourth-largest (12%) Asian group. States with largest populations are California, New York, New Jersey, Illinois, and Texas; cities are New York, Chicago, Los Angeles, San Francisco, and Washington, DC.

- **History of immigration**. First wave came to U.S. as laborers in the 19th and 20th centuries, mainly Punjabi Sikhs who worked in lumberyards, farming, and railroad construction, and at steamship companies. Organized labor successfully lobbied Congress to bar Asian immigration in 1917. From 1920–30, 3,000 East Indians left U.S. because of lack of work. By the time the ban was lifted in 1946, only 1,500 East Indians remained in U.S. In 1965, immigration reform abolished quotas, after which immigration and diversity in social and geographical origin increased. Highly educated, technically trained East Indians entered U.S., raising "brain drain" concerns in India. Since the 1987 Immigration Act eased the process for obtaining visas, more than 20,000 have come to U.S. annually.

SPIRITUAL/RELIGIOUS ORIENTATION

- **Primary religious/spiritual affiliations**. Nearly all religions are represented in India. Although 83% of Indians are Hindus, there are 120 million Muslims (12%), one of the world's largest Muslim populations. Others are Christians, Sikhs, Jains, Buddhists, Parsis, Zoroastrians, and Jews. Each religious group maintains distinctly different customs and traditions that influence lifestyle and health practices. For example, Jains strictly believe in nonviolence and observe vegetarian dietary practices in U.S.
- **Usual religious/spiritual practices**. Hindus worship many gods and goddesses, in temple (*mandir*) or at home, and read from holy scriptures (Vedas). Hindus believe in the caste system hierarchy of four social classes: Brahmins (priest class), Kshatriyas (warrior class), Vaishyas (merchant class), and Sudras (laborer class). Individuals inherit their class from parents; believe that birth in a particular caste is predetermined by karma from previous lives. While legally abolished for many years, the caste system still influences social relations. Sikhs believe in one God and equality of all people. Guru Granth is their holy scripture; they sing hymns from Guru Granth in congregation at a Sikh temple and offer prayers daily. Christians believe in Christ as the living God, worship in churches, and pray regularly.
- **Use of spiritual healing/healers**. Accept western biomedical practices along with faith and spiritual healing. For example, Hindus believe that reciting charms and certain ritual acts will eliminate diseases, enemies, sins, and demons. Many believe that yoga eliminates certain physical and mental illnesses. Christians believe in faith healing and pray for it based on God's promises revealed in the Bible. They may have priests, elders, deacons, and/or members of the congregation visit the hospital and pray for the sick.
- **Holidays**. Christians celebrate Christmas and Easter. Hindus celebrate *Diwali* (week of November 1), the festival of lights, which remembers the return of their god Rama and his wife Sita after 14 years of exile in the forests; *Holi* (week of March 1), the festival of colors, which commemorates the Hindu god Krishna playing with Gopis; *Pongal* (January 14), the harvest festival, which includes decorated cows and a procession, and is celebrated in Tamil Nadu and Andhra Pradesh states; *Onam* (10 days in late August), a festival commemorating the golden era of King Mahabali (whose spirit is said to visit during the festival), celebrated with traditional cuisine, dance, decorations, exchange of gifts, feasts, and music, including brightly decorated and exciting snake boat races; and, among Hindus, *Durga Puja* (four days in late September or early October), which symbolizes the goddess Durga fighting and winning over evil. All of these religious holidays are celebrated in U.S. Secular holidays include New Year's Day (January 1), Independence Day (August 15), celebrating independence from British rule; Republic Day (January 26), when India became a republic, celebrated with lavish parades all

over India; and Mahatma Gandhi's birthday (October 2) and the day he was assassinated (January 30). Independence Day widely celebrated in U.S. Some groups observe other secular holidays.

COMMUNICATION
ORAL COMMUNICATION

- **Major languages and dialects**. Immigrants to U.S. and Canada speak more than 20 languages and more than 200 dialects. For most, language identifies their origin. For example, people from the Gujarat region speak Gujarati. Other common languages are Bengali, Malayalam, Tamil, Telugu, Kannada, Marathi, Punjabi, Urdu, Hindi, Kashmiri, Assamese, Oriya, Sindhi, and Sanskrit. As English is the official language of India, young immigrants, other visa holders, all professionals, and those with higher education write, read, and speak English when they arrive. Elderly immigrants or visitors may not be fluent in English.
- **Greetings**. Press hands together in front of chest and say, *"Namaste"* (Hindus and Christians) or *"Sasriyakal"* (Sikhs), a graceful gesture that represents both welcome and respect. Shaking of hands among men adopted during British rule. Persons of same or younger age address each other by first names. Older persons prefer to be addressed by titles. Examples are *Didi* (Hindi), *Kochamma* (Malayalam), or *Acca* (Tamil) for a woman of an older sister's age, and *Bhayya/Achayan/Anna* for a man of an older brother's age; *Amman/ Valiyamma/Patti* (female) and *Baba/Valiappan/Thatha* (male) for those of grandparents' age; and, in Malayalam and Tamil, *Chachi/Ammachi* (female) and *Chacha/Appachen* (male) for persons of parents' age. Each ethnic/religious group uses such titles to show respect, especially when greeting parents, older relatives, teachers, religious leaders, and persons of higher status. In some situations, greeting may be a simple nod or smile.
- **Tone of voice**. Expect to be spoken to in soft tone. May interpret loud voice as disrespect, rudeness, or lack of anger control. Acceptable to raise one's voice to correct and guide younger persons, but older persons are spoken to respectfully and politely at all times.
- **Direct or indirect style of speech**. Acculturated persons welcome direct questions during health care interviews, but older persons may view direct questions as rude or disrespectful. Often unassertive and unwilling to question clinician about disease, medications, and treatment. Many do not initiate discussions about genitals, breasts, and sex, but young, educated persons are more receptive to discussing personal topics. Silence or brief response indicates agreement and cooperation.
- **Use of interpreters**. Elderly immigrants may need interpreter; most prefer a close family member of same gender and older age to interpret and offer advice. Privacy and confidentiality important. Highly educated and/or professional persons may prefer an interpreter of same gender who also is a

health professional of the same or older age. Interpreter who speaks same language/dialect desirable.

- **Serious or terminal illness**. Prefer to have physician disclose serious diagnosis and prognosis first to a close family member. Then family members decide whether to disclose information to patient. Sometimes patient may not know about his/her condition until close to death.

WRITTEN COMMUNICATION

- **Literacy assessment**. Immigrants of urban and rural origin likely to be fluent and literate in English. Because education of males receives more emphasis, some women may be less fluent in English. Young children speak native language at home but learn English in schools and colleges. Appropriate for clinician to assess written and verbal English skills by asking patient to respond to direct questions or a brief checklist.
- **Consents**. When asked for consent, patient may want a close family member present for moral support and consultation. Traditionally value verbal consent; once East Indians give their "word," they do not change it, so some feel uncomfortable with written consent. Clinician fosters trust and cooperation by explaining a procedure in simple terms. Patients may not be keenly interested in research evidence for procedures; many focus on their own health issues and rely completely on health professionals, whom they highly respect, to make decisions.

NONVERBAL COMMUNICATION

- **Eye contact**. May consider direct eye contact rude or disrespectful, especially with elderly. May not sustain eye contact with strangers and older persons. Unrelated men and women do not sustain eye contact.
- **Personal space**. Unrelated men and women, boys and girls maintain greater distance (about 3 feet). Preference varies by level of acculturation, gender, age, and relationship. To ensure a comfortable distance and that patient's personal space is not violated, clinician should explain purpose of contact (e.g., history-taking vs. pelvic exam). In social situations, men and women usually stay in separate groups or rooms. Traditional churches seat men on one side and women on the other. Men and women eat in separate areas. In U.S., these practices are gradually changing.
- **Use and meaning of silence**. May indicate acceptance, approval, and/or tolerance or reluctance to confront or oppose. Recognize silence, modesty, humility, and tolerance as good qualities, particularly in women. Second generation in U.S. more assertive and verbal in communicating ideas and disagreements.
- **Gestures**. Usually use hand gestures while conversing. Consider it disrespectful for women to sit with legs crossed or apart. Some gestures may be confusing to non-East Indians. For example, to express remorse or honesty

in India, one grasps his/her earlobes, a gesture servants use when scolded. East Indians do not point with one finger (use that gesture with inferiors); rather, use full hand or point with chin. Show respect by offering an item to, or receiving an item from, someone with right hand; person of lower status should receive item with both hands. Younger persons may be less strict about or overlook these customs. In India, offensive to step on someone's toes or brush him/her with foot, even accidentally; one should apologize immediately. A form of apology is to touch the other's shoulder or toes briefly with fingertips, then tap own forehead, which means the offender seeks forgiveness. This gesture also expresses utmost respect. For example, before marriage, bride uses this gesture when seeking her parents' blessing.

- **Openness in expressing emotions**. East Indians do not often freely express fear, sadness, or anger to family members or close friends. Acculturated persons also may repress their feelings, as a way to feel in control of the situation. May avoid openly expressing feelings to health care professionals and strangers. However, facial expressions may be revealing. Younger persons may be more open with siblings, parents, and friends.
- **Privacy**. Very important, especially personal private space and protecting personal information from anyone other than a close family member. Often unwilling to share personal information and issues with health care providers, unless it is relevant to care. May disclose necessary information only to close family members and/or friends with whom they share problems. Close family members expect to receive information about a patient's condition so they can help.
- **Touch**. Not common, particularly between unrelated men and women. Express love and caring through eye contact and facial expressions rather than kissing or hugging. Best if clinician explains what he/she is about to do and asks permission before touching patient, particularly in examination of private parts. Helpful to ask patient if there is any part of the body clinician should avoid touching.
- **Orientation to time**. Future-oriented. Incorporate past experiences and present situations to meet future goals and commitments. May not be very time-conscious, especially in social gatherings, and do not like to monitor every minute of daily life. However, quite aware of importance of keeping health care appointments and being on time for professional responsibilities.

ACTIVITIES OF DAILY LIVING

- **Modesty**. May prefer health care professionals of same gender. Men may be comfortable with hospital gown and pajama bottoms, but women may prefer not to wear gown because it is not modest enough. Hindu and Christian women new to U.S. may wear a *sari* (long dress for adult); most Sikh women prefer loose pants (*shalwar*) and a top (*kameez*) that extends below the knees.

Some cover their head and chest with a rectangular, 3-by-6-foot cloth (*chader*).

- **Skin care**. Most East Indians shower daily. But persons with a cold or respiratory tract infection, and those who have undergone surgery, prefer a bed bath. Use lots of running water when bathing; need it for washing long hair. Also consider water a symbol of purity. Sometimes prefer perfumed soaps, such as sandalwood, and herbal products for cleansing skin. Immigrants very careful to maintain healthy skin; may use both Eastern and Western methods of care. They wash hands and feet with soap and dry them carefully. Wash after work.

- **Hair care**. Some Hindu castes take infants to temple for first haircut and offer hair to the gods. Similarly, adults shave head ceremoniously and offer long hair. South Indian women, in particular, consider long hair a sign of beauty. East Indians usually wash hair daily or once or twice weekly. Do not wash hair when ill, believing that wet hair or a bath exposes them to cold and makes illness worse. Women massage scalp with coconut or mustard oil daily or weekly, and comb and braid hair daily. Traditional Sikh males not allowed to cut hair or shave beard; hair usually secured in turban. Hindus and Christians do not restrict cutting or shaving of body hair.

- **Nail care**. Cut nails short and keep them clean. Consider nails to be body parts that must be disposed of properly. Cutting nails at night discouraged; once clipped, nail parings should be thrown on the roof or in sink with running water.

- **Toileting**. Prefer private toilet but accept bedpan, urinal, or bedside commode when necessary. Like thorough peri-wash with water after elimination, so a pint-size, plastic water pitcher should be placed near commode. East Indians must use left hand to wash and wipe perineal area, and must wash hands with soap and water after toileting.

- **Special clothing or amulets**. High-caste Hindu men wear a sacred thread (*poonul* in Malayalam) tied around their body. Health care providers must never remove it without patient's or family member's permission. Baptized Sikh men and women wear a piece of cloth (*kirpan*) around their chests, a wooden comb (*kanga*), and an iron bracelet (*kara*) that must never be removed. Clothing varies by age and level of acculturation. Syrian Christian women from southern India always wear a wedding chain with small, gold-cross pendant (*minnu*) and a wedding ring; married women are buried with the *minnu*. Clinician should not remove these items unless necessary for surgery.

- **Self-care**. In many Indian hospitals, family and friends provide care. In U.S., patient and family expect caregiver or a family member to assist patient with personal hygiene and meals. Prefer that someone stay with hospitalized patient so he/she feels close family support and so family feels reassured that patient is OK. Given adequate explanation and support, patients participate in self-care.

FOOD PRACTICES

- **Usual meal pattern**. Usually 2–3 meals a day. Big meal at lunch, small meal at supper. Most also take afternoon tea with snacks, and supper in late evening.
- **Special utensils**. Hindus prefer metal utensils—copper, brass, stainless steel, and iron—for cooking and eating, as they consider them to be sacred. Christians and Sikhs have no such preferences. In southern India, serve meals on banana leaves at banquets. In U.S., East Indians use cooking and serving utensils brought from India or available in Indian stores. Many eat with right fingers. Wash hands before touching food and after eating.
- **Food beliefs and rituals**. Most Indian religions greatly respect food. People must eat with love and compassion, and be thankful to God for giving food that alleviates hunger and nourishes body and mind. Avoid any form of distraction while eating, such as watching television, reading, or excessive talking. Hindu, Sikh, and Christian religions discourage overeating, as it is believed to reduce one's life span. Carefully adhere to "hot/cold" (humoral) balance in selecting food, particularly for sick persons and women after childbirth. When hospitalized in U.S., may prefer food prepared with some spice.
- **Usual diet**. In U.S., combination of Western and Indian cuisine. Most common staples are rice or flat, baked, whole wheat bread (*chapati*) with meat, fish, vegetable, or lentil curry. Do not regularly eat sweet dishes but serve such dishes lavishly at special celebrations. Unhealthy practices include cooking with lots of oil and clarified butter (*ghee*).
- **Fluids**. Water or buttermilk (*lassi*) is beverage of choice. Believe *lassi* helps digestive processes. Drink tea instead of coffee, and usually water with meals. Alcohol uncommon at home. Children drink milk, juice, or water. May use ice in hot weather.
- **Food taboos and prescriptions**. When acutely ill, may like bland, easily digested foods. Hindus usually refrain from eating any kind of meat and fish; some avoid eggs. Some families permit alcohol but only in moderation. East Indians may fast one day a week or month, either totally abstaining from food and fluids or only eating pure foods—e.g., fruit, yogurt, and nuts. In U.S., many second-generation Hindus eat meat and fish. Vegetarian mothers may ask nonvegetarian women to teach them to cook meat for their children. Some Sikhs fast or refrain from eating meat products and smoking; they generally discourage alcohol. Hindus, Sikhs, and some Muslims and Christians who use Ayurvedic medicine—including people in U.S.—classify foods as "hot" or "cold." They prescribe hot foods in winter for such cold diseases as arthritis, respiratory tract infection, gastrointestinal problems, and circulatory problems, and for fever and surgery. Hot foods include meat and fish, eggs, yogurt, honey, most oils, nuts and seeds, most herbs, and spices. Prescribe cold foods (e.g., milk, butter, cheese, most vegetables and fruits, and some grains and legumes, such as wheat, rice, barley, and lentil) in hot

weather. Believe that certain foods are incompatible and will produce toxins when eaten together (e.g., fish and milk, meat and milk, and sour fruits and milk). Recommend fasting for fever, cold, constipation, or arthritic pain. Advise a warm-water fast one day a week for healthy persons to rest the digestive system.

- **Hospitality**. An extremely important value. Always welcome visitors and treat them respectfully, offering them the best meals and comforts available, including feasts prepared with traditional East Indian food. Families excited when relatives or other visitors come. They spend more than they can afford and give up their beds to visitors, then ask them to stay longer. Difficult to maintain such hospitality in U.S., so East Indians modify practices to fit the circumstances.

SYMPTOM MANAGEMENT

East Indians do not usually use numerical scale to quantify pain but can do so without difficulty. Numbers to quantify other symptoms may be more difficult; may prefer words.

- **Pain** (*darad*, *vali*, and *vedana*, depending on language). Accept narcotics. Some prefer intramuscular analgesics. Prefer prescribed analgesics for surgical pain or chronic illnesses (e.g., cancer and arthritis) but home remedies to manage acute muscle pain and joint inflammation from trauma. Common pain remedies include mustard-paste poultice or herbal leaves and oils applied to painful muscle, and turmeric paste warmed and applied with gauze to painful joint and wrapped with bandage.

- **Dyspnea** (*sans ukhrna* and *swasam muttal* [breathlessness]). May become very anxious and frightened, and hyperventilate; consider dyspnea a sign of death. Accept oxygen without hesitation. Some use home remedies such as licorice and ginger tea.

- **Nausea/vomiting** (*ulti/chardil*). Believed to be caused by toxins in the stomach that must be eliminated. Sometimes induce vomiting as therapy for chest congestion, asthma, indigestion, ingestion of poison, and edema. Encourage ill person initially to refrain from eating to rest gastrointestinal tract; sometimes offer herbs and spices, such as black pepper and/or dill seeds. Ill person may also drink Coke™ or ginger ale. In severe cases, may seek help from homeopathic, Ayurvedic, or Western practitioners. May accept IV or other medications.

- **Constipation/diarrhea** (*kabz* or *malabundham* [constipation], *gulab* or *vayarilakam* [diarrhea]). Believe that constipation causes abdominal distention and discomfort, headache, and bad breath. To relieve constipation, take one teaspoon of clarified butter (*ghee*) mixed with hot milk at bedtime. Generally accept enemas if necessary. For diarrhea, mix fresh-ginger paste with buttermilk and take orally. Also believe that black coffee, cumin, or nutmeg, or other combinations of herbs and spices, cure diarrhea. In severe cases, seek clinician's help.

- **Fatigue** (*thakan lagna* or *kshinam*). Give it serious attention—considered a sign of poor health. East Indians believe that a hot bath or shower and drinking a warm glass of milk with sugar just before bedtime promote sleep and alleviate fatigue, as does proper diet. Drink Ayurvedic tonics (special preparations with vitamins and iron) to overcome fatigue and build body strength. Recommend special preparations of liver with herbal medicines for anemia.
- **Depression** (*dil uddas hona* [Hindi, Urdu, Punjabi, and Gujarati], *manasika rogam* [Malayalam]). Not a clearly recognized diagnosis and condition. East Indians may consider it a sign of spiritual unhappiness. Some deal with depression by praying and meditating. Those who believe in Ayurvedic therapy may perform yoga exercises to feel better. In psychotic depression, may consult psychiatrist, spiritual healer, or, in some cases, a healer who deals in witchcraft. Usually delay reporting depression, due to stigma attached to mental illness. Very hesitant to discuss it with extended family and friends.
- **Self-care symptom management**. Usually respond promptly to symptoms causing discomfort. May rely on home remedies to alleviate symptoms but usually seek medical advice after trying such remedies. Accustomed to receiving care from family, friends, and community when sick. Those in U.S. are learning about self-care, such as self-monitoring for diabetes and hypertension, and about additional helpful resources.

BIRTH RITUALS/CARE OF THE NEW MOTHER AND BABY

- **Pregnancy care**. Consider pregnancy a healthy state. Pregnant woman's mother and mother-in-law play important advisory roles. Expectant mother allowed to perform usual tasks, except heavy lifting. She usually is protected from emotional stress and shock. Those who believe in Ayurvedic practices consider pregnancy a "hot" state and encourage eating "cold" foods, such as milk products, fruits, and vegetables. Some believe that mother must avoid hot foods, especially during first trimester, because they cause miscarriage. In U.S., those who are educated and those who have health insurance use prenatal care. Almost all young pregnant couples attend childbirth preparation classes.
- **Preferences for children**. In many regions, prefer boys to girls because sons carry the family name forward. Daughters marry and move in with husband's family. Sons are expected to stay home with their parents and provide for elderly parents. Historically, average family size was 6–8 children; in U.S., average is 2–3 children, mainly for economic reasons and because extended family provides limited child care.
- **Labor practices**. Encourage mother to walk to help dilatation of cervix and descent of fetus. Mother eats light meals. Usually discourage pain medications, as they may delay delivery.
- **Role of the laboring woman during birth**. Her modesty is protected. Laboring woman usually wants to know what will happen and follows instruc-

tions of health care providers and family members. Primipara may be frightened and anxious, and request pain medication. Moaning, grunting, and screaming acceptable. More recently, educated women have been exploring the Internet for childbirth options, initiating discussions with health care providers, and assuming a very active role in choosing birth process and anesthesia. Sex of baby may not be revealed to mother until placenta delivered because some families favor boys; a girl's birth may cause sufficient emotional upset to interfere with uterine contractions and delay delivery of placenta.

- **Role of the father and other family members during birth**. Women want their own mothers, sisters, or in-laws with them during labor for emotional support. Father usually waits outside labor room, but this trend is changing; many husbands stay with wives during labor and delivery, depending on level of education and acculturation. Traditional rituals at time of birth vary by religion. For example, in southern India, grandparents place a drop of gold in honey on baby's tongue soon after birth as a blessing.
- **Vaginal vs. cesarean section**. Prefer vaginal delivery but accept cesarean if necessary.
- **Breastfeeding**. East Indians value breastfeeding as important to infant growth and development, and to emotional attachment between baby and mother. Encouraged for at least six months. Occurs on demand for up to 2–3 years. Working mothers may combine breastfeeding with bottle-feeding.
- **Birth recuperation**. Typically expect new mother and baby to remain at home for 40 days, but Syrian Christians in southern India expect 56 days, during which time mother and baby not allowed to leave home for any reason; family and friends may visit with gifts. During recuperation, expect mother to get adequate rest and offer special foods to her. These include *katlu* (Gujarati)/*panjiri* (Punjabi), prepared by frying whole wheat flour in butter and adding sugar, almonds, pistachios, and a powdered mixture of herbs from an Indian grocery store. Most of the ingredients have "hot" effects that are believed to restore energy the mother lost during birth. Back massages with warm oil also common. Some groups strongly emphasize keeping mother warm. She may take a full bath only weekly but take partial baths and wash perineal area with warm water after elimination. Christian women in southern India use Ayurvedic medicine to cool the body after delivery. Take hot baths with medicinal leaves (*vedu*) every day for first 10 days.
- **Baby care**. Expect grandmothers to assist with new baby until mother recovers—2–6 months after delivery. Baby bathed every morning and its muscles and joints are gently massaged with oil. Baby kept warm, comfortable, and always close to the mother, including overnight. In U.S., practices similar to what clinicians recommend. Mothers and grandmothers try to combine the best of both worlds for health of mother and baby.
- **Problems with baby**. Grandmothers or other older women helpful in observing baby carefully and preventing problems. In India, fathers not usu-

ally involved in baby care. If problems with baby arise in hospital, mother should be told first. If illness is serious, father or mother-in-law may be notified first. Accept nurses' advice about managing problems.

- **Male and female circumcision**. Hindus, Sikhs, and Christians may allow male circumcision for health reasons. Female circumcision never practiced.

DEVELOPMENTAL AND SEXUAL ISSUES

- **Celebration of menarche or becoming a man**. Varies by religion and sub-culture. In several Hindu castes, special rituals celebrate girls' transition into womanhood and boys' into manhood. In some areas, girl is dressed in a *sari* (long dress for adult) and family holds a celebration when she starts menstruating. Parents and adolescents do not discuss puberty and sex openly. Girls usually approach the mother when they begin menstruating and do not mention it to male family members. In U.S., families talk about it more openly.
- **Attitudes about birth control**. Most married women use contraceptives to control number of pregnancies, although Catholics have restrictions. All birth control methods available in India, but East Indians mostly use oral contraceptives or intrauterine devices. In U.S., some single, young women use contraceptives in secret.
- **Attitudes about sexually transmitted infection (STI) control, including condoms**. Consider prevention of STIs very important; immigrants emphasize family values in that regard. East Indian culture discourages multiple sexual partners. Health education, including use of condoms, helps young persons understand and prevent STIs. Generally resist using condoms; think it is unnecessary, as multiple sexual partners are uncommon.
- **Attitudes about abortion**. View abortion negatively, based on health, religious, and social concerns. Married women seek abortion to limit number of children and to space pregnancies, or for health or financial reasons. Teen abortion infrequently performed in North America; community generally disapproves of it.
- **Attitudes about unwed sexual experimentation**. Parents of all religious backgrounds forbid it among boys and girls—strong cultural sanctions against dating, premarital sexual activity, and childbearing. Parents strongly oppose contraception and abortion as a health hazard and as a source of shame for family and guilt for the girl. Unacceptable to put unwed mother's baby up for adoption. In U.S., second-generation youth who are single keep their sexual activity secret.
- **Sexual orientation**. Christianity and other religions do not approve of homosexuality. Gay and lesbian persons hide their orientation from family and community out of fear of being disowned.
- **Gender identity**. Expect gender-appropriate behaviors. Very clear feminine identity for girls and masculine identity for boys. In India, transsexuals or individuals with ambiguous sex organs are not identified as such in social sit-

uations. Health care providers do not deal with their needs adequately. In U.S., attitudes are less negative.

- **Attitudes about menopause**. Most women have little difficulty coping with it. Extended family helps if there are problems. Hot flashes and emotional changes usually not serious; women typically ignore symptoms. Herbal remedies and Ayurvedic treatments available. Some women in U.S. use hormone replacement therapy based on clinician recommendations. Women generally do not talk freely about menopause; consider it embarrassing.

FAMILY RELATIONSHIPS

- **Composition/structure**. Importance of extended family—grandparents, their sons and families, and unmarried daughters—ingrained in East Indians. Daughter usually moves in with husband's family after marriage. In U.S., some prefer to live in nuclear families. Family members are interdependent and always cognizant of family obligations—even place them above obligations to their own spouse and children. Do not allow same-gender marriages.
- **Decision-making**. Male—usually father or eldest son—has decision-making power. Mother and other family members consulted before final decision made. Oldest male member in extended family consulted regarding major family decisions, such as a child's marriage.
- **Spokesperson**. Father, eldest son, or any other male in family. In their absence, senior member of family.
- **Gender issues**. Gender roles well-defined. Men primarily responsible for all activities outside the home, women for all activities within. In U.S., men are traditionally the breadwinners, but roles may be reversed due to lack of job opportunities. When women work, unemployed husbands have difficulty managing household chores. Some men expect their wives to handle household responsibilities as well as full-time employment, but attitudes vary depending on education and acculturation. Fathers usually discipline children; mothers guide and comfort them.
- **Changing roles among generations in U.S.** Early immigrants have acculturated yet retain many customs and values, such as East Indian food preferences and religious and social customs. East Indians acknowledge, but do not fully accept, gender equity, which has been difficult to implement. Second generation has grown up with a mix of U.S. and East Indian values. First- and second-generation family members may clash on philosophic, economic, religious, social, and health issues, with conflicts related to dating, arranged marriage, divorce, and children's traditional support of older parents. Many immigrant women older than 30 have difficulty finding husbands of their choice, due to lack of single, acculturated, and educated Indian men in U.S. who also respect traditional customs and values.
- **Caring roles**. Mother, wife, daughter, or other adult female relative usually cares for children and elders. If a child or elderly parent is chronically ill

and requires constant care, female family member is expected to care for him/her at home.

- **Expectations of and for children**. Expect children to obey parents, work hard at school, behave well, respect others (especially elders), and be God-fearing. Parents and extended family treat them affectionately. Acceptable in India to physically punish children for misbehavior. Children rarely make decisions independently; are guided by parents or older siblings, often relying on parents' decision or advice about career choice. Nearly all families in U.S. value higher education. Both boys and girls usually live at home until marriage, but young, single persons may live alone for employment or education.

- **Expectations of and for elders**. Highly respect elders; expect younger family members to stand up when parents or grandparents enter room. An elderly family member in the home considered to be a blessing from God. Younger generations grateful because elderly previously provided for them. Fulfill demands of elderly parents or grandparents even if it means sacrificing their own wishes. Elders usually live with children (preferably married sons) and grandchildren. Sometimes they babysit and teach cultural values and religion to grandchildren. In U.S., most young parents have their parents live with them; grandparents care for the grandchildren while parents work.

- **Expectations of hospital visitors**. Close female family member usually stays with patient (including overnight in patient's room or in lounge) and participates in care if necessary. Other family members and many friends visit frequently, sometimes unannounced, and may bring homemade food. Patient and family appreciate visits. Clinician can advocate for patient by telling relatives to be considerate of his/her need for rest.

ILLNESS BELIEFS

- **Causes of/attitudes about physical illness**. Hindus and Sikhs believe that disease is due to karma, the result of one's actions in past lives that determine his/her body constitution and susceptibility to disease in the current, reincarnated life. Ayurvedic philosophy attributes illness to an imbalance in bodily humors, which creates circulating toxins that accumulate in weaker areas of body. For example, if the joints are weak, accumulated toxins cause problems such as arthritis. Naturalistic causes of illness include bacteria, stress, and weather. Supernatural causes include the evil eye and evil spirits.

- **Causes of/attitudes about mental illness**. Believe that psychosis occurs when an enemy casts a spell or the body falls prey to an evil spirit. Ayurvedic explanation is that a person's constitution influences his/her susceptibility to mental problems. Cultural factors and stigma attached to mental illness inhibit people from seeking counseling or psychotherapy. In U.S., stigma remains; families do not discuss the situation openly and seek help only when absolutely necessary. Other families are reluctant to arrange a marriage with a family that has a mentally ill member. Traditionally, some East Indians sought remedies against witchcraft or shut an uncontrollable psychotic person in a room.

- **Causes of genetic defects**. Those who believe in karma think that hereditary or congenital problems occur because the afflicted individual inflicted pain on helpless animals or persons in past lives. Many folk beliefs regarding genetic defects (e.g., that certain behaviors of women during pregnancy cause defects). Chromosomal aberrations, cleft lip and palate, and congenital heart defects common in India.

- **Attitudes about disabilities**. Most often believed to occur with God's knowledge. Disabled person accepts and lives with disability. Parents and/or family members love and care for him/her. Traditionally keep disabled family members at home or, in some cases, in institutions (orphanages). However, awareness of the possibility and need for disabled persons to live independently has increased in India, although resources are inadequate. In U.S., East Indians seek and use such resources very effectively.

- **Sick role**. Sick persons usually passive. Expected to rest and have family members relieve them of responsibilities. Family member is assigned to look after person's needs. If mother is sick, members of extended family or friends offer assistance.

- **Home and folk remedies**. Most use home and folk remedies before consulting a physician, believing that substances found in nature cure many ailments. Boil spices and herbal remedies and use them internally to treat conditions such as a cold, congestion, heart problems, and sinusitis. Folk remedies passed down from generation to generation. Elders recommend and prepare home remedies, which include turmeric paste as an antiseptic for wounds, ginger and lime juice with sugar for stomach upsets, buttermilk kept overnight in iron utensils for treating anemia, a particular plant juice that provides iron for treating anemia, and rubbing the whole body with certain leaves in silence to get rid of the evil eye. May use alternative therapies concurrently with pharmaceuticals (e.g., chelation and Ayurvedic herbal treatment to remove blockage of coronary arteries).

- **Medications**. Use herbal, Ayurvedic, homoeopathic, and Western medicines. Generally compliant, but elderly taking multiple medications may get confused about timing. Recommend Ayurvedic tonics for those recovering from illness, children, and pregnant and postpartum women as a way of maintaining "hot"/"cold" balance. May not disclose other therapies to clinician—depends on patient's education and degree of acculturation.

- **Acceptance of procedures**. Generally quite receptive to surgery and transfusion but may prefer to receive blood from persons in their own family, caste, or religion. May fear donating blood, believing it causes loss of strength. Seek organ transplants in life-threatening situations. Many uncomfortable with organ donation due to religious or philosophical orientation.

- **Care-seeking**. Accept and respect Western biomedical practice; use it in

India when herbal, natural, homeopathic, and Ayurvedic approaches do not succeed. In U.S., some consult homeopathic and Ayurvedic experts concurrently. Some consult a spiritual healer and use prayer in conjunction with biomedicine. Many travel to southern India to receive Ayurvedic treatment and massage therapy for joint or back pains or for general rejuvenation. Homeopathy very popular in India. In U.S., travel long distances to consult homeopathic practitioners for treatment of ailments such as cancer and skin conditions.

HEALTH ISSUES

- **Concept of health**. Ayurvedic medicine influences many to think that the body is healthy when digestive fire (*agni*) is balanced; bodily humors are in equilibrium; waste products (urine, feces, and sweat) are at normal levels and in balance; senses are functioning normally; and body, mind, and consciousness harmoniously work as one. Wholeness is an important concept. Some believe that the spiritual state of health, attained through fasting, prayer, and meditation, supercedes all physical ailments and that a person can function despite ailments.
- **Health promotion and prevention**. Consider health a precious gift that must be enjoyed. Adopt practices that preserve, maintain, and protect health. Recommend getting adequate rest and sleep (rise before sunrise, retire early), bathing/showering daily, eating in moderation, and exercising and praying regularly. Unhealthy practices include too much sex and negative emotions, such as hate, anger, greed, jealousy, fear, and worry. In U.S., the young and elderly are becoming aware of the role of proper nutrition and exercise in preventing disease, and attempting to avoid chronic illnesses that afflict others in U.S. population.
- **Screening**. Consent to all screening procedures, except vaginal exams for unmarried, virginal women. Generally beginning to accept need for annual physical exams. Younger, educated persons undergo screening more regularly.
- **Common health problems**. East Indians have very high prevalence and risk of coronary artery disease (prevalence is triple that of U.S. population as a whole), which develops earlier in them than in other ethnic groups. Elevation of lipoprotein should be monitored in East Indians along with other conventional risk factors. Type 2 diabetes very common, attributable to genetic propensity for insulin resistance and hypertension.

DEATH RITUALS

- **Beliefs and attitudes about death**. Conceive of death in context of religious beliefs. Hindus and Sikhs believe that the body dies but the soul remains alive and is immortal. Both religions also believe in reincarnation. For Christians, those who believe in Christ will be resurrected after death and have eternal life.

- **Preparation**. Clinician should tell family members first about approaching death and let them decide whether to tell patient. When death is near, father, husband, or other responsible person informs all relatives and friends so they can gather before death. Christians arrange for a priest to visit, provide holy communion, and pray for salvation of the person's soul.
- **Home vs. hospital**. Strongly favor death at home with all family members present. Family may perform religious rituals at time of death. Hospice acceptable if absolutely necessary.
- **Special needs**. If death imminent, family members and relatives must be called and allowed to stay at bedside; important to have at least immediate family with dying person. Some families wish to call spiritual leader, who prays for dying person and gives a drink of holy water to purify body internally just before death. Surviving family members express grief openly by crying.
- **Care of the body**. Body is washed and dressed, candles are lit, and funeral services are held before a Christian burial. Among Hindus and Sikhs, body is washed by close family members, dressed in new clothes, and prepared for cremation. Hindus save ashes of cremated body until they can be thrown into the Ganges, a sacred river in India.
- **Attitudes about organ donation**. Hindus, Sikhs, and Christians prohibit organ donation. May be exceptions, but they are mostly reluctant to allow it in U.S.
- **Attitudes about autopsy**. Most East Indians do not agree to autopsy unless absolutely necessary.

SELECTED REFERENCES

Assanand, S., Dias, M., Richardson, E., & Waxler-Morrison, N. (1993). The South Asians. In N. Waxler-Morrison, J. Anderson, & E. Richardson (Eds.), *Cross-cultural caring: A handbook for health professionals in Western Canada* (pp. 139–180). Vancouver: UBC Press.

Helweg, A. W., & Helweg, U. M. (1990). *An immigrant success story: East Indians in America*. Philadelphia: University of Pennsylvania Press.

Jha, P., Enas, E. A., & Yusuf, S. (1993). Coronary artery disease in Asian Indians: Prevalence and risk factors. *Asian American and Pacific Islander Journal of Health*, 1, 163–175.

Kolanad, G. (1993). *Culture shock! India. A guide to customs and etiquette*. Portland, OR: Graphic Arts Center Publishing.

Lad, V. (1994). *Ayurveda: The science of self-healing*. Delhi: Motilal Banarsidass.

Zachariah, R. (2002). South Asians. In P. St. Hill, J. G. Lipson, & A. I. Meleis (Eds.), *Caring for women cross-culturally* (pp. 263–285). Philadelphia: F. A. Davis.

AUTHOR

Rachel Zachariah, DNSc, RN, is associate professor at Bouvé College of Health Sciences, School of Nursing, at Northeastern University in Boston.

She holds a bachelor of science degree in nursing and a midwifery diploma from the Christian Medical College and Hospital, College of Nursing, at the University of Madras in Vellore, southern India; a master's in nursing from the University of California-Los Angeles; and a doctorate in nursing from the University of California-San Francisco. Zachariah's practice and research focus on women's health. She has planned and provided health care for rural and urban populations in southern India.

CHAPTER 13

ETHIOPIANS AND ERITREANS

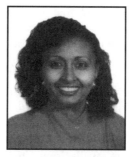

Yewoubdar Beyene

CULTURAL/ETHNIC IDENTITY

- **Preferred term(s)**. Ethiopian and Eritrean, which represent national and political entities. Until May 1993, when long-standing and bitter internal conflict that had divided the country was politically resolved, Ethiopia included Eritrea. All existing literature and community studies consider Ethiopians and Eritreans to be from the same cultural groups. However, both nations are multiethnic and multireligious, with many political factions and considerable regional variation. Despite tremendous diversity, similar core cultural values influence the behavior of most Ethiopians and Eritreans. People in northern Ethiopia and Eritrea speak the same language and have stronger cultural similarities.
- **Census**. Ethiopian and Eritrean community in the U.S. is relatively new and its exact size unknown. In 1999, a joint report by the U.S. Ethiopian and Eritrean Catholic Apostolate estimated the total population to be 250,000–350,000. Based on other community data, the total could be as high as 500,000. Lack of reliable numbers will remain a problem well into the next decade because in the 1990 and 2000 Census, Ethiopians and Eritreans were subsumed under "other" and "foreign-born."
- **History of immigration**. Before 1974, 95% of an estimated 3,000 Ethiopians/Eritreans were students who expected to return to their homeland after completing their studies. The other 5% were diplomats or persons affiliated with international organizations. Large numbers came to the U.S. in the 1980s and 1990s after 1974, when a Marxist government rose to power in Ethiopia and there was a brutal civil war in Eritrea and Tigray. Many who were residing in the U.S. decided not to return home, choosing instead to seek asylum. Most who have arrived since 1980 came as refugees under a pro-

vision of the 1990 Immigration Act that increased the number of countries whose citizens qualified for permanent visas. U.S. Immigration and Naturalization Service statistics for 1999 indicate that 14% of 33,740 African immigrants admitted to the U.S. were Ethiopians/Eritreans—the second largest group, following Nigerians—and that between 1981–99, they were the largest group of refugees/asylees from Africa. Most had urban backgrounds and resided predominantly in large cities on the East and West coasts. Young, single adults dominate: 70% are younger than 40 years. Sixty-six percent are male, 34% female. Their employment spans the job spectrum—from low-paying, "dead end" positions to esteemed positions in academia, medicine, and the high-tech electronic and computer-engineering fields.

SPIRITUAL/RELIGIOUS ORIENTATION

- **Primary religious/spiritual affiliations**. Predominantly Coptic Orthodox Christians and Muslims. Also a few Catholics, Protestants, and Jews.
- **Usual religious/spiritual practices**. Families may say prayers, read the Bible, rub patient's forehead and body with holy water, and place religious icons close to the bed or hang them above the headboard to protect patient from evil spirits and promote healing. Older patients may want a priest to visit.
- **Use of spiritual healing/healers**. No traditional Ethiopian/Eritrean healers in U.S. Healing usually the domain of older persons and religious leaders. However, the recent development of several Ethiopian and Eritrean Orthodox churches in major U.S. cities offers some access to spiritual healing by Coptic priests.
- **Holidays**. Ethiopian calendar, similar to the Coptic Egyptian calendar, has 13 months. The first 12 months have 30 days each (from September to August) and the 13th month (*Pagumiene*) has five days (six days in leap year). Ethiopian calendar runs seven or eight years behind the Gregorian year, depending on the month. The difference between calendars creates problems translating Ethiopian/Eritrean birth dates, especially among elderly immigrants. New Year's Day is either September 11 or 12 in leap years. Other holidays include Coptic Christmas (January 7); Epiphany (January 19), a Coptic religious celebration of the baptism of Christ by St. John the Baptist; and Feast of the True Cross (*Meskel*) (September 27), a specifically Ethiopian and Eritrean Coptic Orthodox religious holiday that commemorates the discovery of a piece of the cross on which Christ was crucified. The holy month of Ramadan is the ninth month of the Muslim calendar, observed by fasting from sunup to sundown.

COMMUNICATION
ORAL COMMUNICATION

- **Major languages and dialects**. Amharic is one of the major languages in Ethiopia, and Tigrigna is the national language of Eritrea and major language spoken in Northern Ethiopia. In U.S., the three major languages are Amharic, Tigrigna, and Oromigna. Most Ethiopians/Eritreans speak English: 81% have some skills, ranging from fluent to some English, but 19% have no English skills at all, particularly the elderly who have had no formal education.

- **Greetings**. Hugging, kissing on cheeks, and touching are very acceptable forms of greeting among family and friends. A woman and man, or two women, kiss on cheeks 3–4 times. Hugging and kissing between men common. Handshakes between unfamiliar persons common. Bowing is a formal, polite greeting for elders and authority figures. Proper to add "Mr." (*Ato*), "Mrs." (*Weizero*), or "Miss" (*Weizerit*) to first name when addressing adults. Names are confusing to providers of health care and social services in U.S. because there is no family name as in Western society. A person's first name is his/her given name and the second name is the father's given name, which indicates paternity. Descent is patrilineal. Only siblings with the same father have the same last name. But father's last name is first name of his father. Women do not change their last names when they marry; therefore, husband, wife, and children in a family all have different last names. To address an Ethiopian or Eritrean woman by her last name is to call her by a male name, as her last name is her father's given name. Because of the inability to understand the relationship of family members without a matching family name, the U.S. Immigration and Naturalization Service has forced some recent immigrants to take their paternal grandfather's name as their last name, confusing the situation further. Ethiopian and Eritrean women married in U.S. must use their husband's last name as their last name for insurance and other official records to avoid challenges.

- **Tone of voice**. Speak very softly, particularly women. Nonconfrontational and polite. Frown upon shouting under any circumstances.

- **Direct or indirect style of speech**. Bluntness not the norm. Most Ethiopians/Eritreans are shy and tend to give short, direct answers to any questions. Patients and family members rarely disagree with treatment procedures if they trust the health care provider. To avoid disappointing a provider, most acknowledge and agree with care regimens even when they have reservations and ultimately do not comply.

- **Use of interpreters**. Immensely important—not only to translate medical history and procedures but to help health care professionals treat patients in culturally appropriate ways. However, most interpreters live in same community as patient, know his/her family or friends, and cannot be neutral. Thus, the interpreter may be caught in an emotional conflict with the patient or in a cultural conflict with the health care provider, sometimes caused by the provider's persistence in asking culturally inappropriate questions or relating distressing information too quickly. Important to match gender of patient and interpreter.

- **Serious or terminal illness**. Communicating openly evokes strong emotional reaction in patients and family, and may even interfere with care of the dying. Vital to choose an appropriate person, time, place, and way to break bad news. Sudden shock should be avoided at all costs because of harmful effects of news on persons with fragile emotional states. Clinicians should communicate little information to patients. Whatever the diagnosis, clinicians are expected to tell bad news to a family member first; that person will decide how and when to inform patient. This varies depending on patient's age, level of understanding, and emotional and physical condition. Clinician should be selective when imparting information (e.g., avoid telling mother or wife, as women are socialized to be fragile). In the absence of a male member of the immediate family, clinician should ask for a close friend. Friendship ties strong among Ethiopians/Eritreans—even stronger when they are away from their homeland; these ties are a substitute for extended family. Ethiopians/Eritreans strongly believe in destiny and in God's power to influence events, especially health events. Their persistence in holding on to hope is tied to their religious belief in God's miraculous powers.

WRITTEN COMMUNICATION

- **Literacy assessment**. Most young persons speak, read, and write English, but some elderly Ethiopians/Eritreans have minimal or no education and need help translating and understanding medical procedures. Health care providers should ask patient if he/she can read and write in English.
- **Consents**. Most have no knowledge of treatment procedures and allow physicians to decide for them. Therefore, consent forms written for middle-class Americans are not useful for immigrants/refugees and may cause anxiety. Informing a patient of the odds of not surviving an operation or, for example, of bleeding risks or anesthesia risks only makes him/her anxious. Even when chances of an adverse outcome are statistically low, patients retain the negative information. Ethiopians/Eritreans look to physicians, nurses, and family for reassurance that they will make it through a crisis; health care providers who cite any evidence of poor prognosis undercut patient's hope and will to fight disease. In Ethiopia/Eritrea, family members sign a consent for surgery, so clinicians might consider having a designated family member sign in order to alleviate patient's anxiety.

NONVERBAL COMMUNICATION

- **Eye contact**. Little direct eye contact when speaking with authority figures. Varies depending on length of time in U.S., level of education, and age and gender.
- **Personal space**. Concept of personal space unknown. People share living space, beds, etc., with family members and friends. When talking, individuals stand closer to each other than what is acceptable in mainstream U.S. culture.
- **Use and meaning of silence**. Very commonly use silence to indicate disapproval, disappointment, and discontent with family members and health care providers.

- **Gestures**. Impolite to stare at others, frown, point finger at someone, or use one finger to beckon someone. Use whole hand to beckon.
- **Openness in expressing emotions**. Mostly stoic and shy. Men unlikely to cry, show anger, or express other emotions to strangers. Women likely to cry but usually reserved in showing anger to health care providers. Ethiopians/ Eritreans often assess physicians and nurses more by warmth of manner than by professional appearance. A few introductory words and a show of concern and interest in patient's background make him/her feel welcome. Knowing and mentioning something, however trivial, about the patient's country of origin or culture breaks the ice.
- **Privacy**. Do not easily reveal personal information, especially upon first clinical encounter. Socialized to believe that it is improper to reveal oneself fully or to disclose personal secrets to anyone other than a close friend, that others are not normally entitled to information about personal matters. Vital that clinician reassures patient about confidentiality and the importance of patient information for treatment. Clinician should discuss with a family member or spokesperson the appropriate approaches for eliciting information from patient.
- **Touch**. Touching and caressing face and hands of sick person are acceptable expressions of care, concern, and love. Touch has a healing effect. However, inappropriate to touch top of an adult's head unless touch is part of a medical procedure or necessary for care.
- **Orientation to time**. Usually late in social and business situations. Have difficulty judging distance, assessing traffic, understanding public transportation schedules, and gauging amount of time they need to get from place to place. Customary for an invitation to state that an event will begin at 6 p.m., for example, when in fact the planned starting time is 7 p.m., as guests are always expected to be late. Important that health care providers emphasize the importance of prompt arrival for appointments and adhering to medication schedule. Instead of telling patients to take their medication three or four times a day, better to give a specific time or say, for example, "Every six hours." Although tardiness illustrates their orientation to the present, Ethiopians/ Eritreans also strongly emphasize the past and future. Teaching children their cultural and family history is an important part of upbringing. They firmly believe in educating children and preventing disease.

ACTIVITIES OF DAILY LIVING

- **Modesty**. Both genders very modest. Clinician should offer hospital robes and gown, and hospital pants to males. Elderly women may wear traditional cotton shawl over gown at all times.
- **Skin care**. Varies by age and length of time in U.S. Recently arrived older patients may not want to shower every day. However, Ethiopians/Eritreans consider bathing relaxing; even older patients do not mind showering daily.

They pay close attention to hygiene and smelling good. Women like to use lotions. Some women, particularly older women, douche in the morning and at night using only lukewarm water.

- **Hair care**. Women wash their hair weekly, depending on length and texture. Those with short hair may wash twice a week. Men wash their hair each time they shower.
- **Nail care**. Men keep nails short. Among women, depends on age and personal preference. Older persons may object to cutting nails at night.
- **Toileting**. Insist on using bathroom for privacy. Bedpan uncomfortable. Worry about creating inconvenience for staff or family members.
- **Special clothing or amulets**. Religious medallions, crosses, figure of Virgin Mary or other saint, and rosary beads. Elderly women like to wear a traditional cotton shawl at all times. Muslim women may wear a special shawl to cover their heads, and amulets containing Koranic verses.
- **Self-care**. Patient performs hygiene when able. Family member or close friend may help. Women accustomed to bathing with other women and assisting each other while bathing. Older women may like assistance if family member is unavailable.

FOOD PRACTICES

- **Usual meal pattern**. Eat three times a day. Breakfast very light. Lunch and dinner are the main meals. Usually prefer very spicy food.
- **Special utensils**. Usually eat with fingers but use silverware for some types of food. Very important to wash hands before and after meals.
- **Food beliefs and rituals**. Prefer warm, soothing foods when ill (e.g., chicken or beef soup, hot oat gruel with honey, hot tea, and hot milk). No ice or cold drinks.
- **Usual diet**. Consists of *injera*, a type of bread or pancake eaten with a meat or legume sauce or with stew called *wot* or *zigni*. Make *injera* mostly from a type of cereal called *teff* but may use a mixture of cereals. Legumes important in diet; usually prepared as a very spicy stew containing a variety of condiments, including onions, garlic, hot chili powder with other spices (*berbere*), cardamom, white and black cumin, basil, and ginger. Do not commonly eat fruit and vegetables, except in larger towns and during religious fasting. Prefer chicken or beef soup, noodles and pasta, and traditional hot oat gruel with honey. Highly recommend drinks made with flax seed to soothe and promote health. Do not like bland foods.
- **Fluids**. Generally do not drink enough water or any other healthy fluids. Prefer drinks at room temperature. Like to drink coffee and to spice tea with cinnamon, cloves, cardamom, and lots of sugar.
- **Food taboos and prescriptions**. Coptic Orthodox Christians and Muslims strictly observe religious taboos that forbid eating the meat of wild animals (including pigs and fowl), snakes, domestic pigs, dogs, horses, and shellfish.

Muslims avoid eating from vessels in which pork may have been served or cooked. Coptic Christians do not eat meat or dairy for 200 days of each year. Religious and elderly groups strictly avoid meat and dairy products for 50 days before Easter, although Ethiopians/Eritreans in U.S. are less likely to observe this proscription than are those in homeland. Some elders follow the strict religious norms of not eating meals until noon and, in some cases, eating only one meal a day, a potential concern for patients who depend on regular food intake or take medications several times daily. Clinician should ask Coptic Orthodox Christian patient if he/she fasts accordingly and remind him/her that the church exempts persons on medication from skipping meals. All major U.S. cities have one or two Coptic churches; if necessary, clinician can refer patient to the head priest for counseling.

- **Hospitality**. Offering visitors food and coffee is an important Ethiopian/Eritrean cultural norm. Offer guests the best seat in the house, the best plate, the best food, etc. Children usually relinquish their beds to guests. Parents relinquish their beds to elderly relatives.

SYMPTOM MANAGEMENT

- **Pain**. Stoic. Have high pain threshold. Patients do not explain symptoms clearly; have difficulty pinpointing symptoms, explain them in very general terms, and do not understand numerical scale for rating pain. Do not like to use pain medication for extended period, due to concern about addiction. Older women usually moan, are passive, and behave as if very helpless. Accept pain medication to relieve acute pain. Commonly use nonpharmacological measures to manage pain.

- **Dyspnea**. Hyperventilate and panic. Family members also panic and hover over sick person. Use oxygen but need reassurance, as they associate oxygen and other major interventions with grave disease. Clinician should explain necessity of oxygen to family members because their panic increases patient's anxiety level.

- **Nausea/vomiting**. May alert family member or nurse before vomiting and ask for medication. Tend to clean up or throw away vomitus. Clinician should explain to patient and family caregiver the importance of waiting for nurse before throwing away vomitus. Traditionally use lemon peel, ginger root, rue, or fennel to control nausea.

- **Constipation/diarrhea**. Disclose these conditions only when asked. Traditional remedies for constipation include herbs, castor oil, Epsom salts, or some form of laxative. For diarrhea, recommend eating rice or drinking rice water. Do not recognize the dehydration associated with diarrhea, so patient should be encouraged to drink fluids.

- **Fatigue**. Older persons like to nap after lunch. Overall, very hesitant to accept sleeping pills for fear of strong effect and future dependency.

- **Depression**. Ethiopians/Eritreans express anxiety and depression somatically and deny any relationship between worries and vague complaints for which there is no apparent physical cause. View psychiatry negatively. Resist seeking help from mental health counselors because of cultural stigma associated with mental illness.

- **Self-care symptom management**. Use home remedies and other means first. Delay seeking professional help until pain is severe. Most do not understand chronic illness well and are not good about taking medications on time, especially in absence of pain.

BIRTH RITUALS/CARE OF THE NEW MOTHER AND BABY

- **Pregnancy care**. Traditionally, consider pregnancy a dangerous state, as fetus could be easy prey for the evil eye and sorcery, which are believed to cause miscarriage, premature delivery, or fetal malformation. Family members and others give expectant mother much attention. She is to avoid excess activity—e.g., carrying heavy loads and climbing stairs—and exposure to emotional situations, such as funerals, fights, and bad news. Encouraged to eat well, get plenty of sleep, and forego day-to-day tasks that require bending and lifting. Ethiopians/Eritreans pay special attention to cravings for particular foods, generally believing that unfulfilled craving will cause miscarriage. Expectant mother is encouraged to walk and move around as due date approaches. Traditionally, she drinks a hot mixture of ground, toasted flax seed and water sweetened with honey or sugar (which is believed to ease labor or act as a laxative) one week before due date.

- **Preferences for children**. Ethiopian/Eritrean families prefer male first-born, due to cultural expectation that eldest son is responsible for looking after siblings economically and protecting family's honor if father dies prematurely. Father congratulated when first-born is a boy. Younger brothers and sisters address an older brother using a special family title that reflects his role as family's protector. Overall, however, this cultural expectation does not make the birth of a girl any less important. Mothers prefer daughters because they are assumed to be emotionally closer to the mother and can help with household chores. Most believe that the number and sex of children is God's will. Others do not look negatively upon a woman who has given birth only to girls. Large families—average of five children—are traditional. Most Ethiopians/Eritreans in U.S. have fewer children.

- **Labor practices**. Self-trained midwife or older, female family member traditionally assists with delivery. Urban women are accustomed to hospital delivery. Expectant mothers tolerate labor pain and prefer female family members and friends to be present to provide comfort and massage their back and feet. May be hesitant to take pain medication. Labor practices among women in U.S. vary depending on education level. Most accept whatever is allowed in birth setting.

- **Role of the laboring woman during birth**. Takes active role. Modesty very important, so she must be kept covered. Low level of moaning or grunting socially acceptable; screaming unacceptable.

- **Role of the father and other family members during birth**. Traditionally, father and male family members not allowed to be with birthing woman. In U.S., young fathers participate in childbirth preparation classes and stay close to their wives during delivery.
- **Vaginal vs. cesarean section**. Prefer vaginal delivery. Many Ethiopians/ Eritreans think American doctors are too quick to perform cesarean sections for what Ethiopians/Eritreans consider to be normal variations in labor. Expectant mothers may wait at home until well into labor to avoid unwanted procedures. Women prefer female doctors and interpreters, especially for childbirth.
- **Breastfeeding**. Traditionally, mothers breastfeed for an average of 23 months or longer. No taboo against breastfeeding in public. Women prefer to breastfeed as much as possible; however, working mothers bottle-feed as well as breastfeed. Women eat special foods and drink milk and gruel made from oats and honey to increase their breast milk.
- **Birth recuperation**. Female family members help new mother care for and bathe baby. Consider both mother and baby to be delicate and make every effort to protect them from disease and harm. Prescribe 40 days seclusion postpartum. Mother fed special foods (e.g., porridge made from barley and other cereals, meat, and chicken stew). Her food and drinks must be warm. Family and friends celebrate childbirth with gifts for mother and baby, and joyous sharing of food.
- **Baby care**. New mother expected to be with baby 24 hours a day. Mothers and female members of family mainly care for infant; female members of extended family available to help. Husbands and other male family members not expected to care for infants, except for short play periods. Young immigrant males in U.S. share infant care responsibilities.
- **Problems with baby**. Best to consult with father or other male family member. Clinician should not tell mother or any female members of immediate family. Should ask spokesperson for advice.
- **Male and female circumcision**. Among Christians, male circumcision traditionally performed eight days after birth. In urban settings and in U.S., common to allow baby boys to be circumcised before hospital discharge. Female circumcision and clitoridectomy practiced throughout homeland. This tradition varies according to regional practices, urban/rural settings, religion, and level of parents' education. Most urban and educated families in Ethiopia/Eritrea do not follow these traditions. Most common procedure among Christians is excision of prepuce seven days after birth. Do not perceive this practice as an initiation or rite of passage; it essentially takes place before the child has an identity. Muslims practice infibulation—removing labia minora and clitoris, sewing the labia majora, and leaving a small hole

for urination and menstruation. This varies according to geographic area, social class, religion, and education.

DEVELOPMENTAL AND SEXUAL ISSUES

- **Celebration of menarche or becoming a man**. No special practices.
- **Attitudes about birth control**. Contraceptives not widely available in Ethiopia/Eritrea, but contraceptive use has increased among younger women in urban areas. Do not openly discuss contraceptives. Many in U.S. readily accept contraceptives, but acceptance varies by level of education, religious beliefs, and length of time in U.S.
- **Attitudes about sexually transmitted infection (STI) control, including condoms**. Have limited knowledge about STIs. Condom use varies depending on education, age, and religious beliefs.
- **Attitudes about abortion**. Abortion is stigmatized and not a common practice in the culture as a whole. For Ethiopians/Eritreans, miscarriage and abortion mean the same thing.
- **Attitudes about unwed sexual experimentation**. Do not allow dating and sexual activity before marriage. Out-of-wedlock pregnancy brings tremendous shame on the family and girl. If the pregnancy is discovered early, girl's parents insist on marriage before it becomes obvious so they can conceal the situation. Ethiopian/Eritrean immigrant youth want to follow the norms for dating in American society, which has become a major cause of intergenerational conflict.
- **Sexual orientation**. Community shuns the very few Ethiopian/Eritrean men and women in U.S. who are openly gay. It does not acknowledge gay and lesbian couples.
- **Gender identity**. Ambiguous gender identity strongly stigmatized and not discussed openly. Child with ambiguous gender identity is assigned a gender at parents' discretion; however, there is no attempt to change the child's identity surgically or otherwise.
- **Attitudes about menopause**. Most women experience menopause after they have fulfilled their reproductive responsibilities. It indicates to them they no longer can bear children. Menopause frees women to attend religious duties without restrictions (menstruating women are not allowed to attend church). Being menopausal does not affect a woman's sexual relations with her husband. In some groups, widowed menopausal women become sexual mentors for young males. Women do not talk about menopause and never refer to it as a health concern. Traditionally, there are no particular associated symptoms. Menopause is not something that requires coping strategies.

FAMILY RELATIONSHIPS

- **Composition/structure**. Extended family is the most important institution. However, among mostly young, single persons in U.S., close friends substitute for extended family. Typical household of Ethiopians/Eritreans in U.S. consists of siblings, cousins, and friends. Common in these groups to introduce a childhood friend or very close friend as a sibling.

- **Decision-making**. Family members make decisions together. Traditionally, father or eldest son plays leading role. In U.S., even if father is living with family, most-acculturated family member leads decision-making.

- **Spokesperson**. Father, eldest son, or daughter. In U.S., the most-acculturated family member is spokesperson. Close friend can substitute in absence of appropriate family member.

- **Gender issues**. Men are in charge of duties such as breaking bad news, making funeral arrangements, arranging religious services, and taking care of financial needs. Although urban women in Ethiopia/Eritrea work in offices, responsibilities such as cooking, cleaning, and caring for family are still theirs. Some married immigrant men persistently adhere to traditional gender roles, a source of family conflict.

- **Changing roles among generations in U.S.** Because children and young immigrants adjust faster than adults do in U.S., parents and older adults whose roles included providing guidance in everyday life now depend on their children as mediators in, and interpreters of, American culture. This role reversal puts children in difficult situations at times; at a very young age, they end up as the main communicators of illness and grave diagnoses to their parents. This is emotionally stressful for both parents and children.

- **Caring roles**. Expect female family members (e.g., mothers, grandmothers, sisters, cousins) or close friends to care for sick person. In absence of close female family member, husbands and brothers provide care. During illness and crisis, Ethiopians/Eritreans rely heavily on family members to help them cope.

- **Expectations of and for children**. Prolong and indulge infancy. Raise children in a highly protective environment. From about age 3, subject children to a discipline regimen. Obedience and politeness are overriding goals in raising children. Discourage physical aggression. Emphasize a quiet, reserved manner of speaking. View noisy, disrespectful children as rude. Strongly emphasize education. Children remain deeply attached to their family and are sensitive to parents' wishes. Children responsible for taking care of elderly parents.

- **Expectations of and for elders**. Children respect and look after their elders. Elders play major role in raising and disciplining grandchildren. Traditionally, elders receive care at home; nursing home or hospice unacceptable.

- **Expectations of hospital visitors**. Friends and family members come throughout the day to visit patient. Ethiopian/Eritrean patients do not like to be left alone. Family and friends want to stay at bedside at all times, especially when patient's illness is grave.

ILLNESS BELIEFS

- **Causes of/attitudes about physical illness**. Have two broad etiological theories of disease: naturalistic and magico-religious. In naturalistic etiology, sickness may result from external factors, such as drinking polluted water, eating unfamiliar or spoiled food, contagion, excess sun exposure, exposure to cold wind, interpersonal conflict, or personal excess (e.g., emotional distress). In magico-religious etiology, attribute illness to God, nature and demonic spirits, magical forces, or breach of social taboos or personal vows. In general, Ethiopians/Eritreans strongly believe in the notion of destiny and in God's power to influence events. Do not readily understand illnesses that have no symptoms.

- **Causes of/attitudes about mental illness**. Traditionally, Ethiopians/Eritreans routinely attributed mental illness and epilepsy to evil spirits. Families do not disclose any kind of mental illness to others for fear of being shunned. Generally, people avoid marrying into families with mentally ill siblings or parents. Mental illness stigma is as strong among immigrants in U.S. as in homeland. Therapy should be active and include the family. Community generally resists psychiatric treatment.

- **Causes of genetic defects**. Accept them as God's will. Expect family members to care for child at home. Frown upon institutionalization.

- **Attitudes about disabilities**. Highly stigmatized. Family cares for disabled member, but he/she is not visible when strangers visit nor taken out in public.

- **Sick role**. Sick person behaves helplessly and passively; totally depends on family members. Customary for family to bring home-cooked, soothing foods to patient. Family members alter their schedules to attend to needs of sick persons, pampering them with attention and services, and protecting them from emotional upsets. Family members do not encourage patient to be independent. Health care providers must stress and reinforce importance of ambulation.

- **Home and folk remedies**. Largely derive pharmacopoeias from the natural world: plants, grains, spices, oil seeds, herbs, and butter. Popular remedies for headache include coffee and lemon tea; for colds, boiling or smelling eucalyptus leaves. Most immigrants rely on Western biomedicine, but some bring medicinal herbs from their homeland. Current popularity in U.S. of herbal medicine is very appealing to them. Best to ask patient if he/she is taking any herbal substances, including teas.

- **Medications**. Because they do not readily understand a disease that has no symptoms, important for clinician to emphasize the need to complete the full course of prescribed antibiotics, and to explain that some conditions, such as hypertension, are risky even if there are no symptoms. If an elder is fasting or takes one meal per day for religious reasons, he/she may miss doses of medications that should be taken multiple times daily. Patient may double or triple doses to make up for those he/she missed.

- **Acceptance of procedures**. Clinician should explain procedures clearly to patient and family members. They rarely disagree if they trust the health care provider. Fear surgery and donating or receiving blood.

- **Care-seeking**. Generally delay seeking medical attention. Consult family and friends about major concerns before seeing clinician. Self-care in households without access to professional healers is common throughout Ethiopia/Eritrea. In U.S., most rely on Western biomedicine and do not have folk healers. However, they consider folk medicine to be better for some illnesses. Some return to homeland for treatment.

HEALTH ISSUES

- **Concept of health**. A state of equilibrium among physiological, spiritual, cosmological, ecological, and social forces. Believe that one achieves well-being by securing a peaceful relationship with the supernatural world. Traditionally, identify illness by the presence of symptoms and measure wellness by their absence.

- **Health promotion and prevention**. Believe that proper function of body depends on physiological balance and adequate food intake. Eating and drinking moderately, avoiding emotional distress, never bathing in cold water, avoiding exposure to atmospheric changes, and cleanliness promote health. Generally discourage a sedentary lifestyle. Although a few immigrants exercise at a gym or on their own, most lead a sedentary lifestyle because of work demands and lack of time.

- **Screening**. In Ethiopian/Eritrean culture, patient-healer relationship is paternalistic and protective; trust is a major component. Generally do not like to visit clinician for routine examination but accept screening when suggested. Modesty may be an issue when they avoid screening.

- **Common health problems**. Long-term effects of malnutrition, war trauma (physical and psychological), and a variety of infectious diseases, including malaria and tuberculosis. High prevalence of hepatitis B, cervical cancer, and sexually transmitted infections. Drastic changes in lifestyle and diet since immigration have increased the risk of high blood-lipid levels, diabetes, and hypertension.

DEATH RITUALS

- **Beliefs and attitudes about death**. Death is the most ritualized of all life stages in Ethiopian/Eritrean societies. Religious traditions shape perceptions of life and death. Overall cultural belief is that God gives and takes away life. But Ethiopians/Eritreans grieve bitterly when death separates them from a loved one, and lament even more the death of a young person who has no offspring. Consider suicide a sin; it does not warrant traditional church ceremonies and prayers.

- **Preparation**. Culturally important *how* tragic news is communicated. Ethiopians/Eritreans disclose news of family member's impending or actual death to close friends before telling family so friends will be there to provide emotional support. Never tell female family member first. Spokesperson may arrange for Coptic priest (where available) or religious figure to administer sacrament to patient.

- **Home vs. hospital.** Traditionally, dealing with death was the domain of older persons, who preferred that loved ones die at home. But in U.S., where immigrants are mostly young and urban, prefer that patient remain in hospital.

- **Special needs.** Ethiopians/Eritreans mostly refrain from emotional outbursts, except when a loved one dies; at such times, they encourage great demonstrations of feeling. Cry loudly and uncontrollably. Women tear their clothes and beat their chests until they become sick with grief. Men permitted to cry out loud and shed tears. Mourning marked by religious prayers and gatherings. Christian women wear black for a year when a close family member dies; some shave their hair or cut it very short, remove jewelry, and avoid make-up. Men wear a black tie and grow a beard. Close family and friends stay together for the first week; food and drinks are brought to the mourning family.

- **Care of the body.** Ethiopian/Eritrean communities in U.S. accept standard preparation of body at morgue. Some family members want to say good-bye before body is taken to morgue, but this is not customary and may vary. Throughout the homeland, people bury their dead. Cremation unacceptable unless specified.

- **Attitudes about organ donation.** Organ donation a new concept for immigrants. Clinician should check with family members. Very few immigrants have had organ transplants and generally are reluctant to donate organs. This attitude varies by age and length of time in U.S.

- **Attitudes about autopsy.** Autopsy unacceptable unless family is convinced it is medically necessary.

SELECTED REFERENCES

Beyene, Y. (1992). Medical disclosure and refugees: Telling bad news to Ethiopian patients. *Western Journal of Medicine, 157,* 328–332.

Gavagan, T., & Brodyaga, L. (1998). Medical care for immigrants and refugees. *American Family Physician, 57,* 1061–1068.

Kloos, H., & Zein, A. Z. (Eds.) (1993). *The ecology of health and disease in Ethiopia.* Boulder, CO: Westview Press.

AUTHOR

Yewoubdar Beyene, PhD, is an associate professor in the Department of Social and Behavioral Sciences in the School of Nursing and in the Department of Anthropology, History and Social Medicine in the School of Medicine at the University of California-San Francisco. She was born and raised in Ethiopia and came to the U.S. as a college student. She studies immigrant and refugee health, with a focus on African immigrants in the U.S.

CHAPTER 14

FILIPINOS

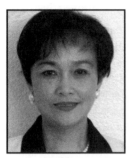
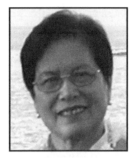
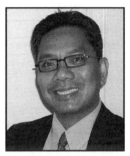

Daisy M.
Rodriguez

Carolina P.
de Guzman

Arthur Cantos

CULTURAL/ETHNIC IDENTITY

- **Preferred term(s)**. Filipino American. Filipino is accepted English spelling, although correct spelling is Pilipino; there is no "F" in the Philippine alphabet.
- **Census**. The 2000 U.S. Census reported 2.4 million Filipinos, including the 1.9 million who described themselves only as Filipino and 500,000 who described themselves as being a combination of Filipino and one or more other races or Asian groups. Sixty-four percent are foreign-born.
- **History of immigration**. First immigrants possibly were men from Manila who deserted Spanish galleons in Mexico and settled in New Orleans in the early 1700s. The first wave of immigration (1903–10) consisted of young, bright Filipino men sponsored by a U.S. government program who attended American educational institutions. The second wave, after World War I, was the Manong generation. (*Manong* is a title of respect for elderly men from the Ilocos region.) These poorly educated male agricultural workers settled in Hawaii and the western U.S. There they experienced low pay and discrimination, and were prevented from owning property, intermarrying, and becoming citizens. The third wave began in 1965 after the U.S. quota system ended. Third-wave immigrants are well-educated and have caused a "brain drain" in the Philippines. These immigrants often work in health care, education, and engineering. They include more women than men.

SPIRITUAL/RELIGIOUS ORIENTATION

- **Primary religious/spiritual affiliations**. Predominantly Roman Catholic, as a result of four centuries of Spanish colonization. Other religions include

Protestantism, Islam (mostly in the southern Philippines), and other Christian sects, as well as sects such as *Iglesia ni Cristo*, *Aglipayans*, and Mormons.

- **Usual religious/spiritual practices**. Most are church-going, pray the rosary, believe in the power of saints, use religious objects, and observe religious holidays. Religious sacraments for the sick or dying are important to Roman Catholics.
- **Use of spiritual healing/healers**. Immigrants come from a country with very limited access to health care, especially in the lower socioeconomic classes. Traditional Filipinos often use faith healers or herbalists (*herbolarios*). More-cosmopolitan Filipinos use Western biomedicine but may still use spiritual healers. Some persons use water obtained from religious icons, believing it can cure diseases. Healers generally do not discourage clients from seeing physicians.
- **Holidays**. Labor Day (May 1), Independence Day (June 12), National Heroes Day (last Sunday of August), All Saints Day (November 1), Bonifacio Day (November 30), and Rizal Day (December 30).

COMMUNICATION
ORAL COMMUNICATION

- **Major languages and dialects**. National language is Pilipino (Tagalog), but different ethnic and subethnic groups speak about 85 other languages and dialects, including Ilocano, Visayan (Cebuano, Ilongo, Boholano), Waray, Bicolano, Pampango, and Ibanag. Filipinos are divided geographically and culturally; each region has distinct traits and dialects. There are about 7,100 islands in the Philippines; the three largest are Luzon, Visayas, and Mindanao. Use English in schools, government, business, and media.
- **Greetings**. Filipinos smile a lot, to greet or acknowledge. May greet with a quick lifting of the eyebrows. Handshake not uncommon but not standard. Respectful greetings of older persons may include a bow or kissing the hand, forehead, or cheeks. Formal address is "Mr.," "Mrs.," or appropriate title with last name. Elders addressed with respectful terms, such as Grandmother (*Lola*), Grandfather (*Lolo*), *Manong* (for an older man), and *Manang* (for an older woman). Other respectful terms common in the Tagalog region of central Luzon are "yes," "yes, sir," and "yes, ma'am" (*po*, *opo*, *ho*, and *oho* are interchangeable).
- **Tone of voice**. Filipinos are typically soft-spoken and uncomfortable giving commands. Can be loud and animated with family. Sensitive to the way they are spoken to and to tone of speaker's voice. May perceive a health care provider who speaks loudly as angry and disrespectful. Prefer a polite request to a blunt command.
- **Direct or indirect style of speech**. Indirect and polite. Mostly avoid confrontation or direct expression of disagreement so as not to give offense and cause loss of face. Emphasize smooth relationships. Show respect for elders

and authorities, including health care professionals. May not question health care providers, even if they do not fully understand an issue. May acknowledge a message or express agreement by nodding head, not verbally. May give brief answers to questions.

- **Use of interpreters**. English proficiency seldom an issue for young persons but may be a problem for older persons educated under Spanish regime. Generally understand English better than they speak it. If necessary, a family member or friend can interpret, help fill out forms, and provide information regarding an illness.
- **Serious or terminal illness**. Discuss prognosis with head of the family, eldest son, or eldest daughter first before disclosing it to patient. Clinician should allow patient's family to disclose prognosis the way it prefers to. Family may request presence of physician, registered nurse, or social worker.

WRITTEN COMMUNICATION

- **Literacy assessment**. Elderly persons and those with minimal or no education may need help reading or writing English. Clinician should ask patient directly if he/she can read and write in English. If an interpreter is necessary, should ensure that he/she speaks same dialect as patient.
- **Consents**. Clinician should avoid medical jargon, encourage questions, and ask patient to confirm his/her understanding.

NONVERBAL COMMUNICATION

- **Eye contact**. Generally avoid direct eye, especially women and particularly with superiors and authority figures. Sustained direct eye contact may mean anger or aggressiveness. Fleeting eye contact with the opposite sex might signal physical attraction.
- **Personal space**. Require little personal space. New immigrants often share living space with family and friends. Patient may be uncomfortable leaving small hospital room. Family members and friends often present at the bedside. Expect outsiders and health care providers to show respect by standing at least an arm's length away.
- **Use and meaning of silence**. May mean approval, disapproval, disappointment, lack of understanding, or aloofness. To avert misunderstanding, clinician should ask patient what silence means.
- **Gestures**. Traditional Filipinos show respect for elders by touching elder's hand to their forehead (*mano*) as a way of greeting. Stand when a person of authority enters room and relinquish seat to older person. May point to an object by shifting eyes toward it or by pursing their lips and pointing with their mouth, rather than pointing with hand. Filipinos may smile as acknowledgment, or raise both eyebrows, instead of responding verbally. Inappropriate, offensive, or disrespectful gestures include pointing a finger directly at someone, putting hands on hips when addressing an older person,

or, for young persons, staring back when an elder admonishes them.
- **Openness in expressing emotions**. To avoid offending others, may say "yes" or nod head in agreement even if they disagree. May not express personal feelings openly for fear of losing face. Men have difficulty acknowledging or expressing emotions. Women express emotions more openly. Family members and close friends express emotions more freely with each other. Openly disagreeing or raising one's voice signals disrespect. Filipinos use silence instead of verbal confrontation.
- **Privacy**. Value privacy in family matters and very often do not verbalize their feelings to outsiders. Privacy related to sensitivity to shame (*hiya*) and preserving self-esteem (*amor propio*). Close family members share feelings and information freely. Strong respect for authority figures enables disclosure of health information. Most Filipinos private about sexual topics, tuberculosis, or other contagious diseases.
- **Touch**. Typically demonstrative when greeting close friends and relatives; they hug and kiss each other on the cheeks. Touching, patting, or putting arms on other person's shoulders is a sign of closeness. Holding hands acceptable among females who have a close relationship. Unacceptable for men to touch women in public. Women demonstrate modesty by avoiding outward demonstration of affection with men. Before touching patient, clinician should ask permission and explain the need to touch. This will avoid embarrassment and protect patient's modesty.
- **Orientation to time**. Oriented to both past and present. Concept of future influenced by an attitude of "God willing" (*bahala na*), which reflects a fatalistic outlook on life. One should unquestioningly accept whatever life brings. Distinguish between social and business time. "Filipino time" means being late to social gatherings. Acculturated persons are prompt for appointments, work, and church. Clinician should emphasize and reiterate importance of being on time for appointments and adhering to medication schedules.

ACTIVITIES OF DAILY LIVING
- **Modesty**. Extremely modest, especially young and unmarried women, who prefer health care provider of same gender. Clinician should ensure privacy when patient toilets and bathes. Should offer robe with hospital gown, and hospital pants to male patients.
- **Skin care**. Women protect skin against the sun, particularly their face. Some use "whitening cream" to lighten face. Prefer to shower daily in the morning. Concerned about hygiene. Some prefer soap and water peri-wash after every bowel movement or urination.
- **Hair care**. Wash and shampoo/condition while showering. Prefer to air dry rather than use hair dryer. Women with longer hair may put it in a bun. Some traditional women believe that cutting hair on Fridays is bad luck. Do not sleep when hair is still wet.

- **Nail care**. Women keep fingernails a bit longer, and some do their own manicure. Women are meticulous about hand and foot care, using lotions and moisturizing cream. Men keep their nails short. Considered bad luck to cut nails at night or on Fridays.

- **Toileting**. Insist on using bathroom rather than bedpan or urinal for privacy and for thorough peri-wash. Health care providers should offer a small plastic pitcher for pouring water. Use bedside commode if necessary but want privacy. If patient unable to get out of bed, caregivers should offer baby wipes or a damp wash cloth so he/she can cleanse perineal area or rectum.

- **Special clothing or amulets**. Possibly religious medallions, rosary beads, or an image of a saint in patient's room. Clinician should ask permission to remove such items if necessary to do so and explain the reason. Some want an object pinned to hospital gown when going into surgery.

- **Self-care**. Patient performs self-care when able, or a family member helps. If no one available to help, patient accepts hospital personnel.

FOOD PRACTICES

- **Usual meal pattern**. Light breakfast and moderate to heavy lunch and dinner. May snack between meals.

- **Special utensils**. Most use fork and spoon. Use spoon rather than fork as primary utensil. In rural areas, some do not use any utensils at all; use hands instead.

- **Food beliefs and rituals**. Prefer soft and warm food when ill. Drink water and other fluids without ice.

- **Usual diet**. Prefer rice with most meals. After surgery, start with rice porridge (*lugao*) until they can tolerate regular diet. May bring food from home. Like salty and fried food, as well as soups. Add salt, fish sauce, or soy sauce to food at the table to enhance flavor. In the morning, many dislike chilled or acidic food, such as fruit juice and fresh fruit. There are regional preferences for recipes and cooking methods. For example, those from northeastern Philippines prefer stewed vegetables cooked in salty anchovy sauce, while those from southern Luzon (Bicol region) prefer cooking with coconut milk and chilies.

- **Fluids**. Lots of water at meals. Also juices, soft drinks, or coffee.

- **Food taboos and prescriptions**. Some Filipinos are lactose intolerant, others may have difficulty digesting wheat bread. Some Catholics do not eat meat on Fridays during Lent. Some believe in humoral theory of balancing "hot"/"cold" foods and in eating moderately to maintain health. Some eat garlic daily for hypertension or drink ginger tea for digestion. Believe that bitter melon prevents diabetes.

- **Hospitality**. Filipinos use food to express themselves, welcome guests, soothe the body, and celebrate. Hospital visitors bring home-cooked meals or food bought at Filipino bakeries rather than flowers. Expect health care providers to partake of some delicacies they bring to hospital.

SYMPTOM MANAGEMENT

- **Pain** (*masakit*). Generally stoic. May refuse pain medication; reluctant to accept narcotics out of fear of addiction. Some understand numerical scale to describe pain level. Generally prefer oral medications to other routes of administration. Often try nonpharmacological methods before going to clinic or hospital.

- **Dyspnea** (*mahirap huminga* or *hindi makahinga*—"hard to breathe" or "cannot breathe"). Clinician may need to explain use of numbers to describe level of dyspnea. Patient may be anxious about using oxygen because it implies more serious illness. May be receptive to relaxation techniques to ease symptoms.

- **Nausea/vomiting** (*nasusuka* or *napapasuka*). Because of modesty and shame, patient alerts health care provider only after vomiting. Some clean up or throw away vomitus. Some ask for nausea medication. Clinician may need to explain use of numbers to describe severity of nausea/vomiting. Usually prefer IV rather than rectal medications.

- **Constipation/diarrhea**. Regular bowel movements enable body to maintain balance. Diarrhea more common than constipation because of prevalence of gastrointestinal diseases. Due to modesty and shame, patient may disclose symptoms of diarrhea or constipation only if health care provider asks. Consider enema a last resort. Accept dietary and other measures to correct alteration in bowel function.

- **Fatigue** (*pagod*—"tired"). May take afternoon naps. Expressions of fatigue may signify a physical or emotional ailment, although patient may not acknowledge an emotional cause. Rather than verbally express depression, anger, sadness, or frustration, may simply withdraw and sleep. Generally hesitant to use sleeping pills, out of fear of addiction, but may use vitamins, herbal formulations, or traditional remedies to combat fatigue, increase energy level, or promote sleep.

- **Depression** (*lungkot*—"sad"). Common among immigrants. May be temporary; prolonged separation may cause pathological symptoms. Filipinos may not verbally acknowledge depression, but it may be manifested by withdrawal and not eating. Marital separation also may cause depression (divorce is illegal in the Philippines). Medication for depression generally unacceptable because of shame (*hiya*) related to stigma of mental illness. Religious persons usually pray.

- **Self-care symptom management**. Usually use herbal and home remedies before seeing a physician, or take them concurrently with prescribed medications. Clinician should emphasize importance of timely medical consultation and make patient aware of possible interaction of herbs and home remedies with prescribed medications. Fatalistic attitude (*bahala na*) may influence self-care in chronic illness. For example, it may hinder willingness to comply with diabetes diet or insulin regimens.

BIRTH RITUALS/CARE OF THE NEW MOTHER AND BABY

- **Pregnancy care**. Traditionally, pregnant woman not allowed to work outside the home. Encouraged to eat well and given a choice of food. Some believe that first trimester food cravings must be satisfied to protect fetus. She is encouraged to get ample sleep and avoid prolonged sitting to avert water retention. Less-acculturated Filipinos may believe that if a pregnant woman encounters a deformed or disabled person or animal that frightens her, it can affect the developing fetus. Encouraged, but not required, to stay indoors. Sexual intercourse taboo during last two months of pregnancy. Near term, traditional woman encouraged to eat fresh eggs (and other slippery food) to facilitate the baby "slipping" through the birth canal.
- **Preferences for children**. Chinese Filipinos have very strong preference for boys, but other families care less. Fathers, in particular, want a boy to carry on family name. Some couples continue to try to produce a male offspring. Sons receive preferential treatment, especially in Chinese Filipino families. Filipinos value all of their children and do not neglect girls. Mothers may prefer girls, who help with household chores.
- **Labor practices**. Traditionally, upon first labor contraction, self-trained midwife (*hilot*) summoned to expectant mother's house. Laboring woman discouraged from eating. She usually takes a shower in early labor. She is encouraged to walk around before the membranes rupture because walking promotes dilatation. *Hilot* stays with her constantly and helps make her comfortable (e.g., by rubbing her back and abdomen during contractions). Noise and commotion kept to a minimum, as they are thought to increase labor pain. If physician absent during labor, *hilot* assists in delivery. Laboring woman may refuse pain medication.
- **Role of the laboring woman during birth**. Verbalizes pain in various ways. Demands attention, pampering, and solicitude from husband and family members.
- **Role of the father and other family members during birth**. Family focuses on the delivering mother. Father generally plays a passive role and is not present during birth unless the couple has taken childbirth preparation classes. Some fathers remain at work or with their male friends for support. A female family member who has given birth serves as labor coach, staying with expectant mother throughout the process.
- **Vaginal vs. cesarean section**. Prefer vaginal delivery. Accept cesarean section when medically necessary.
- **Breastfeeding**. Breastfeeding on demand is an expectation of all Filipino mothers, especially rural Filipinas—sometimes until child is a toddler. Some mothers may mix breast- and bottle-feeding because of work demands outside the home, but breastfeeding continues until child is at least 1 year old.
- **Birth recuperation**. New mother stays with baby 24 hours a day. Her mother, a sister, and the baby's father or her in-laws share most care and

household tasks. Traditional practice is bed rest for one week to one entire month postpartum, during which the mother is freed from heavy housework. Fear that if the new mother does heavy work too soon, she may experience a "relapse" that manifests as extreme tiredness, weakness, and chronic headache. She is given nourishing soups made with meat and vegetables that are believed to promote lactation. Traditionally, new mother does not bathe for 10 days after giving birth. Perineal care involves washing with soap and water, adding some drops of vinegar to the warm water, or using a warm solution made from boiled guava leaves and ashes from the cooking stove. In Philippines, midwife (*hilot*) visits new mother daily to give her a whole-body massage, with special emphasis on the uterus. Uterine massage and use of a pelvic girdle are believed to help in involution of uterus. Critical for new mother to avoid cold drinks and exposure to cold breezes during postpartum period. Her room window should be closed and she should wear socks, long skirt, and long-sleeve shirt or sweater. Exposure to cold believed to predispose mother to arthritic conditions.

- **Baby care**. Mother is most important caregiver. Maid or nanny is second most important caregiver for infants and toddlers in families that can afford such care. Otherwise, a female member of extended family who lives with the family usually helps with child care. In U.S., fathers take active part in child care if no members of extended family live in the home.
- **Problems with baby**. Best to consult with father and other family support persons, such as woman's mother, before breaking the news to new mother. Physician must be the one who informs her.
- **Male and female circumcision**. Male circumcision traditionally performed at puberty, not at birth. Some parents allow circumcision before discharge from hospital. Female circumcision never practiced.

DEVELOPMENTAL AND SEXUAL ISSUES

- **Celebration of menarche or becoming a man**. No formal ritual to celebrate menarche. Several folk practices at first menses are believed to make future menstruation easier. Jumping off the bottom three stairs limits menstruation to three days; sitting on a banana leaf prevents blood-stained clothing even during heaviest days; stepping over a blooming flower three times while clutching a cotton ball ensures a fragrant smell and prevents feeling heavy/burdened during menstruation. Girl is asked to take a bath to ensure she will be able to bathe during all future menses without getting sick. In Philippines, many rural women prohibited from bathing lest they go insane. Traditionally, male circumcision performed on boys at puberty, when hair growth and voice changes begin. In rural areas and among those who cannot afford to have the procedure done in a clinic, a trained male member of the community (*manunule*) performs circumcision.
- **Attitudes about birth control**. Catholicism strongly influences norms in

Philippines. Abstinence from premarital sex highly valued; therefore, birth control for unmarried women not usually discussed. Only acceptable and most commonly used birth control method is natural family planning (rhythm method and fertility awareness). Degree of acculturation significantly influences Filipinos' decision to use contraceptives.

- **Attitudes about sexually transmitted infection (STI) control, including condoms**. Some awareness of STI control among educated Filipinos, but sexual health education is unavailable to less-educated persons and those in rural areas. In Philippines, inadequate condom supplies and affordability can pose barriers to condom use. In U.S., some immigrant men continue having unprotected sex and some may dislike using condoms, as evidenced by the high incidence of HIV/AIDS.
- **Attitudes about abortion**. Uncommon in Philippines—illegal and against laws of the Catholic Church. Culture is child-centered. Abortion evokes strong reactions even in liberal Filipino Americans. Some support the right to an abortion in the abstract but may experience difficulty and guilt in exercising this option. In U.S., more-acculturated women access abortion services without the knowledge and consent of family.
- **Attitudes about unwed sexual experimentation**. In Philippines, adolescent dating not sanctioned. Reportedly, first sexual experiences typically occur at age 18 among both genders. In U.S., first sexual experience among adolescent and unmarried Filipino women may occur at a younger age because social environment is generally more tolerant regarding sex.
- **Sexual orientation**. Filipino family usually tolerates, and is supportive of, a gay or lesbian child or sibling.
- **Gender identity**. Usually accept a child whose gender identity is ambiguous or opposite to his/her birth gender. Parents who are aware of gender identity problem may pressure child by reminding him/her to behave in a manner appropriate for his/her birth gender.
- **Attitudes about menopause**. No socially sanctioned behavioral or clothing restrictions for middle-age women in perimenopausal transition. Women recognize a decline in sexual interest but do not believe that sexual relations cease at that time. Tend to have a positive attitude toward menopause and aging, viewing menopause as a natural life stage. Many Filipinos believe that menopause causes one to become "nervous" and "irritable" in mid-life. Do not consider these conditions to be serious; often resolve over time. Hormone replacement therapy uncommon in Philippines, but in severe cases, women may seek help from herbalists (*herbolarios*).

FAMILY RELATIONSHIPS

- **Composition/structure**. Filipinos strongly oriented to family, which usually includes members of extended family. Even unrelated persons are considered to be "part of the family." In rural areas of Philippines, six children is average. Procreation an important life focus. Catholic ban on contraception, illegality of abortion, and unmet needs for contraceptive services contribute to large family size. Immigrant couples and their children constitute the basic social unit in a household, but a couple's parents or first-degree cousins may live with them. Very commonly, three generations reside under one roof.

- **Decision-making**. Usually an internal family affair. Entire family typically makes decisions regarding serious matters, especially those pertaining to health care, finances, and other family matters.
- **Spokesperson**. Usually the father or eldest son or daughter.
- **Gender issues**. Women traditionally have equal rights and share authority with spouses, although they may defer to husband's decisions as head of the family. Women responsible for mothering and housekeeping, and caring for ill family members. Men usually handle financial matters and children's education and discipline. In U.S., common for both men and women to work outside the home.
- **Changing roles among generations in U.S.** Gender roles related to when immigrants arrived. First immigration wave comprised mostly single and poorly educated men who lived as bachelors because antimiscegenation laws prohibited marriage outside of one's race. Second wave included more women, who cared for house and children; a small number entered the workforce. Third wave comprised educated and urban-dwelling Filipinos. Women in this group joined the workforce in greater numbers. Modern Filipino women are regarded as wage earners equal to men. Currently, women play a leading role in family and society at large, although traditional families still defer to the father and eldest family member in decision-making. In acculturated families, the most-educated members play key role in family decision-making, especially about health care and financial matters. Younger generation has a greater say than in the past.
- **Caring roles**. Generally expect women to care for sick family member. Eldest daughter is caregiver for father or mother; in her absence, other female family members fill that role. Patient pampered with attention and services. Family members protect patient and may not support early ambulation, self-care, or rehabilitation.
- **Expectations of and for children**. Children reared in highly protective environment. Filipinos emphasize negative sanctions—frightening, teasing, and shaming—to discourage misconduct (e.g., "If you leave your room, the boogie man will get you."). Teach children to be quiet, avoid direct confrontations when there are personal differences, contain emotions, and be obedient, respectful, and shy. Strongly emphasize education, particularly college.
- **Expectations of and for elders**. Respect for elders a cornerstone of Filipino values, demonstrated by deference in body language, tone of voice, and verbal response. Common for parents to live with their adult children. Children expected to care for elderly parents to repay their debt of gratitude (*utang na loob*).

- **Expectations of hospital visitors**. Hospitals in Philippines allow family members to stay with patients 24 hours a day. In U.S., entire families may visit, including young children.

ILLNESS BELIEFS

- **Causes of/attitudes about physical illness**. Caused by imbalance of "hot"/"cold" and air elements in body. Filipinos may associate illness with bad behavior or punishment. Prevent illness by avoiding inappropriate behaviors that cause imbalance, and cure illness by restoring balance. Some believe that overeating, poor diet, or excessive drinking causes illness. Many believe that illness is God's will. Some believe in supernatural causes, such as ghosts or evil spirits, and may wear talismans, amulets, a cross, a scapular, or other protective objects.
- **Causes of/attitudes about mental illness**. Filipinos may believe in Catholicism and mystical causation simultaneously. Believe that mental illness occurs when harmonious function of the whole individual and spiritual world is disrupted. Four categories of cause: mystical (contact with a person or stronger life force); supernatural (life force in all objects manifesting as ghosts [*multo*] or souls of the dead); naturalistic (wind, vapors, diet, body-organ shift, and stress); and Western (physical and emotional strain, sexual frustration, unrequited love, and inherited constitution). Mental illness stigmatizes the individual and family, and is not readily reported. May deny rather than acknowledge mental illness in a family member.
- **Causes of genetic defects**. Tend to accept a loved one's genetic defect, believing it is God's will or punishment for bad behavior. Some attribute genetic defects to what the mother ate or did during pregnancy. Family cares for severely affected child at home.
- **Attitudes about disabilities**. Accepted as God's will. Treat disabled persons with kindness and pity (*awa*), especially the elderly. Relatives often help disabled family members with chores. Helping disabled persons is considered a worthy sacrifice in the eyes of God; turning one's back is considered cruel and can cause misfortune.
- **Sick role**. Usually pamper sick family members, who often are passive. Others make decisions for them, give them the best treatment, and protect them from undue exertion, fatigue, or discomfort. Special food usually prepared and brought to the bedside. Walking and other physical activities discouraged, as they might cause a relapse. Use healing ointments and rubs to comfort the sick.
- **Home and folk remedies**. Chinese influence on herbal medicines. Both folk medicine and Western biomedicine prevalent. Acculturated persons may combine home remedies with Western medicine, while those with poor access to health care mainly use herbal and home remedies. Herbalist (*herbolario*) prescribes treatments for ailments such as fever, stomach pain, and

headache. *Herbolario* also performs a ritual to cast away evil spirits. Patients may not divulge use of home remedies to clinician for fear of ridicule or embarrassment.

- **Medications**. Common home remedies include oils, liniments, and ointments to ease body aches. In recent years, medicinal plants, parts of trees, and herbs have become popular for treating various ailments. They include bitter melon (*ampalaya*), a special shrub (*lagundi*), aloe vera, guava leaves, and leaves from a native tree (*banaba*), which are available in tea form. May use these in conjunction with prescribed medicine.

- **Acceptance of procedures**. Some Filipinos are more fearful of donating than receiving blood because they believe that donating will cause a health imbalance. Family may want to donate blood only for loved ones. Do not accept surgical procedures until they have consulted with family members. May not consider organ donation, preferring to keep body intact for burial. More-acculturated persons may consider accepting donated organs.

- **Care-seeking**. Filipinos believe concurrently in modern and folk medicine. Believe that Western biomedicine makes some conditions worse. If unable to obtain relief from Western medicine, consult folk healers. Some believe in healers who can placate or exorcise spirits and ghosts.

HEALTH ISSUES

- **Concept of health**. The result of balance (*timbang*) or harmony between the person and nature/supernatural forces. Associate health with good appetite, strength (*malakas*), and ability to carry out everyday activities. Religious Filipinos derive spiritual strength from prayers and frequently ascribe healing to God's will. Traditional Filipinos consider being overweight, especially in children, a sign of well-being, good socioeconomic standing, and contentment.

- **Health promotion and prevention**. Maintaining balance promotes health. Three practices underlie health promotion and prevention: Flushing rids the body of debris and impurities, heating maintains internal temperature balance, and protection guards the body from harmful external influences. Eating well (not necessarily eating balanced meals) promotes good health. Consider rice, the main dietary staple, essential for maintaining health. Covering the head prevents illness caused by exposure to cold and outside air. Avoiding supernatural causes also prevents illness. For most Filipinos, exercise is not a regular part of health promotion.

- **Screening**. Generally not accustomed to regular Pap smears, breast exams, mammograms, and physical exams. Do not readily answer questions about sexual and marital practices. However, disclose medical information out of respect for health care providers. Generally accept and follow suggestions about regular physicals, colonoscopy, diabetes screening, etc., if health insurance coverage is not an issue.

- **Common health problems**. May be related to diet, living conditions, and stress. High incidence of hypertension may be associated with high intake of salty foods. Dealing with difficulties of separation from loved ones, low socioeconomic status, and lack of opportunities to improve quality of life contribute to many psychosomatic problems. Very high incidence of hepatitis and liver cancer. Other common diseases are diabetes, gallstones, gastrointestinal diseases, pulmonary diseases, arthritis, and osteoporosis. Filipinos are lactose sensitive, which accounts for typical absence of milk in diet. Tuberculosis prevalent in lower socioeconomic groups.

DEATH RITUALS

- **Beliefs and attitudes about death**. Largely influenced by religious beliefs. Filipinos see death as part of God's divine plan, but acceptance differs depending on age of deceased. View death of a young person as a tragedy, that of an elderly person as "going back to God" after living a long life. Catholics believe that most souls go to purgatory to cleanse their sins before going to heaven. Those who have done evil deeds will suffer in hell. Souls or spirits of the dead stay around to watch over their loved ones and sometimes reveal themselves to certain persons.
- **Preparation**. Head of family (usually a parent or eldest child) is notified of death. Clinician should deliver news gently and privately using respectful language and demeanor. Strong belief that family members should be present when someone dies; clinician should tell family members of imminent death so they can say good-bye and hear the dying person's last words. Do-not-resuscitate decision usually very difficult; close family members typically consulted.
- **Home vs. hospital**. If diagnosis is terminal and there is no hope of recovery, generally prefer to die at home. Acculturated Filipinos may bring their loved one to hospital to die but still prefer to be at bedside when that happens. Those who are unable to care for a dying loved one at home may seek hospice or nursing home care. However, family may feel guilty about "abandoning" a loved one.
- **Special needs**. A priest and/or spiritual adviser must be present to minister to the dying person and provide support for the family. Usually keep religious relics, rosary beads, medallions, holy water, and figurines of Christ, saints, and the Holy Family at patient's bedside while family members and friends pray for recovery, even when patient is terminal. Usually, many visitors pay their respects to the dying.
- **Care of the body**. Death is a major spiritual event. It is also an opportunity for family members to gather and make amends to the dead person and to each other. Modern Filipinos prefer to keep the remains of their loved ones in the mortuary instead of at home. Cremation uncommon. Viewing of body important. Body dressed in formal attire, such as a suit, wedding dress, or gown. Most common is the *barong*, a special cloth made of fibers from native plants, such as pineapple, banana, and ramie. Catholics place rosary beads,

crucifix, medallions, and other religious objects on body. Burn candles to keep vigil over body. Place flowers around coffin and may display picture of deceased. Muslims believe that the remains should be buried immediately after preparation of body because the soul will face final judgment right after burial; delaying burial increases spiritual agony of the deceased.

- **Attitudes about organ donation**. Not quite accepted in Philippines, due to respect for body and preference for keeping it intact for burial. May con- sider donation if recipient is a relative, especially in a life-or-death situation.
- **Attitudes about autopsy**. Rarely request it, due to respect for body and preference for keeping it intact for burial. Generally consider autopsy only when there is suspicion of foul play or family is uncertain about cause of death. Needing to know cause of death may stem from guilt or vindication of long-held ideas regarding the events that brought about the person's death. When autopsy is legally required, as in coroner cases, family should be noti- fied. If a physician requests autopsy, he/she should explain reason for the request, using an interpreter if necessary. Whole family should be involved in resolving this sensitive issue.

SELECTED REFERENCES

Berg, J. A., De Guzman, C. P., & Rodriguez, D. M. (2003). Filipinos. In P. St. Hill, J. G. Lipson, & A. I. Meleis (Eds.), *Caring for women cross-culturally* (pp. 156–171). Philadelphia: F. A. Davis.

Dela Cruz, F. A., McBride, M. R., Compas, L. B., Calixto, P., & Van Derveer, C. (2002). White paper on the health status of Filipino Americans and rec- ommendations for research. *Nursing Outlook, 50*, 7–15.

Orque, M. S. (1983). Nursing care of Filipino American patients. In M. S. Orque, B. Block, & L. A. Ahumada-Monrroy (Eds.), *Ethnic nursing care—a multicultural approach* (pp. 149–181). St. Louis, MO: C. V. Mosby.

Vance, A. R. (1995). Filipino Americans. In J. N. Giger & R. E. Davidhizar (Eds.), *Transcultural nursing: Assessment and intervention* (2nd ed.) (pp. 417– 438). St. Louis, MO: Mosby-Year Book.

AUTHORS

Daisy M. Rodriguez, MN, MPA, RN, is an administrative nursing supervisor at the San Ramon Regional Medical Center in California. She received her bachelor's and master's degrees in nursing from the University of the Philip- pines, and a second master's degree in health services from the University of San Francisco. She is past president of the Philippine Nurses Association of Northern California, president of the University of the Philippines Nursing Alumni Association of Northern California, a member of the executive board of the Philippine Nurses Association of America, and a member of the Sigma Theta Tau International Honor Society.

Carolina P. de Guzman, MSN, CPAN, RN, is a trainer for the National Asian Women's Health Organization. She obtained her bachelor's degree in nursing from the University of the Philippines and a master's in nursing from Sonoma State University in Rohnert Park, CA. She taught at the Philippine General Hospital School of Nursing before emigrating to the U.S. De Guzman retired after 32 years of nursing practice. She is past president of the Philippine Nurses Association of Northern California and the University of the Philippines Nursing Association of Northern California, which she founded.

Arthur Cantos, RN, returned to the Philippines as the CEO of Bayani Consulting, an international nurse recruitment firm. He was an assistant nurse manager in the cardiothoracic unit at the University of California-San Francisco Medical Center for more than a decade before he switched to nursing informatics and worked for various information technology companies. He has worked as a clinical engineer at a software development company, as a clinical educator and product designer at a telemedicine company, and as a clinical product manager at a Web portal. He also was a television news anchor at Filipino American Report, a daily newscast on KMTP in San Francisco.

CHAPTER 15

GERMANS

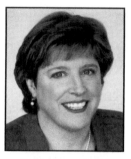 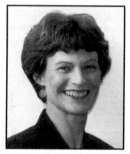

Catherine Dodd   *Petra Eggert*

CULTURAL/ETHNIC IDENTITY

- **Preferred term(s)**. German. Also Amish, German Baptist, German American.
- **Census**. In the 2000 Census, more than 57.9 million people claimed to be solely or partially of German ancestry. About 98% were born in the U.S. Of the foreign-born, 88% entered the U.S. before 1980.
- **History of immigration**. More than 7 million Germans have emigrated to the U.S. since 1608. Germans were among the first settlers at Jamestown. In 1683, German Quakers and Mennonites (including Amish sect) arrived in Pennsylvania seeking religious freedom. In the 1700s, the British Colonies were settled by small, German-speaking, religious groups often called "Pennsylvania Dutch," which refers to *Deutsch*, the German language. Pennsylvania Dutch include Amish, German Baptists, and other Mennonite sects. Biggest Amish immigration was between 1727–70. Largest Amish populations are in Pennsylvania and Ohio, but there are Amish communities in 20 states and Ontario, Canada. German Baptists fled persecution and settled in Pennsylvania around the time of the Revolutionary War. There was continuous immigration during the 1800s; some immigrants came for political reasons, others were seeking economic opportunity or religious freedom. In 1924, after World War I and the spread of anti-German hysteria, an immigration law limited the number of German entrants (there were 386,634 in the 1920s and only 119,107 in the 1930s), who included thousands of intellectuals and Jews fleeing the Nazi holocaust. After President Franklin Roosevelt's national conference in 1938 on Jewish immigration, the U.S. agreed to accept 130,000 German Jewish immigrants. Annual immigration declined in the following decades to a low of 55,800 in the 1990s.

SPIRITUAL/RELIGIOUS ORIENTATION

- **Primary religious/spiritual affiliations**. Most immigrants are Lutheran, Jewish, or Catholic, but many—such as Mennonites, specifically Amish—have been of nonconformist Protestant faiths. Catholics came primarily from southern Germany and Lutherans from northern Germany. Lutheran Church began in Germany based on the teachings of Martin Luther, originator of the Protestant Reformation. German immigrants in the U.S. founded the Lutheran Church, Missouri Synod, in the 1830s out of frustration with conservatism and state controls on Lutheran Church in Germany. Most Jews who came in the mid-19th century supported the Reform Judaism movement that started in Germany; another wave of Orthodox Jews arrived at the end of that century. Christian Moravians settled in Pennsylvania. German Baptists are scattered throughout the country, with large populations in Ohio and Pennsylvania. There are about 60 Amish communities in North America divided into four independent orders, with variations in faith practices and daily living activities. Amish accept Christ as the Savior. They emphasize obedience and yielding to God, the church, and others. Most distinctly, they strive to preserve traditional ways of life and separation from the outside world, avoiding modern technology. Amish are not permitted to attend school beyond eighth grade; because of this, there are no Amish health professionals. They shun members who leave their community. There are about 11,000 German Baptists in the U.S. who are among several religious sects that religious scholars describe as "plain people." In appearance, they resemble Amish or Mennonites but are distinct in terms of doctrine and practice. For example, German Baptists dunk members three times during baptism, do not shun the outside world, drive, and use telephones. But they avoid certain "evils," such as television, radio, computers, and newspapers, that they believe would erode their way of life. In 1881, the Brethren Church split into Old German Baptist Brethren, who retain original church practices and dress, and a more modern group called the Church of the Brethren. Every year on Pentecost, the Old German Baptist Brethren hold a national meeting that draws thousands to make decisions about their way of life.
- **Usual religious/spiritual practices**. Amish, German Baptists, Catholics, and Lutherans celebrate Christian holidays and worship on Sundays. Amish Church is decentralized; services rotate among several dozen families every other Sunday. Communion services are held in spring and fall; the faithful prepare for these by washing each other's feet. Amish believe in adult baptism. Religious celebrations include baptisms, usually in August or September; weddings in November; communion during Sunday services; and funerals. Daily worshippers pray and read the Scriptures. Lutherans' and Catholics' practices are similar—worship Christ as the Son of God, seek grace through the Holy Spirit, baptize infants, and take communion. Catholics practice sacraments of confession, confirmation, marriage, and absolution. They also

believe in purgatory, where unbaptized souls go after death, and pray to to the Virgin Mary and saints beatified by the Pope. Jewish practices depend on whether family is reform, conservative, or orthodox. Many Jews go to synagogue/temple on Friday night and some on Saturday morning, as the Sabbath begins at sundown on Friday and ends at sundown on Saturday. They commonly have a Friday evening Sabbath meal after saying a prayer while lighting candles. Orthodox Jews do not work or drive during Sabbath.

- **Use of spiritual healing/healers**. Only the Amish use religious or spiritual healers, who are women knowledgeable about the use of herbs and poultices. Healers pass down their knowledge to the next generation.
- **Holidays**. Christian holidays include Epiphany (January 6, at the end of 12 days of Christmas), Good Friday (*Karfreitag*), Easter Monday, Ascension Day (40 days after Easter) (*Christi Himmelfahrt*), Pentecost (*Pfingsten*), Corpus Christi (50 days after Easter) (*Fronleichnam*), Assumption of the Virgin Mary (August 15), All Saints Day (November 1), Day of Prayer and Repentance (Wednesday before Advent), and Christmas (December 25–26) (*Weihnachten*). The Amish solemnly celebrate Christ's birth on December 25 and hold family dinners and visits on December 16. Jewish holidays include *Purim* (celebrating religious freedom); Passover (*Pesach*); and the autumn high holidays of Jewish New Year (*Rosh Hashanah*), Day of Atonement (*Yom Kippur*), and *Hanukkah*. Secular holidays include New Year's Eve (*Sylvester*), New Year's Day (*Neujahr*), Labor Day (May 1), *Oktoberfest* (end of September), Day of Unity (October 3, reunification of East and West Germany) (*Tag der Deutschen Einheit*), Reformation Day (October 31) (*Reformationstag*), St. Nicholas Day (December 5–6) (*St. Nikolaustag*), and Memorial Day (third Sunday in November). Many of these holidays are not celebrated in U.S.

COMMUNICATION
ORAL COMMUNICATION

- **Major languages and dialects**. The great majority of Germans in U.S. speak English. Some communities highly value their bilingualism. Amish and German Baptists speak a dialect of German in everyday life and high German at church services. Because Amish do not use electricity, it is inappropriate to explain procedures or provide health information via computers or videos. Some older Jews speak Yiddish, which originated in 1100 A.D. as a blend of several German dialects in central European ghettos and spread with Judaism throughout the world.
- **Greetings**. Family and friends use familiar names, but strangers should address adults using "Mr.," "Mrs.," "Miss," or "Ms.," especially when the adult is elderly. Handshakes common; person entering a group may need to shake everyone's hand. Family members and good friends may kiss on each cheek. Younger generations and those who are more-acculturated are less

formal. Clinician should ask patient how he/she prefers to be addressed. Should address Amish using *Herr, Frau*, or *Fräulein*. Amish and German Baptists greet friends of same gender with kiss on the lips.

- **Tone of voice**. Do not use loud tone. Amish women and children very reserved.
- **Direct or indirect style of speech**. Same as in dominant culture, with emphasis on verbal rather than nonverbal communication. Value precise, explicit, and direct communication.
- **Use of interpreters**. Older family members appropriate. Most adult Amish speak English. Amish very modest regarding sex and pregnancy issues, so clinician should ask a family member of same gender to translate.
- **Serious or terminal illness**. Clinician should tell patient and family members together as soon as illness becomes known.

WRITTEN COMMUNICATION

- **Literacy assessment**. Most German Americans literate in English. Clinician should politely ask Amish and older Jews if they read English before asking them to read forms or instructions. Amish have only a grade-school education, so information must be simply stated.
- **Consents**. Willing to sign consent forms for tests and procedures after these are explained.

NONVERBAL COMMUNICATION

- **Eye contact**. Direct eye contact typical. Amish women may avoid eye contact when speaking with husband or father.
- **Personal space**. Varies according to relationship and gender. In general, 1.5–3 feet appropriate with family and friends; closer distance appropriate when necessary for physical care. With strangers, personal space may be more than an arm's length. Amish increase the social distance between themselves and non-Amish "outsiders."
- **Use and meaning of silence**. Similar to that of others with northern European heritage.
- **Gestures**. Nodding means approval. Rude or disrespectful behaviors include chewing gum, not removing sunglasses when meeting others, cleaning one's fingernails in public, talking or shaking hands with one hand in pocket, and using the middle finger to "flip the bird." A good-bye gesture is raising hand upward with palm out and waving fingers up and down. Waggling hand back and forth means "no."
- **Openness in expressing emotions** (non-Amish). Among family and friends, express emotions openly, both verbally and nonverbally, but this depends on generation and age. Older and more traditional persons may be uncomfortable expressing emotions to strangers, fearing loss of control and vulnerability. Much more comfortable debating social, political, and philo-

sophical issues than sharing feelings. Younger generation more willing to share thoughts and feelings with others.

- **Privacy**. Highly value privacy, but this varies among individuals and families. Often consider feelings to be private. A closed door protects privacy and requires a knock and permission to enter. Amish very private about sexual and pregnancy issues.
- **Touch**. Acceptable when necessary for care. Before clinician touches patient's breasts or genitals, very important to explain intent and importance. Touch for comfort varies among individuals. Often frown upon public displays of affection.
- **Orientation to time** (non-Amish). Very punctual. May be intolerant of others who are late or who do not adhere to schedule. Orientation to past illustrated by Germans' attention to heritage and historical events. Focus present actions on ensuring a better future. Amish and German Baptists often set clocks slower or faster by one-half hour. Other German Americans set their clocks ahead so they are on time without being rushed. When clinician schedules appointment, should determine if Amish/German Baptist patient uses slow or fast time.

ACTIVITIES OF DAILY LIVING

- **Modesty**. Gender of clinician not an issue. Orthodox Jewish women prefer female physician if possible and require special attention after childbirth. Amish are very modest. Women's clothing is long enough to cover ankles.
- **Skin care**. Some do not bathe daily. May prefer sponge bath. Amish bathe less frequently because they must heat the water on a stove. In some households, father bathes in tub first, then mother and children in birth order. But this practice is rare in U.S. Orthodox Jews do not allow tattooing; clinician should explain why tattoos are necessary for radiation treatments.
- **Hair care**. Orthodox Jewish women cover their hair because they consider hair sensual; allow only husbands to see it. Older Germans and Amish do not wash hair daily and never wash it before going to sleep or outdoors for fear of catching cold. Some Amish women do not cut their hair. All Amish and German Baptist women part hair in the middle and put it in a bun at back of head, covered with white organdy cap. Orthodox Jewish men grow sideburns long; some cut sideburns along the jaw bone, others grow and curl them. Amish men cut hair such that it has bangs and is even with earlobes; no part. Amish and Baptist men do not cut their beards but shave their mustaches.
- **Nail care**. Neatly trimmed or manicured.
- **Toileting**. Accept use of urinals, bedpans, and commodes. Keep toileting implements very clean and covered. Some German Americans use only small amounts of toilet paper; think large crumpled bunches of toilet paper are wasteful.
- **Special clothing or amulets**. German women wear wedding ring on right

hand and prefer not to remove it if possible. Amish dress plainly; children dress exactly like adults. Women wear black bonnets and single-color dresses with white aprons. Fasten dresses only with straight pins, no buttons or zippers. Men wear plainly cut black suits and flat, brimmed hats of black felt or straw. Men fasten their clothing with straight pins and hooks and eyes. German Baptists dress simply, but women's dresses are colored and bonnets are white. Orthodox Jewish men wear a small head covering (*yarmulke*) and prayer shawl (*tallit*).

- **Self-care**. Willing to do all self-care or most self-care with help from a family member or nursing staff.

FOOD PRACTICES

- **Usual meal pattern**. Three meals a day. Older Germans may prefer the main meal at midday, and coffee and cake in late afternoon. Light supper of cheese and bread is common.
- **Special utensils**. None.
- **Food beliefs and rituals**. Food symbolizes celebration and love, and may be one of the few cultural traditions passed down through generations of German Americans. Many like having abundant food on hand at home. Traditional foods for holidays or weddings may require weeks of baking ahead of time.
- **Usual diet**. German diets are high in fat and starch, and include rich pastries, fried foods, and gravies. Often serve eggs with toast for breakfast. Serve sausage and cheese for breakfast and evening meals. Pork common among non-Jews. Chicken is popular. Cornmeal mush, eggs and cereal, bread, meat, cabbage, potatoes, rutabagas, and Brussels sprouts are common. Often overcook vegetables. Desserts with chocolate, whipped cream (*Schlag*), and cinnamon and sugar are favorites. Most Amish have no electricity and very few have freezers. They prepare food from scratch using home-grown vegetables and fruit.
- **Fluids**. Tea a common beverage. Chamomile tea a very popular remedy. Caffeine ill-advised during illness. Germans do not use ice in beverages. Coffee, beer—including dark beer (*Dunkelbier*)—and flavored spirits (*Schnapps*) are popular. Consider *Sprudel*, a natural soda, to be healthful. Children drink primarily milk and water.
- **Food taboos and prescriptions**. For illness, prefer warm or hot foods, toast, and tea. Some eat garlic and onions daily to prevent heart disease. Other food prescriptions reflect those of dominant culture (e.g., prune juice for constipation, ginger ale for upset stomach). Main food taboos are Jewish. Orthodox Jews strictly avoid pork and shellfish, and adhere to kosher (*kashrut*) laws. For example, they do not cook meat and dairy together or eat them at same meal (use different sets of dishes and cookware for each), and meats are specially butchered. Kosher packaged foods identified by "K" or "U" in a circle on the label. Some conservative Jews also observe these tra-

ditions. In planning patient's diet, clinician should ask family about its level
of keeping kosher.

■ **Hospitality**. Germans welcome visitors. Offer a beverage, snack, or meal,
which may include large servings and second helpings. Amish isolate themselves from larger society and do not welcome outsiders into their homes and
communities; are required to socialize among themselves.

SYMPTOM MANAGEMENT

Germans generally understand numerical scales for symptom level after they
are taught how to use them. Do not always report symptoms without being
asked. Accept IV, oral, and rectal medications.

■ **Pain** (*Schmerz*). Tend to be stoic and may not report pain or ask for pain
medication. Jews see suffering as a byproduct of illness; accept anything that
will ease their suffering. Amish are stoic about pain and believe that it is
God's will.

■ **Dyspnea** (*Atemnot*). May get anxious. Use of, and response to, nonpharmacological treatments vary.

■ **Nausea/vomiting** (*Übelkeit/Erbrechend*). Accept toast and tea. Do not use
ice chips.

■ **Constipation/diarrhea** (*Verstopfung/Diarrhöe*). Regular bowel movements
very important. Older Germans describe what bowel movements look like.
Consume prune juice or laxatives. Enemas common. Take medications for
diarrhea after consuming tea and toast.

■ **Fatigue** (*Ermüdung* or *Müdigkeit*). Commonly recommend rest and sleep.
Illness-related fatigue (*Erschöpfung*) is different. Sleep and fresh air important. Many Germans not comfortable sleeping (especially when ill) unless a
window is open, but one should never sleep in a draft.

■ **Depression** (*Tiefstand*). Recognize and accept mental illness, as Freud was
German. Most accept medication, but psychotherapy is less common. A
1990 study found more-frequent "stress-related feelings" among Amish
women than among their non-Amish counterparts; such feelings are associated with the Amish culture of great responsibility. Amish culture with
deeply held Christian values is the basis of social support for families.

■ **Self-care symptom management**. Usually rely on self-care before seeking
medical attention. Amish and German Baptists do all they can to help themselves, getting advice from family and friends and using herbs and home
remedies. Those raised in Germany are accustomed to taking medications
because medical care and pharmaceuticals there are free.

BIRTH RITUALS/CARE OF THE NEW MOTHER AND BABY

■ **Pregnancy care**. Motherhood an important role in society. Pregnant
women should get plenty of fresh air, exercise, and extra food. Germans
expect regular prenatal care and childbirth preparation classes. Some Amish

women do not seek prenatal care until sixth month of pregnancy, but most have first birth in hospital. Lack of insurance limits subsequent hospital births, although communities maintain a mutual aid fund for care. Amish must hire a driver and car if hospital is far away. Orthodox Jewish women prefer female physicians.

- **Preferences for children**. Orthodox Jews believe that the Old Testament calls upon them to have at least two children, a boy and a girl. Amish and German Baptists believe that children are gifts from God; they hope to have many children (average is seven). Amish have the highest incidence of twins of any population. Among acculturated German Americans, preference for gender and number of children resembles that in dominant culture.
- **Labor practices**. Women go to the hospital when in labor. Amish and German Baptist women may undergo labor and give birth at home. No special labor practices. Women cooperate with staff's suggestions.
- **Role of the laboring woman during birth**. Follows instructions of physician or midwife.
- **Role of the father and other family members during birth**. Varies among families. Father and woman's mother participate if available.
- **Vaginal vs. cesarean section**. For most, choice does not involve any special values. Among some Amish, cesarean section is against teachings of the community's bishop; C-section may result in excommunication from community. Consider mother's and/or baby's death as God's will.
- **Breastfeeding**. Important. German society supports 1–2 years of breastfeeding. Expect mothers to consume foods that increase milk supply, including beer. Amish women breastfeed for eight months, on average; many breastfeed beyond 18 months. They supplement breastfeeding with water, juice, and cow's and goat's milk. Research in one Amish community documented failure to thrive in 35% of infants. Clinicians should monitor weight, length, and head circumference at well-child visits and promote pasteurized vs. raw milk, complementary iron-fortified foods, and vitamin supplements for infants 6–18 months old.
- **Birth recuperation**. German grandmother (*Oma*) often stays with new mother to help for a few months. New mothers encouraged to exercise and breathe plenty of fresh air. Amish and German Baptist communities provide support for new mothers; they consider new babies to be gifts from God.
- **Baby care**. Grandmother, father, and older siblings help.
- **Problems with baby**. Consult with relatives and take baby to physician. Amish seek physician's advice after they have exhausted other remedies. Clinician should tell parents about a problem together as soon as any information becomes available.
- **Male and female circumcision**. Generally do not circumcise male babies, but acculturated German Americans may not object to it in hospital. Jewish boys are circumcised eight days after birth in a religious ceremony (*Brit*) per-

formed by a person who is religiously authorized (*Mohel*). Bury foreskin in the garden or a planter. Amish and German Baptists do not circumcise males. Female circumcision never performed.

DEVELOPMENTAL AND SEXUAL ISSUES

- **Celebration of menarche or becoming a man**. After intensive study and at age 13, Jewish boys are eligible for *bar mitzvah*; girls who are 12 years old celebrate *bas mitzvah*. These celebrations formally acknowledge an obligation to observe the commandments and rights associated with helping to lead religious services, form binding contracts, testify before religious courts, and marry. In U.S., the ceremonies usually are held in a synagogue and feted with food and dancing, although no ceremony is required. Catholic boys and girls usually observe the sacrament of confirmation at or around age 12 or 13. At age 16 in some Amish communities, some teenagers begin a period of "running free" (*rumspringa*), during which they have enormous freedom to explore the "English" (non-Amish) world before deciding whether to undergo baptism and join the Amish Church. Also at this age, Amish teenagers begin searching for a spouse.
- **Attitudes about birth control**. Jews permit birth control and consider it a couple's private affair, guided by tenets of their branch of Judaism. Orthodox Jews may use birth control as long as the couple is committed to eventually fulfilling their duty to be fruitful and multiply—to have at least a boy and a girl. Most accept the pill, but Orthodox Jewish law does not permit methods, such as condoms, that destroy or block the passage of the seed. Amish Church doctrine forbids birth control; German Baptists prohibit it as well. Catholics permitted to use only natural methods, such as withdrawal and timing intercourse to avoid fertile days.
- **Attitudes about sexually transmitted infection (STI) control, including condoms**. Jewish law permits condoms to prevent the transmission of AIDS or similar diseases, based on priority of preserving the life of the uninfected spouse. Catholics, Amish, and German Baptists consider condoms a form of birth control; therefore, they forbid condoms for any purpose. Consider sexual relations outside of marriage to be a sin, and believe that STIs are contracted outside of a monogamous relationship. Acculturated German Americans use condoms.
- **Attitudes about abortion**. Most religions accept therapeutic abortion to save mother's life. Exception is Catholicism, which permits it only indirectly (e.g., to remove uterine cancer). Catholics, Lutherans, Amish, and German Baptists prohibit abortion by choice.
- **Attitudes about unwed sexual experimentation**. Generally disapprove of pregnancy out of wedlock, but more-acculturated persons and younger generations are less disapproving. Catholics, Lutherans, Amish, and German Baptists forbid unwed sexual experimentation. Jewish law also forbids sexual

contact short of intercourse and prohibits male masturbation because it "destroys the seed." Jews generally frown upon female masturbation as "impure thoughts." Catholic and Lutheran laws prohibit male and female masturbation because it separates sexual satisfaction from intercourse within the marital union.

- **Sexual orientation**. Acceptance of gay, lesbian, bisexual, transgender, and uncertain sexual orientations varies among individuals and families. Middle-age and older persons may fear exposure because of Nazi history of extreme harassment and punishment. Jewish law forbids sexual acts between men; however, it does not forbid different sexual orientations, as Jews focus on actions rather than desires. Jewish law does not forbid female homosexual relations. Catholics, Lutherans, Amish, and German Baptists believe that teachings in Bible prescribe heterosexual lifestyles only and that homosexual orientations are sinful.
- **Gender identity**. Acceptance of different gender identities varies among individuals and families. Catholics, Lutherans, Amish, German Baptists, and Orthodox Jews believe that God assigns gender identity at birth.
- **Attitudes about menopause**. View it as a normal phase in woman's life. No negative attitudes. Women discuss menopause with each other and use home remedies to control symptoms.

FAMILY RELATIONSHIPS

- **Composition/structure**. Nuclear families are the norm among acculturated German Americans. Traditionally, father is head of household, although in U.S. and among acculturated persons, this is changing and varies among families. Father is head of household in Amish and German Baptist communities, which have very large families. All family members nurture children, who create bonds beyond the single-family unit. Intergenerational responsibility is a basic tenet of Amish life. Because Amish society is closed, entire community is essentially an extended family.
- **Decision-making**. Varies among families and depends on generation and religious affiliation. Amish fathers make decisions, although women are respected for their opinion and even deferred to for some final decisions. In Orthodox Jewish families, the father, then eldest son have authority.
- **Spokesperson**. Traditionally, in older German families (including those that are Jewish, Amish, or Baptist), father is spokesperson. This is changing and varies among families.
- **Gender issues**. Roles of men and women vary within the family depending on acculturation, economics, and children.
- **Changing roles among generations in U.S.** Catholic, Lutheran, and Jewish German Americans become more Americanized with each new generation. Attitudes about sex, sexual orientation, and family roles are influenced by how strictly they adhere to religious traditions. Today in Germany, as in

U.S., divorce and teen pregnancy rates are high, which indicate tolerant social mores regarding sex and sexual experimentation. In contrast, Amish and German Baptists continue to separate themselves from the modern world. Amish culture emphasizes the welfare of the community over that of the individual (*Gelassenheit*). It also values being reserved, modest, calm, and quiet; submission to God's authority; serving and respecting others; and social communities that are small and simple. Amish take vow of separation from the outside world; also vow to remain close to nature.

- **Caring roles**. Women are main care providers in all German subcultures, although men also participate. In Amish families, husbands accept responsibility for child-rearing and supervision. Amish are committed to caring for community members throughout life.
- **Expectations of and for children**. All religions cherish children. Germans expect children to respect elders, do what they are told and not talk back to adults, be polite, work hard in school, and stay out of trouble. There is deep respect for education among mainstream German Americans; most have a high-school or postsecondary education. Amish children acquire work skills early in childhood. Amish strongly believe that children learn from adult role models, that God expects children to obey parents. Children's games are related to Amish lifestyle. German Baptist children are permitted more play activities. While adult Amish do not permit photographs, they allow children to be photographed because children are not baptized into Amish faith until adulthood.
- **Expectations of and for elders**. First- and second-generation German Americans maintain close relationships with parents and grandparents, although family mobility affects their ability to do so. Seek advice from elderly, whose children help them stay in their own homes as long as possible. Amish and German Baptists view family relationships as reciprocal throughout life. In these communities, grandparents usually live with their children or move from child to child during the year.
- **Expectations of hospital visitors**. Visitors, including pastors and rabbis, are important. With exception of spouse, visitors usually abide by visiting hours. Family tries to spread out visitors so there are not too many at one time. Visitors bring flowers rather than food.

ILLNESS BELIEFS

- **Causes of/attitudes about physical illness**. Most believe that poor nutrition, stress, and inadequate rest cause illness. Amish attribute illness to God's will.
- **Causes of/attitudes about mental illness**. Some view mental illness as a flaw and a stigma on the family, which may discourage seeking psychotherapy or hospitalization. This view was more prevalent in the past. Jews, Lutherans, and Catholics do not believe that mental illness is punishment

for not following the rules of their faith. Amish and German Baptists believe that mental illness is God's will; however, they are willing to seek help. Because Amish society is insular, the community is essentially a closed genetic population; mental retardation and mental illness are common.

- **Causes of genetic defects**. Perceive defects as hereditary or just an accident. Jews and Amish have some specific genetic risks. Tay-Sachs disease is 10 times more prevalent among Ashkenazi Jews (those from Germany) than among non-Jews. This enzyme defect first appears in the startle reflex at age 6 months. Affected children gradually lose their ability to make purposeful movements, have seizures and vision loss, and, by age 2, enter a vegetative state. No treatment. Germans keep Tay-Sachs children comfortable and provide good nutrition. Genetic DNA testing via amniocentesis enables diagnosis before birth; Jews are receptive to genetic testing. A rarer condition is Canavan disease, which impairs the brain's ability to communicate. No cure, but gene therapy can slow its progression. Because Amish Church forbids marriage outside the community, this genetic population has been closed for more than 12 generations. Intermarriage has resulted in twice the risk for some diseases compared to general population in U.S. These diseases include dwarfism, mental retardation, and four autosomal recessive disorders: glutaric aciduria type 1, juvenile-onset glaucoma, cystinosis, and cystic fibrosis. Each is treatable if identified early. Clinician should encourage parents to undergo DNA screening to enable early treatment, although Amish reject prenatal testing, as abortion is forbidden.

- **Attitudes about disabilities**. Generally accepting of persons with physical disabilities. Disabled persons participate in public life. Amish and German Baptists attribute disabilities to God's will. Amish have special schools for children with disabilities. Care of disabled persons is community's responsibility.

- **Sick role**. Expect sick persons to rest and recuperate, although work ethic is so strong that some insist on working despite pain. When sick persons cannot care for themselves, family members provide care. Amish miss Sunday services only if they are very, very ill.

- **Home and folk remedies**. Amish home remedies include herbs, teas, ointments, tonics, salves, liniments, and poultices. *Brauch* is a folk health art that involves laying on of hands and sometimes massage and manipulation. Amish seek a *Braucher*'s help before they seek non-Amish medical care, due to religious beliefs and cost of medical care. Chiropractic also common among Amish. Jewish home remedies include chicken soup. Germans also frequently use hot and cold compresses, and believe that warm mineral springs have healing powers.

- **Medications**. Comply with Western medications and advice of physicians but also use home remedies/herbs at same time.

- **Acceptance of procedures**. As in dominant culture, Germans accept most suggested medical procedures, such as blood transfusions, surgery, and organ transplants. Amish question procedures and often are concerned about cost; accept procedures if convinced they will restore health.

- **Care-seeking**. Seek biomedical care after trying home remedies. Amish actively participate in both folk and professional health care systems.

HEALTH ISSUES

- **Concept of health**. Mainstream, acculturated German Americans believe that health is the ability to work hard, take time to relax, and have fun. Amish believe that the body is God's temple, good physical and mental health is a gift from God, illness is God's will, and that illness affects the entire community and must be endured with faith and patience. Amish are very health-conscious; place high value on health because it is essential for work. Orthodox Jewish teaching includes the importance of taking care of the body.

- **Health promotion and prevention**. One can promote health and prevent illness by getting enough rest/sleep and drinking sufficient water. Saying "*Gesundheit*" after someone sneezes means "good health." Amish believe that each person is responsible for promoting health and well-being, and that hard work, clean living, and a well-balanced diet contribute to good health. Clinician should ask about status of children's immunizations.

- **Screening**. Orthodox Jews and Amish prohibit prenatal genetic screening because they strictly forbid abortion. Many Amish do not take children for immunizations and check-ups because they believe that exposing children to the outside world and the high esteem of physicians may encourage them to leave the community. Also, they do not have health insurance—must pay for services. Amish often need careful explanation of need for screening and treatment because they are reluctant to spend money. Germans generally accept regular screenings and examinations.

- **Common health problems**. Heart disease, stroke, arthritis, and diabetes. Amish are frequently the victims of accidents on roads when horses and buggies collide with motor vehicles or other buggies; accidents frequently result in disability and death. Clinician should urge Amish to use reflective tape on buggies. Farm accidents also common, especially among children, who help with chores and operate farm equipment beginning at a young age. Some of these accidents result in serious injury or death. Clinician should encourage Amish parents to participate in farm safety workshops. Should also ask about child's responsibilities at home. Old Order Amish drink from wells contaminated with total coliform bacteria and *E. coli* because wells are poorly constructed and maintained. Lack of refrigeration and faulty canning equipment for food preservation often result in bacterial infections that cause diarrhea.

DEATH RITUALS

- **Beliefs and attitudes about death**. Judaism does not view death as a tragedy but rather as a natural process, even when death occurs early in life or is a result of unfortunate circumstances. Jews believe that those who have lived a worthy life will be rewarded in the afterlife. Amish and German Baptists believe that death is God's will and part of life. Catholics, Lutherans, Amish, and German Baptists believe in eternal life after death (heaven). Religion influences life-support decisions (e.g., Jewish families decide in consultation with rabbi). Generally, when death is imminent and patient is suffering, Jewish law permits ending artificially prolonged life. Catholics, Lutherans, Amish, and German Baptists oppose euthanasia. However, Catholics and Lutherans allow administration of sedatives and analgesics to alleviate pain even when such medication reduces patient's ability to reason or shortens his/her life.

- **Preparation**. Spouse or adult children should be told so family can gather. When Jews are near death, they should receive as much attention as possible from family, friends, community, and rabbi; this is one of the most important commandments. Persons about to die are encouraged to read a confessional and say the *Shema*, a prayer of faith. If they cannot talk, someone says it for them. Catholics, even those who are not devout, may request that a priest administer last rites (Sacrament of Extreme Unction) near death. It involves anointing eyes, ears, nostrils, lips, hands, and feet with oil blessed by the bishop, along with a prayer and final confession of sins, which the priest forgives. This ritual is lengthy, but when death is imminent or has just occurred, a single unction (e.g., on forehead) is sufficient. If this sacrament is administered months before death, many Catholics want it to be repeated.
- **Home vs. hospital**. Preference varies among individuals and families. Generally accept hospice. Amish prefer to die at home.
- **Special needs**. When Jewish parents or close relatives hear of the death, they tear their clothing as an expression of initial grief. Mourners are responsible for caring for the deceased and burial preparation. After burial, a close friend or relative prepares the first meal for the mourners, consisting of eggs and bread for family only. After this meal, condolence calls acceptable. Mourners sit *shiva* for seven days in home of deceased or principal mourner. Customs include covering mirrors, burning large candle for seven days, and providing basin of water next to unlocked door so visitors can enter and wash hands without disturbing family members, who sit on cushions or low chairs that symbolize being struck down by grief. Relatives and friends bring food and family members refrain from virtually all usual activities during those seven days.
- **Care of the body**. Traditionally, cremation unacceptable among Jews, Catholics, Lutherans, Amish, and German Baptists, although many are cremated today. After an Orthodox Jew dies, the eyes are closed, body is laid on the floor and covered, and candles are lit next to body, which is never left alone until after burial. Those who sit with body (*shomerim*) may not eat or drink in the presence of the dead because the deceased no longer can

eat or drink. In preparation for burial, body is thoroughly cleaned, wrapped in a plain linen shroud or simple clothing, and placed in coffin. Traditionally, body was not to be viewed; viewing acceptable at some modern funerals. Also traditionally, body was not embalmed and was buried directly in the ground ("earth to earth") without coffin. Today, however, except for Orthodox Jews, most bodies are embalmed and buried in coffin, although coffin should have holes drilled in it so body has contact with earth. Amish burial usually takes place three days after death. Local funeral director from outside the community assists by embalming and sometimes providing coffin and hearse. As in life, there is simplicity in death: Amish coffins are wooden and plain. Viewing the body expected. Deceased women are dressed in apron they wore on their wedding day. Funerals do not include eulogies but rather admonitions for the living. Hymns are spoken, not sung; there are no flowers, and grave is dug by hand in an Amish Church district cemetery. Tombstones are simple and similar because Amish believe that in death, as in life, everyone is equal and no one should be elevated above anyone else.

- **Attitudes about organ donation.** Catholics and Lutherans do not object to organ donation. Most Jews permit it. In Orthodox families, rabbi is extremely important in all decisions regarding body. Amish have no religious prohibition against organ donation but generally do not participate.
- **Attitudes about autopsy.** Catholics and Lutherans do not object to autopsy. Jews may view it as desecration of the body but permit it when medically necessary or local law requires it, as long as autopsy is minimally intrusive and all body parts are buried. Autopsies seldom done on Amish but are permitted when medically necessary or legally required.

SELECTED REFERENCES

Adams, C. E., Leverland, M. B. (1986). The effects of religious beliefs on the health care practices of the Amish. *Nurse Practitioner*, 11, 58 and 63–67.

Breaking New Ground Outreach Program. (2002). Proceedings of the Plain Communities Conference, Purdue University. Retrieved June 15, 2004, from http://www.breakingnewground.info

DeRue, D. S., Schlegel, R., & Yoder, J. (Spring 2002). Amish needs and mental health care. *Journal of Rural Community Psychology*. Retrieved June 11, 2004, from http://www.marshall.edu/jrcp/sp2002/amish.htm

Hendricks, M. (1994). A doctor who makes barn calls. *Johns Hopkins Magazine* (electronic ed.), November. Retrieved June 2, 2004, from http://www.jhu.edu/~jhumag/1194web/barndoc.html

JAMARDA Resources Inc. *The Amish.* Retrieved June 11, 2004, from http://www.jamardaresources.com/JMDA%20Sample%20CD/WebHelp/amish.html

Merrill, P. C., and Reichmann, E. (1998). Religious denominations and religious communities in German-American life. Lesson outline from the Max

Kade German-American Center. Retrieved June 2, 2004, from http://www. ulib.iupui.edu/kade/merrill/lesson7.html

Shea, R. German and German-American customs, traditions, origins of holidays. Retrieved June 15, 2004, from http://www.serve.com/shea/germusa/customs.htm

Shenberger, P. (1995). Cultural diversity: Eating in America. Amish. Ohio State University Extension Fact Sheet. Retrieved June 2, 2004, from http://ohioline.osu.edu/hyg-fact/5000/5251.html

Steckler, J. A. (2003). People of German heritage. In L. D. Purnell & B. J. Paulanka (Eds.), *Transcultural health care: A culturally competent approach* (2nd ed.) (compact disk). Philadelphia: F. A. Davis.

Wenger, A. F. (1995). Cultural context, health and health care decision-making. 1994. *Journal of Transcultural Nursing, 7*, 3–14.

AUTHORS

Catherine Dodd, RN, MS, is a graduate of the University of California-San Francisco School of Nursing. She is currently a PhD student at UCSF working in the area of health policy, and the congressional district director for Rep. Nancy Pelosi, the House Democratic leader. She is a second-generation German American.

Petra Eggert, DC, PT, was born in Germany and now lives in Cupertino, CA. She currently practices independently as a chiropractor and physical therapist at Intrahealth (see www.intrahealth.net). Her family still lives in Germany.

ACKNOWLEDGMENT

Catherine Dodd thanks her cousin, Gernot Kaiser, MD, who is a recently retired family practice physician from a rural area of Germany, where his family has provided medical care for more than a century.

CHAPTER 16

GREEKS

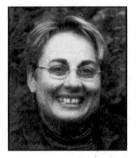

Joanne B. Genet

CULTURAL/ETHNIC IDENTITY

- **Preferred term(s)**. Greek or Greek American.
- **Census**. According to 2000 U.S. Census, there are nearly 1.2 million people of Greek ancestry in the U.S., of whom 142,896 are foreign-born. Largest populations are in New York, California, Illinois, Massachusetts, and Florida. There are more Greeks in the U.S. than anywhere else in the world outside of Greece.
- **History of immigration**. Greeks aspire to improve their economic status and will emigrate to do so. In 1763, first wave of 1,400 Greeks settled in New Smyrna, FL. When their homeland was under Turkish rule from 1453–1853, Greeks were forbidden to practice their religion or speak their language; however, language, cultural, and religious programs continued clandestinely. Turkish rule prompted some emigration. A large wave arrived in U.S. between 1901–24. These immigrants left Greece because of poverty resulting from the 400-year occupation by Turkey and subsequent emancipation from Turkish rule, war in the Balkans, and World War I. Most were laborers whose brides from arranged marriages in Greece followed them to the U.S. As families became established in the U.S., they sent money home to help other family members join them. Consequently, many related Greeks from the same geographic areas settled in the same parts of the U.S. Panhellenic organizations reminded immigrants of their heritage and tried to persuade them to return to Greece to help its ailing economy. Congress legislated restrictions that severely limited immigration for the next three decades. Another large immigration wave occurred between 1961–80 after a military junta took control in Greece. This wave included students and educated professionals. By 2001, about 732,000 Greeks had immigrated.

SPIRITUAL/RELIGIOUS ORIENTATION

- **Primary religious/spiritual affiliations**. More than 90% are Greek Orthodox. The Orthodox Church split from the Roman Catholic Church in 1054 A.D. Greek Orthodox religion in U.S. is more conservative than that in Greece. Leader of the Orthodox faith is the Patriarch, located in Greece. There is a hierarchy of archbishops, bishops, and priests. The head of each community church is a priest called "Father." Other religious affiliations are Jehovah's Witnesses, Judaism, and Evangelical Christianity.
- **Usual religious/spiritual practices**. Attend high church services on Sunday, which include a choir and burning of incense. Faith is more important than Bible reading or study. Greeks ask for intercession of saints to provide guidance in spiritual matters. Most homes have a shrine (*ikonostasion*), located in the eastern corner of master bedroom or a child's bedroom, to signify God's presence in the home. Some Greeks pray daily to saints. Believe that God is the center of the material and spiritual universe, so church is an important cultural and religious center. For example, it provides Greek language schooling for children and other activities, such as Greek dancing, cooking classes, and events for seniors, after church.
- **Use of spiritual healing/healers**. Consult priests for spiritual guidance when ill. Priests may provide communion or last rites in home or hospital. Greeks light candles at church entrance for loved ones who are ill or who have died. Priests may say blessings from the pulpit for those who are sick or deceased. Believe in evil, in the devil's parasitic power that seeks to control, and in demonic possession. Exorcism of satanic powers is called *vaskania*. Many also believe in the evil eye (*matiasma*) whereby an envious person can cause illness in another. An old woman removes such a curse through ritual "magic."
- **Holidays**. Celebrate religious holidays according to the Orthodox calendar, which is different from the mainstream Gregorian calendar. Families often celebrate according to both calendars. Easter is most important holiday. It begins with a large church ceremony on Friday evening. The main celebration is Holy Saturday evening: Church goes dark at midnight and the congregation lights candles to celebrate the resurrection, a ceremony that continues into early Easter Sunday morning. Most of the faithful have not eaten meat for two weeks, so the ceremony ends with a feast to break the fast. Dye Easter eggs only red to represent death and rebirth. Cook the eggs into a circle of bread eaten at the feast, along with lamb, pilaf, and feta cheese and cucumber salad (*ensalada*). Greeks celebrate Christmas on January 8, but it is low-key. Families celebrate name days (the day of the saint for which a person was named). Every summer, each church holds a large festival or picnic. As an example of how culture and religion intersect, Greek Independence Day (March 25) is the chief secular holiday and also one of the holiest days for Greek Orthodox Christians: the annunciation of the *Theotokos*.

On this day, the archangel Gabriel announced to Mary that she would bear a child. Greeks celebrate the day with family and at church. Greek immigrants and those born in U.S. also celebrate secular American holidays.

COMMUNICATION
ORAL COMMUNICATION

- **Major languages and dialects**. Demotic Greek, which is different from ancient Greek in word usage but shares same alphabet. Dialects vary by region, each having slightly different pronunciation and vernacular. However, the same basic language allows communication across regions. Written Greek is uniform.
- **Greetings**. Very formal. New acquaintances shake hands. Establish familiarity very quickly. As familiarity increases, persons may greet one another with a kiss on each cheek. Highly respect elders and greet them as "Mr."/ "Mrs." or "Aunt"/"Uncle," even when there is no blood relationship. More-acculturated persons may use first names.
- **Tone of voice**. Tend to be loud and use lots of hand gestures, even in pleasant conversations. Talk over one another.
- **Direct or indirect style of speech**. Respectful of, and indirect with, health care personnel. To keep relationships smooth, older adults and less-acculturated persons may verbally agree with caregivers even if they do not accept a suggested procedure or instructions. May reply to questions with stories rather than short, direct answers.
- **Use of interpreters**. Typically seek a family member to interpret. Reluctant to have strangers interpret; they do not trust strangers to communicate accurately or honestly, and believe that family issues should remain within the family. May ask children to interpret but not when the issue is sexual, a private family matter, or a life-threatening illness.
- **Serious or terminal illness**. Family and friends become very anxious when they have little or no information about a disease process and/or prognosis. Family often does not want to communicate the seriousness of an illness to patient. Clinician should speak with the eldest male family member or eldest adult child if no other adult is available. If ill person is elderly or a child, should notify family members first; they will decide whether to tell patient. In cases of terminal illness, family usually favors doing everything possible to preserve life, regardless of cost. Do not generally provide advance directives or do-not-resuscitate orders. Both patient and family accept imminent death as God's will.

WRITTEN COMMUNICATION

- **Literacy assessment**. Appropriate for clinician to ask immigrants directly about their literacy level. Older adults may have limited education and English skills. Most recent immigrants are well-educated, multilingual professionals who read English proficiently. Ninety percent of all immigrants have received some type of education, can read Greek newspapers, and know about past and current political events.

- **Consents**. Clinician should approach eldest male to find out who is family spokesperson. Eldest male often guides family discussion (which may include a priest) regarding consent. Best if clinician explains procedures, tests, and treatments in family's presence, and provides ample time for questions and discussion. If there is no health-professional friend or family member they can consult, Greeks typically follow physician's suggestions without question. Willingly sign consents for medical procedures. Less likely to participate in research.

NONVERBAL COMMUNICATION

- **Eye contact**. Sustained eye contact acceptable, except with authority figures, such as physicians and priests.
- **Personal space**. Close contact with members of immediate and extended family acceptable (closer than in dominant culture). Keep greater distance with health care providers, although proximity diminishes as familiarity grows.
- **Use and meaning of silence**. Silence infrequent. May use silence to express disapproval.
- **Gestures**. Often use hand gestures in conversation. Slight nod indicates agreement or approval. Raised eyebrows indicate a negative response or doubt. Most other gestures similar to those in dominant culture.
- **Openness in expressing emotions**. Tend to be rather stoic with outsiders. Especially reluctant to express depression or anxiety. Openly express anger. Show emotions within family but shield children and ill family members from emotional upset.
- **Privacy**. Family members very protective of one another with regard to privacy and other matters. May not trust health care providers; thus, family vigilance can be intrusive. Do not easily share private information with persons outside the family.
- **Touch**. Warm and affectionate with everyone. Touching and hugging very common. Acceptable to touch "public" areas of the body (e.g., to put a hand on someone's arm). Breasts and genitalia are "private" areas. Clinician should describe procedure and ask for permission to touch.
- **Orientation to time**. Greeks acknowledge schedules but commonly arrive at social functions 30 minutes to two hours late. The more social the event, the later one may arrive. Never consult clocks about when to get out of bed. May observe Greek time for social occasions and U.S. time for business appointments, when punctuality is valued. At health care appointments, may become impatient and demand immediate help if they perceive a problem as severe. If they do not receive immediate attention or believe they are

being ignored, most Greeks become verbally explosive. Accept a sufficient explanation for the delay. Orientation to the past is illustrated by elderly persons' regard for historical events, such as those that took place in ancient Greece, as important lessons for younger generations. Value the present as a means to an end (i.e., working hard today will lead to better times). Perceive the future as a time to rest and reap the rewards of a lifetime of hard work.

ACTIVITIES OF DAILY LIVING

- **Modesty**. Very modest. Prefer own nightgown/pajamas, robe, and slippers. Women and men both prefer help from person of same gender, but both also have the most confidence in White male physicians. Most prefer that all family members leave the room while they receive care.
- **Skin care**. Prefer to bathe daily but adjust according to level of illness. Elderly may prefer sponge baths to daily showers. Women may wear makeup in hospital to look good for family members.
- **Hair care**. Do not wash hair daily for fear of exacerbating illness. Women frequently have their hair done (prefer to look well-coifed) and may not want to shampoo while in the hospital. Men shampoo frequently.
- **Nail care**. Women get frequent manicures and pedicures in accordance with fashion trends. Men keep nails short; fashionable for those with old-world ties to leave nail of the little finger of right hand about one-half inch long.
- **Toileting**. Prefer bathroom with door closed. Use urinal or commode if necessary. Usually wash hands afterward.
- **Special clothing or amulets**. Married women wear wedding ring at all times. Both men and women may wear a Greek Orthodox cross and/or pendant of the Virgin Mary at all times. Children often have a small cross or small pendant of the Virgin Mary pinned to inside of undergarment. May use worry beads or a crucifix, and are likely to have a picture of Christ or a crucifix nearby. Clinician should not touch or remove items without permission. Family members surround and comfort patient with religious or secular items they bring.
- **Self-care**. Patient or family member may perform personal hygiene. Most patients allow someone of same gender to help if they are unable or a family member is not present. Women are far more receptive to help from nurses and nursing assistants than are men. Most patients want to participate actively in their healing and follow staff recommendations.

FOOD PRACTICES

- **Usual meal pattern**. Usually three meals a day. Breakfast typically light (e.g., bread with jam or honey and coffee). Lunch usually heaviest meal. It traditionally begins with pasta or rice with tomato or meat sauce, soup, or a specialty dish, such as macaroni and cheese with meat (*pastitsio*) or eggplant casserole (*moussaka*), followed by meat or fish. Often serve green salad or boiled greens, such as dandelion, collard, or mustard greens, with main dish. Sweet desserts include *baklava*, a pastry, followed by fresh fruit. Usually serve white resinated wine (*retsina*) with main meal and Greek coffee afterward. Do not normally serve evening meal before 8:30. This meal may be as large as lunch if lunch was light. If lunch was heavy, dinner may consist of tomato cucumber salad, fresh bread with feta cheese, black olives, and *retsina*. May precede the meal with *ouzo*, an anise-flavored aperitif. Meal pattern and foods of acculturated Greeks in U.S. are more similar to those in dominant culture.

- **Special utensils**. None, except for Turkish coffee maker for special coffee at home.
- **Food beliefs and rituals**. Believe that eating meals with family has a healing effect. Not eating implies serious illness. Healing foods include macaroni and cheese with meat (*pastitsio*), rice pudding (*rizogalo*), baked custards, cream pie (*galaktoboureko*), and yogurt.
- **Usual diet**. Typically a lot of rice, fish, boiled greens, lamb, bread, olives, and feta cheese. Meat very important in diet, especially lamb, but acculturated persons may substitute beef for lamb.
- **Fluids**. Coffee, resinated wine (*retsina*) with meals, anise-flavored aperitif (*ouzo*). Intake of other fluids, such as water and fruit juices, similar to that in dominant culture, although Greeks drink less soda. Alcoholism lower in Greece than in other European countries.
- **Food taboos and prescriptions**. No prohibitions. Special holiday foods include Easter pastries and Christmas breads. Greeks prepare a special bread for funerals and small, individual cakes for weddings. When ill, they prefer hot teas, such as chamomile and "mountain" tea with lemon and honey, and light broths, boiled rice with lemon, and dry toast. "Greek penicillin" is egg and lemon chicken soup (*avgolemono*). Many cultural foods bring enjoyment and special comfort when someone is sick. These include *ensalada*, macaroni and cheese with meat (*pastitsio*), rice pudding (*rizogalo*), baked custards, cream pie (*galaktoboureko*), and yogurt.
- **Hospitality**. Always offer food and drink to visitors, even if family is poor or host is very ill. Consider it unfriendly if health care provider refuses an offer of food.

SYMPTOM MANAGEMENT

- **Pain** (*ponos*). Reluctant to admit pain. Stoic when expressing pain. Understand numerical scales but may underestimate pain level. May refuse pain medication, especially morphine, out of fear it will affect consciousness and lead to addiction. Prefer oral medications. After getting permission from family spokesperson, clinician may want to consult priest about providing guidance to patient.
- **Dyspnea** (*duspnoia*). Manage symptoms same way as dominant culture does. Use words better than numerical scale to describe activity limitations. Likely

to accept opiates for dyspnea because they believe that opiates cure it. May use prayer as a nonpharmacological treatment.

- **Nausea/vomiting** (*nautia/emetos*). Embarrassed about vomiting; may try to clean up before calling nurse. May underestimate the severity of nausea and the number of times they vomit. May prefer to eat boiled rice with fresh lemon. May use prayer as nonpharmacological treatment but also accept pharmacological modalities.
- **Constipation/diarrhea** (*diskilia/diarroia*). Embarrassed about diarrhea; may try to clean up before calling nurse. Use boiled rice soup or prayer as non-pharmacological treatments. Otherwise, manage symptoms as dominant culture does.
- **Fatigue** (*koposi*). May underplay level of fatigue. Use words better than numerical scale to describe fatigue. View rest and sleep as necessary for recovery. Accept medication if physician recommends it. May use prayer as non-pharmacological treatment.
- **Depression** (*katathlipsi*). Greeks deny depression, viewing it as disharmony between one's spirit and God. Use words better than numerical scale to describe depression. Patient has difficulty accepting medication even if physician recommends it. Prefer prayer and consultation with priest as non-pharmacological treatments.
- **Self-care symptom management**. Attempt self-care with over-the-counter medication and home remedies before seeking medical advice. In hospital, patient may be passive and expect family members to care for him/her, or participate in self-care and expect help from women family members. Families may have to coax or coerce men to seek professional advice regarding symptoms.

BIRTH RITUALS/CARE OF THE NEW MOTHER AND BABY

- **Pregnancy care**. Much family celebration of pregnancy, which is central to Greek culture. Women generally obtain prenatal care. Allow pregnant women to work outside the home, unless primary care doctor imposes restrictions. Expect a pregnant woman to eat large quantities, especially protein and foods high in iron, and to satisfy cravings; otherwise, baby may be born with birthmark. Woman's mother may help with daily household chores and may live with her. Discourage heavy lifting and intense physical activity during pregnancy. Attend childbirth preparation classes.
- **Preferences for children**. Prefer males, although all children are well-loved. Want large families—more than two children is the norm. Number of children depends on family's economic situation.
- **Labor practices**. If physician unavailable for delivery, accept midwife. Many families have stories of beloved midwives in their past. Discourage expectant mother from taking any pain medication during delivery out of fear it will harm her or baby. Acceptable for her to walk around, eat, and shower.

- **Role of the laboring woman during birth**. Generally passive. May be vocally expressive during delivery. Follows clinician's commands.
- **Role of the father and other family members during birth**. Expect father to attend birth. Family members usually remain nearby but may not attend birth, considering it to be private.
- **Vaginal vs. cesarean section**. The more natural the process, the better. Accept cesarean section if necessary.
- **Breastfeeding**. Common, as mothers are aware of benefits for baby, and spouses support breastfeeding. Some women delay showering for the first few days, believing that it can make infant allergic to milk. Breastfeed in seclusion to maintain modesty and privacy.
- **Birth recuperation**. Expect mother to be up and care for child soon after birth. Family members likely to assist. Traditionally, expected mother and infant to stay at home and not attend church for 40 days, believing she was ritually impure (*lahoosa*) and particularly susceptible to illness. After 40 days, mother and baby receive a ritual blessing in church. Maternal grandmother often stays on for six weeks to eight months to help with household chores.
- **Baby care**. Important to keep baby warm and its head covered at all times. Prevent illness by protecting baby from the elements and possible curse of the evil eye. Otherwise, same as in dominant culture.
- **Problems with baby**. Physician should inform mother; she tells the family. Often request a priest.
- **Male and female circumcision**. Traditional Greeks do not circumcise boys, but second generation often does. Girls never circumcised.

DEVELOPMENTAL AND SEXUAL ISSUES

- **Celebration of menarche or becoming a man**. Neither celebrated.
- **Attitudes about birth control**. Greek Orthodox Church teaches that birth control is immoral and that sexual expression is fulfilled in marriage, the purpose of which is to procreate. Birth control pills disrupt the relationship with one's body and, therefore, the relationship with God. Use of birth control related to religious practices and degree of acculturation.
- **Attitudes about sexually transmitted infection (STI) control, including condoms**. Perceive condoms similar to the way they perceive other birth control methods. Believe that monogamy will prevent STIs.
- **Attitudes about abortion**. Immoral and unacceptable. Women do undergo abortion but keep it very private or secret, especially from their family.
- **Attitudes about unwed sexual experimentation**. Sinful. Sexual relations do occur, but there is great social pressure to abstain and marry.
- **Sexual orientation**. Greek Orthodox Church views gay or lesbian orientation as immoral. Such a person still considered to be part of the family, especially if he/she is heterosexually married and has children. Society ignores the additional homosexual relationship or treats it with distaste. Greeks

view openly gay and lesbian persons, especially those without children, as sinners who are not contributing to family and are in disharmony with God. More accepting of gays and lesbians who have children.

- **Gender identity**. Church and family strictly enforce gender and social norms. Censure females who are masculine and males who exhibit feminine behaviors. Families pressure them to change.
- **Attitudes about menopause**. A natural phase in women's lives. Accept it stoically. Is a private matter. Women unlikely to take medication. If symptomatic, some pray.

FAMILY RELATIONSHIPS

- **Composition/structure**. Patriarchal. Multiple generations live together or close to each other. Children participate in all family activities. Little place for single persons, especially single women. Very difficult to divorce—considered a sin.
- **Decision-making**. Immediate family usually discusses choices that will have major impact on family. Eldest male or oldest adult makes all decisions related to the family and handles disputes that cause family rifts.
- **Spokesperson**. Eldest male or, if none, the oldest adult.
- **Gender issues**. Expect men to work outside the home and financially support the family. Many Greek women still work primarily within the home. Men discipline children, women nurture and care for them.
- **Changing roles among generations in U.S.** As Greeks become more acculturated, they may begin to ignore their heritage and values; family structure becomes more like that in dominant culture. However, divorce still less common.
- **Caring roles**. Women most often provide care. Men do so if there is no woman to provide it.
- **Expectations of and for children**. Greeks cherish and indulge young children. Expect adult children to take on culturally appropriate family roles, such as caring for elders. Emphasize religious training. Social activities are centered on church rather than school. Strongly emphasize education and getting ahead for both boys and girls. Expect men to be financially successful and women to marry well. Families influence the choice of career and marital partner. Expect babies to be baptized in Greek Orthodox Church; baptism is a major life event and cause for much celebration. Choose a dear friend (*coumbada*) or family member to be the godmother or godfather (*nouna* or *nouno*), who provides life-long spiritual guidance. Young adults may live at home until they marry, then live nearby.
- **Expectations of and for elders**. Elderly women have a higher standing and more power within the family than younger women do, and are expected to live with or near adult children, especially daughters. Oldest man in family is the patriarch and oldest woman dominates, especially if widowed.

- **Expectations of hospital visitors**. Some patients prefer having family members at bedside at all times to intervene on their behalf. Friends also may stay at bedside and be overprotective. Priest may visit. Staff should consult with family spokesperson regarding patient care or safety. Family and friends may try to circumvent severe restrictions on visitation. Most believe that their support is necessary for the patient's recuperation and that the presence of loved ones will enhance recovery.

ILLNESS BELIEFS

- **Causes of/attitudes about physical illness**. Naturalistic causes of illness include specific disease processes, poor hygiene, genetic predisposition, stress, lack of proper food, and catching a wind or cold. Supernatural causes are God's will, punishment for sins, or being nonreligious. Social causes include the evil eye (*matiasma*) either intentionally or unintentionally cast by a jealous person, not respecting parents, leaving the family or other bad behavior, and neglecting work or school.
- **Causes of/attitudes about mental illness**. Almost invisible in the community. Greeks consider mental illness shameful, something the family keeps to itself and deals with. Some view it as demonic possession or as "having a nervous breakdown." Perceive mentally ill person as weak and sinful. Emphasize individual's responsibility for mental illness. Greeks may be very reluctant to seek help; when they do, more likely to seek spiritual than psychiatric help. Patients may present with dizziness or other somatic symptoms. Accept medication. Mental illness less stigmatized than drug addiction and alcoholism.
- **Causes of genetic defects**. Evil eye may cause genetic problems. Most Greeks attribute genetic illness to sins of previous generation. Genetic counseling before marriage appropriate because it helps couples gauge suitability for marriage and risk of genetic defects in offspring. If amniocentesis indicates genetic abnormality, abortion not ethically or spiritually acceptable. Women may choose to abort without family's support or conceal abortion by describing it as miscarriage.
- **Attitudes about disabilities**. Disability is routine part of family life and of family member's role as caretaker. Greeks consider disabled persons, who attend church and other events, to be part of the community. May enroll disabled persons in life-skills or related programs.
- **Sick role**. May not want to go out even if able. Women may take to bed; men unlikely to do so. Expect sick persons to rely completely on family for care and constant support.
- **Home and folk remedies**. May massage rubbing alcohol into ailing body part. Also may use cupping (*vendouzes*) to draw out fever and for colds, hypertension, or backache. In cupping, a vacuum is created by lighting a cotton swab on a fork in an inverted glass or cup, then placing it on patient's

back. Herbal remedies (*praktika*) include chamomile for stomach problems or abdominal cramps, raw garlic for warding off colds, and cooked garlic for high blood pressure and heart disease. Place cucumber on forehead for headache and use menthol to open up chest during a cold. Use various amulets or charms to prevent the evil eye, but only an elderly, "knowing" woman can remove the evil eye by performing a ritual.

- **Medications**. Comply well if they understand how to take a medication and why it is necessary. May not pose questions to physician for fear of challenging authority; do not want to appear uninformed or uneducated.
- **Acceptance of procedures**. Consider human life to be God's gift. However, Greeks do not have any religious objections to skin grafts, blood transfusions, or most organ donations. Some may object to heart transplants due to Greek Orthodox belief that the heart is the seat of the soul.
- **Care-seeking**. Acculturated persons seek care like those in dominant culture. Some Greeks do not trust health care professionals; first seek family or community advice about home or folk remedies. May delay seeking professional care even if they have adequate health insurance.

HEALTH ISSUES

- **Concept of health**. Healthy persons feel strong, joyful, content, and free of pain, and can care for themselves. Body and spirit are inextricably bound in religious beliefs. Priest and physician roles are closely linked through beliefs and faith in healers.
- **Health promotion and prevention**. Good food and healthy eating necessary for good health. Understand that exercise is beneficial, but older men and women are unlikely to exercise. Health promotion and prevention among Greeks similar to that in dominant culture.
- **Screening**. Important for preventing illness. Older, less-acculturated women may not obtain Pap smear or breast cancer screening; they do not think these tests are useful, believing that the related areas of their bodies no longer function after menopause.
- **Common health problems**. Lactose intolerance in adults, thalassemia, diabetes, heart disease, obesity, and high cholesterol. Increasing incidence of heart disease and cancer, especially among women. However, among European Union countries, Greece has the third-lowest rate of death from all cancers and the fewest breast cancer deaths. Very common for men—and increasingly common for women—to smoke.

DEATH RITUALS

- **Beliefs and attitudes about death**. View death as part of life. According to Greek Orthodox religion, there is a heaven, resurrection of the body (considered to be sacred), and redemption of the soul. Baptism necessary to reach heaven after death. Suicide is sinful; funeral for someone who has died

by suicide cannot be held in the church and he/she cannot be buried in consecrated ground.

- **Preparation.** Clinician should inform family of imminent death. Family members typically remain in room. Family calls priest or church. Priest visits and gives communion and last rites.
- **Home vs. hospital.** Family initially prefers patient to be hospitalized, hoping for a miraculous cure. When it finally accepts terminal illness, prefers to have patient die at home in family's care. Accept hospice, but pain medication may pose a problem due to belief that it can hasten death.
- **Special needs.** Immediate family and priest should be present. Religious beliefs and practices dictate behavior during bereavement. Public displays of grief acceptable. Adults and children wear dark, somber colors.
- **Care of the body.** Do not believe in cremation because it desecrates the body. Funeral home embalms body and prepares it for burial. Traditional wake in funeral home on one evening (*trisagion*). Viewing of body may last 1–3 days. Funeral, generally with an open casket, takes place the day after the viewing. Priest performs last rites over the body in solitude at end of funeral.
- **Attitudes about organ donation.** Acceptable for preserving life, unacceptable for scientific research. Attitudes are changing. Clinician should discuss donation with family before death and with patient. Unlikely that family will donate heart, due to belief that it is the seat of the soul.
- **Attitudes about autopsy.** Unacceptable, unless medically necessary, as autopsy desecrates the body.

SELECTED REFERENCES

Harakas, S. S. (1980). *For the health of body and soul: An Eastern Orthodox introduction to bioethics.* Brookline, MA: Holy Cross Press.

Makedon, A. (1998). *The social psychology of immigration: The Greek-American experience.* Chicago: Chicago State University.

Papadopoulos, I., & Purnell, L. (2003). People of Greek heritage. In L. D. Purnell & B. J. Paulanka (Eds.), *Transcultural health care: A culturally competent approach* (2nd ed.) (compact disc, pp. 56–69). Philadelphia: F. A. Davis.

Tripp-Reimer, T. (1983). Retention of a folk-healing practice (*matiasma*) among four generations of urban Greek immigrants. *Nursing Research, 32,* 97–101.

Tsemberis, S. J., Psomiades, H. J., & Karpathakis, A. (Eds.). (1999). *Greek American families: Traditions and transformations.* New York: Queens College of the City University of New York.

World Health Organization. (1997). *Highlights on health in Greece.* Retrieved July 16, 2004, from http://www.who.dk/document/E62336.pdf

AUTHOR

Joanne B. Genet, PA, MLS, is the granddaughter of Greek immigrants and was raised in a Big Fat Greek Family. She has been a physician assistant for more than 22 years, specializing in women's health. Her current work in the Public Health Division of Contra Costa Health Services in Northern California targets low-income and immigrant populations. It includes improving access to care and helping to eliminate health disparities.

ACKNOWLEDGMENT

Several portions of this chapter are based on a chapter about Greeks that Z. JoAnna Papadakos prepared and submitted in 1997 to the editors in hopes that it would be included in a second edition. Despite numerous attempts, the editors were unable to locate Papadakos but nevertheless want to thank her for her assistance.

CHAPTER 17

HAITIANS

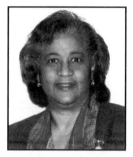

Jessie M. Colin

CULTURAL/ETHNIC IDENTITY

- **Preferred term(s)**. Haitian or Haitian American. Haitians in U.S. strongly resist acculturation, taking pride in preserving traditional cultural, spiritual, religious, and family values.
- **Census**. According to 2000 U.S. Census, 548,199 Haitians live in U.S.; however, there are probably well more than 1 million. Foreign-born Haitians represent 1.3% of the total foreign-born population in U.S. Largest numbers live in Miami, New York, Boston, Chicago, and Los Angeles.
- **History of immigration**. Before 1920, Haitians traveled to U.S. only for educational purposes. They learned a profession and returned to Haiti to practice it. Since 1920, most emigration has been linked directly to political crises in Haiti. First wave of immigrants came to U.S. that year because of atrocities associated with the American occupation of Haiti (1915–34). This group is believed to have settled in Harlem and assimilated into American society. In 1957, Francois Duvalier became president of Haiti, prompting the first official emigration of Haitians. Among them were politicians whose aim was to organize the overthrow of Duvalier's regime while in exile, and educated professionals in search of a better life; they set-tled in U.S. and quickly sent for their families. Duvalier was elected presi-dent for life in 1964, which led to a significant number of Haitians fleeing the island, primarily relatives of politicians who opposed the Duvalier regime. Most of those who had emigrated up to that time entered U.S. legally. In 1971, Duvalier died and was succeeded by his 19-year-old son, Jean-Claude, also appointed for life. Meanwhile, Haiti was suffering from economic deprivation, which spurred another major exodus consisting of urbanites and peasants, many of whom came covertly through the under-

ground. During the political crisis and armed uprising against President Jean-Bertrand Aristide in February 2004, the number of interdictions by the U.S. Coast Guard peaked; it dropped to zero in the weeks after Aristide left the country.

SPIRITUAL/RELIGIOUS ORIENTATION

- **Primary religious/spiritual affiliations**. Catholicism. Since 1970s, 15–20% of Haitians have been Protestant. Voodoo (also spelled *voudou, vodoun,* and *vodun*) is an important religious component, an African spirit religion closely related to Catholicism, including trance-enhanced communication with ancestors, saints, or deities. All Haitians, not just the lower class and unlettered persons, take voodoo very seriously.
- **Usual religious/spiritual practices**. Often receive holy communion. Pray using rosary beads and they practice novenas. May pray to a particular saint and wear only colors associated with that saint for a predetermined time period. Believe in power of prayer to physically heal. Strongly believe in all sacraments; very fearful of sacrament of the sick, which Haitians equate with death. In voodoo, Haitians gather to worship deities or spirits (*loa*) who are believed to have received their powers from God.
- **Use of spiritual healing/healers**. Female voodoo priest (*mambo*), male voodoo priest (*hougan*), and practitioners of black magic (*bokors*). Believers seek these practitioners when they must worship the spirit to be relieved of illness. Some believe it is important to maintain this relationship for protection or to avoid any harm.
- **Holidays**. Widely celebrate three feasts: Carnival (which lasts a week, although only one day is an official holiday), Good Friday, and Easter. Other religious holidays include the Epiphany (January 6, Catholic), the Annunciation (March 25, Catholic), feeding of the dead (April 30, voodoo), feeding of different deities (*loa*) (May 12, voodoo), *Notre Dame de Lourdes* (August 15, Catholic), All Saints Day (November 1, Catholic), All Souls Day (November 2, Catholic), Immaculate Conception (December 6, Catholic), feeding of the sea (December 12–14, voodoo), and Christmas (December 25). Secular holidays include Independence Day (January 1), Ancestors Day (January 2), Agriculture and Labor Day (May 1), Flag Day (May 18), anniversary of the death of Jean-Jacques Dessalines (October 17), United Nations Day (October 24), and Battle of Vertieres Day (November 18). Haitians in U.S and Haiti celebrate all of these holidays.

COMMUNICATION

ORAL COMMUNICATION

- **Major languages and dialects**. Two official languages in Haiti: French and Creole, designated by 1987 Haitian Constitution. Creole is the national language spoken by entire population of Haiti and by people of Haitian descent born or living abroad. Educated and upper-class persons also speak French. Haiti has an oral culture, with a long tradition of proverbs, jokes, and stories reflecting on philosophy. Haitians use these as educational tools to pass on unwritten knowledge. Those who recently immigrated do not speak English, but those from middle and upper classes understand, and may be able to communicate in, English. Haitians are frequently subsumed in the African American population.

- **Greetings**. Very friendly. In informal situations, embrace and kiss as a sign of affection and acceptance. In formal encounters, handshake greeting may be composed and stern. Gender also plays significant role in formal situations. For example, a man does not embrace a woman, even if they are friends. A handshake is the polite and respectful salutation. Friends address each other by first name and family members by nickname, but health care providers should address patient/family using "Mr.," "Mrs.," "Ms.," or "Dr." Children refer to adult friends as "Auntie" or "Uncle."
- **Tone of voice**. Haitian language very rich and expressive. Voice intonation conveys emotions. Pitch is high or low, depending on message. Tone expresses joy or sadness, happiness, or deceit. Haitians are very expressive and tend to be loud.
- **Direct or indirect style of speech**. Generally direct, except regarding personal or religious matters. Communication with health care providers reserved and polite. Some Haitians, rather than risk conflict or disagreement with a person of higher socioeconomic status or authority, indicate agreement even when they disagree. Communication with friends animated and expressive.
- **Use of interpreters**. Mistrust interpreters, believing that they generally do not accurately convey the intended message. Prefer to use family members rather than friends because the former are very keen on maintaining confidentiality. In absence of a family member, prefer a professional interpreter with whom they have no relationship and will likely never see again.
- **Serious or terminal illness**. Expressed as "I am very sick" (*Moin malad anpil*), meaning in critical condition, or "I will never be well again" (*Moin pap refe*), meaning terminal and death is imminent. Haitians first inform closest family member or person who patient designated as the one to be informed in case of problems; that person informs patient if he/she thinks it necessary. This also applies in cases of surgery, especially abdominal surgery, which Haitians generally fear.

WRITTEN COMMUNICATION

- **Literacy assessment**. Haiti is a nonliterate culture. Eighty percent or more of Haitians neither read nor write. Educational materials about health should be visual and oral (e.g., video and radio programs). Illiteracy rate in U.S. also high. Health care professionals can assess literacy by offering to clarify information. Directly asking patient if he/she can read embarrasses patient and makes him/her reluctant to ask for other assistance.

- **Consents**. Haitians generally imply they do not want to know about a procedure and do not want informed consent. Trust experts, believing that they have patient's interests at heart, are more knowledgeable, and have authority to dictate what should be done. To obtain consent, important for clinician to indicate clearly the importance of a procedure and the absolute need for consent. Clinician should ask a family member the patient has chosen to be present throughout the interaction.

NONVERBAL COMMUNICATION

Affectionate and polite but shy. Uneducated Haitians generally do not show their lack of knowledge to non-Haitians; rather, they keep it to themselves and avoid conflict, sometimes projecting a timid attitude. More comfortable with immigrants who do not speak English, especially islanders, with whom they feel a common bond.

- **Eye contact**. Traditional persons avoid direct eye contact as much as possible, especially with authority figures, as they consider it insolent. More-acculturated adults make eye contact with each other, but children may avoid direct eye contact with adults.
- **Personal space**. Interactions are very close, 1–2 feet. Sharing personal space not much of an issue among family and friends. Keep a comfortable distance with health care professionals. Adults prefer not to share space with children, believing that children should not participate in adult conversation and should not be within hearing distance of a group of adults.
- **Use and meaning of silence**. Generally means disapproval, disappointment, or possibly disagreement.
- **Gestures**. Haitians use many hand motions while talking. There are no particular gestures that may lead to misunderstanding.
- **Openness in expressing emotions**. Smile a lot. Among family and friends, hand gestures generally accompany animated and loud conversation as a means of reinforcement or emphasis, especially when Haitians discuss issues of particular interest (e.g., politics). Do not express emotions to health care provider unless they have a trusting relationship with him/her. May cry if something really bothers them or express fear of the unknown or of procedure and test outcomes. To express major disapproval, may fold arms across their chest, roll their eyes, or look away or up at ceiling.
- **Privacy**. Very private. Disclose information only when absolutely necessary and, even then, only if they are ready to. Concept of shame is strong: Their bodies are not to be exposed. Private even with themselves. For example, women are not supposed to touch their own bodies, which means it may be very difficult to teach breast self-examination. Haitians do not appreciate it when a health care worker talks about their condition with a friend or family member if patient has not given permission. Will not out-

wardly express their disapproval in such cases but will automatically sever their relationship with health care worker.

- **Touch**. Haitians freely touch family and friends. May touch health care providers to let them know they are being spoken to. Appreciate providers' supportive touch.
- **Orientation to time**. Not committed to time or schedule. Perception of time is flexible. Not impolite for Haitians to arrive late for an appointment; everyone and anything can wait. Compensate by manipulating the timing of activities. For example, a wedding invitation may indicate a starting time of 6 p.m., though the actual starting time is 7 or 7:30. This practice is pervasive in Haitian society. May be on time for medical appointments if health care provider has emphasized importance of punctuality. Haitians from poor or lower-class backgrounds are more past- and present-oriented; those who are educated and upper-class tend to be present- and future-oriented.

ACTIVITIES OF DAILY LIVING

- **Modesty**. Both genders very modest. Men embarrassed to wear hospital gowns, so they should be offered pajamas. If hospital stay is planned, patients bring their own gowns or pajamas. Gender important in health care interactions: Physicians should be male, nurses female. Haitians highly respect and trust both physicians and nurses. Although Haitians are puzzled by male nurses, they accept care provided by opposite gender.
- **Skin care**. Shower daily, preferably in the morning. Women perform thorough peri-care with soap and water at night before bedtime. Better-educated Haitians may use lotion.
- **Hair care**. Women shampoo weekly. Use rollers at night to maintain style. Use oil-based pomades to replenish scalp and keep hair from drying. Men shampoo daily while showering.
- **Nail care**. Less-educated women keep nails short and unpolished for hygiene. More-educated women can afford weekly manicures and pedicures, which enhances their positive self-care image.
- **Toileting**. Insist on using bathroom, as privacy is very important. If family member can assist, patient may use bedpan or urinal. Perform peri-anal care after using toilet—pour water on perineal area and anus, wash with soap, and dry thoroughly. Staff should provide small pitcher in bathroom.
- **Special clothing or amulets**. Catholics often have religious medallions, rosary beads, or a figure of a saint to whom they are devoted. Saints worshipped by Catholics are same as those in voodoo but have different names and functions. Therefore, picture of a saint in patient's room may have double meaning, but generally it is there for protection. Clinician should not remove articles from patient's room unless they interfere with care; should ask permission before removing them.
- **Self-care**. During initial stages of illness, family members want to help with

patient's hygiene, due to privacy. They wait for directions regarding the care they should provide. Clinician should be specific but also offer assistance whenever possible. Patients want to be clean, feel clean, and smell clean. Because Haitians fear surgery, patients limit self-care activities, believing that any physical strain may negatively affect their body. Clinician must strongly encourage them to cough, breathe deeply, and ambulate to avoid complications.

FOOD PRACTICES

- **Usual meal pattern**. Lunch is typically largest meal. Breakfast generally consists of bread with butter and coffee, and dinner is soup or hot cereal. Some Haitians have adjusted to U.S. routines. For example, dinner may be their largest meal.
- **Special utensils**. None.
- **Food beliefs and rituals**. Haitians believe that exposing the body to an imbalance of "hot" (*cho*) and "cold" (*fret*) factors causes illness. For example, eating tomatoes or white beans after childbirth induces hemorrhage, and cold orange juice should be avoided during menstruation. Haitians also assess food in terms of heavy or light qualities; one should eat heavy foods, such as cornmeal mush, broiled plantain, or potato, during the day to provide energy for work. One should eat light foods, such as hot chocolate milk, bread, or soup, for dinner because they are easily digested. Method of preparation also important: Boiled green plantains are heavy, but fried yellow/ripe plantain is light.
- **Usual diet**. In hospital, prefer fasting to eating non-Haitian food—afraid such food may make them sicker. Prefer rice, beans, plantain, spicy braised meat with gravy or stewed vegetables, and chicken. Haitians generally do not eat yogurt, cottage cheese, or runny egg yolks.
- **Fluids**. Drink lots of water and homemade fruit juices, cold fruity soda, coffee in the morning, and tea only when sick.
- **Food taboos and prescriptions**. Food prohibitions are related to particular diseases and life stages. For example, to avoid acne, teenagers should not drink citrus juices, such as orange or lemon. After strenuous activity or any activity that makes the body hot, one should not eat cold food because that will cause an imbalance (*chofret*). For example, eating cold pineapple after excessive walking could cause gastric hemorrhage. When ill, Haitians like pumpkin soup, bouillon, or a special soup of green vegetable, meat, plantain, dumplings, and yam. Also like all kinds of porridge, oatmeal, and *akasan*, a cornmeal cream prepared with milk, sugar, cinnamon, vanilla flavoring, and a pinch of salt.
- **Hospitality**. Haitians are very hospitable. Welcome guests to their home with food, refusal of which is impolite. May offer child's bed if guest stays overnight. Family offers most comfortable space to guest.

SYMPTOM MANAGEMENT

Haitians can use numerical scales for symptoms if the scales are explained.

- **Pain** (*doule*). Have very low pain threshold. Whole demeanor changes. Very verbal about what hurts. Sometimes moan. Usually very vague about location of pain, believing that whole body is affected; because disease travels, location of pain not important. Prefer injections. In lieu of injections, order of preference is elixir, tablets, and capsules. Accept alternative pain treatments.

- **Dyspnea**. A primary respiratory ailment is *oppression*. Haitians use this term to describe asthma, but it includes more than that. Also seems to describe a state of anxiety and hyperventilation. Consider *oppression* (like many respiratory conditions) a "cold" state. Patient says, "I am suffocating" (M *ap toufe*) or "I cannot breathe" (M*wen pa ka respire*). Clinician should offer oxygen only when absolutely necessary, as Haitians associate it with serious disease.

- **Nausea/vomiting** (*Lestomak-mwen ap roule* or *Ke mwen tounin* means "My stomach is churning"; *Lestomak-mwen chaje* means "I feel nauseous"; M *santi m anvi vomi* means "I feel like vomiting"). More-educated Haitians express their discomfort as nausea. Because of modesty, they dispense of vomitus immediately so as not to upset others. Hospital staff should provide specific instructions about keeping the specimen.

- **Constipation/diarrhea** (*konstipasyon*). Treat with laxative or some herbal teas. Sometimes use enemas (*lavman*). Diarrhea not a major concern among adults. However, Haitians consider diarrhea to be very dangerous in children and sometimes interpret it as a hex on the child. They try herbal medicine, seek help from a voodoo priest (*hougan*), and, if all else fails, may seek a physician. Very important for clinician to assess child carefully because he/she may have been ill for quite some time. If a stranger offers food to a child, parents very reluctant to accept it. They question a health care practitioner who does so—want to make sure physician approves.

- **Fatigue**. Haitians think fatigue signals a physical weakness known as *febles*, caused by anemia or insufficient blood. Generally attribute symptoms to poor diet. Patients may suggest a need for special care—i.e., eating well, taking vitamins, and resting. To counter *febles*, eat liver, pigeon meat, watercress, bouillon made from green leafy vegetables, cow's feet, and red meat.

- **Depression** (sometimes *depression nerveuse*). Stigma attached to mental illness is so strong that Haitians do not readily admit to depression. According to voodoo, depression indicates possession by malevolent spirits or is punishment for not honoring good, protective spirits. Also may view depression as a hex put on someone by a jealous or envious person. Factors that may trigger depression are memories of family in homeland, thinking about spirits in Haiti, dreams about dead family members, guilt and regrets about abandoning family in Haiti for abundance in U.S., and loneliness in U.S. Clinician needs to be sensitive to root cause of problem and ascertain need for comfort within particular religious beliefs. For example, clinician may want

to summon priest or pastor if depression is related to something spiritual. If depression severe, patient accepts therapy with caution.
- **Self-care symptom management**. Haitians try home remedies first; at the outset, clinician should ask about them and herbal treatments. Patient may gauge his/her symptoms and institute treatment based on another Haitian's experience with the same illness. Haitians consider health to be a personal responsibility, so patient may tell clinician what illness he/she has rather than describe symptoms, and seek confirmation of self-diagnosis. Sometimes use biomedical terms inappropriately. Therefore, very important for clinician to elicit symptoms and history.

BIRTH RITUALS/CARE OF THE NEW MOTHER AND BABY
- **Pregnancy care**. Some seek prenatal care at private physician's office or clinic, but many women do not seek prenatal care. View pregnancy as a happy time for entire family, not as a health problem. Pregnant woman is expected to fulfill her work obligations throughout pregnancy. Pregnant women experience an increase in salivation and rid themselves of the excess in places that may seem inappropriate. Sometimes carry a spit cup with them; not embarrassed to use it. Do not believe they should swallow their saliva. Pregnant women are restricted from eating spices, as spices may irritate fetus. However, are permitted to eat vegetables and red fruits, believing that these will build up fetus's blood. Are encouraged to eat large portions because they are eating for two.
- **Preferences for children**. Perceive all children as key to their culture and values; celebrate them as a gift from God. Welcome large families. Prefer first-born be a boy; if it is a girl, implies father is not *macho* enough and others tease him about his sperm not being sufficiently strong. He has what Haitians refer to as "weak kidney" (*rein faible*). Having a son is extremely important because it means he will carry on the family name. Large families also welcome female children because they help with household chores and care of siblings.
- **Labor practices**. May walk, pace, sit, squat, and rub their belly. Do not request analgesics.
- **Role of the laboring woman during birth**. Active role. Talks loudly, may scream or curse, and sometimes even becomes hysterical. Some are stoic—only moan or grunt.
- **Role of the father and other family members during birth**. Father does not participate, believing that birth is a private event best handled by women. Laboring woman not coached; however, female family members help as needed if midwife involved.
- **Vaginal vs. cesarean section**. Vaginal delivery more common, as natural childbirth is the norm. Women in higher social strata quicker to have cesarean. Fear C-section because it is abdominal surgery.

- **Breastfeeding**. Encouraged for up to nine months postpartum. Believe that milk of lactating woman can be detrimental to both mother and child if it becomes too thin or too thick. If too thin, believe that milk has "turned" and may cause diarrhea in the child, and headache and possibly postpartum depression in the mother. If milk is too thick, may cause impetigo (*bouton*). In rural areas, mothers continue to breastfeed children before going to, and after returning from, working in the fields. If child develops diarrhea, immediately discontinue breastfeeding. Commonly accept a combination of breast- and bottle-feeding, especially if mother works. Bottle-feeding apparently more prevalent now, as more women in Haiti and U.S. work. Based on "hot"/"cold" theory, do not use formula—consider it to be hot; may use whole milk, as it is cold. Herbal tea an integral part of the feeding. Routinely use herbs such as marjorlaine for colicky infants.
- **Birth recuperation**. Very important period for Haitian women. Take active role in their own care, dress warmly, take sitz baths (*vapors*), and drink tea to rejuvenate. Believe that during first three days postpartum, new mother should be on bed rest, avoid drafts, and not venture out at night. A common practice during this period is "three baths": Special leaves are boiled in preparing water for hot bath. New mother encouraged to drink tea brewed from these same aromatic leaves, which include papaya, sour orange, sour soup (*corossol*), mint (*ti baume*), anise, bugleweed, and eucalyptus. These relax and tranquilize the mother, and cause her muscles to tighten. About one month postpartum, she takes a cold bath; it enhances healing and tightens muscles and bones loosened during delivery. Believe that after childbirth, women are particularly susceptible to gas (*gaz*) entering the body. They can prevent *gaz* by wearing a tight belt or piece of linen around the waist, a practice that also tightens bones loosened during childbirth. Avoid white foods, such as white lima beans, lobster, and milk, which they consider to be "cold," believing that such foods increase vaginal discharge and/or hemorrhage. Acceptable foods include cornmeal mush or porridge, red bean sauce, rice, beans, and plantain.
- **Baby care**. Name the baby after one month of confinement. Keep infant wrapped to avoid drafts. May place nutmeg, castor oil, or spider web on umbilical stump. May use belly bands.
- **Problems with baby**. Pediatrician should communicate with both parents if they are available. Mother relies heavily on husband to make final decision about care of child. If mother is a single parent, pediatrician should ask if there is an elder family member she wants present during discussion. At home, maternal grandmother is first person summoned if problems arise. Haitians try home remedies first.
- **Male and female circumcision**. Do not encourage male circumcision, believing that it reduces sexual satisfaction. Females not circumcised.

DEVELOPMENTAL AND SEXUAL ISSUES

- **Celebration of menarche or becoming a man**. No special rituals. Caution girls about their fertility and the risk of having sex. Boys are free to explore and initiate sexual activity.
- **Attitudes about birth control**. Inappropriate and undesirable. Consider children to be a blessing from God.
- **Attitudes about sexually transmitted infection (STI) control, including condoms**. Very sensitive and suspicious when topic of discussion is STIs and HIV because, in 1982, Haiti was the first developing country blamed for the origin of AIDS. Today, Haitians still endure stigma of "Haitians are AIDS carriers." Do not recognize male partner's responsibility in preventing conception. Males resent condom use, believing that condoms reduce sexual pleasure.
- **Attitudes about abortion**. Not socially sanctioned. However, it is not unusual for middle- and upper-class women to have an abortion to avoid the shame and disgrace of an unwanted pregnancy or pregnancy out of wedlock. May drink herbal teas during first trimester to induce abortion. An herbal leaf called *boule ti mas* produces a tea that has anticoagulant and abortive properties.
- **Attitudes about unwed sexual experimentation**. Believe that teenage girls should not engage in premarital sexual intercourse because they will lose their self-respect and be perceived as "loose" or even as prostitutes. Girls should prepare themselves for marriage and learn about sexual intercourse from their partner. This view is less strict in rural areas; there, it is more acceptable for young girls to engage in premarital sex with older men because it helps secure the family's economic well-being. Permit teenage boys to have premarital sex as part of their "training." Male sexuality closely associated with prestige; it also affirms manhood.
- **Sexual orientation**. Homosexuality taboo in Haitian culture. Gay and lesbian persons remain closeted. Haitians do not acknowledge or discuss homosexual relationships. Do not overtly display sexual behavior.
- **Gender identity**. Very private issue, not openly discussed. Taboo to deviate from normal male and female identities. Pressure masculine girls and feminine boys to conform to societal rules of female and male behavior.
- **Attitudes about menopause**. Believe that menopause is a natural occurrence. Generally welcome it as liberation from pregnancy. Drinking herbal teas an integral part of strategies for dealing with hot flashes and other symptoms. In U.S., women may accept hormone replacement therapy if husband or partner agrees.

FAMILY RELATIONSHIPS

- **Composition/structure**. Close, tightly knit nuclear family and extended family. Sometimes, three generations and extended-family members live together under one roof and in small quarters.

- **Decision-making**. Men influence and sometimes direct family decisions, although behind the scenes, women are highly influential; men allowed to believe that they are head of household.
- **Spokesperson**. Depending on situation, spokesperson may be father, mother, or an elder kinsman/person in position of authority in that family unit.
- **Gender issues**. Haitian society projects image of male chauvinism. Men relinquish all responsibilities for managing household and caring for children; they are expected to be financial providers and to discipline children. Fathers are distant figures with great authority. However, women are the family unit's real backbone.
- **Changing roles among generations in U.S.** Haitian society in U.S. is very much in flux. Many intergenerational conflicts as a result of Haitian parents holding views different from those of their children growing up in U.S. These conflicts create tension regarding sex, reproduction, peer affiliations, and roles within the family. There are also male/female role conflicts in family relationships. Traditional Haitian culture is highly paternalistic, one in which women play a subservient role. Haitian American women, in contrast, make overt decisions about their lives, challenging their partners and expecting equality in relationships. This change has come about because many Haitian American women work and generate income, and also because they see that male-female interactions in various U.S. cultures differ from those in their native culture.
- **Caring roles**. Women generally responsible for care. Haitians expect men to project an image of strength and not display emotion.
- **Expectations of and for children**. Expect children to be respectful, caring, and obedient, and to become self-sufficient and competent at an early age. Both parents provide emotional care, but mothers take care of the day-to-day task of raising children in a highly protective, secure environment. Expect children to be high achievers, especially in education. May send children to boarding school.
- **Expectations of and for elders**. Highly respect elders. Children should care and provide for them. Elders are the family advisers, babysitters, historians, and consultants. Haitians usually care for elders at home, despite the challenges posed by children who work outside the home. Small percentage reluctantly decide to place elders in nursing homes.
- **Expectations of hospital visitors**. Encourage visits by close family members and friends. They help maintain comfort of patient around the clock until they think he/she is ready to be independent. If patient is on a strict hospital diet, clinician should inform family members, as they will bring in home-cooked meals. Haitians are very traditional—do not enjoy American food. Would rather go hungry than eat hospital food.

ILLNESS BELIEFS

- **Causes of/attitudes about physical illness**. Haitians have a fatalistic view of illness, reflected in the expression, "God is good" (*Bondye Bon*). Whatever happens is God's will. They think of illness as a continuum from "I do not feel well" (*Kom pa bon*) to "I am dying" (*Moin pap refe*). Perceive illness as punishment, an assault on the body that may have natural or supernatural etiologies. Natural illness, known as "disease of the Lord" (*maladi Bondye*), is of short duration. It may occur frequently and is caused by such environmental factors as food, air, cold, heat, and gas. Other causes of natural illness are movement of blood within the body, "hot"/"cold" disequilibrium, and bone displacement. Supernatural illness is very serious; Haitians attribute it to the anger of spirits (*loa*). This happens when a body inhabited by a spirit deceives it. Voodoo priest must find out what the spirit advises for a cure. A folk condition is fright (*sezisman*), in which bad news, a frightful situation, or an indignation as a result of unjust treatment disrupts normal blood flow. Haitians believe that *sezisman* makes blood move to the head, causing partial loss of vision, headache, increased blood pressure, and/or stroke.
- **Causes of/attitudes about mental illness**. Highly stigmatized and shameful for the family. Topic is taboo. Haitians typically believe that mental illness has supernatural causes, such as a hex or punishment for not honoring protective spirits with feasts. Accept treatment and hospitalization only in cases of severe mental problems.
- **Causes of genetic defects**. An angry spirit, perhaps enlisted by an enemy, causes physical deformity. Persons with genetic defects are viewed as a curse on the family. Receive care at home and sometimes are hidden from society. No institutional placement in Haiti. Because both parents work outside the home in U.S., institutionalization may be acceptable; it also maintains the silence about this shameful aspect of their life.
- **Attitudes about disabilities**. View a disabled child as punishment or as a condition caused by a supernatural force. Mother feels extremely guilty, wondering what she is being punished for or what she has done to deserve it. Parents attempt to determine if the disability is due to the influence of a powerful spirit who has been neglected or to a spirit who is being malicious. If their search confirms their belief, they participate in all types of prayer services or voodoo ceremonies in hopes of placating the spirit. If that does not work, they seek medical care. Adults who become disabled may follow these same steps. Disabled family member is loved, sheltered, and cared for at home. Disability not shameful for family.
- **Sick role**. Sick person assumes passive role and allows others to care for him/her. All family members participate in providing care.
- **Home and folk remedies**. Usually the first line of treatment. May include tea, massage, hot bath with boiled leaves (*benye fey cho*), or poultice. Immigrants may ask friends or relatives to send medications from Haiti. Such

medications may consist of roots, leaves, and products made in Europe.

- **Medications**. Some Haitians stop taking prescription medicine when symptoms abate rather than continuing full course. Haitians are self-diagnosticians: They have home remedies for particular ailments and take medicines prescribed for others. May take herbal and prescribed biomedicines concurrently. Barriers to medications include lack of health insurance and affordability.
- **Acceptance of procedures**. Greatly fear surgery, especially abdominal surgery, because of its seriousness. Also fear blood transfusions for that reason and because of potential HIV transmission. Organ donations rare; Haitians believe that a body should be buried intact. May not accept transplant, fearing that the organ will bring in some of the donor's personality. Clinician should explain procedures clearly and slowly. Use of a trusted interpreter essential.
- **Care-seeking**. Very strong belief in God's power and His ability to heal. God works through various media, including dreams and both traditional and medical means. Haitians seek medical care when it becomes clear that an illness requires attention.

HEALTH ISSUES

- **Concept of health**. Maintaining equilibrium and praying are essential for good health. Achieving a healthy balance requires good spiritual habits. A healthy person is strong and plump, has good color, and is without pain.
- **Health promotion and prevention**. To maintain health, Haitians believe that one must eat right, sleep right, keep warm, exercise, and keep clean. Eating right means balancing food in terms of "hot"/"cold," acidic/nonacid, and heavy/light. The most important exercise is walking, which is so ingrained in daily activity that it is not viewed as exercise. Haitians self-treat as a way to promote health or prevent disease. For example, a person who suspects a venereal disease may buy penicillin and have someone administer it, or to treat a minor cold, they may take antibiotics supplied by a friend. In summer, parents promote the health of their children by, for example, giving them *lok*, a mixture of bitter tea leaves, juice, sugar cane syrup, and oil. Also give their children enemas (*lavman*) to ensure cleanliness. Enemas also rid the bowel of impurities and refresh it, prevent acne, and rejuvenate the body.
- **Screening**. Haitians do not admit to diseases, especially contagious diseases. Very respectful of doctors and nurses; follow their suggestions for screening. Health promotion and disease prevention are not first and foremost in Haitians' minds. Believe that the more one visits a doctor, the more problems one attracts.
- **Common health problems**. Prone to hypertension and diabetes, due to Haitian diet and genetic predisposition. High incidence of cancer and heart disease related to high-fat diet. Sickle cell anemia seems to be highly preva-

lent, although there are no statistics demonstrating this. Sexually transmitted infections and tuberculosis also are common.

DEATH RITUALS

- **Beliefs and attitudes about death**. Haitians greatly fear and misunderstand death. Death of an old person more acceptable than that of a young person: An old person lived his/her life, but a young person did not accomplish life goals or mission. Death of a young person may have supernatural connotations.
- **Preparation**. Health care providers should tell family spokesperson when death is imminent so family members can assemble at the bedside. The whole extended family is mobilized; it prays and cries uncontrollably, even hysterically. Family members try to meet spiritual needs of dying person by bringing religious medallions, pictures of saints, or fetishes/talismen for protection or as good luck for a peaceful death and restful afterlife. Dying person's elder kinsman usually makes arrangements, including notifying all family members wherever they may be; their travel plans will influence funeral arrangements. Kinsman also arranges preburial activities (e.g., purchase of coffin and prayer services before funeral) and funeral and burial services.
- **Home vs. hospital**. Generally prefer to be cared for, and die, at home. However, since immigrating to U.S., Haitians have accepted death at the hospital because of the heavy burden that terminal illness imposes on family. No hospice care in Haiti, so this concept is foreign to immigrants and must be carefully explained.
- **Special needs**. Because of Haitians' deep respect for the dead, they keep body until all family members can be present for the service. *Dernie priye* is a special service consisting of seven consecutive days of prayer. Usually takes place in the home. Purpose is to facilitate passage of the soul from this world to the next. On the seventh day, there is a mass called *prise de deuil*, which begins the official mourning process. Each of these activities concludes with a reception/celebration in memory of the deceased.
- **Care of the body**. Family member gives deceased a final bath. Health care providers should allow family to participate in postmortem care if this is not too disruptive for nursing unit. Cremation unacceptable because of Haitians' deep respect for the body and their belief in resurrection and paradise.
- **Attitudes about organ donation**. Neither acknowledge nor encourage donation.
- **Attitudes about autopsy**. Very cautious about this procedure. However, if Haitians suspect foul play or an unnatural death, request autopsy to ensure that patient is really dead. The practice of zombification—creating a zombie out of malice or greed—is more prevalent among persons of rural origin. Haitians believe that zombies are persons whose spirits have been captured and are brought back from the dead. In that postmortem state, such individ-

uals are in a trance and aware of their surroundings and what is happening to them, but they cannot react. A master, the one who made the person a zombie, directs the zombie mentally. Zombies have listless eyes, speak in a nasal voice, and walk very stiffly. They are conscious but deprived of will, which indicates their "other world" origin. Fear of zombiism prompts some families to poison the body to ensure that the deceased is truly dead. Haitians consider zombification the supreme punishment, as it reduces an individual to slave—precisely the condition that voodoo evolved to counteract.

SELECTED REFERENCES

Colin, J., & Paperwalla, G. (2003). Haitians. In P. St. Hill, J. G. Lipson, & A. I. Meleis (Eds.), *Caring for women cross-culturally* (pp. 172–187). Philadelphia: F. A. Davis.

Colin, J. M., Paperwalla, G. (2003). People of Haitian heritage. In L. D. Purnell & B. J. Paulanka (Eds.), *Transcultural health care: A culturally competent approach* (2nd ed.) (pp. 517–543). Philadelphia: F. A. Davis.

Laennec, H. (1995). *Voodoo: Search for the spirit.* New York: Harry N. Abrams.

Laguerre, M. S. (1981). Haitian Americans. In A. Harwood (Ed.), *Ethnicity and medical care* (pp. 172–210). Cambridge, MA: Harvard University Press.

U.S. Department of Commerce. (2000). Economic and statistics administration: U.S. Census Bureau. Retrieved March 30, 2003, from http://www.uscensus.gov

AUTHOR

Jessie M. Colin, PhD, RN, is an associate professor of nursing and director of the PhD program at Barry University in Miami Shores, FL. A Haitian American, she emigrated to the U.S. as an adolescent. She is co-founder of the Haitian Health Foundation of South Florida, and a member and past president of the Haitian American Nurses Association of Florida. Her research interests are multicultural health and vulnerable populations, particularly Haitian women and children.

CHAPTER 18

HAWAIIANS

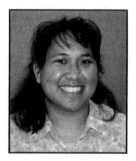

Donna-Marie Palakiko

CULTURAL/ETHNIC IDENTITY

- **Preferred term(s)**. Native Hawaiian, part Hawaiian, Hawaiian, and *Kanaka Maoli* (a traditional term that refers to a full-blooded, indigenous, Hawaiian man). Hawaiians are sensitive about issues concerning their identity, passionate about their culture, and respectful of others. Native Hawaiian (upper case "N") includes all persons of Hawaiian ancestry, regardless of blood quantum. In the 1970s, the U.S. Government defined Native Hawaiians as those having ancestry in the Hawaiian Islands before 1778. The term native Hawaiian (lower case "n") refers to individuals with 50% or more Hawaiian blood. The Native vs. native distinction determines eligibility to entitlements and benefits according to blood quantum, including, but not limited to, land ownership and health care benefits. Current legislation would give federal recognition to Native Hawaiians.
- **Census**. According to the 2000 Census, 401,162 Hawaiians live in U.S., about 240,000 of them in the State of Hawaii. There has been no significant emigration, but the population declined from 1 million in 1778 to 40,000 in 1893, the year the monarchy was overthrown.
- **History of migration**. Hawaiians are the original, sea-faring people who arrived in and settled the islands in 500 A.D. From 500–1400 A.D., migration back and forth between the Hawaiian Islands and Tahiti took place. Early Hawaiian culture developed, none of which was carried forward until fairly recently. In 1400, a second group of settlers—led by Paao, a high priest and famous navigator—came from Tahiti and introduced the *kapu* system of taboos and laws that governed Hawaiians. From 1400–1778, Hawaiians had no contact with outsiders; they and their culture continued to thrive. In 1778, Captain James Cook rediscovered the Hawaiian Islands. His crew introduced

foreign diseases that decimated the Hawaiian population. Christian missionaries settled in Hawaii in the 1800s. That and the arrival of the whaling industry introduced more foreign diseases. Asian immigrants began arriving during
those years to work the land crops. In 1893, Hawaii's monarchy was overthrown. Hawaii became the 50th U.S. state in 1959. From 1778 until today,
Hawaiian culture has waxed and waned and almost became extinct. The
1970s saw a renaissance of Hawaiian culture that is celebrated to this day.

SPIRITUAL/RELIGIOUS ORIENTATION

- **Primary religious/spiritual affiliations**. Hawaiians have a deeply rooted
  spiritual connection. Historical stories (*mo`olelo*) describe the connection
  among man (*kane*), god (*akua*), fellow man (*kanaka maoli*), and the land
  (*aina*). Spirituality was based on maintaining *lokahi* (unity, balance, harmony), essential to the welfare of the people. *Lokahi* often is symbolized in the
  center of a triangle with *akua* at the top and fellow man and land at the sides.
  Spiritual energy or power (*mana*) is the essence of all living things. Manifes-
  tations of disruption in balance include ill fortune, illness, and disharmony.
  Hawaiians believed in dualism, such as good/evil, male/female, and "hot"/
  "cold". This dualism is evident in creation stories. Hawaiians brought their
  traditional religion from central Polynesia. It contained a pantheon of gods.
  The general population worshipped four main gods: Kane, Ku, Lono, and
  Kanaloa. Hawaiians also prayed to their ancestors (*aumakua*) for guidance.
  Calvinist missionaries arrived in 1820. About 1,300 Hawaiians converted to
  Calvinism in the first 17 years. During the so-called Great Revival (1837–
  1840), 20,000 Hawaiians converted. Calvinists were followed by other religious orders, such as the Church of the Latter Day Saints (Mormons), who
  established a Hawaiian branch of Brigham Young University. Today, religions
  represented in Hawaii include Christianity, Mormonism, and Buddhism.
- **Usual religious/spiritual practices**. Pray to God (*akua*) daily. Maintain
  balance (*lokahi*) through proper self-care (healthy lifestyle), care of the family (*ohana*), care of the land (*aina*), and prayer (*pule*). Christians pray to God
  and attend church.
- **Use of spiritual healing/healers**. Spirituality is the source of healing in all
  traditional healing modalities, including massage (*lomilomi*), setting right
  (*ho`oponopono*), and herbal medicine (*la`au lapa`au*). Some Hawaiians con-
  tact their church elders or priest (*kahu*) for guidance. Traditional healers
  practice one modality, but some receive training in a complementary modality. Trainers are elders (*kupuna*) who in turn were trained by their family
  keeper of secrets/medicine person (*kahuna*) and granted permission to practice. Hawaiians make contact with traditional healers through families and
  word of mouth. *Ho`oponopono*, a counseling style designed to mend relation-
  ships, is rooted in spirituality; it treats symptoms as well as underlying problems, such as stress, anxiety, and worry. One technique in *ho`oponopono* is

"talk story," a conversation style that encourages openness, honesty, and truthfulness and that requires active listening in order to learn. Participants share their experiences, which teach a lesson.

- **Holidays**. Observe state and federal holidays. Celebrate Prince Jonah Kuhio Kalanianaole Day (March 26), which honors the Hawaiian statesman who fought for Hawaiians' rights, and King Kamehameha Day (June 11), which honors the man who united the islands into one kingdom.

COMMUNICATION
ORAL COMMUNICATION

- **Major languages and dialects**. Before 1778, Hawaiian was the only spoken language, including dialects. English was introduced that year, but Hawaiian remained the common language. Missionaries developed the Hawaiian alphabet, which led to a written language. This language nearly disappeared in subsequent years, but the 1970s saw a re-emergence of the Hawaiian language and creation of Hawaiian language schools. The spoken language today is different from that of long ago. Hawaiian is the official language of the State of Hawaii, although English is most commonly spoken.

- **Greetings**. *Aloha*, which means hello and signifies hospitality, unconditional love, and respect, and a handshake with a hug and kiss on the cheek. Some older Hawaiians practice *honi*—literally, to touch noses. It traditionally symbolized the exchange of breath (*ha*), as greeters touch the side of each other's nose. Calling older persons "Aunty" or "Uncle" shows respect. Prefer first names unless otherwise indicated. *Mahalo* means good-bye, thank you. To build rapport, Hawaiians establish common ground by linking their family genealogies, acknowledging common social relationships, or simply having a common interest.

- **Tone of voice**. Discourage loud tone. Prefer calm, soft tone when requesting something and in conversation.

- **Direct or indirect style of speech**. Hawaiians enjoy stories. They learn how to tell them with words and gestures. Dance (*hula*) is a dramatic example of illustrating a story with gestures. People communicate through "talk story," a dialogue with no formal beginning, middle, or end. Verbal communication is tightly integrated with nonverbal cues (e.g., tone, length of silence, eye contact, and hand gestures) that provide the message. To understand the message, observing these cues is critical. "Talk story" respects all participating persons. Elders speak first in a conversation; young children should not speak unless spoken to. Older persons can express their disagreement, but younger adults and children refrain from saying what they think out of respect for elders. With a nod or word, family members acknowledge someone who is speaking; nodding means they are listening, not necessarily that they understand or agree.

- **Use of interpreters**. There are a few fluent, native speakers who may need an interpreter. However, English is the primary spoken language.

- **Serious or terminal illness**. Clinician should inform the eldest family member and patient using simple medical terms. Best to inform family early so it can make arrangements for others to be present for recovery or death.

WRITTEN COMMUNICATION

- **Literacy assessment**. Schools in Hawaii teach English. Many elders did not receive formal education and are self-taught. Others cannot read or write in English. Even if persons can write their name, they may not be able to read or write. Clinician should ask who in the family is able to fill out forms. Clinician can assess a patient's literacy by having him/her read a statement out loud. Asking the patient directly about literacy may shame him/her.

- **Consents**. Hawaiians trust authority figures and those who are knowledgeable. Therefore, verbal agreement may not always signify understanding. Clinician should be culturally sensitive when seeking consent; best to use "talk story," establish rapport, clearly explain a procedure, and use simple medical terms. Patient may refuse to sign forms. Clinician should not ask why, which may seem threatening, but rather carefully explain the need for patient's signature. Hawaiians do not sign consents just to be polite. May be hesitant to participate in research, although community-focused research (e.g., focus groups, interviews, and surveys) is less threatening than clinical trials are. May want to discuss elective surgery or participation in study with a family member before deciding.

NONVERBAL COMMUNICATION

- **Eye contact**. Direct eye contact customary, depending on situation. In a group, respectful to look at all persons present. Some Hawaiians make direct and sustained eye contact while talking. Fleeting eye contact shows disrespect.

- **Personal space**. Traditionally, the space in front of a chief (*ali`i*) was taboo (*kapu*). If the shadow of an *ali`i* fell upon a commoner, he/she was punished by death. Hawaiians believed that bodies possess great power (*mana*); stealing *mana* (e.g., through contact with shadow or acquiring someone's personal trimmings or excrement) would empower the thief to inflict harm or illness. Today, when interacting with strangers, appropriate social space is about an arm's length, or 18–20 inches. Personal space between family members may be less than 12 inches.

- **Use and meaning of silence**. Signifies agreement or attempted compliance with requests or orders, whether or not they are fully understood.

- **Gestures**. Appropriate gestures include handshakes, talking with hands (such as drawing a picture in mid-air or pointing to an object), removing shoes before entering a house to show respect for family, and smiling when greeting or being greeted by others. The *shaka* sign, a form of greeting that also means "OK," like a thumbs-up, involves sticking thumb and little finger out and folding the other three fingers down. May be inappropriate to greet patient with a kiss or by touching noses (*honi*).

- **Openness in expressing emotions**. Easily express emotions to family, friends, and others they trust and to those with whom they have good rapport, such as physicians, dentists, and priests. Smile frequently. Show contentment, acknowledgment, and warm expressions of welcome. Subdue or internalize anger and fear. Discourage violent actions.
- **Privacy**. Guard personal information, including health information; share it at their discretion. Share health information with persons they trust, such as clinicians. Share family surnames and genealogies with others to establish a common link.
- **Touch**. Handshake or touching shoulder acceptable. However, out of respect, best to ask permission. Touching head unacceptable, as it is the source of power (*mana*) and knowledge.
- **Orientation to time**. Traditionally, Hawaiians are present-oriented. Tend to work on "Hawaiian time"—keep their own schedule and arrive at their convenience. Often trust in God to get people where they need to be on time, but transportation issues may cause tardiness for appointments. Orientation to past illustrated by ancient dance (*hula kahiko*), modern *hula* (*hula auwana*), and sharing stories (*mo`olelo*). Little orientation to future, although some Hawaiians are adopting preventive health concepts to perpetuate the bloodline. Hawaiians tend to do things before sunset, such as preparing food, bathing, trimming hair or nails, making decisions, or ending discussions.

ACTIVITIES OF DAILY LIVING

- **Modesty**. Hawaiians are modest. Both men and women prefer a health care provider of same gender. Nudity can be embarrassing to both genders.
- **Skin care**. Hawaiians generally are very clean. Traditionally, they bathed 2–3 times a day. Modern Hawaiians clean themselves daily; more-frequent bathing is at their discretion. If hospitalized, prefer shower.
- **Hair care**. By individual choice. Typically wash hair daily, do not use special soaps or lotions. Prefer not to wash hair late at night. Traditionally, Hawaiians believed that hair possessed power (*mana*) and they took great care when disposing of cut hair. Today, they still pay attention to how their trimmings are discarded; health care provider should ask patient about his/her preference.
- **Nail care**. Keep nails short, unless they need long nails to play an instrument, such as a guitar or ukulele. Traditionally, Hawaiians believed that nails possessed power (*mana*) and took great care when disposing of trimmings. Today, they still pay attention to how their trimmings are discarded; health care provider should ask patient about his/her preference.
- **Toileting**. Modest and private. Prefer bathroom to bedpan or urinal. If a commode or bedpan is necessary, health care provider should close curtain, place call light within reach, and explain in clear, simple terms the impor-

tance of calling if patient needs help. Provider should check on patient to offer assistance.

- **Special clothing or amulets**. None.
- **Self-care**. Hawaiians may not trust Western biomedical care, due to history of high death rates after foreign illnesses were introduced in Hawaiian Islands. Some consult traditional practitioners to treat common ailments. If able, they prefer to be independent in self-care and daily activities; if unable, family members help. Hospitalized patients expect whole family or a family member to spend the night with them.

FOOD PRACTICES

- **Usual meal pattern**. Prefer three meals daily. Largest meal is dinner. Snack between meals.
- **Special utensils**. None.
- **Food beliefs and rituals**. Hawaiians serve elders before youth. Younger persons may have to prepare food and serve it to older persons. Typically pray before eating. Traditionally, men and women ate separately. Before 1819, women were not allowed to eat foods that possessed supernatural forms (*kinolau*), but this taboo (*kapu*) came to an end when Kamehameha II overturned the *kapu* system. Modern Hawaiians have no *kapu*. A *lu'au* is a traditional Hawaiian feast that brings together an entire family and community for special occasions, such as first birthdays, graduations, marriages, and other milestones. ("*Lu'au*" refers to the leafy tops of young taro plants cooked in coconut milk, one of a variety of traditional foods served.) Food is cooked in an underground pit oven (*imu*) covered with hot rocks and leaves. Traditionally, Hawaiians drank a narcotic drink made from kava root (*awa*) during special ceremonies.
- **Usual diet**. Traditional diet encompassed complex carbohydrates, minimal amounts of protein, and very little fat. Native diet now uncommon. Western influences popularized convenience foods and plate lunches (e.g., rice, macaroni salad, and a main dish). Hawaiians consume large amounts of processed foods, such as Spam™ and corned beef. Asian and mainland American dietary practices influence modern Hawaiian diet. Rice, an Asian staple, has replaced mashed taro root (*poi*), a traditional Hawaiian staple.
- **Fluids**. Prefer cool water or sweet drinks. Consume lots of carbonated drinks.
- **Food taboos and prescriptions**. Traditionally, there were restrictions (*kapu*) on certain foods for women, due to beliefs that those foods represented particular gods or body parts. For example, women were not allowed to eat pig, banana, coconut, and some types of seafood. Hawaiians do not practice these restrictions today. They practice healthier living by eating certain foods, such as *poi* and fish, and balancing their diet.
- **Hospitality**. Always offer refreshments (food and beverage) to guests. Greet the eldest family member first. Show respect for elders or head of family. Pro-

vide chairs for elders. Expect children to leave room and/or sit on floor. Family members honor overnight guests by providing them a place to sleep and relax. Relinquish their bedrooms to guests.

SYMPTOM MANAGEMENT

- **Pain** (`eha*). Stoic. Do not complain. Accept pain medication, but clinician should ask before administering it. Use massage (*lomilomi*) to alleviate discomfort. Hawaiians understand numerical pain scale but may rate pain lower than it actually is. Clinician should encourage patients to express pain in words.
- **Dyspnea** (*ka`apa ka hanu I ka houpo*, or "pant for breath"). Believe that dyspnea or severe shortness of breath may be caused by someone stealing their breath (i.e., their life source or spirit). Patients may not report dyspnea; health care providers should look for respiratory distress. Patients may use words and/or number ratings to express dyspnea. Clinician can offer oxygen after explaining its purpose and the potential outcome. Patients may accept medication if they cannot "catch their breath." Hawaiians encourage nonpharmacological treatments, such as relaxation, prayer, and meditation.
- **Nausea/vomiting** (*pailua/lua`i*). Believe that loss of power (*mana*) or an imbalance causes nausea/vomiting. May want to rest after periods of vomiting. May treat nausea with traditional medicine, such as the *lau kahi* plant. Report nausea/vomiting to caregivers in words or numbers. Accept pharmacological intervention, but clinician should ask patient's permission. Nonpharmacological interventions may include relaxation and massaging a pressure point.
- **Constipation** (*kukae pa`a*)**/diarrhea** (*hi* or *palahi*). Change in bowel function may signal disharmony, discontent, or loss of power (*mana*). There is some evidence that Hawaiians in earlier times used enemas; the individual disposed of excrement. Today, no concern about disposal of wastes. May request traditional medicines, such as hibiscus (*hau*) for constipation and guava for diarrhea. If asked, patient reports changes in bowel function; does not volunteer the information. May acknowledge nutritional controls but not adopt them.
- **Fatigue** (*maluhihuli*—tiredness or weariness; *ho`omaluhiluhi*—to cause fatigue). Believe that a loss of power or energy (*mana*) causes fatigue. Other possible causes are overexertion, heat, illness, depression, or stress. Traditionally, Hawaiians napped when the sun was at its highest point. Foreigners interpreted this habit as laziness. To determine cause of fatigue, clinician should use "talk story" with patient. Hawaiians report fatigue in words. Prefer nonpharmacological interventions (e.g., counseling or therapy) first. Accept pharmacological interventions as a last resort.
- **Depression** (*kaumaha*). Traditionally, Hawaiians believed that depressed persons were spiritually imbalanced, a condition that healers treated. Modern Hawaiians believe that depression is a state of mind and may result from

a loss of power (*mana*). They approach the problem holistically, addressing all issues and/or concerns. Patient must be ready for treatment and/or counseling, and external support system should be in place; otherwise, treatment/counseling may fail.

- **Self-care symptom management**. Older family members may use traditional medicines to treat minor ailments. Younger/modern persons seek medical treatment if necessary. Hawaiians mostly treat their ailments independently; self-medicate with over-the-counter drugs for common colds and minor aches or pains. Treat chronic illnesses, such as diabetes, hypertension, and high cholesterol, with biomedical drugs. Older Hawaiians may use traditional medicines, such as the herbs *mamaki* for hypertension and *pukiawe* for headache, and coconut water for diabetes. Others make lifestyle changes, such as balancing regular exercise, healthy nutrition, and relaxation.

BIRTH RITUALS/CARE OF THE NEW MOTHER AND BABY

- **Pregnancy care**. Prenatal care essential. Women not allowed to wear necklaces during pregnancy, and some may not be allowed to eat certain foods. Pregnant women should avoid lifting heavy objects. They are expected to rest and care for themselves and the unborn child. Parents may attend free childbirth preparation classes.

- **Preferences for children**. Traditionally, Hawaiians encouraged large families. Today, society frowns upon large families; typical number of children is 2–3. No preference for girls or boys.

- **Labor practices**. Walking is common. May use massage (*lomilomi*) to alleviate pain. Generally tolerate pain but may request pain medication. Eating before delivery permissible. No special meals. Showers help relax expectant mother.

- **Role of the laboring woman during birth**. May reposition herself for comfort. Takes active or passive role in labor. May remain stoic and refrain from loud noises.

- **Role of the father and other family members during birth**. Father and family members are present. Normally, father is birthing coach; however, other family members may assume that role. Expect immediate family members to attend birth.

- **Vaginal vs. cesarean section**. Prefer vaginal delivery but accept cesarean if medically necessary.

- **Breastfeeding**. Prefer breastfeeding. However, if mother cannot produce sufficient milk or infant cannot latch on, bottle-feeding is an option. Breastfeeding lasts 6–12 months. If mother goes back to work, she pumps and freezes the milk, and baby gets breast milk from bottle.

- **Birth recuperation**. Mother is expected to rest during first month postpartum. She and/or family members care for baby. Family members typically help with housework and cooking during recuperation.

- **Baby care**. Mother is expected to care for baby, but modern Hawaiians share that responsibility. Grandparents also may take an active role. Duration of baby care by others varies. Some grandparents babysit until child is ready for preschool.
- **Problems with baby**. Clinician should tell parents immediately if something is wrong with baby. Modern Hawaiians consult pediatrician or family physician; others seek advice from family elder. Treat some problems with traditional therapy (e.g., massage [*lomilomi*] for a "turned stomach" [*huli*]). Allow biomedical physician to treat other problems.
- **Male and female circumcision**. Not practiced.

DEVELOPMENTAL AND SEXUAL ISSUES

- **Celebration of menarche or becoming a man**. No special practices.
- **Attitudes about birth control**. Depends on family's values. Single persons use birth control. Adolescents may use birth control if parents approve.
- **Attitudes about sexually transmitted infection (STI) control, including condoms**. Hawaiians are knowledgeable about STIs, including HIV/AIDS. They educate adolescents in high school and through various community agencies. Both adults and adolescents may use condoms for birth control.
- **Attitudes about abortion**. Not widely accepted. Abortion performed at discretion of patient and depending on circumstances (whether, for example, the pregnancy is unwanted or a result of rape). Patient may not want to disclose abortion to her family, preferring to keep the matter private. Families care for children born out of wedlock.
- **Attitudes about unwed sexual experimentation**. Tolerated but not widely accepted.
- **Sexual orientation**. Some families accept a gay or lesbian member, others deny same-sex orientation.
- **Gender identity**. In ancient times, Hawaiians accepted transgender persons. The term *mahu* (males who identify as female or have female tendencies) applies to male-to-female transgender orientation or to males who sleep with males. Acceptance is family-based. Some families accept transgender orientation, others deny or hide it.
- **Attitudes about menopause**. Accept it as part of the life cycle. Women continue to live normal lives while adjusting to changes associated with menopause. They treat symptoms, preferably with nonpharmacological methods, such as adapting to changes in body temperature, eating a healthier diet, and exercising. Women may seek hormone replacement therapy, but medical treatment for menopause is uncommon.

FAMILY RELATIONSHIPS

- **Composition/structure**. Family (*ohana*) includes nuclear and extended members. Extended family includes blood relatives, persons related by marriage, adopted persons, and friends. Hawaiians believe that the power of the collective, including *ohana*, is more important than the individual. *Ohana* is at the foundation of all other Hawaiian values.

- **Decision-making**. Depends on situation. Preparing for burial of a parent or sibling requires the family's collective authority and decision-making, with the family elder assuming the role of spokesperson. Patient makes decision when the issue is private and he/she does not want to involve family.

- **Spokesperson**. Clinician should communicate only with eldest member of family, who will inform everyone else and facilitate discussion. Prefer that spokespersons be men (*kane*) rather than women (*wahine*). Clinicians should address eldest male; if none, eldest female. Some families may tell health care provider who is the spokesperson.

- **Gender issues**. In earlier times, Hawaiians were matriarchal. Modern Hawaiians are patriarchal. Men are primarily responsible for family's livelihood, women for household and upbringing of children. In the younger generation, men and women share household responsibilities and both earn incomes.

- **Changing roles among generations in U.S.** Gender roles have shifted in last few decades. Modern Hawaiians are patriarchal, yet women continue to excel, earn college degrees, and seek professional careers. Both parents rear the children, perhaps with help of grandparents.

- **Caring roles**. Whole family may care for sick person or family may designate a member—adult man or woman, oldest child, cousin, aunt, or uncle—to provide such care.

- **Expectations of and for children**. Expect children to learn through observation and, above all, to respect elders, who set expectations for them. As children mature, they may be allowed to voice their own expectations. Hawaiians also expect children to be polite, clean, honest, educated, and career-bound. Modern Hawaiians value education; families expect children to attend college. If a child is not college-bound, he/she is expected to join a trade or find a job after high school.

- **Expectations of and for elders**. Family unit often includes three or four generations. Elders often live with their children; may provide child care and educate the grandchildren. Independent elderly couples live alone, although an elder who becomes disabled or frail may live with the family, which cares for him/her. Long-term-care and skilled-nursing facilities are last resorts.

- **Expectations of hospital visitors**. Hospitalized patients want family members to stay with them, including overnight. Visitors stay for a long time, keeping the patient company and "talking story." May bring food from home or a favorite restaurant for patient and staff. Expect family members to participate in patient's care (i.e., help with activities of daily living).

ILLNESS BELIEFS

- **Causes of/attitudes about physical illness**. According to ancient beliefs, the body is a vessel for God and a house for spirits. Disharmony, loss of power (*mana*), or loss of balance between a person and god, other humans, and the land are causes of illness (*ma`i*). One regains balance through prayer, *ho`oponopono* (setting right, counseling), correcting the cause of the illness, and herbal medicine. A curse or a jealous outsider's or evildoer's wish for ill harm also may cause illness. Hawaiians treat modern illnesses, such as diabetes and cancer, with modern therapies. They may treat common ailments, such as sore throat, nausea, and constipation, with family remedies and/or traditional medicine.

- **Causes of/attitudes about mental illness**. A person's disharmony causes mental illness. This disharmony may be a result of discord or disunity with fellow man, God, or the land. Modern mental illness also may be the result of stress, such as that caused by work, family, or peer pressure. Hawaiians acknowledge mental illness, but it is stigmatized. Persons with severe mental illness seek biomedical treatment and/or counseling. If biomedicine is not an option, patients may turn to traditional remedies, such as *ho`oponopono* (setting right, counseling).

- **Causes of genetic defects**. God's will. The family accepts a person with genetic defects and cares for him/her.

- **Attitudes about disabilities**. Traditionally, disabled persons were outcasts. Today, families care for disabled relatives and accept them as active community members.

- **Sick role**. All family members care for a sick person. A person who has a minor ailment, such as a cold, the flu, or headache, is expected to be active and get well; he/she is not excused from work or household chores. A post-surgery patient is expected to rest and recuperate, and is excused from work or chores. As patient gets stronger, he/she is expected to take an active role in getting well.

- **Home and folk remedies**. Treat illness with massage (*lomilomi*), herbal medicine (*la`au lapa`au*), or *ho`oponopono* (setting right in order to mend relationships). However, Hawaiians may not divulge such treatments out of fear that health care providers will ridicule them. *Lomilomi* practitioners assess the client for blocked energy. A complaint of muscle ache or "knots" may be a manifestation of other problems, such as stress, anxiety, worry, or conflict. Aim of *lomilomi* is to restore flow of energy throughout the body by working muscle. *La`au lapa`au* practitioners comprehensively assess a client's complaints, which may not be medical in nature (e.g., stress manifested as an upset stomach or headache). Practitioner prescribes herbal remedies to treat the symptoms and give the client an opportunity to "talk story." *Ho`oponopono* practitioners first assess a problem by talking to all parties involved. If they agree to perform *ho`oponopono*, treatment begins.

- **Medications**. Older persons may question the use of medication; compliance could be an issue. Patient may not understand importance of taking a full course of antibiotics and assume that when symptoms go away or improve, he/she can stop medicating. Also may not understand how to take medication, how much to take, or when to take it. For compliance, clinician may have to explain these things clearly, write down the medication schedule, and remind the patient by telephone. Hawaiians may use traditional medicine alone or in conjunction with biomedicine. Clinician should inquire about which treatment the patient prefers and explain it in simple medical terms.

- **Acceptance of procedures**. Hawaiians may be leery of procedures, such as organ transplants or surgery, because of the fear and stigma associated with hospitals and physicians. Accept procedures if they are explained satisfactorily. Transfusions acceptable if situation is life-threatening. Some may opt for nonmedical intervention, such as iron supplements for anemia.

- **Care-seeking**. Foundation of healing is spirituality. Hawaiians may identify a problem first and try to work through the problem/ailment before seeking biomedical care. Practitioners of herbal medicine (*la`au lapa`au*) ask clients to refrain from biomedical treatment while using traditional medicine. Some Hawaiians seek both traditional and Western healers.

HEALTH ISSUES

- **Concept of health** (*ola*). Traditionally, Hawaiians took a holistic approach to staying healthy: One maintained his/her health through unity, balance, and harmony (*lokahi*), which provided a connection with God, people, and the land. Hawaiians believed that their bodies had power (*mana*), which is the connection with God (*akua*). They considered breath (*ha*) to be the essence of life. Today, some Hawaiians retain this concept of health.

- **Health promotion and prevention**. Traditionally, promoting health and preventing illness involved healthy eating and regular exercise. The preventive practices of both younger and older modern Hawaiians tend to be health education and lifestyle modifications similar to those in dominant culture.

- **Screening**. Accept procedures such as Pap smears, prostate exams, mammograms, and cholesterol/glucose tests when such tests are conducted in the community. May avoid more-invasive screenings, such as colonoscopy. Health screeners must use "talk story" approach and need to explain clearly why screening is necessary. Hawaiians prefer that family members be screened at same time.

- **Common health problems**. State of Hawaii has highest prevalence of cancer, diabetes, cardiovascular disease, hypertension, and obesity.

DEATH RITUALS

- **Beliefs and attitudes about death**. Traditionally, Hawaiians believed that death was the end of the life cycle and the time when the spirit (*uhane*) left the body (*kino*). There were taboos (*kapus*) associated with the death of family members. For example, family members and their residence were placed in strict *kapu*; they could not have contact with others until the deceased was buried. A priest/keeper of secrets (*kahuna*) lifted the *kapu*. Modern Hawaiians no longer practice these *kapus* but still believe that upon death, the *uhane* leaves the *kino*. Also believe it is important to allow the soul to escape a patient who has died in the hospital.

- **Preparation**. Regarding an impending death, clinician should inform eldest family member and/or family spokesperson early so he/she can tell other family members, who then begin grieving. Family members want to be present at time of death.
- **Home vs. hospital**. Prefer home. Accept home hospice.
- **Special needs**. Catholics may want a priest called to deliver sacrament of last rites. Priest, ministers, and family members comfort the dying person and his/her family. After death, family members want to view body in private. Grieving process includes an unspecified period of mourning. Family support is common.
- **Care of the body**. Modern Hawaiians rely on mortuary to prepare body. Some families still practice the traditional custom of preparing the body, including bathing, dressing, and laying it in state.
- **Attitudes about organ donation**. Traditionally, Hawaiians believed that organs contained a person's power (*mana*) and that the body should be buried intact. However, modern Hawaiians may opt to donate organs. Appropriate for clinician to ask the medical guardian or next of kin. Patient may have stipulated organ donation on his/her driver's license or in a living will; may have made that decision independently, without family's knowledge.
- **Attitudes about autopsy**. Traditionally, Hawaiian priest/keeper of secrets (*kahuna*) performed autopsies. Modern Hawaiians do not request autopsy unless they perceive the death as unintended or a physician recommends it. Clinicians should consult the eldest family member.

SELECTED REFERENCES

Blaisdell, R. K. (1989). Historical and cultural aspects of Native Hawaiian health. In E.L. Wegner (Ed.), *Social process in Hawaii* (pp. 1–21). Honolulu: University of Hawaii Press.

Handy, E. S., & Pukui, M. K. (1972). *The Polynesian family system in Ka`u, Hawaii*. Tokyo: C. E. Tuttle.

Marsella, A. J., Oliveira, J. M., Plummer, C. M., & Crabbe, K. M. (1994). Native Hawaiian (*Kanaka Maoli*) culture, mind, and well-being. In H. McCubbin & E. Thompson (Eds.), *Stress and resiliency in racial and ethnocultural minority families in America* (pp. 93–113). Madison, WI: University of Wisconsin.

Office of Hawaiian Affairs. (2002). In *Native Hawaiian data book* (pp. 333–336). Honolulu: Office of Hawaiian Affairs.

AUTHOR

Donna-Marie Palakiko, RN, MS, had several years of acute-care nursing experience before she received her master's degree in community and cross-cultural health from the University of California-San Francisco School of Nursing. She currently is an administrator for Ke Ola Mamo, a community-based organization on the Hawaiian island of Oahu. There, she manages an assortment of programs and staff that focus on chronic disease management/prevention and community research in Native Hawaiian communities.

CHAPTER 19

HMONG

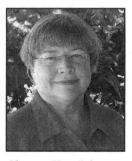 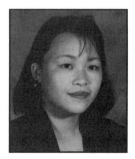

Sharon Kay Johnson   *Ae Lee Hang*

CULTURAL/ETHNIC IDENTITY

- **Preferred term(s)**. Hmong ("H" is silent). It means "human being" in English. Diverse beliefs and perspectives among individuals, even within families. Many Hmong are acculturated and highly educated. Because clinicians may encounter the greatest communication difficulties with older, recent immigrants who are more traditional, this chapter describes traditional beliefs and practices. Clinicians should assess individual and family beliefs.

- **Census**. According to the 2000 Census, 186,301 Hmong live in U.S. Largest numbers are in California (65,095), Minnesota (41,800), and Wisconsin (33,791). Fifty-six percent are 18 years old or younger. Average household size per housing unit is 6.27. An additional 15,000–20,000 immigrants (half younger than 14 years old) are expected to arrive in U.S. as last refugee camp in Thailand closes.

- **History of immigration**. Hmong reside in southern China, Laos, Vietnam, Burma, and Thailand, primarily in high mountainous areas. Because of geographical isolation, they have retained their own unique language and customs. Immigration to U.S. began in 1975 after the Vietnam War. There is secondary migration within U.S. as families move to be with extended families. Those in U.S. are originally from Laos and most lived many years in Thai refugee camps. During the Vietnam War, they fought for U.S. against Communists and took significant risks to rescue downed American pilots. When the war ended, Communists who controlled Laos targeted Hmong for genocide. Many continue to suffer from past war injuries and long-term physical and emotional effects of exposure to biological and chemical warfare. Recent immigrants generally illiterate, uneducated, and lack modern work skills. Long-time residents and young

Hmong born in U.S. have achieved various levels of education and higher socioeconomic status.

SPIRITUAL/RELIGIOUS ORIENTATION

- **Primary religious/spiritual affiliations**. Hmong may be Christian and simultaneously hold animistic beliefs. An estimated 75% practice traditional animistic religion. Others are Buddhist. The Catholic, Missionary Alliance, Baptist, and Mormon churches are among those with Hmong members.
- **Usual religious/spiritual practices**. Hmong traditionalists (animists) believe that spirits inhabit many places in the world, including objects and natural settings (such as trees, springs, and mountains), and that if a person's soul does not receive proper ceremonies and burial, it could wander the earth causing harm. In animistic religion, believers worship ancestors with ceremonies and offerings of animal sacrifice so the ancestors' spirits will bring good fortune and protect the family from harm. Among the beliefs and practices of Christians and Buddhists are karma and reincarnation, the power of prayer, the eight-fold path to right living and thinking, and memorial services for ancestors.
- **Use of spiritual healing/healers**. Christians want their ministers or priests to visit them in the hospital. Hmong who retain traditional beliefs need a shaman for the purpose of communicating with the spirit world. Shamans are mostly men who believe that spirits selected them (usually after a serious illness) to become shamans. Shamanism is not a profession but rather a calling. Once an individual believes he has been selected, he seeks an apprenticeship with a shaman to learn the basics, although spirits teach him the healing process. During the healing ritual, members of the sick person's family gather at home and the shaman rides an imaginary horse to the spirit world to learn why that person is ill and what sacrifice is necessary to make him/her well again. A healing ceremony follows, usually involving the sacrifice of a chicken, pig, or cow. Sacrifice sends the animal's spirit to the other world in place of the ill person's spirit, which has been stolen or has wandered away. The animal's spirit protects the ill person from further harm. During the ceremony, the sick person receives amulets that provide these protective powers for as long as he/she wears them. A shaman may visit a patient in the hospital, but rituals are not performed there. Ritual food, a sacrificed animal, and a contribution to the shaman can cost thousands of dollars. Ceremonies usually last 3–4 days, during which time all family members must remain secluded at home and no outsiders enter. Because of the cost and time commitment, such ceremonies generally are reserved for very serious illnesses. Christian Hmong do not practice shaman healing rituals.
- **Holidays**. Major holiday is Hmong New Year, celebrated for a week between Christmas and New Year's. Families celebrate together, meeting friends,

feasting, and participating in traditional ceremonies. Hmong also celebrate U.S. holidays, mostly because they are off work and out of school. Christian Hmong celebrate Christian holidays.

COMMUNICATION
ORAL COMMUNICATION

- **Major languages and dialects**. Many elders speak only Hmong. Two dialects: White and Green (sometimes called Blue).
- **Greetings**. Handshakes, smiles, introductions, and brief eye contact appropriate. Older women usually retain their own surname after they marry, while younger women may adopt husband's surname. Clinician should ask patient which title he/she prefers.
- **Tone of voice**. Should be modulated. Hmong speak in a normal or soft tone.
- **Direct or indirect style of speech**. Tend to communicate indirectly. Try to present a positive image. Exchange pleasantries upon introduction. Hmong consider it rude to begin interviews with direct questions. They often think Americans' communication styles are blunt and rude. Many say "no" outright or "I'll think about it" when in fact they do not want to do something. "Yes" not necessarily an affirmative response; may also mean "I hear you."
- **Use of interpreters**. Prefer interpreters who are Hmong health care professionals. Otherwise, many want a bilingual adult relative they trust. May distrust Hmong interpreters employed by hospital, believing that such interpreters' first loyalty is to hospital. Children lack adequate Hmong language skills; it is inappropriate and disrespectful for them to know about elders' health care concerns. Patient and interpreter should be of same gender; men and women may not discuss or admit to intimate problems when interpreter is of opposite gender. Because Hmong language structure is so different from Indo-European languages, interpreter must have an entire sentence, paragraph, or thought so he/she can accurately interpret the patient's intent. Many English terms, such as those regarding sexual topics, lack a comparable Hmong word, and Hmong has almost no medical or internal-anatomy terms. Persons may use metaphors to describe physical symptoms. For example, they may describe a developing viral rash as a "crop that is growing" and a man's impotence as "being like a woman." "Saving face" important. Interpreter may not tell clinician that he/she did not understand what the clinician said. Clinician should talk with interpreter beforehand to assess his/her level of knowledge, comfort with the topic, and understanding of the clinician's questions and discussion. The difficulty of translating medical procedures and diagnoses may result in a very rudimentary or erroneous translation. Incorrect translation may cause patient and/or family to become concerned, confused, or hostile.
- **Serious or terminal illness**. Hmong present a positive attitude in presence of seriously ill patients. When visiting someone they know is dying, they

nevertheless assure the patient that he/she will get well soon. Visitors do not mention possibly serious outcomes because patient and family might construe such mention as a cause of those outcomes. Factual information the clinician presents abruptly may cause the shocked patient to leave and never return. Better to discuss serious diagnoses, sensitive issues, and potential complications with family privately and to ask how this information would best be conveyed to patient.

WRITTEN COMMUNICATION

- **Literacy assessment**. Written Hmong language was not developed until 1950s. Most elders have had no formal schooling and are illiterate in their own language or English. Younger persons are literate in English but may not be able to read Hmong, although the community provides traditional language classes. Christian Hmong are more literate in Hmong because their Bible is in the Hmong language. Clinician should ask patient directly what language he/she prefers to use or read.
- **Consents**. Many are suspicious of consent forms if they cannot read them. Also afraid that the form does not contain what was explained to them verbally. Rumors persist that American doctors "practice or experiment" on Hmong people because they are uneducated about Western medical system. Patient and family may be suspicious of health care professionals' motives, especially if students or residents provide the care. Patient often wants elder male family members to review consent forms before he/she will sign. May use the unavailability of an elder as a delaying tactic when family either needs more time to make decision or does not want the surgery yet feels it would be rude to say "no." Women want husbands or other adult male relatives to participate in consent process. The family rather than the patient generally makes health care decisions.

NONVERBAL COMMUNICATION

The Hmong are very polite and reticent. Very aware of disrespectful and prejudicial behavior but do not protest such behavior to health care professionals. A friendly facial expression that connotes patience and respect communicates the health care professional's caring attitude to Hmong patient and family, and builds trust.

- **Eye contact**. Both prolonged, direct eye contact and no eye contact are rude. Health care provider should take clues from patient and avoid sustained, direct eye contact. Fleeting glances more appropriate.
- **Personal space**. Similar to that in dominant culture.
- **Use and meaning of silence**. Similar to that in dominant culture.
- **Gestures**. Hmong pat or rub the heads of children as an affectionate gesture. Patting or rubbing an adult's head is disrespectful. Pointing a finger at an adult is rude.

- **Openness in expressing emotions**. Women generally are emotionally expressive. Men tend to be more stoic. Hmong do not exaggerate emotions they express.
- **Privacy**. Adult women are modest and uncomfortable with physical exam. Clinician must clearly explain purpose of exam and obtain consent. Women often refuse pelvic exams by male health care providers; more likely to accept them if practitioner is female and they understand the need for exam. Males are especially sensitive to topics such as impotence; they deny this problem even if a male Hmong interpreter is present. Sometimes, clinician can obtain sensitive information if he/she first explains that "this is a common problem for all people who have your diagnosis, and I am wondering if this also might be a concern of yours."
- **Touch**. Hmong neither show physical affection nor touch in public. Acceptable for health professionals to touch patient while providing care, but they should first explain the procedure and the need for it. Should ask permission to touch genital areas.
- **Orientation to time**. Most older Hmong are present-oriented. Hmong in rural Laos rarely use calendars and clocks. Persons born there may not know their birth date. Many birth dates were assigned in refugee camps, resulting in some errors; individuals may actually be younger or older than their given age. Often difficult for Hmong to keep appointments. Patients may arrive in early morning on the day of their medical appointment. This occurs less often as children socialize their families to Western system. Social events in Hmong communities may start several hours after the stated time.

ACTIVITIES OF DAILY LIVING

- **Modesty**. Women's perspectives regarding their bodies can vary considerably. Older women are modest about their genitals, but, because of past breastfeeding, they may not be concerned about baring their breasts. Men are modest but accept examination of their genitals by female health care professionals.
- **Skin care**. In Laos, bathing infrequent because water is available only from wells or streams. In U.S., daily bathing more common.
- **Hair care**. Varies. No apparent restrictions.
- **Nail care**. Varies. No apparent restrictions.
- **Toileting**. No apparent restrictions or concerns.
- **Special clothing or amulets**. Hmong may wear amulets on their neck, wrists, waist, and/or ankles. These may be gold necklaces or bracelets, a white or red string, fabric bands, or chains. May attach small amulet pouches in the belief that amulets have special powers to hold the soul in and keep evil spirits out. Caregivers should not remove amulets without permission. Persons who have undergone a shaman ritual to treat illness may put blood of sacrificed animal on their clothing. May place animal parts, such as nails or teeth, in a pocket on their back or sew them onto

clothing. Patient may not want this clothing removed; spirit of dead animal provides protection.

- **Self-care**. Hmong perceive wellness as the ability to fulfill one's role and meet responsibilities. They try to perform their usual duties even when ill, though they may expect female family members to care for them. Patients may resist self-care practices. For example, family members may be expected to administer insulin injections.

FOOD PRACTICES

- **Usual meal pattern**. Usually 2–3 meals a day. Among those who customarily eat two meals a day, first meal is usually at around 9–10 a.m. Second is in late afternoon or early evening.
- **Special utensils**. None.
- **Food beliefs and rituals**. Eat special foods when ill or not feeling well. Suspicious of store-bought chicken and meat, believing these contain unhealthy chemicals. Many prefer to kill their own chickens and other animals or to purchase fresh meat. Small vegetable gardens are common even among Hmong who live in apartments.
- **Usual diet**. Main staple is rice, with small amounts of meat, fish, and green vegetables. Noodle dishes and soups also are favorites. American favorites are sweets and soda. Often use generous quantities of MSG. Food usually is bland, but Hmong may add hot chili condiments and salty sauces at the table according to individual taste. Rarely eat fruit. Adults rarely consume dairy products, such as milk and cheese, but enjoy ice cream and pizza. Hmong eat the same types of food at each meal.
- **Fluids**. Avoid iced drinks. May request warm water. Soft drinks and sodas are favorites at special occasions.
- **Food taboos and prescriptions**. May prohibit fried foods or those that have a strong odor, such as garlic and onions. Illness and perinatal foods include plain, boiled rice soup, which may contain small amounts of chicken. Family may want to bring in food to hospitalized patient, as hospital food does not fit into cultural illness practices.
- **Hospitality**. In the home, Hmong offer food to guests, who are expected to refuse at first, then accept after the host has offered several more times.

SYMPTOM MANAGEMENT

- **Pain** (*mob* ["b" is silent]). Hmong do not use pain scales well. Better for clinician to ask if pain is mild, moderate, or severe. Tend to be stoic, but they request pain medication if aware of its availability and if they can communicate their desire to caregiver. In Laos, Hmong traditionally grew and used opium as an analgesic. Readily accept analgesic medications but may take more than prescribed to find pain relief.
- **Dyspnea** (*txog txog siav*). May describe shortness of breath as "tired" or "dif-

ficulty breathing." Incidence of asthma increasing among adults and children. Patients infected with human lung fluke (paragonimus) or exposed to biological/chemical warfare may have lung disease. Instead of using numerical scale, clinician should ask patient if dyspnea is mild, moderate, or severe.

- **Nausea/vomiting** (*xeev siab*). Gastrointestinal disturbance common. Patients freely discuss distress and request relief from symptoms. Clinician should ask patient if nausea/vomiting is mild, moderate, or severe.
- **Constipation** (*cem quav* or *quav tawu*)/**diarrhea** (*lawv plab, raws plab,* or *thoj plab*). Constipation frequent due to poor intake of roughage, but Hmong may not report it to health care professionals unless specifically asked. Receptive to advice about changing diet to control symptoms. Consider diarrhea a distressful symptom. Request medication to control it.
- **Fatigue** (*nkees*). Often a presenting symptom of depression. Hmong say "tired" to indicate physical illnesses; sometimes, families use the Hmong word for "tired" to indicate that someone is near death. Instead of using numerical scale, clinician should ask patient if fatigue is mild, moderate, or severe.
- **Depression** (*nyuajsiab*). Post-traumatic stress disorder common. Women often express their marital discord as depression if they feel helpless about changing their situation. Men become depressed due to physical limitations from war injuries and their sense of powerlessness since immigrating to U.S. Unemployment is high among older adults who are not fluent in English. Hmong sometimes accept suicide, interpreting it as going to a "better world." Acculturation stresses and conflicts between older and younger generations have generated a high incidence of suicide among young Hmong.
- **Self-care symptom management**. Often try home remedies, including cupping, coining, pinching, massage, herbs, and shaman rituals, before seeking biomedical care. Some purchase pharmaceuticals in Mexico or at swap meets, or obtain them from friends and family. Rarely, among these medications are intramuscular and intravenous preparations. Use herbs extensively. Recent evaluations of imported herbs used by Hmong have detected arsenic in some and potent pharmaceuticals in others.

BIRTH RITUALS/CARE OF THE NEW MOTHER AND BABY

- **Pregnancy care**. Prenatal care becoming more widely accepted, although some may not seek it until third trimester because they do not consider pregnancy an illness. Older Hmong women have as many as 10–12 pregnancies.
- **Preferences for children**. Prefer boys, but acculturated Hmong desire boys and girls, and fewer children.
- **Labor practices**. Labor can progress very rapidly for multiparous women. Labor practices vary. Some women prefer to walk about and others prefer to lie in bed. Husband and/or family members provide support for Hmong women during labor.
- **Role of the laboring woman during birth**. Older Hmong women often

quiet during labor, although behavior may vary. Younger women are aware of analgesics and may request them during labor.

- **Role of the father and other family members during birth**. Traditionally, father delivered baby by reaching under skirt of squatting mother to avoid full exposure of genital area. If there are problems, in-laws may help, as the birthing couple usually lives with in-laws. Since immigration and the practice of giving birth in hospitals, father usually present, but his assistance during labor and delivery varies. Some men do not want to be present. Husband usually at hospital; he expects to participate in all decisions regarding surgical options.
- **Vaginal vs. cesarean section**. Prefer vaginal delivery. Often refuse cesarean section.
- **Breastfeeding**. Declining in practice. Bottle-feeding becoming standard within Hmong community, even though health care professionals encourage breastfeeding. Many women think American women do not breastfeed, as they never see it in public. Breastfeeding more acceptable among young, educated Hmong women.
- **Birth recuperation**. New mothers remain on a restricted diet of chicken and white rice for 30 days after delivery. Desire fresh chicken, preferably killed by father. May eat store-bought chicken if fresh chicken unavailable. Rice must be soft and white. No other foods allowed during this time. New mothers allowed to drink warm water but not iced water. New mothers shower and perform usual self-care. They are expected to rest after delivery and not do any housework.
- **Baby care**. Mother-in-law and husband help.
- **Problems with baby**. When clinician notices problems, should tell parents and other family members who are present. If problems develop and extended family cannot handle them, parents/family members seek medical care.
- **Male and female circumcision**. Neither practiced.

DEVELOPMENTAL AND SEXUAL ISSUES

- **Celebration of menarche or becoming a man**. No special ceremonies or responsibilities. Girls are marriageable when they get "plump," which usually occurs at puberty. Males are not considered to be adults until they marry.
- **Attitudes about birth control**. Hormonal birth control methods not widely accepted due to fear of side effects. Younger women are more accepting of birth control and may use many different methods. May use abstinence, withdrawal, and douching.
- **Attitudes about sexually transmitted infection (STI) control, including condoms**. Men rarely use condoms; acculturated young men may. Hmong are aware of STIs but consider them a taboo subject, except with health care professionals. Misunderstandings about STIs common. For example, they may believe that STIs can spread when a person sits in a chair previously occupied by someone with an STI.

- **Attitudes about abortion**. Accept abortion if the family feels it is best.
- **Attitudes about unwed sexual experimentation**. Believe that sexual intercourse should occur only in marriage. Young, single persons most likely have sexual intercourse outside of marriage, but this is not discussed. Teen pregnancy common because girls often marry very young—during pubescence is not unusual. Marry only through Hmong ceremonies, so they are not subject to U.S. age requirement for obtaining marriage license.
- **Sexual orientation**. Hmong in Laos unfamiliar with homosexuality. A few in U.S. have identified themselves as gay or lesbian. Hmong community does not easily accept these orientations. Family and clan generally ostracize gays and lesbians.
- **Gender identity**. Hmong community does not acknowledge transgender and gender-ambiguous persons.
- **Attitudes about menopause**. Older women welcome the transition. It means no more menstruation, no more pregnancies. Younger, nonpregnant women who stop menstruating become very distressed because menstruation means their body is functioning properly. For this reason, Hmong women avoid hormonal treatments that interfere with normal menstrual patterns.

FAMILY RELATIONSHIPS

- **Composition/structure**. Immigrant families large and patrilineal, with well-organized hierarchy of decision-making. Younger and U.S.-born Hmong have fewer children than their parents did. Grandparents and/or siblings, their wives, and children usually live with young couples. Head of family generally is an older male. There are 18 Hmong clans. All members of a clan have same last name. All clan members with same name are considered to be related and thus prohibited from intermarrying, even though they may not actually have a close biological relationship. Consider cousins in same generation to be brothers and sisters. Expect sons to marry and bring wives to live in family's home. Daughters marry and become part of husband's clan, though they may retain the birth clan's name as their surname. In Laos, men may have more than one wife. Plural marriages still occur in traditional families. But because such marriages are not legal by U.S. standards, they are not bigamous. Hmong community considers plural marriages legitimate. All of a man's wives and children have equal status.
- **Decision-making**. Women may express opinions, but father/husband makes final decisions regarding major family issues. If an older woman's husband dies, eldest adult male is expected to make decisions for her. Major decisions may be made at family meetings. Younger, acculturated persons are more independent and may make their own decisions.
- **Spokesperson**. Most likely someone who speaks English. But this person may not have decision-making power.
- **Gender issues**. Women subservient to men. Women take care of the house-

hold and family. Men traditionally provided for their family as farmers in Laos, where the whole family worked together on the farm.

- **Changing roles among generations in U.S.** Inactivity and lack of meaningful work for older Hmong adults create stress. Recent immigrants have difficulty coping with American practice of working outside the home. Children become powerful in the family, as intermediaries between it and American society, because of their acculturation and fluency in English. This role reversal creates great tension in families. When a young woman is evaluated as a potential mate, her reputation as a "hard worker" is part of her value as a bride. After she marries, she is expected to cook and clean for her in-laws. This role expectation persists even though the daughter-in-law may have a job or attend school.

- **Caring roles**. Women are the caretakers in sickness and in health. Hmong expect daughters-in-law to care for ill in-laws.

- **Expectations of and for children**. Hmong highly value children. The more children one has, the higher one's status in the community. Expect children to obey parents, other adults, and older siblings. May make decisions for children about schooling and career. Believe that such decisions are in best interest of family; individual's desires are secondary to family's needs. Stress arises when children want to engage in sports, extracurricular activities, and social events. Parents do not understand such activities and often disapprove of them. Some children sign their own school permission slips and report cards because their parents do not understand these documents and cannot write.

- **Expectations of and for elders**. Elders take on child-rearing roles when they no longer are able to work outside the home. Hmong community respects the elderly and looks to them for advice. Families care for, rather than institutionalize, the elderly.

- **Expectations of hospital visitors**. Hmong expect all family members to visit hospitalized patient. Hospital may be overwhelmed by visitors, as families can be quite large and extended-family members have close ties. Family members want to stay in patient's room to help.

ILLNESS BELIEFS

- **Causes of/attitudes about physical illness**. Believe that illness can have natural or supernatural etiologies, although Hmong are beginning to understand infectious-disease etiologies. According to traditional beliefs, illness may be caused by a lost soul or an ancestral spirit trying to get that person's attention and remind him/her that honor ceremonies have not been sufficiently performed. Christians may have illness beliefs similar to those of other Westerners or believe that illness is God's will. Those who have recently converted to Christianity may believe that illness is retribution by ancestral spirits for abandoning traditional ways.

- **Causes of/attitudes about mental illness**. No word for mental illness in

Hmong, except one that means "crazy" in English. Depression common and not concealed. Post-traumatic stress disorder (PTSD) with depression and flashbacks is common among those who experienced war. Hmong accept those who have PTSD and depression because these conditions are so prevalent, though severe mental illness with symptoms such as bizarre behavior and hallucinations is stigmatized. Readily accept mental health counselors and antidepressants for PTSD and depression.

- **Causes of genetic defects**. Believe that spirits cause genetic defects because the parents did something wrong or the child did something wrong in a former life. Concerned about defects and disabilities because they may render a child unmarriageable.
- **Attitudes about disabilities**. Extremely important to be able to function normally and to be healthy and whole. Although disabilities are stigmatized, disabled persons are well cared for. Disabled family members, including those who need assistive devices, stay home and do not participate in community events. A disabled child may not be marriageable.
- **Sick role**. Ill persons expect family members to provide illness care, even insulin injections, but not usual self-care. Family relationships can be strained by prolonged illnesses or insufficient help.
- **Home and folk remedies**. Traditionalists who retain animist beliefs use shaman rituals to treat disease. Christians may use traditional medical practices except shamanism. Skin treatments directly over painful or affected area release evil spirits or illness-causing toxins from the body and result in ecchymosis. Darkness of the bruise indicates seriousness of illness. "Cupping" involves burning cotton or tissue in a small glass jar. After flame dies, jar is placed over painful area and remains until air in jar has cooled, producing a vacuum and round ecchymotic area. "Coining" involves lightly stroking the skin with a coin, spoon, or other object that has a rounded edge until an oval bruise with an irregular border appears. In "pinching," skin is squeezed until a bruise appears. Bruise is usually narrow, such as that between the eyes of a person treated for headache. Common practice is to puncture ecchymotic area with a sewing needle and express blood, thereby releasing the cause of the illness. Needle is rarely sterilized and may be used on several persons. Hmong in Laos and U.S. frequently use herbs. Many traditional herbs unavailable, but some are imported from Laos. Chinese herbs are popular. May use U.S. plants and roots that resemble herbs in their homeland.
- **Medications**. Expect a medicine to work immediately. If antibiotic does not relieve pain, patient stops taking it or may increase dosage. Interpret side effects as the medicine being "too strong" and may not take the full dose. Clinician should explain that an antibiotic will not make someone feel better for at least three days. Hmong with chronic disease stop medicating if there are no symptoms and the medicine causes side effects. Clinician must

teach patient or family about the chronic disease and explain why he/she must take the medicine. Sliding-scale and tapered dosing are extremely difficult for Hmong to understand, and should be avoided if possible. Because Hmong respect clinicians, they usually do not reveal that they have not followed recommendations. Rather than asking patients directly how much medication they are taking, clinician should request that they bring in medicine bottles so the frequency and date of refills can be compared with the number of remaining pills. Checking medicine bottles may prevent inappropriate increase in dosage and identify medications that might cause overdose (e.g., prescriptions for both furosimide and Lasix.) Patients who make medication errors need additional instructions, but a clinician who berates the patient (which is disrespectful) may prompt him/her not to return.

- **Acceptance of procedures**. Generally do not accept invasive procedures. Surgery was rarely available in Laos, so patients may be afraid of surgical procedures they do not understand. Some do not want blood drawn when they feel ill because they think it will make them "too sick." Many complain if they have "too many" blood tests, due to a belief that blood is not regenerated. Others request blood tests because they think such tests release "bad blood" and that they will feel better afterward.

- **Care-seeking**. Hmong often try home remedies and traditional medicine before going to a biomedical physician. Sometimes this practice enables diseases to become well-advanced before Western practitioners intervene.

HEALTH ISSUES

- **Concept of health**. Equate health with being whole and able to perform routine duties. Great distress occurs when someone cannot perform these duties.

- **Health promotion and prevention**. Health promotion with a Western focus is not a priority. Hmong are beginning to recognize the importance of a nutritious diet and exercise. Practice some healthy behaviors and avoid others because of widespread beliefs that certain Western foods or medical procedures will cause harm. Most parents have their children immunized if reminded or if immunization takes place during routine visits. To ensure compliance, clinicians may need to remind patients by telephone or mail.

- **Screening**. Most do not visit health care providers strictly for screening. Do not accept routine procedures, such as sigmoidoscopy, if there are no symptoms to justify them. Most screening is done when ill patients seek treatment. Screens such as Pap smears, breast examinations, and mammograms are gaining acceptance as a result of women's greater awareness of breast cancer.

- **Common health problems**. Obesity, as a result of adopting a sedentary Western lifestyle and a diet that has excess calories. Hmong also are prone to type 2 diabetes, hypertension, hyperlipidemia, and cardiovascular diseases. Renal disease and kidney failure are increasing.

DEATH RITUALS

- **Beliefs and attitudes about death**. Believe in afterlife and reincarnation, that spirits of ancestors are always with them, and that spirits wishing them harm co-exist with ancestor spirits. Many traditional ceremonies and amulets protect them from spirits. Hmong elders are greatly revered; their funerals are elaborate and last many days, compared to the very short funerals for small children.

- **Preparation**. Best if clinician advises family when a person is near death. Unacceptable for Hmong to say "dying"; rather, "tired" is code word they use to communicate the seriousness of patient's condition. Extremely inappropriate to speak about impending death with a patient who is terminal. This may be due to the belief that evil spirits cause illness; if clinician discusses complications or potentially fatal outcomes with patient, indwelling evil spirit will know how to make patient sicker. Elders in family/clan meet regarding any decisions to be made about the dying person. A traditional religious belief is that the deceased enters the next world appearing as he/she did at time of death. In preparation for burial, both Christian and traditional families dress the deceased in finest traditional Hmong clothing, as it is shameful to enter the next world poorly dressed or unclothed.

- **Home vs. hospital**. May accept dying at home or in hospital. Decision always based on what is best for dying person. Welcome hospice care if patient is at home.

- **Special needs**. Health care providers should not remove amulets from body. Hmong may perform shaman rituals at home in attempt to cure dying person. They consider these rituals to be less effective if performed in hospital. After death, Hmong perform specific rituals over several days to help send spirit of deceased to the afterlife.

- **Care of the body**. Family usually prepares body at funeral home for burial. Some families believe that the deceased will suffer if hard objects are buried with his/her body; they may ask that indwelling metal plates, bullets, and shrapnel be removed. Deceased cannot be buried with buttons, zippers, or metal closures on clothing, and screws and nails must be removed from inside of coffin. Dress body in traditional Hmong or Western clothing, and place extra finery in coffin. Do not bury Hmong metal amulets or jewelry with body.

- **Attitudes about organ donation**. Hmong accept donated organs. However, it is unacceptable for a person who was ill to donate to another family member, as the recipient also may become ill.

- **Attitudes about autopsy**. Unacceptable.

SELECTED REFERENCES

Barrett, B., Shadick, K., Schilling, R., Spencer, L., del Rosario, S., Moua, K., et al. (1998). Hmong/medicine interactions: Improving cross-cultural health care. *Family Medicine, 30,* 179–184.

Culhane-Pera, K. A., & Vawter, D. E. (1998). A study of healthcare professionals' perspectives about a cross-cultural ethical conflict involving a Hmong patient and her family. *Journal of Clinical Ethics, 9,* 179–190.

Davis, R. E. (2001). The postpartum experience for Southeast Asian women in the United States. *American Journal of Maternal and Child Nursing, 26,* 208–213.

Fadiman, A. (1997). *The spirit catches you and you fall down.* New York: Farrar, Straus and Giroux.

Henry, R. R. (1999). Measles, Hmong, and metaphor: Culture change and illness management under conditions of immigration. *Medical Anthropology Quarterly, 13,* 32–50.

Johnson, S. K. (2002). Hmong health beliefs and experiences in the Western health care system. *Journal of Transcultural Nursing, 13,* 126–132.

Levenick, M. (2001). Hmong and prenatal care. *Journal of Cultural Diversity, 8,* 26–29.

Plotnikoff, G. A., Numrich, C., Wu, C., Yang, D., & Xiong, P. (2002). Hmong shamanism: Animist spiritual healing in Minnesota. *Minnesota Medicine.* Retrieved July 27, 2004, from http://www.mmaonline.net/publications/MNMed2002/june/Plotnikoff.html

AUTHORS

Sharon Johnson, RN, FNP, PhD, is a graduate of the University of California-San Francisco School of Nursing. In her dissertation, "Diabetes in the Hmong Population," she examined the emergence of diabetes among Hmong individuals, including health beliefs, practices, and perspectives that influence diabetes management. She is director of the associate-degree nursing program at Santa Rosa Junior College in Santa Rosa, CA.

Ae Lee Hang, RN, MSN, FNP, is a graduate of the California State University-Fresno School of Nursing. Her senior project was "Elder Hmong's Beliefs, Practices, and Perceptions of Western Healthcare." She is a mentor for college-level students who are interested in a health care profession. She also provides primary care at the Fresno Family Practice Center, specializing in chronic pain management.

CHAPTER 20

IRANIANS

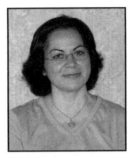

Homeyra Hafizi

CULTURAL/ETHNIC IDENTITY

- **Preferred term(s)**. Use Persian and Iranian interchangeably. Most adopt a Persian cultural identity rather than a Muslim identity. They are not Arabs. Iran is ethnically diverse and secular, but the sense of nationalism is strong. Vast intragroup diversity. Heterogeneous religion, language, and regional practices, as well as time of immigration, acculturation, ethnic identity, gender roles, socioeconomic status, and education.
- **Census**. The 2000 U.S. Census estimates 338,000 Iranians. However, other unofficial estimates range from 1–3 million.
- **History of immigration**. First wave, before the 1979 revolution in Iran, comprised mostly students, elites, and professionals. Second wave, which coincided with Iran-Iraq war (1980–90), comprised immigrants of more diverse socioeconomic and educational backgrounds. Most families fled as refugees mainly to Scandinavian countries and U.S. In contrast with earlier immigrants, those in second wave were more like refugees; they abandoned their financial resources, social status, and professions. Many still resist acculturation, given the uncertainty of their immigration status and finding meaningful employment.

SPIRITUAL/RELIGIOUS ORIENTATION

- **Primary religious/spiritual affiliations**. Majority are Muslims, mostly Shi'ites. In U.S., religious minorities, including Baha'is, Jews, Christians, and Zoroastrians, have been more active than Muslims have in establishing cultural organizations and networks.
- **Usual religious/spiritual practices**. Muslims pray either individually or as a group, either at home or at mosque, and directly to one God (Allah). Reli-

gious practices rare in hospital setting, except for silent prayers at bedside. Prayer gatherings outside the hospital by and for women (*sofre'*) are intended to return the patient to health. Other forms of spiritual or religious practices abroad and in U.S. may involve giving alms to needy families.

- **Use of spiritual healing/healers**. Achieve spiritual healing through prayer and support of family and friends. Do not use specific spiritual healers or expect any to visit hospitalized patient.

- **Holidays**. New Year's (*Norouz* or *Norooz*), a secular holiday marking spring equinox and beginning of calendar year. Regardless of religious differences, all Iranians celebrate this most-recognized national holiday with family gatherings, visits, and good food. Adults give money—traditionally, brand new bills—to children and teenagers. Particular religious communities observe specific holidays.

COMMUNICATION
ORAL COMMUNICATION

- **Major languages and dialects**. Farsi (Persian) is national language. However, nearly half of the country's population speaks other languages or dialects, reflecting vast ethnic variation. U.S.-born Iranians are in their teens and early twenties, and speak English. Their command of the Persian language varies, depending on exposure and formal language training.

- **Greetings**. May prefer use of last name, at least on first meeting. Appropriate greetings are handshake, slight bow, and even standing when someone enters room. Generally greet elderly first as sign of respect. Kissing and embracing common among close relatives.

- **Tone of voice**. In presence of family, tone of voice may become loud, emotional, and animated. Among strangers, may be more restrained. Requests to care providers polite; may use apologetic tone.

- **Direct or indirect style of speech**. Complex and less direct than in dominant culture. Avoid forwardness in expressing true feelings or thoughts; strongly value being polite, pleasant, and keeping social relationships smooth. May communicate negative feelings or disagreements through metaphor or humor. In health care, depending on how personal the topic is, communication can be "careful" rather than "open and direct." Greater acculturation, trust, and severity of illness lead to more direct conversation with clinician.

- **Use of interpreters**. Generally choose someone (relative or friend) who can discuss sensitive issues. Prefer interpreter of similar age and same gender. Family may validate medical information by tapping into network of Iranian health care professionals or the many broadcasts on satellite Persian TV and radio, which convey information to previously isolated Iranian immigrant enclaves.

- **Serious or terminal illness**. Clinician should disclose news about a serious health condition in guarded manner, often little by little. Best to assess family dynamics and patient's state of mind. Traditionally, Iranians keep bad news hidden from patient to maintain his/her hope and promise of life. Best if clinician tells spouse or older adult child first. Patient may selectively choose to communicate news about a serious illness. Some Iranians, particularly those who are less-acculturated, older, and less-educated, are fatalistic, believing in God's will in life and death as a predestined journey (*tagdir* or *ghesmat*).

WRITTEN COMMUNICATION

- **Literacy assessment**. Older immigrants either do not speak English or speak in simple words and sentences. This does not reflect their literacy in Farsi, as many are highly educated. Clinician should directly ask patients about their ability to read and write in English. Health information materials translated into Farsi give the elderly more autonomy and self-respect in their encounters with health care system.
- **Consents**. Clinician should explain procedure or treatment to family spokesperson or interpreter if patient does not speak English. Some families believe in protecting a loved one by not mentioning potential complications or by disclosing only some of the facts so patient does not lose hope. When patient gives informed consent, he/she does so willingly.

NONVERBAL COMMUNICATION

- **Eye contact**. Direct eye contact acceptable, especially between equals and intimates.
- **Personal space**. Generally closer than that among North Americans.
- **Use and meaning of silence**. May use silence in situations where respectability and maintaining a good appearance could be compromised, as in a disagreement with a health care professional of high status or in a situation that might publicly expose the family or sensitive personal issues.
- **Gestures**. Thumbs-up inappropriate, as it means the same as a raised middle finger in dominant culture. Hands and body language highly expressive and animated in close circles but more restricted in public.
- **Openness in expressing emotions**. May guardedly express emotions, depending on situation and degree to which such expression will publicly expose a family's sensitive personal issues. A hierarchy of relationships, age, gender, education, and socioeconomic status influences communication. Iranians very cautious about disclosing feelings or personal thoughts to those with whom they are not intimate; seek to avoid external judgment. May mask inner feelings to keep social relationships smooth.
- **Privacy**. May be sensitive about sharing personal information. Iranians' respect for professional caregivers makes them more likely to release information regarding health care. Concept of shame (*haya*) influences their decision about whether to share information that may be embarrassing. This

trait may be more evident in older generation. Women share information more readily than men do.

- **Touch**. Modesty and shame underlie who may touch whom and in what setting. For example, sisters may touch each other frequently when conversing, but couples may refrain from showing affection in public. Touch related to health care is acceptable. Iranians are most cooperative if clinician explains a procedure or treatment and asks permission to touch.
- **Orientation to time**. Iranians' orientation to future enhances the effectiveness of health education and maintaining health. However, their fatalistic beliefs hinder complete understanding and compliance. Refugees and those experiencing difficult adjustments in U.S. may live and relive many memories. May be flexible about social time but observe on-time demands of dominant culture in business and health care.

ACTIVITIES OF DAILY LIVING

- **Modesty**. Varies by age, traditional values, and degree of acculturation. As a whole, population is modest regarding clothing. May be more comfortable with a caregiver of same gender.
- **Skin care**. If ill, may refrain from daily shower, as Iranians believe that dampness and draft accentuate weakness and malaise. However, important to cleanse with water after every urination or defecation.
- **Hair care**. No particular preference.
- **Nail care**. Varies as in dominant culture.
- **Toileting**. More inclined to use bathroom for privacy and to wash; may insist on it. Often prefer washing in addition to, or instead of, using toilet paper. Caregiver should provide a small water pitcher in bathroom.
- **Special clothing or amulets**. No special clothing, but modesty and privacy are important to older immigrants. May wear wrist chains and gold charm on neck. Some may read prayers quietly at bedside using prayer beads.
- **Self-care**. Family and friends are an important part of care. Patient may seem less involved in self-care. Some families expect nurses to handle all minor care and activities of daily living but take over willingly if given permission and instructed what to do.

FOOD PRACTICES

- **Usual meal pattern**. Usually three meals a day and possibly snacks, especially fresh fruit. Prefer to eat with family. May eat dinner late in evening.
- **Special utensils**. Fork and spoon.
- **Food beliefs and rituals**. Food classification of "hot"/"cold" based on humoral theory, which sometimes corresponds to high- and low-calorie foods. Balancing these two food categories is key. For example, to treat symptoms of weakness and vomiting after eating too many cold foods, such as plums or cucumbers, one must eat hot foods, such as walnuts, onions, or

honey. Iranians believe that women are more susceptible to digestive problems caused by eating too much cold food. Food and food combinations play
an important role in balance of Iranians' social and physiological lives.

- **Usual diet**. Prefer fresh rather than frozen or canned foods. Use some dry
  herbs, due to unavailability or cost of fresh herbs. Fast food less common
  among Iranians, who believe that it lacks nutritional value. Most common
  starches are rice and bread, which accompany most meals. Vegetables, beans,
  and legumes prepared in different mixtures and served with rice make up
  large part of diet. Dairy products, such as feta cheese, yogurt, eggs, and milk,
  also are staples. Meat favorites include beef, chicken, fish, and lamb. Sometimes eat shellfish. Enjoy and often consume leafy green vegetables and
  fruits. Also serve fruit for dessert. Strongly believe that properly balanced
  nutrition promotes healing and prevents disease.

- **Fluids**. Serve tea after each meal and with snacks when guests arrive. Like
  warm tea sweetened with hard candy. Believe that herbal teas have medicinal properties. Avoid ice-cold water when ill.

- **Food taboos and prescriptions**. Must balance "hot"/"cold" foods. Strict
  Muslims believe in permitted (*halal*) and forbidden (*haram*) foods based on
  Koran. *Haram* food and drinks include pork and alcohol. Patient and family may desire or provide homemade food during short- and long-term hos-
  pitalizations.

- **Hospitality**. Iranians greatly value hospitality as a social and personal
  virtue. Revere and care for visitors to the best of their ability. A driving factor is preservation of "face" and social stature. They even sacrifice something
  else when inadequate finances might preclude providing a lavish meal.

SYMPTOM MANAGEMENT

- **Pain** (*dard*). Express pain variously with facial grimaces, guarded body posture, moans, and even soft cries. Iranians use the body as a metaphor to
  express feelings and thoughts, especially those that are not socioculturally
  sanctioned for public disclosure. Persian phrases that describe pain provide
  vivid images of the body and a person's reaction to the experience of pain
  (suffering). Somatization, an expression of social and personal problems
  through bodily reactions and complaints, is common. Iranians do not have
  difficulty understanding any of the commonly used pain scales, although
  they define pain in more qualitative terms. Clinician should offer pain medications (patients may prefer intramuscular meds initially) and provide alternative means of relief, such as warm or cold compresses.

- **Dyspnea** (*tange-nafas* or *nafas-tange*—"tight breath"). May overtly show signs
  of anxiety. Readily accept medication and oxygen to control dyspnea and to
  relieve accompanying fear. Clinician should reassure patient and family that
  dyspnea can be controlled to a degree. Should also suggest relaxation exercises.

- **Nausea/vomiting** (*tahavo/estefrog*). Readily accept medication for symptom

relief. Some complement biomedicine with herbal teas. No particular practice in terms of reporting or cleaning up after vomiting. Privacy essential, as
Iranians are embarrassed by, and shameful of, any bodily function that is
unpleasant or that they consider unclean.

- **Constipation/diarrhea** (*yobousat/eshaul*). May attribute any alteration in
bowel function to pathology and/or imbalance of food categories. Some Iranians first try to treat pathology or food imbalance with humoral remedies
rather than Western medications. Accept medications and use them in conjunction with humoral remedies. Though not prevalent, modesty may interfere with reporting of a health condition to care provider.

- **Fatigue** (*khasteh*—"tired"; *beehall*—"without energy"). Has nonphysiologi-
cal origins, as somatization is an acceptable illness behavior. Iranians understand numerical scale for rating fatigue but may deem it irrelevant, given
that symptoms also serve as metaphors for sociocultural problems. Accept
medications. However, clinician should be cautious and assess the source of
fatigue if disease pathology does not correspond.

- **Depression** (*afsorde*). "Existential depression," a manifestation of a deeper
understanding of human mortality, is common among the elderly and likely
to manifest as somber mood. Clinical depression presents as sleep and
appetite disturbances and frequent complaints about diffuse aches and pains.
Narahati is a general term that refers to a wide range of unpleasant emotions
or physical feelings, such as depression, disappointment, anxiety, fatigue, and
unease. Iranians may express *narahati* in various nonverbal ways, such as
through silence, quiet isolation, or reduced interaction, all of which are
acceptable illness behaviors.

- **Self-care symptom management**. Attempt to cure an ailment with home
and herbal remedies before seeking medical care. Ultimately, Iranians use a
combination of both to achieve a desired outcome.

BIRTH RITUALS/CARE OF THE NEW MOTHER AND BABY

- **Pregnancy care**. Prenatal care depends on financial resources and access to
medical care; family provides help and support. Expectant mother encouraged to balance her diet, rest adequately, and refrain from heavy work
throughout pregnancy. Pregnant women generally agree to take childbirth
preparation classes.

- **Preferences for children**. Some families prefer boys rather than girls. Family economics, education, and level of acculturation affect family size.

- **Labor practices**. Midwife or physician of either gender acceptable at childbirth. Encourage walking before delivery. Mostly prefer hospital rather than
home delivery. Showering common soon after birth.

- **Role of the laboring woman during birth**. Depends on woman's personality rather than a cultural norm. Some moan and grunt during labor, others
may become hysterical. Accept either natural or reasonable medical inter-

ventions. Modesty may exert a controlling influence on woman's role.

- **Role of the father and other family members during birth**. Fathers who are more-acculturated take active role. Female family members are supportive and may be present.
- **Vaginal vs. cesarean section**. No preference. Health of mother and baby are determining factors.
- **Breastfeeding**. Preferred, but bottle-feeding is acceptable. May use homemade, softly pureed food as an adjunct at age 6 months; prepackaged baby food far less common. Do not typically mix breast- and bottle-feeding unless mother works. Breastfeeding may last as long as one year.
- **Birth recuperation**. Rest, proper diet, hygiene, and emotional comfort are essential. In the past, new mother recuperated for 30–40 days, but today, it depends on her health, the child, family's economic status, and other factors. Mother, sister, or female family member and friends provide support and guidance for baby care.
- **Baby care**. Families use grandparents, other female family members or friends, or childcare centers; prefer the first two options. If a parent stays home, it is most often the mother. Infants go to childcare center beginning at about age 1 year. Iranians believe it is important for infant to spend first year with the family or in a home setting.
- **Problems with baby**. If baby is diagnosed with an ailment, clinician should approach the parents together, assess the emotional state of both parents, always provide a hopeful message, and discuss treatments.
- **Male and female circumcision**. Male circumcision always performed, female circumcision never. Procedure is done either in the hospital or at a later date, depending on baby's health. Some families mark the occasion with festivities.

DEVELOPMENTAL AND SEXUAL ISSUES

- **Celebration of menarche or becoming a man**. No particular ceremony or celebration to mark either event. Girls learn about menarche and discuss related hygiene only with older sisters, mother, or other close female relatives. Most Iranian women do not openly discuss sexuality but may discuss it with spouse in context of marriage. Globalization and acculturation have increased openness in discussion of such issues.
- **Attitudes about birth control**. Immigrants and people in Iran use birth control. In both populations, it is more acceptable for married couples. Encourage marriage at a young age as a compromise, given the cultural expectation that girls remain virgin until married. These guidelines do not hold for young males. Single women who are openly or secretly sexually intimate use various types of contraceptives.
- **Attitudes about sexually transmitted infection (STI) control, including condoms**. In U.S., level of acculturation affects knowledge, norms, and

beliefs regarding STI control. Younger adults have a more scientifically based understanding of the issues and protection methods. Typically in Iran, birth control is the woman's responsibility, so condom use is uncommon. In U.S., more-open discussion of sex, health, and gender equality may facilitate a greater potential use of condoms.

- **Attitudes about abortion**. Practiced to some degree. Religious belief less influential than are practices related to a woman's rights.
- **Attitudes about unwed sexual experimentation**. Sexual activity remains traditionally forbidden for unmarried women. However, acculturated women may practice sexual freedom without disclosing it to family. Iranian society is more tolerant of males' sexual activity outside of marriage.
- **Sexual orientation**. Gays and lesbians either do not disclose or selectively disclose their orientation to family, friends, and community. Others, especially traditional families, may disown them.
- **Gender identity**. Social and parental expectations of women are such that, in contrast to men, women must restrain their overt behaviors; refrain from being loud, vocal, or animated; and be more prim and proper. A son or daughter whose gender identity is ambiguous or opposite to his/her birth gender may encounter difficulties in his/her family and community. Estrangement possible.
- **Attitudes about menopause**. Modesty and embarrassment hinder open discussion of sexual or other gender-related topics. Regard menopause as a normal life process and sometimes even welcome it as a contraceptive and mark of maturity. Women discuss their symptoms and treatment choices with sisters and close women friends. Far easier for women to discuss menopause than menarche.

FAMILY RELATIONSHIPS

- **Composition/structure**. Iranian culture is highly family-oriented. Relationships are complex and transcend many generations. Men and oldest persons have the most influence. Close and regular contact with family and friends is a source of strength and, at times, distress. Many unmarried adult children live at home until they marry. Parents remain involved in the lives of their adult children even after they marry and form their own nuclear families.
- **Decision-making**. This mostly patriarchal society respects the eldest male member of both the nuclear and extended family. In some families, father/husband is the sole decision-maker.
- **Spokesperson**. Clinician should identify family spokesperson and use him/her as an interpreter of both language and culture. Spokesperson is not necessarily male; could be an educated, female family member.
- **Gender issues**. In traditional patriarchal society, father ruled the family and expected obedience from wife and children. His role was protecting and providing for the family and handling finances and other outside matters. Mother was responsible for care of household and children. Gender roles

have changed, influenced by acculturation, education, and socioeconomic status, which mitigate the Islamic influences of male superiority and paternal hierarchy. Many women immigrants, encouraged by equitable family laws abroad, acculturate faster than do male Iranians, who tend to remain traditional in their family relationships. However, men may acculturate faster in arenas such as competitive business ventures. Intrafamily stress still occurs when immigrant men realize they have less power in U.S., particularly if they lost social status as a result of relocating.

- **Changing roles among generations in U.S.** Family hierarchy may change according to speed with which family members acculturate, learn English, and secure meaningful employment. Children adjust and acquire English skills faster and easier than their parents do, which increases children's power in family affairs. Elderly parents find themselves dependent on their adult children or grandchildren. The new structure is stressful for all parties as the lines of authority become more ambiguous.

- **Caring roles.** Family members play an important role in caring for and supporting the patient, and may be expected to serve as care providers. While traditional patriarchal ideology characterizes women as direct care providers and men as protectors and controllers, clinicians should not generalize. Men have proved they can assume the role of care provider with extreme finesse and attention.

- **Expectations of and for children.** Families expect children to be clean, well-behaved, and serious students. Parents are willing to sacrifice for their children's welfare, particularly for their education. Iranians rarely use boarding schools. The defining term is family interdependence—mutual dependence, respect, and responsibility. Even if a child interprets for the family, it still expects him/her to behave respectfully.

- **Expectations of and for elders.** Aging denotes experience and knowledge. Iranians respect and care for most elderly, regardless of kinship. Rarely use nursing homes.

- **Expectations of hospital visitors.** Allow family members and other visitors to stay for extended periods. To control number of visitors, clinician should work with family spokesperson and look for cues from patient. Family members can be an asset in patient care and education if clinician approaches and instructs them. Social interaction with visitors helps patient recover. Clinician should not under- or overestimate the power of family in spiritual healing. If possible, patient should have private room to allow for better crowd control. Family members generally accept visiting limitations if they are medically necessary and part of hospital policy.

ILLNESS BELIEFS

- **Causes of/attitudes about physical illness**. Discuss and challenge illness. Solicit remedies and advice. View body in terms of its relationship to society, God, nutrition, family, and other factors. When someone feels discomforting symptoms, Iranians first inquire if the individual ate something that did not agree with his/her humoral temperament (*mezaj*). If answer is no, they do not investigate further. Accept both Western biomedical diagnoses and their own cultural illness categories.

- **Causes of/attitudes about mental illness**. Somewhat stigmatized. Iranians may present with somatic symptoms when they are under emotional stress. Consider psychopharmacology to be more effective than psychotherapy; however, more-acculturated immigrants are becoming more comfortable with psychotherapy. May use their body as a metaphor to express depression, fear, sadness, isolation, and other mental health issues. Clinician should assess patient for degree of somatization.
- **Causes of genetic defects**. View defects both scientifically and as God's will, depending on family beliefs. Some care for the affected child at home and others institutionalize, depending on the severity of the defect, the degree of support, and family's sense of social shame.
- **Attitudes about disabilities**. God's will and an act of nature. Iranians do not discriminate against persons with disabilities. Iran-Iraq War was an awakening for the population; it created many physically and psychologically disabled veterans. Parents, siblings, or other family members may care for the disabled person. May institutionalize persons who have a severe mental or physical disability.
- **Sick role**. Expect patients to be passive. Protect them from bad news; may not inform them at all or only gradually. Everyone treats and cares for patient. Sick persons may receive care at home if intensity and level of care are not too acute. Never lose hope. Among immigrant Iranians, a sense of personal responsibility for health is emerging.
- **Home and folk remedies**. Iranians always look for an herbal and humoral cure while simultaneously visiting a physician. Solicit advice and treatment regimens from others (e.g., mint tea for intestinal distress). Western medicine complements home remedies and traditional cures.
- **Medications**. Mostly take Western medications as prescribed. Use folk and herbal remedies in conjunction with such medications. High cost of medications may limit their use.
- **Acceptance of procedures**. Iranians respect education and authority figures, including most health care professionals. Patients generally accept clinicians' suggestions for procedures, including surgery, blood transfusions, and organ transplants, if these are explained well. Gender, race, or religion of donor are not limiting factors in blood or organ donations.
- **Care-seeking**. Iranians may initially seek home remedies, including humoral remedies and/or herbal medicine. Prefer Western medicine but use it along with alternative treatments. Economic status and access to care are determining factors.

HEALTH ISSUES

- **Concept of health**. Health is harmony of the mind and soul, a state that depends on the interplay and balance of factors both within one's control and beyond it. This is a strongly holistic view. Health is a diffuse, deeply rooted, cultural concept. Health and maintaining it are continuous daily concerns that Iranians deal with mainly on the subconscious level. For example, balancing one's intake of "hot" and "cold" foods is a daily consideration, although it is not articulated daily.
- **Health promotion and prevention**. Preventive medicine is not a foreign concept to Iranians because they practice humoral medicine. In both Western and Iranian health promotion, they give careful consideration to the choice, combination, and preparation of foods and their compatibility with a person's temperament. Also emphasize physical activity and adequate rest.
- **Screening**. Screening not practiced in Iran. May be a foreign concept to new immigrants and the elderly. If Iranians are educated about screening, accept it for chronic conditions. More receptive to screening if health care professionals respect their modesty and privacy, and if practitioner is of same gender.
- **Common health problems**. Cardiovascular disease, hypertension, arthritis, gastrointestinal disorders, and cancer. Thalassemia not uncommon in some regions of Iran. Among immigrants, adjustment disorders and mental health issues may arise, especially if they are related to immigration concerns, social support/isolation, and financial instability.

DEATH RITUALS

- **Beliefs and attitudes about death**. View death as a form of beginning, not an end, in which mortal life gives way to spiritual existence, a cherished state that solidifies one's relationship with God. Iranians assess family and individual beliefs before death approaches. If medical care becomes futile, clinician should discuss do-not-resuscitate options. In general, not very difficult for Iranians to reach a do-not-resuscitate decision.
- **Preparation**. Clinician should tell family spokesperson about impending death so family and friends can be notified. All family and friends typically gather to provide support and assistance. Sometimes family needs more preparation time if local mortuaries are not sufficiently familiar with Muslim customs.
- **Home vs. hospital**. Prefer hospitalization in cases of acute illness requiring lots of care. In cases of chronic ailments, family may opt to provide care at home. Families may be receptive to hospice care.
- **Special needs**. Families prefer to gather in larger numbers at home and in fewer numbers at hospital when death occurs. Praying or crying softly at bedside common. Family members control noise level among themselves so patient can be peaceful. Health care providers should allow family to visit the body; some may decline.

- **Care of the body**. Family may wish to prepare body in ritual manner—wash it with soap and water, close orifices, pack orifices with cotton—if a properly trained person is unavailable. Family preparation of body in hospital or funeral home is less necessary than in the past because now there are more persons who have been trained to perform the washing ritual. Iranians "let go" more easily than do people in dominant culture but grieve more publicly and longer. Do not view body after it is washed. Do not practice embalming or cremation.
- **Attitudes about organ donation**. Socially and culturally acceptable. Organ donation practiced in Iran.
- **Attitudes about autopsy**. No specific rules, but body must be respected. Most families accept autopsy if the need for it is fully explained and if it is medically necessary to identify cause of death.

SELECTED REFERENCES

Bozorgmehr, M. (1997). Internal ethnicity: Iranians in Los Angeles. *Sociological Perspectives*, 40, 387–409.

Daneshpour, M. (1998). Muslim families and family therapy. *Journal of Marital and Family Therapy*, 24, 355–368.

Darvishpour, M. (2002). Immigrant women challenge the role of men: How the changing power relationship within Iranian families in Sweden intensifies family conflicts after immigration. *Journal of Comparative Family Studies*, 33, 271–296.

Emami, A., Benner, P., & Ekman, S. L. (2001). A sociocultural health model for late-in-life immigrants. *Journal of Transcultural Nursing*, 12, 15–24.

Emami, A., Benner, P. E., Lipson, J. G., & Ekman, S. L. (2000). Health as continuity and balance in life. *Western Journal of Nursing Research*, 22, 812–825.

Ghaffarian, S. (1998). The acculturation of Iranian immigrants in the United States and the implications for mental health. *Journal of Social Psychology*, 138, 645–654.

Hojat, M., Shapurian, R., Foroughi, D., Nayerahmadi, H., Farzaneh, M., Shafieyan, M., et al. (2000). Gender differences in traditional attitudes toward marriage and the family: An empirical study of Iranian immigrants in the United States. *Journal of Family Issues*, 21, 419–434.

Hojat, M., Shapurian, R., Nayerahmadi, H., Farzaneh, M., Foroughi, D., Parsi, M., et al. (1999). Premarital sexual, child rearing, and family attitudes of Iranian men and women in the United States and in Iran. *Journal of Psychology*, 133, 19–31.

Moghissi, H. (1999). Away from home: Iranian women, displacement cultural resistance, and change. *Journal of Comparative Family Studies*, 30, 207–217.

AUTHOR

Homeyra Hafizi, RN, MS, LHRM, immigrated to the United States from Iran at the age of 16. She graduated from the University of California-San Francisco

School of Nursing in 1991 and currently serves as adjunct faculty at Brevard Community College in Florida. She is a licensed health-care risk manager and an occupational health nursing specialist/consultant at Dynamac Corp.

ACKNOWLEDGMENT

I offer my gratitude to my dear friend, Maryam Sayyedi, PhD, for her extensive assistance in reviewing and updating this content. I also thank her for her graceful responses to the barrage of e-mails I generated from my residence in Florida to hers in California.

CHAPTER 21

IRISH

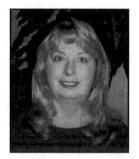

Fonda K. Barnard

CULTURAL/ETHNIC IDENTITY

- **Preferred term(s)**. Irish or Irish American.
- **Census**. According to the 2000 U.S. Census, more than 33 million people reported Irish ancestry and an additional 5 million reported Scottish-Irish ancestry; 165,440 were foreign-born. Undocumented persons are likely to avoid the Census, so numbers may be significantly understated.
- **History of immigration**. In the 1700s, the first wave of predominantly Presbyterian Scots-Irish emigrated from the north of Ireland to seek opportunities in the New World. These settlers generally were self-sufficient and financially secure; some were indentured servants. The second wave included Catholics from southern Ireland who emigrated as a result of the Great Potato Famine of the 1840s. These immigrants were poor, desperate, and left their country reluctantly. There was a steady stream of Irish immigrants from 1846 to 1985, more than half of whom were women. Many decided to emigrate during "The Troubles," a period of violent conflict in Northern Ireland beginning in the late 1960s that culminated in the political resolution known as the 1998 Good Friday Agreement. Computer technology and the electronics industry fueled Ireland's economic recovery in the mid-1980s; opportunities in Europe also became available. The 1990s, the era of the so-called "Celtic Tiger," saw the return of numerous Irish Americans to their homeland, although many remain in the U.S., with the largest populations in California, New York, Pennsylvania, Florida, and Illinois.

SPIRITUAL/RELIGIOUS ORIENTATION

- **Primary religious/spiritual affiliations**. Protestant and Catholic.
- **Usual religious/spiritual practices**. The Irish Catholic and Protestant

churches, as well as the spirituality of Celtic Paganism, have served as sources of community and individual comfort and strength. Practices vary, depending on tradition and the religiousness of individuals. Irish Americans consider prayer to be a private matter. Catholics may attend mass daily; some carry rosary beads and wear religious medals as protection from sickness.

- **Use of spiritual healing/healers**. Many spiritual healing customs are derived from Catholic practices. In the event of a serious illness or imminent death of a Catholic, a priest may perform the sacrament of the sick. Priests offer oils, prayers, and blessings during healing rituals.
- **Holidays**. Most holidays are religious. The two major holiday seasons are Christmas and Easter. Among Catholics, Christmas is preceded by a four-week period of preparation called Advent. A Christmas tradition is placing a candle in the window of the home to welcome Mary and Joseph, who are searching for shelter. Sometimes the youngest member of the household lights the candle and a girl in the family named Mary extinguishes it. A heavily laden table traditionally includes a loaf of caraway-seed and raisin bread, and a pitcher of milk to welcome travelers. A ring of holly may adorn the front door. Easter celebrates the resurrection of Christ; among Catholics, it is preceded by the season of Lent, a six-week period of special prayers and some types of fasting (e.g., not eating meat). St. Patrick's Day (March 17) celebrates Ireland's patron saint, who is credited with bringing Christianity to the island. Celebrants wear green clothing or shamrocks, drink green beer or ale, and eat corned beef and cabbage. Many Irish Americans participate in commemorative parades in the U.S. Americans who are not overtly Irish also celebrate this popular holiday. The Irish also have a female patron saint, St. Brigid, who founded the first convent in Ireland. February 1, the day she died, is a feast day in Ireland; reeds are fashioned into St. Brigid's crosses.

COMMUNICATION
ORAL COMMUNICATION

- **Major languages and dialects**. The national language is Irish, also called Erse or Irish Gaelic. Irish was not written in the Latin alphabet until the 5th century, when the language was introduced into Ireland as Christianity spread. About 5,000 elderly persons residing in the U.S. remain fluent in Irish. There are efforts to revive the language to maintain respect for Irish culture and history. English is the first language of most Irish Americans. It is unlikely that any of today's Irish immigrants do not speak English.
- **Greetings**. Friendly and informal. Younger Irish Americans are comfortable being greeted by their first name. To show respect, an elder should be addressed as "Mr." or "Mrs."/"Miss" followed by surname.
- **Tone of voice**. Health care providers should use a friendly and calm tone when speaking to patients. Although the Irish can be vocally passionate when discussing topics of moral or political importance, the proper tone of

voice in ordinary conversation is controlled and relaxed. May interpret loud vocal intonations as hostile.

- **Direct or indirect style of speech**. May enjoy playing with language and using many words; can be very indirect when communicating. Because they traditionally are very private and do not divulge their thoughts and feelings, Irish tend to speak in euphemisms and metaphors. The English use the expression "speaking Irish" to refer to someone's ability to talk all around a subject and avoid saying anything at all. Clinician may need to ask several direct questions to clarify an indirect response; some patients avoid saying "no," instead saying "perhaps" or "I will let you know."
- **Use of interpreters**. In the rare event of a language barrier (e.g., when the patient is an elderly, Irish-speaking immigrant from western Ireland), a son or daughter may be able to help explain the medical condition and treatment, and to elicit important information.
- **Serious or terminal illness**. A patient who is informed of the prognosis will confide in a close family member, such as a sibling, son, or daughter, if the patient is able to confide in anyone at all. When communicating information about a patient's medical condition, the clinician should consider asking a sibling, son, or daughter to be present. Seriously or terminally ill Irish often are stoic; they do not like to talk about their illness or how they feel. An Irish Catholic's priest might provide helpful support during this time.

WRITTEN COMMUNICATION

- **Literacy assessment**. Adult literacy rate in Ireland is 98%, so most Irish Americans have a reasonable ability to read and write. A patient who has difficulty may not reveal it willingly because of privacy, independence, and perhaps embarrassment and shame. Clinician should observe a patient's skills and ask questions to assess his/her reading and writing proficiency.
- **Consents**. Make their own decisions about health care but may need the support of close family members when weighing medical options. Because the patient may not be expressive or explicit about treatment preferences, particularly in cases of serious illness, the clinician may need to encourage the patient to verbalize his/her wishes about intensity of care, especially regarding a living will, do-not-resuscitate orders, or other treatment preferences.

NONVERBAL COMMUNICATION

- **Eye contact**. Direct eye contact can communicate honesty and sincerity, but in certain cases the Irish may interpret it as hostility. May perceive someone who diverts his/her eyes as shifty or untrustworthy. May avoid eye contact in order to hide strong emotions, so clinician may need to ask patient to clarify his/her feelings.
- **Personal space**. Conversational distance is greater than that between other Northern European Americans. The Irish are uncomfortable when their per-

sonal space is entered and may back away to preserve distance.

- **Use and meaning of silence**. Comfortable with silence, which allows them to conceal uncomfortable feelings.
- **Gestures**. Use few gestures; there is little body movement while speaking. Therefore, clinician must closely observe cues from facial expressions.
- **Openness in expressing emotions**. Tend to conceal their true feelings. Avoid expressing emotions and affection in public, which would embarrass them and their family.
- **Privacy**. Irish culture places high value on preserving privacy. To protect itself from ridicule, family does not talk about a family member's failure.
- **Touch**. The Irish are not very tactile when communicating with family and friends. When meeting or greeting, a handshake is appropriate. Hugging is less common, even between close family members. Such touch would be embarrassing and uncomfortable for many.
- **Orientation to time**. Some Irish are not likely to adhere to a schedule; may perceive time as flexible. Orientation to past is evident in their strong sense of history, tradition, and allegiance to ancestors. Also present-oriented. Future orientation reflected in strong work ethic, saving money, and investing in education.

ACTIVITIES OF DAILY LIVING

- **Modesty**. Both men and women highly modest. Caregivers should avoid exposing patient's body unnecessarily. Irish do not speak freely about sex and other sensitive subjects, which they find embarrassing.
- **Skin care**. Americans of Irish descent usually have a fair and pale complexion, so they should avoid prolonged sun exposure. Skin care should include sun screen and moisturizer. The Irish may not spend much time on skin care.
- **Hair care**. Hair is typically straight. The Irish traditionally place little emphasis on hair care. Women may wear their hair pulled back in a clasp. Second- and third-generation Irish Americans are more likely to emphasize and style their hair according to current fashion.
- **Nail care**. Spend little time on appearance or anything that would draw attention to themselves. May view time-consuming nail care as frivolous and wasteful. Younger Irish Americans more frequently get manicures and pedicures.
- **Toileting**. Observe great privacy in toileting. Health care providers should respect privacy needs.
- **Special clothing or amulets**. In ancient Ireland, common attire included a shirt (*leine*), trousers (*trews*), and a long cloak fastened with a brooch. Today, the Irish wear black clothing to and following funerals to express grief. Alternatively, they may wear a black armband. Catholics may carry rosary beads or wear a crucifix or medal of a saint on a necklace. A scapular is a type of necklace that hangs down both in front and in back, with a small, flat, rectangular pendant of cloth at each end. An older Catholic may pin a scapular to his/her clothing; staff must take care not to lose it.

- **Self-care**. Patients prefer to perform activities of daily living independently. They may not ask for, and may even refuse, assistance in an effort not to be a burden on other family members.

FOOD PRACTICES

- **Usual meal pattern**. May have coffee or tea and oats for breakfast, a midday meal, and an evening meal. Some continue afternoon tea with a light sandwich or cookies and have a later evening meal.
- **Special utensils**. None.
- **Food beliefs and rituals**. Mealtime traditionally is a family occasion. May say prayers at the start of meals. Traditionally celebrate Catholic holidays with food. Catholics may give up certain foods during Lent and eat fish instead of meat on Friday. Consume lots of food and drink at wakes. On St. Patrick's Day, all Irish typically eat corned beef and cabbage.
- **Usual diet**. View bread as the "staff of life"; serve it with most meals. Soda bread and oatmeal are traditional foods. Typical meals consist of meat, potatoes, and vegetables. Although potatoes are not native to Ireland, they are a dietary staple and prepared in various ways. Other common dishes include pot pies (pastry crusts filled with meat and potatoes) and shepherd's pie, a ground-meat and mashed-potato dish.
- **Fluids**. Tea and coffee. In addition to ale, the Irish consume alcoholic beverages such as stout (dark beer with a foamy head) and whiskey. Children drink nonalcoholic beverages such as tea and soft drinks. The national minimum age for alcohol consumption in Ireland is 16 in restaurants; the minimum age for alcohol purchases is 18. These lower age limits demonstrate greater cultural acceptance of alcohol consumption by youths. Long-standing stereotypes portray the Irish as prone to excessive drinking. One recent study found that, compared to others, Irish American men in New York City have higher lifetime prevalence rates in terms of excessive alcohol intake, alcohol tolerance and/or dependence, physical or psychological problems associated with alcohol misuse, and social and/or occupational problems associated with such misuse.
- **Food taboos and prescriptions**. During Lent, the 40 days before Easter, Irish American Catholics may eliminate meat from their diet. For colds and other illnesses, the Irish may drink a "hot toddy," made with Irish whiskey, sugar, lemon, and cloves. Other traditional, common food remedies are hot tea with honey and lemon, and hot soups.
- **Hospitality**. The Irish are hospitable and friendly to strangers. They are accommodating and willing to share meals but do not insist that guests eat. Irish pubs and parties feature music and merrymaking. There is a lot of encouragement to join in the celebration by drinking and dancing.

SYMPTOM MANAGEMENT

The Irish tend to ignore their own bodily symptoms as long as possible. Clinicians must encourage patients to describe symptoms. Numerical scales for rating pain and other symptoms may help clinician assess symptom severity.

- **Pain**. View pain as something to be endured and a part of life. Patient may be stoic and reluctant to ask for pain relief or other assistance. Irish men see pain as weakness; do not complain for fear of ridicule or because they deny feelings of vulnerability. Women more frequently express feelings of pain or discomfort. The Irish may use willow-bark tea (the bark is the origin of aspirin) as a home remedy. Health care providers should carefully explain the reasons for, and benefits of, pain medication and its importance in the healing process.
- **Dyspnea**. Commonly describe dyspnea as shortness of breath or an uncomfortable awareness of breathing. Traditional home remedies include herbs such as angelica, coltsfoot, horehound, and thyme, all of which are expectorants. The Irish add licorice tincture to tea to dilate the bronchi and break up phlegm.
- **Nausea/vomiting**. May be embarrassed by nausea/vomiting. May attempt to clean up vomitus to avoid being a burden to others. Folk medicine includes ginger or peppermint tea.
- **Constipation/diarrhea**. View these as a private matter. May be embarrassed to report constipation/diarrhea symptoms or may describe them in very vague terms. May use various herbal compounds as treatments.
- **Fatigue**. Reluctant to report symptoms, even when they may indicate a more serious illness. Want to remain independent and not burden others. May use stimulants such as tea or coffee to counteract fatigue in the morning and afternoon.
- **Depression**. The Irish may have little understanding of mental illness. Men are more likely than women to view depression as a sign of weakness and to feel shameful or embarrassed about reporting symptoms. Ireland has a comparatively high suicide rate; more than three-fourths of suicides occur among men. The stigma surrounding depression prevents discussing symptoms. Denial may interfere with a patient's acceptance of counseling and treatment for depression.
- **Self-care symptom management**. May neglect symptoms or choose to use home remedies. Need a goal-oriented approach to treatment. May participate in self-care if clinician offers encouragement and reinforcement.

BIRTH RITUALS/CARE OF THE NEW MOTHER AND BABY

- **Pregnancy care**. Use regular prenatal care and abide by physician recommendations during pregnancy. Second- and third-generation Irish and acculturated immigrants may take childbirth preparation classes. Expect women to eat a well-balanced diet during pregnancy and after birth to ensure baby is healthy. Traditional pregnancy taboos include avoiding hares or rabbits out of fear that the unborn child will develop a harelip, and not entering cemeteries, as a woman may turn her ankle and bear a child with clubfoot. According to traditional beliefs, a child born at night can see ghosts and fairies, one born after the death of his/her father has special powers, and a birth on Sunday is unlucky. Some Irish have used charms, such as holy water and devices, to prevent fairies from stealing babies.

- **Preferences for children**. Birth rate is higher among Catholic Irish Americans than it is among many other immigrant groups, probably due to teachings of the Catholic Church and a preference for larger families. However, the Irish accept and respect persons who are unmarried and childless. Many women choose not to have children. In 2003, the birth rate in Ireland (1.89) was lower than that in U.S. (2.07). Traditionally, the Irish had large families; their true desire was to have healthy male and female children. Having a boy (preferably as the first-born) is important to parents so he can carry on the family name. Younger Irish Americans do not have large families, but they still desire healthy children and a first-born male.

- **Labor practices**. Women respect medical authorities and prefer to deliver in modern medical facilities. Second- and third-generation Irish and acculturated immigrants are receptive to childbirth preparation techniques and alternative home-birthing practices.

- **Role of the laboring woman during birth**. During labor and birth, she may be reluctant to express pain or may feel ashamed of, or embarrassed about, her utterances during contractions. May want lots of privacy and to avoid exposing her body. Generally trusts physician and accepts his/her directions.

- **Role of the father and other family members during birth**. Women traditionally prefer to labor and deliver in private, with few or no other family members present. A second- or third-generation Irish American woman may want the father to be an active participant in labor and birth.

- **Vaginal vs. cesarean section**. Generally accept the physician's recommendation without question. A nurse or midwife should explain the risks of both options.

- **Breastfeeding**. Increasingly, Irish American women are encouraged to breastfeed instead of bottle-feed. Breastfeeding typically is of short duration after birth. Because many Irish women receive little assistance from members of their extended family, they need extra support and instruction from health care providers.

- **Birth recuperation**. Traditionally, the new mother's mother or aunt helped care for first-born. However, the recuperation period was short; that way, the new mother could learn how to integrate the infant into her daily responsibilities. After the birth of additional children, she had very little recuperation time, given her need to care for family. Irish expected older children to help care for new baby or younger children. Today, recuperation for some first-time mothers is difficult in the context of short hospital stays because they go home with little or no support from members of their extended family. Clinician should focus his/her efforts on helping the new mother arrange adequate support after she returns home.

- **Baby care**. If mother and father care for the baby with little help from members of the extended family, clinicians should instruct new parents on proper care of newborn. Irish American parents are receptive to day care or babysitters when they must work outside the home.

- **Problems with baby**. If a problem develops in the hospital, clinician should inform both parents in a timely manner and privately, away from family and friends. Should use neutral language, as the Irish tend to have a strong sense of responsibility and may blame themselves. Also should give new mothers instructions and telephone numbers to call for support and assistance.
- **Male and female circumcision**. Males customarily circumcised after birth in hospital. Females never circumcised.

DEVELOPMENTAL AND SEXUAL ISSUES

- **Celebration of menarche or becoming a man**. No special acknowledgment of puberty in girls or boys. Onset of menarche is a private issue and seldom discussed. After special teachings, Catholic girls and boys coming into adulthood undergo a confirmation ceremony when they are 8–15 years old. A bishop or priest administers the sacrament of confirmation, which confirms the faith one received as an infant at baptism.
- **Attitudes about birth control**. Irish culture considers men to have a stronger sexual drive than women do, and to have less control over urges. Therefore, women are expected to bear the burden of, and responsibility for, abstinence or pregnancy prevention. Catholics adhered to traditional teachings until the Second Vatican Council in the 1960s, when the Catholic Church changed some of its practices. Since then, many Catholics in the U.S. have questioned the infallibility of the church position on birth control and have become more amenable to using it.
- **Attitudes about sexually transmitted infection (STI) control, including condoms**. Contracting an STI causes guilt and brings shame to the family. Despite modesty about private issues such as this, the Irish are receptive to using condoms for preventing infections and pregnancy.
- **Attitudes about abortion**. The Irish are divided regarding this issue. Although the Catholic Church opposes abortion, many believe in more latitude since the Second Vatican Council in the 1960s. Protestants commonly do not oppose abortion. Currently in Ireland, one must travel to another country to obtain an abortion.
- **Attitudes about unwed sexual experimentation**. Catholic Church prohibits sexual activity by single persons, but since the Second Vatican Council, unwed sexual experimentation has become acceptable to many Irish. It is common but typically not condoned. The Irish still frown upon unwed pregnancy; it brings shame to the family.
- **Sexual orientation**. Traditionally condone only male-female relationships, which Catholic teachings reinforce. Gay or lesbian orientation could bring shame or embarrassment to the family. Recently, same-sex relationships have

become more acceptable among younger Irish Americans.

- **Gender identity**. Little tolerance for, or acceptance of, ambiguous or opposite-gender identity. Those with strong Catholic beliefs do not support alternative gender identity. Family members' feelings of guilt and embarrassment may discourage an individual's openness. Younger or acculturated Irish Americans may be more receptive to gender-reassignment surgery and accept differences in gender identity.

- **Attitudes about menopause**. Irish women view the last decades of their lives as a time of decline, and menopause as a consequence of aging. They do not openly discuss this private bodily function. Clinicians should question women of menopausal age about symptoms and discuss potential treatments.

FAMILY RELATIONSHIPS

- **Composition/structure**. Families are mostly nuclear. The Irish have a strong sense of obligation to members of extended family even when they are not emotionally or geographically close. For example, individuals may attend holiday get-togethers and family celebrations out of a sense of duty and respect, and immigrants in U.S. may provide financial help to relatives in Ireland. Although the Irish are known for being clannish and having strong family ties, relationships may not be close. Ties are closest between mothers and sons and between siblings of the same gender, while mothers and daughters may have stormier relationships. Family roles may be hierarchical and discreet (e.g., strongly patriarchal) but may include a family matriarch (e.g., a grandmother or older maiden aunt who is the female head of the family).

- **Decision-making**. In the past, the male head of the family made decisions, but recently women have begun to play a more prominent role. Consultation with, or permission from, a matriarch may be necessary for health care or treatment decisions. Clinician should ask discreetly who makes decisions in the family.

- **Spokesperson**. Varies among families; could be father, matriarch, or sibling. Among more-acculturated Irish Americans, an adult child may serve as spokesperson.

- **Gender issues**. Two different patterns: (1) husband dominates wife and children, whom he expects to respect, serve, and help him in his work (also expects wife to be responsible for the children and house); and (2) wife dominates husband and sons, who have been dependent upon her. Immigrant Irish women became more dominant when men had to take labor-intensive, menial jobs that frequently kept them away from home; women helped support the family. Traditionally, there is a lack of intimacy between spouses, with sexual relations based on duty to husband or responsibility to procreate. Catholic teachings may underlie these attitudes. However, due to acculturation, most Irish American men and women accept greater equity between genders.

- **Changing roles among generations in U.S.** Irish Catholics in U.S. faced significant discrimination before World War I. The wages they earned from menial jobs were very low. Both world wars encouraged assimilation as men fought for, and proved their loyalty to, the U.S. Subsequently, Irish nationalism began to disappear. Irish men returning from World War II took advantage of the G.I. Bill to become better educated; they entered skilled-labor, white-collar, or professional fields. Women extended their family-caregiver roles to become nurses and teachers. As a result of education, acculturation, and participation by women in the work force, gender roles have become more blurred and equitable.

- **Caring roles**. Women are family caretakers. Irish mothers raise the children and keep the family together. Daughters or daughters-in-law take care of ill family members and willingly attend caregiver support groups.
- **Expectations of and for children**. Raise children to be independent, self-reliant, and self-disciplined. Expect them to respect and obey their parents and elders, and to be loyal to the family. In the past, the Irish expected children to marry within their religion and ethnic group, but there is considerable intermarriage now. Believe that children should be educated so they will have good occupations/professions and achieve economic respectability.
- **Expectations of and for elders**. Respect elders and seek their advice and help with decisions. Mothers are held in high esteem because they made sacrifices in raising their children. Acculturated Irish have endured a breakdown of the extended family. Elderly parents may feel isolated and may lack support from family members.
- **Expectations of hospital visitors**. Family members may visit dutifully— i.e., make an appearance to show respect and concern, then depart. Only a sibling, daughter, or son generally remains at the bedside.

ILLNESS BELIEFS

- **Causes of/attitudes about physical illness**. Believe that human fate involves suffering, which one bears as a natural consequence of living. In the past, the Irish viewed physical illness as God's will (beyond individual control) or they attributed it to sin or guilt. Today, older Irish Americans still view sickness as God's will, while younger persons attribute it to natural causes.
- **Causes of/attitudes about mental illness**. Many in Ireland know little about mental illness, which is stigmatized. Mentally ill persons face discrimination but generally are not blamed for their affliction, although those who have a drinking problem, drug addiction, or eating disorder may be faulted. Family may prefer to care for patient at home. Willingly accept physician recommendations regarding hospitalization and treatment.
- **Causes of genetic defects**. Attribute them to God's will. Affected person receives compassionate care from family, which views the burden as God-given. Persons with Irish, Scottish, or British heritage have a high risk of carrying the gene mutation for hemochromatosis (excess iron absorption).

About 1 in 50 Irish Americans carries the gene for Tay-Sachs, an inherited, neurodegenerative disease.

- **Attitudes about disabilities**. The Irish value independence and have high regard for those who attempt to overcome adversity. Although individuals do not want to be a burden on others, they are compassionate toward disabled persons. Disability is not stigmatized. Family is willing to care for a disabled family member at home. Clinicians can assist families by referring disabled persons to programs that encourage personal development and independence.
- **Sick role**. Typically stoic; do not complain about illness. Attempt to maintain independence and perform self-care as long as possible. May feel embarrassed, guilty, or ashamed about being a burden to other family members. Family excuses a sick member from obligations and provides care until he/she can function again.
- **Home and folk remedies**. May try these before seeking medical care. Numerous folk remedies have given way to biomedicine and medications synthesized from herbs. The Irish chew foxglove leaves (digitalis) for chest pain, and use garlic (*gairleog*) as an antiseptic and to help clear fatty substances (perhaps cholesterol) from the blood. Salad containing garlic is said to protect against the common cold. The Irish boil nettles like spinach, serve them as porridge, and use them in tea to purify the blood and provide iron and stimulants. They use Irish spurge, a plant, to treat warts and corns, and comfrey in a plaster to set bones and as an ointment for psoriasis and wounds. The Irish have used dandelion to treat liver complaints and to stimulate the release of bile from the gallbladder. They have used dandelion leaves as a tonic, blood purifier, and treatment for eczema, warts, and corns. Wild valerian is useful for nervous disorders and migraines.
- **Medications**. Medication compliance is better among Irish American women than it is among men. Women respect medical authority, while men do not want to be perceived as weak.
- **Acceptance of procedures**. Slow to seek medical care but regard physicians as authority figures. Likely to accept procedures that physicians recommend. No cultural or religious taboos against blood transfusions, surgery, or organ transplants.
- **Care-seeking**. May first seek family advice regarding home remedies. Tend to ignore symptoms as long as possible before seeking care. Men may view illness as a sign of weakness; may minimize symptoms and be reluctant to complain about health problems, suffering in silence until illness becomes more serious. Women are more willing to seek medical care.

HEALTH ISSUES

- **Concept of health**. The ability to function independently. Place great emphasis on independence and privacy in health matters.
- **Health promotion and prevention**. Men more often than women are slow

to seek assistance for health problems, but both genders follow clinician recommendations. To prevent illness, the Irish eat a balanced diet; take vitamins; get sufficient rest, fresh air, sunshine, and exercise; maintain their religious faith and a strong, loving family; and focus on goals. Folk prevention practices include wearing religious medals, wearing a bag of herbs around the neck during flu season, and keeping closet doors closed to prevent evil spirits from entering the body.

- **Screening**. Women obtain regular screening. Men are receptive to screening if a physician recommends it.
- **Common health problems**. Irish men have a high rate of premature death, likely due to risky behaviors such as heavy drinking and smoking. Lack of early screening for prostate and testicular cancer may be problematic. Immigrants may have more mental illness than second- and third-generation Irish Americans do, including schizophrenia, depression, and suicide, possibly related to heavy drinking, an inability or unwillingness to express feelings, or a fatalistic world view of humans as subject to the harshness of nature.

DEATH RITUALS

- **Beliefs and attitudes about death**. The Irish view death as inevitable, a result of God's will. Also may greet it with Celtic denial and humorous ridicule. Catholics believe that when someone dies, the soul leaves the body and goes to heaven, purgatory, or hell. After death and subsequent preparation of the body, women "keen," a wailing lamentation. By tradition, keening should not take place until the body has been prepared. After this lamentation, mourning should cease and the wake should begin. The wake is a celebration of the deceased person's life, during which participants tell humorous stories about him/her and may consume large amounts of food and alcohol. Wakes can last for days and feature music, dancing, and merriment. A traditional belief is that excessive mourning is not good for the dead.
- **Preparation**. The devoutly Catholic prepare spiritually for death. Family members should be informed of impending death so they can stay with the dying person and be present for the funeral. When death is imminent, a priest is summoned to perform sacrament of the sick.
- **Home vs. hospital**. May prefer to die at home but do not want to be a burden. May stay at home as long as possible and then go to the hospital to avoid burdening family members. Today, the Irish are more commonly amenable to hospice to assist with pain control and other terminal care.
- **Special needs**. Near death, the family needs ample space to remain at the patient's bedside. Catholic patients may request a priest to visit and offer prayers. Privacy from other patients and staff is desirable for mourning and keening (wailing by female mourners).
- **Care of the body**. Treat body with respect and modesty. Dress it in semiformal attire or, occasionally, in a sleeping gown for a woman. Traditionally, the

body was wrapped in a white garment and laid on a table or bed for viewing. Family members and friends attend the wake out of respect for the deceased. Today, Irish Americans observe modern funeral practices; body is taken to a mortuary where it is prepared and embalmed for the wake. Cremation is by individual choice.

- **Attitudes about organ donation**. Support donation of organs to those in need. Ireland has one of the highest rates of organ donation in the world.
- **Attitudes about autopsy**. Consider the body to be like an empty shell after death. Do not oppose autopsy if it is necessary.

SELECTED REFERENCES

Beaumont Hospital. The National Organ Procurement Service. Retrieved September 4, 2004, from http://www.beaumont.ie/depts/support/transplant/organ_procurement.html

Friend, P. All about Irish. Retrieved September 4, 2004, from http://allabout irish.com

Haggerty, R., & Haggerty, B. Irish culture and customs. Retrieved December 12, 2004, from http://www.irelandnet.com/culture_history.html

Johnson, P. B. (1997). Alcohol-use-related problems in Puerto Rican and Irish-American males. *Substance Use and Misuse, 32,* 169–179.

Klenk, E. (2000). Common genetic disorders in the United States. Retrieved December 12, 2004, from http://journalofscience.wlu.edu/archive/Spring2000/GeneticDisorders.html

McCaffrey, L. J. (1976). *The Irish diaspora in America.* London and Bloomington, IN: Indiana University Press.

McGoldrick, M. (1996). Irish families. In M. McGoldrick, J. Giordano, & J. K. Pearce (Eds.), *Ethnicity and family therapy* (2nd ed.) (pp. 544–566). New York: Guilford Press.

MedMedia. Irish attitudes to mental illness. Retrieved September 4, 2004, from http://irishhealth.com

AUTHOR

Fonda K. Barnard, BBA, RN, has a nursing degree from Kaskaskia College in Centralia, IL, and a bachelor's degree in business administration from the University of South Florida-Tampa. She is pursuing a master's degree in health sciences, with a concentration on health services administration, at Florida Gulf Coast University in Fort Myers. Her heritage is Irish Protestant, English, and German.

ACKNOWLEDGMENT

Thanks to Linda Garratt Slezak, RN, MS, for reviewing and commenting on this chapter.

CHAPTER 22

ITALIANS

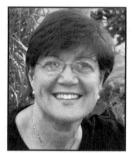
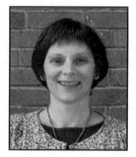
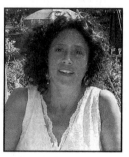

| Cynthia Ruocco Miceli | Karen Lucas Breda | Maria Esposito Frank |

CULTURAL/ETHNIC IDENTITY

Italian Americans constitute a rather heterogeneous group. Their beliefs and practices are influenced by age, region of origin, education, socioeconomic status, place of residence, and year of immigration. Due to the long history of immigration from Italy, Italian American beliefs and practices in the U.S. vary considerably.

- **Preferred term(s)**. Italian or Italian American.
- **Census**. In the 2000 U.S. Census, more than 15.7 million people identified their ancestry as Italian. Most immigrants live in the northeastern U.S.
- **History of immigration**. There have been three distinct waves of Italian immigration. The first wave (1880–1920) comprised mostly immigrants from southern Italy. They came by the millions looking for work. By the time the second wave arrived (after World War I), Americans had become suspicious of foreigners. This sentiment led to passage of the National Origins Act of 1920, which imposed quotas on visas for southern Europeans and severely limited the number of Italians allowed to enter the U.S. The Hart-Celler Act of 1965 abolished national-origin quotas and fostered a third, albeit smaller, wave of immigration. Since then, many Italian professionals have come to the U.S. seeking job and career advancement.

SPIRITUAL/RELIGIOUS ORIENTATION

- **Primary religious/spiritual affiliations**. Most are Roman Catholic. Some are Jewish, Pentecostal, or have other religious affiliations. Although church attendance has declined, Catholicism remains a strong influence for many older Italians. Pray to God, Christ, and many saints who are patrons of various life events and protectors against illness and other adversities. Believe that God is both a benevolent being who bestows favors and a severe judge who punishes.

- **Usual religious/spiritual practices**. Catholics honor Christ's death and resurrection at church masses on Saturday evening, Sunday morning, and during religious holidays; some churches have daily masses. Catholics observe seven sacraments: baptism, communion, reconciliation, confirmation, marriage, holy orders, and illness. Older Italians may carry and use rosary beads to pray for the dead as well as ill family members and friends. Especially devout Italians pray to patron saint of their home town.

- **Use of spiritual healing/healers**. Family usually contacts Catholic priest when someone is very ill so he/she can confess sins and receive sacrament of the sick, which provides spiritual strength for healing or death. During this sacrament, sick person is anointed and given a blessing and small wafer, or eucharist. Health care providers should facilitate privacy and inform priest if ill person has difficulty swallowing. While spiritual healers are less common than in the past, older Italian Americans may seek one to alleviate physical or emotional distress. They also may combine customary religious practices and magical beliefs. Catholic patron saints have healing powers. For example, Santa Lucia, whose feast day is December 13, is patron saint of the blind.

- **Holidays**. Immigrants have stopped celebrating many Italian national holidays. In U.S., Columbus Day (October 11) is a major national holiday attributed to an Italian. Religious holidays remain a central focus of Italian American life. Observe seasonal holidays, such as Advent (Christmas season), Lent (Easter season), and feast days of the saints, Christ, and Mary (*la Madonna*), during religious, cultural, and family events. Honor Italian patron saints in special ways. Some children are named for a patron saint associated with their day of birth. Some older Italian Americans and more recent immigrants celebrate their name day (*onomastico*) in recognition of the patron saint.

COMMUNICATION
ORAL COMMUNICATION

- **Major languages and dialects**. Italian. Numerous regional dialects. Other languages still spoken in Italy include French and Provençal (northwest peninsula), German (Alto Adige region), three varieties of Ladino (Swiss border, northeastern Dolomites, Friuli), Slovene (Alpi Giulie), and Albanian (small southern towns, Sicily). An archaic form of Greek survives in some areas of Salento and Calabria. Residents of three towns in Molise region speak Serbo-Croatian. On island of Sardinia, people speak two varieties of Sardinian, also Catalan. In U.S., numerous Italian dialects and Americanized derivations of dialects are spoken in Italian American enclaves. Most third-generation Italian Americans are completely acculturated; may know only a few words of Italian. Some older immigrants may have limited knowledge of formal Italian.

- **Greetings**. Greet friends and relatives with a kiss on each cheek while gently shaking hands, or they embrace openly. Health care providers should extend a hand to shake. Italians are very respectful; believe that one should never disgrace the family. Health care providers can unknowingly offend someone of Italian ancestry by not showing appropriate respect during treatment. They should acknowledge elderly men and women first and address them formally using titles and surnames. Second-generation, third-generation, and young immigrants may be more inclined to use first names, but clinicians should err on the side of caution and address them formally.
- **Tone of voice**. Conversations among family members may appear to be volatile. Discussions can be passionate and loud, with several family members talking simultaneously.
- **Direct or indirect style of speech**. Some feel vulnerable in uncertain or unfamiliar situations and may need time to get acquainted. Clinician should proceed slowly and give patient a small amount of information while establishing a trusting relationship. Patient may not directly refuse; to be polite, may agree outwardly, avoid answering a question, or delegate a family member to answer. Italians rarely tell stories to strangers.
- **Use of interpreters**. Clinician should assess patient's level of education and communication skills to determine amount of information he/she needs, and use diagrams to convey information. Italians usually designate an educated family member as interpreter or family spokesperson—someone who is familiar with patient's dialect. Some family members may not reveal all relevant information, hoping to shield patient from worry, pain, and suffering.
- **Serious or terminal illness**. When clinician discloses serious illness or a bad prognosis, should reserve ample time to remain with patient. Family members expect to be included in discussions about treatment plans. However, Health Insurance Portability and Accountability Act (HIPAA) requires health care providers to consult with patient about who should receive information. Depending on patient's preference, family members may offer advice regarding when to tell patient about serious illness and who should tell him/her. Once a serious or terminal illness is diagnosed, family members may avoid further discussion to protect patient from emotional suffering. Clinician should evaluate effectiveness of family's support system and patient's adjustment to serious illness before planning treatment.

WRITTEN COMMUNICATION

- **Literacy assessment**. Literacy rate among both genders in Italy is nearly 97%. English replaced French as the preferred second language taught in Italian public schools. Immigrants' command of English depends on level of education; those with only a few years of formal education may not be able to read or write in English or Italian. Acceptable for clinician to ask directly or indirectly about literacy.

- **Consents**. First-generation Italians and newer immigrants with limited English skills may be relatively passive when making health care decisions. Clinician should explain procedure or treatment plan to patient and reinforce the information while family spokesperson or interpreter is present. To assess patient's understanding of information, clinician should ask him/her to repeat it.

NONVERBAL COMMUNICATION

Italians are passionate about many things; communicating their feelings is one. Frequently embellish conversations with colorful gestures and facial expressions. To fully understand meaning, clinician must observe both verbal and nonverbal cues. Gestures contain many subtleties—easy for non-Italians to misconstrue their meaning.

- **Eye contact**. Direct eye contact conveys sincerity and an interest in the conversation. Italians may perceive avoiding eye contact as boredom, dishonesty, rudeness, or disrespect.
- **Personal space**. Italians stand or sit closer to one another than persons in dominant culture do.
- **Use and meaning of silence**. Family members may sit quietly with sick person to keep him/her company. In this context, silence not viewed negatively.
- **Gestures**. Often incorporate gestures into nonverbal communication for emphasis. For example, dragging one's thumb in a straight line, from below the eye to the jaw line and down the middle of the cheek, means someone is sly (*furbo*). Pointing index and little fingers toward body wards off evil, similar to "knocking on wood." However, in other contexts, that same gesture carries an entirely different message: cuckoldry.
- **Openness in expressing emotions**. Openly express feelings with family members; more reserved with strangers. May perceive health care providers who hold in their emotions as cold and uncaring.
- **Privacy**. Usually share information about illness with family members. Make decisions behind closed doors among family members. Out of respect for family, do not share family problems with outsiders. Family chooses spokesperson to provide such information.
- **Touch**. Frequently touch each other when talking with family and friends. Clinician should use appropriate forms of touch (e.g., touching arm or shoulder) after asking patient's permission.
- **Orientation to time**. Value relationships and spending time together more than they value clock time. Eating a meal in Italy can take several hours. First-generation and newer immigrants tend to be present-oriented; may not adhere to clock time. Acculturated second- and third-generation Italians more inclined to adhere to clock time.

ACTIVITIES OF DAILY LIVING

- **Modesty**. Women usually more comfortable with female clinicians. Most men and women are modest and prefer that health care providers use discretion during bathing, treatments, and procedures. Modesty and embarrassment can hinder discussions about sex. Younger women may discuss their symptoms and treatment choices with close female friends or relatives (e.g., aunts, sisters, or cousins).

- **Skin care.** Usually meticulous about hygiene and personal appearance. Many believe that a draft can cause illness, such as a cold, so sick person may avoid bath or shower. In such cases, prefer to sponge bathe in a warm room without any drafts.
- **Hair care.** Historically, Italians used olive oil to clean their hair and prevent the spread of lice and other parasites. This is the origin of the pejorative term "greaser." Italians pride themselves on well-groomed hair. Many second-generation Italian American women enjoy having their hair washed and set weekly at the beauty salon. Younger immigrants follow regional Italian dress and hair fashion.
- **Nail care.** Newer and younger women immigrants may routinely have manicures/pedicures. Men keep nails trimmed.
- **Toileting.** Perineal hygiene important. Some first-generation homes may be equipped with a bidet to wash after urination or defecation. Very ill patients probably will use urinal or commode; otherwise, prefer bathroom for privacy.
- **Special clothing or amulets.** Some Italians still wear horn (*corno*), an amulet, to protect against the evil eye (*malocchio*). Older Italians may carry and use rosary beads and often wear religious medals or carry a wallet-size religious card bearing a prayer or picture of a saint. Older women may wear black or navy blue when mourning the loss of a husband or child.
- **Self-care.** Family plays important role in patient's care. Men may prefer to have their wives bathe and care for them. Family members care for the sick and encourage inactivity so patient can preserve energy and recover.

FOOD PRACTICES

- **Usual meal pattern.** Coffee for breakfast. Older and newer immigrants may still eat the customary noontime meal, the major meal of the day, and a light evening meal. Although acculturated persons have altered the meal patterns typical in Italy, family meal on Sunday and holiday meals remain very important.
- **Special utensils.** None. Prefer not to eat with hands.
- **Food beliefs and rituals.** Recite a prayer (grace) before meal and wish everyone at the table a good appetite (*buon appetito*). Have a close relationship with food; it is a source of comfort and provides an emotional connection among family members. An Italian who disagrees with an outsider may say, "They don't eat at my table" (i.e., one is accountable only to those who eat a meal together, usually other family members). Make every attempt to eat in company of others; family members often join someone eating alone.

Believe that food is important for healing. May bring home-cooked or specialty foods to ill person.

- **Usual diet**. Has not changed much among first-, second-, and third-generation Italian Americans. Lots of complex carbohydrates, little meat and protein. Nutritional deficiencies rare. Staples are pasta, cheese, vegetables, bread, fruit, and dessert. Prefer fresh food to frozen or canned food; gardening is popular. View fast food as unhealthy; eating fast food may insult a woman who cooks. Discourage eating a lot of snack foods, such as potato chips or candy.
- **Fluids**. Believe that water is healthy; may drink mineral water. Traditional persons do not use ice, believing it causes stomach cramps and interferes with digestion. View wine as an extension of food. Often serve wine with meals, sip it slowly. During family meal, may give children wine diluted with water or soda to acclimate them to the taste. Do not routinely drink sodas. Stimulate appetite with alcoholic and nonalcoholic aperitifs. Often drink herbal, fruit, or nut-based liqueurs as digestive aids after meals. Other drinks include *espresso, cappuccino,* or *latte macchiato* (warm milk with a splash of espresso coffee).
- **Food taboos and prescriptions**. As a form of repentance, certain religious holidays (e.g., Fridays during Lent, Ash Wednesday, and Good Friday) require fasting between meals and abstinence from meat. Some Italians avoid meat on Fridays throughout the year. Even though the elderly and sick are excused from fasting and abstinence, some find it difficult to change life-long patterns.
- **Hospitality**. Italians pride themselves on hospitality and serving elaborate meals, good food, and wine to guests. Offers of food are genuine; if possible, health care providers should accept them.

SYMPTOM MANAGEMENT

- **Pain** (*dolore*). View pain as evil, unnatural, something that deprives one of life and living. Greatly fear pain. Openly express pain verbally and nonverbally. Older persons may chant, "Poor me, poor me" (*Povera me, povera me*) when feeling emotional or physical pain. May be reluctant to complain to family members so as not to worry them. Depending on literacy level, may understand numeric scale for rating pain. Some may describe their pain as depression or loss of energy.
- **Dyspnea** (*manca il respiro, non posso respirare,* or *manca il fiato*). May equate difficulty breathing or need for oxygen with dying. In most cases, readily accept oxygen but may fear artificial means of respiration. Clinician should reassure patient and family, and educate them about the need for, and use of, respiratory treatment.
- **Nausea/vomiting** (*nausea, vomito,* or *mal di stomaco*). Use various regional home remedies to treat symptoms. May treat upset stomach with a boiled herbal remedy called *canarino*, which is made with boiling water, lemon rind,

and bay leaves. Others use *brioschi*, a store-bought remedy consisting of lemon-flavored granules with fizz, like Alka Selzer.™

- **Constipation/diarrhea** (*non posso andare di corpo, stitichezza* [constipation]/ *diarea* [diarrhea]). May appear to be overly concerned with digestive system, complaining about it much like other elderly Americans do. May use lemon juice and water to control diarrhea.

- **Fatigue** (*faticata* or *fatica*). May describe it as depression. Treat fatigue with rest or reduced activity.

- **Depression** (*sono depressa* or *mi sento giu'*). May use "depression" or "feeling blue" to describe the effects of pain, fatigue, or other illnesses. No clear boundaries necessarily between physical and emotional disorders. Many Italian Americans less inclined than other Americans to seek mental health counseling or attend support groups; confide in, and accept support of, family members and close friends.

- **Self-care symptom management**. Older Italians may rely on proven home remedies before seeking biomedical care. Numerous home remedies and treatments are associated with particular areas in Italy.

BIRTH RITUALS/CARE OF THE NEW MOTHER AND BABY

- **Pregnancy care**. Pregnancy-leave benefits in Italy, instituted in 1912, clearly illustrate how Italians view pregnancy care and childbirth. Pregnant women receive five-month, paid maternity leave starting two months before mother's due date and ending three months after birth. During pregnancy, families are supportive and may seem overprotective of expectant mother. Mother often cares for her pregnant daughter and encourages her to refrain from too much activity. Acculturated Italian women readily attend childbirth preparation classes and obtain regular prenatal care. To establish a spiritual bond and evoke God's protection, families may use religious medals, holy cards or objects, and holy water or religious gestures, such as prayer and the sign of the cross, to keep unborn child safe. According to some traditional beliefs, a pregnant woman's unsatisfied cravings and accidental liquid spills (e.g., of coffee or wine) may cause baby to have birthmarks or defects. Believe that large babies are healthy and a reflection of mother's parenting ability. May name baby after a grandparent or special person in the family who died; some believe that the child will take on strong characteristics of the deceased person.

- **Preferences for children**. May slightly prefer boys. Women also want daughters who will remain close as adults. Italy has zero population growth, but Italian Americans follow typical American pattern in terms of family size.

- **Labor practices**. Most women deliver in hospitals. Labor practices among Italian American women same as those in dominant culture.

- **Role of the laboring woman during birth**. Expresses pain loudly. Accepts medical interventions. Takes active role and follows instructions of health care providers. May be modest during labor.

- **Role of the father and other family members during birth**. Second- and third-generation fathers take active role in birth process and attend delivery. Expectant mothers may want a female relative present during labor and birth.
- **Vaginal vs. cesarean section**. Prefer vaginal delivery. In recent years, rate of cesarean births in Italy has been rising.
- **Breastfeeding**. Uncommon among Italian Americans during 1950s due to modesty, embarrassment, or exposure to marketing campaigns promoting formula. Today, women accept breastfeeding. Typical duration of breastfeeding same as that among other American women. Women returning to work typically pump breast milk and supplement it with formula.
- **Birth recuperation**. When possible, new mothers are cared for by their own mother or another female relative for several weeks after delivery. In Italy, full-time working mothers are entitled to a two-hour rest period per day, and part-time working mothers to a one-hour rest period per day during first year after delivery.
- **Baby care**. Pierce ears of female babies. Women primarily responsible for children. Female relatives help with, and provide guidance about, care of new baby. Italians prefer that mother or another family member, rather than day care center, care for baby.
- **Problems with baby**. Clinician should discuss problems with both parents.
- **Male and female circumcision**. In U.S., male circumcision performed in hospital. In Italy, circumcision not as common as in U.S. Female circumcision not performed.

DEVELOPMENTAL AND SEXUAL ISSUES

- **Celebration of menarche or becoming a man**. No particular ceremonies.
- **Attitudes about birth control**. Take pride in their ability to conceive; fertility desirable. Some use rituals to promote fertility and pregnancy if a couple does not conceive after marriage; others worry that something is wrong. Today, most couples readily accept birth control when they do not want children. Birth control is an individual choice among singles, similar to dominant culture.
- **Attitudes about sexually transmitted infection (STI) control, including condoms**. Men take responsibility for carrying condoms. There is shame (*vergogna*) associated with STIs; a family member with an STI disgraces the family. Young Italians may be reluctant to seek treatment or may try to self-medicate.
- **Attitudes about abortion**. Italy passed a liberal abortion law in 1978. A referendum by the Catholic Church to make abortion illegal was overwhelmingly defeated in 1981. Religious Italian Americans who have an abortion may feel guilty and ashamed, and may conceal it from family members. May use abortion in cases of unwanted pregnancy or rape, and for young teenagers.

- **Attitudes about unwed sexual experimentation**. Second- and third-generation Italian American teenagers have freedom to date. Girls do not acknowledge nor openly discuss premarital sex. Teenage boys may be more willing to discuss sexual experiences with male friends or family members than with female health care providers.
- **Sexual orientation**. View gay or lesbian family member as a family disgrace; other family members may disown or ridicule him/her. May use the derogatory term *finocchio* to refer to a male homosexual.
- **Gender identity**. Many Italian Americans do not fully understand or accept gender ambiguity. Sexual reassignment surgery is performed in Italy, against teachings of the Catholic Church. Families do not pressure young masculine girls or young feminine boys to change; may pressure them when older.
- **Attitudes about menopause**. Accept *il cambiamento* as a natural part of aging. Many Italian women feel liberated from fear of pregnancy. May treat symptoms with home remedies or tolerate symptoms.

FAMILY RELATIONSHIPS

- **Composition/structure**. Traditional Italian American family consists of a mother and father married in Catholic Church and their children. Father, mother, and then eldest son are the most-respected family members. Disrespectful to criticize parents or elders. Sacrifice individual rights for the good of the whole family, in contrast to the individualism emphasized by U.S. Constitution and society.
- **Decision-making**. Hierarchy and status important in decision-making process. Italians greatly respect power and age.
- **Spokesperson**. Eldest male or educated family member, male or female.
- **Gender issues**. Women primarily responsible for children, family finances, food, family gatherings, and ill family members. Men handle most external business transactions. While most women run the family and household finances, they may give the appearance that husband is in charge.
- **Changing roles among generations in U.S.** Italian Americans have assimilated in many ways while keeping old traditions. For example, family meals remain important. Have not given in to the convenience of fast food. Although traditional roles remain strong in first and second generations, the composition and structure of families are changing to resemble those in dominant culture. Recent immigrants reflect contemporary Italian values and norms. On average, these immigrants have more education and a higher quality of life than earlier immigrants do.
- **Caring roles**. Female family members usually are the caregivers; they care for ill family members and friends.
- **Expectations of and for children**. Teach children to respect women, parents, and the elderly. Also teach them to assist with household chores and care for others, such as younger siblings and grandparents. Expect teenagers

to work and help the family financially or help pay for their college education. Families are proud of children who attend college or receive professional training. Problems may arise if higher education interferes with family roles and responsibilities, or if an educated family member wants to relocate for job advancement. Some young adults may leave home, then return
if they have financial or emotional difficulties. Some may stay home beyond
the age of 18 if they are in school, but most of those in U.S. do not.

- **Expectations of and for elders**. Most elderly prefer to maintain their own
  home close to their children's. Italians attempt to keep an ill or older family
  member at home as long as possible. Adult children may be primary caregivers for aging parents and move them into the children's home when the
  elderly cannot care for themselves. Do not readily accept institutionalization
  for sick or old family members. If a family must place a parent in an assisted
  living facility, it carefully selects a facility in terms of adequate staffing,
  cleanliness, and proximity for frequent visits.
- **Expectations of hospital visitors**. Family and friends frequently visit sick
  person and bring home-cooked food. Family member likely to be present at
  patient's bedside throughout the day or night.

ILLNESS BELIEFS

- **Causes of/attitudes about physical illness**. Traditional families may
  attribute illness to external factors (e.g., God's will, the evil eye, cold air or
  currents, genetics, or contamination) and internal factors (e.g., human
  causes, guilt, anxiety, or suppression of emotions). Acculturated families subscribe to standard biomedical explanations for illness.
- **Causes of/attitudes about mental illness**. Many traditional Italians may
  attribute mental illness and nervousness to an evil spirit or the evil eye (*malocchio*). Acculturated Italians accept biomedical explanations for mental illness. May have difficulty with hospitalization or therapy but take medication.
- **Causes of genetic defects**. Traditional Italians may believe that genetic
  defects are God's will and beyond one's control. Acculturated Italians subscribe to current medical explanations.
- **Attitudes about disabilities**. Family members feel it is their duty to care
  for a disabled family member at home. Italian Americans may be more
  accepting of a physical disability than mental illness or HIV/AIDS. Usually
  do not share information about a disabled family member with those outside
  the family and conceal him/her from society.
- **Sick role**. Take pride in working and being productive. Illness may cause
  feelings of guilt. Many do not readily accept sick role; some try to hide their
  illness from family members. Once ill persons accept their sick role, they are
  receptive to others' care.
- **Home and folk remedies**. In the past, Italians (particularly those from
  southern Italy) had many home remedies and folk practices for treating

physical and mental illness, some based on religious and magical beliefs. Today, they are less likely to consult traditional healers. The home remedies they still use come from plants and byproducts that are plentiful in Italy, such as lemon juice, olive oil, vinegar, and garlic.

- **Medications**. Older Italians and newer immigrants may prefer medication by injection or suppository, as they consider the stomach to be sacred and reserve it for food. Contemporary Italians, including health professionals, believe that the stomach poorly absorbs medication, so they tend to use other routes if possible. Many Italians self-treat (e.g., self-medicate or stop taking medication when symptoms subside); for compliance, they may need supervision and assistance.

- **Acceptance of procedures**. Many factors can influence acceptance of procedures such as blood transfusions, surgery, or organ transplants. Italians prefer to let nature take its course and avoid invasive procedures if possible. Those who have sufficiently self-treated with home remedies and folk practices may be leery of high-tech biomedical care. Health care providers should offer families information to alleviate their fears, allow them to participate in care planning, respect their beliefs and practices, promptly alleviate patient's pain, and promote his/her comfort.

- **Care-seeking**. A proverb summarizes a common belief among traditional Italians: "If the patient dies, the doctor has killed him, but if he gets well, the saints have saved him." They may rely on their faith in God and folk remedies to cure physical and mental illness rather than seek biomedical care. Also may defer seeking treatment until a crisis develops or until a medical problem interferes with relationships, work, or physical activity. Acculturated families accept biomedical care.

HEALTH ISSUES

- **Concept of health**. The ability to enjoy life without chronic pain or the restrictions of a debilitating illness.

- **Health promotion and prevention**. Italians have always practiced self-care. For example, many in Italy vacation at resorts and hot springs for therapeutic mineral baths or to drink the water to flush impurities from their bodies. Italian Americans pray to patron saints for help with specific illnesses and to the patron saint of their region or town in Italy for healing and protection from illness. May generally subscribe to dominant ideas, such as sufficient sleep, cleanliness, and exercise, but make exceptions for food. For example, they prepare eggplant the traditional way (by frying it), use lots of salt in cooking, and do not accept "healthy" pizza containing tofu.

- **Screening**. Older women may be reluctant to examine their breasts or undergo routine Pap smears or mammograms because of embarrassment or fear of uncovering serious illness. Others accept regular or specific screening suggested by clinician after consulting a friend or family member.

- **Common health problems**. Genetic diseases, such as thalassemia major (Cooley's anemia), and minor and familial Mediterranean fever. Italians have a higher risk of multiple sclerosis and tumors of the nasopharynx, stomach, liver, and gallbladder than other groups do. Cardiovascular disease, hypertension, arthritis, gastrointestinal disorders, and cancer are more common among Italians.

DEATH RITUALS

- **Beliefs and attitudes about death**. Many do not fear death but respect and view it as a rite of passage. Believe in life after death. Families often want to be with the dying person and may want to take him/her home to die. Realistic about death; often purchase a family burial plot in advance. Children often attend wakes and funerals. Remember their deceased loved ones in many ways. Close relatives and friends may carry a card commemorating someone's death. Some families burn a votive candle by the deceased's photograph on the anniversary of his/her death and ask priest to say a special celebratory mass in remembrance. Some families believe that suffering before death earns passage into heaven.
- **Preparation**. Clinician should inform family spokesperson of impending death. Typically, close relatives and friends want to see the person before he/she dies. Usually summon parish priest so dying person can receive sacrament of the sick for spiritual strength.
- **Home vs. hospital**. Many older Italians prefer to die at home in their own beds. Acculturated Italians may prefer hospital. May use hospice as a last resort when death is imminent or elderly spouse is physically unable to provide care.
- **Special needs**. More likely to seek support from other family members or parish priest than grief counseling offered by hospital. When death occurs, close family and friends gather at home of the deceased person's family. An extended network of family, friends, and co-workers visit funeral home during calling hours. Priest holds a short service during calling hours and prayers are recited over body. The next day, hold a full service, including funeral mass, in church followed by burial and then a social gathering. Calling hours and funeral may be delayed until distant family members arrive.
- **Care of the body**. If family is not present at time of death, it may want to visit the deceased in the hospital before he/she is taken to morgue. May want to touch and hold body of deceased. Most have a funeral home prepare body. Before embalming, older or new immigrants may want to carefully choose clothes, jewelry, religious objects, photos, and flowers for the deceased. When possible, view body in open casket.
- **Attitudes about organ donation**. Slowly gaining acceptance in Italy, but first-generation immigrants usually do not donate. Donation may be more acceptable among acculturated Italian Americans.

- **Attitudes about autopsy**. Do not readily accept it in most cases. Consider body to be a sacred vessel. View autopsy as invasive and unnecessary.

SELECTED REFERENCES

Bruhn, J. G., Philips, B. U., & Wolf, S. (1972). Social readjustment and illness patterns: Comparisons between first, second and third generation Italian-Americans living in the same community. *Journal of Psychosomatic Research*, 16, 387–394.

Carangelo, A. (2001). Italian-American women and changing childbirth practices. *Midwifery Today with International Midwife*, 60, 48–51.

Eisenbruch, M. (1984). Cross-cultural aspects of bereavement. II: Ethnic and cultural variations in the development of bereavement practices. *Culture, Medicine and Psychiatry*, 8, 315–347.

Lassiter, S. M. (1995). *Multicultural clients: A professional handbook for health care providers and social workers*. Westport, CT: Greenwood Press.

Lipton, J., & Marbach, J. (1984). Ethnicity and the pain experience. *Social Science and Medicine*, 19, 1279–1298.

Mangione, J., & Morreale, B. (1993). *La storia: Five centuries of the Italian American experience*. New York: Harper Collins.

Mathias, E. The Italian-American funeral: Persistence through change. Retrieved July 5, 2004, from http://www.italianancestry.com/mathias

New advent. Retrieved June 1, 2004, from http://www.newadvent.org

Purnell, L. D., & Paulanka, B. J. (Eds.). (2003). *Transcultural health care: A culturally competent approach* (2nd ed.). Philadelphia: F. A. Davis.

Ross, H. M. (1981). Societal/cultural views regarding death and dying. *Topics in Clinical Nursing*, 3, 1–16.

Westbrook, M. T., Legge, V., & Pennay, M. (1993). Attitudes towards disabilities in a multicultural society. *Social Science and Medicine*, 36, 615–623.

AUTHORS

Cynthia Ruocco Miceli, BSN, RN, received her bachelor of science in nursing from the University of South Florida in Fort Myers and has completed courses for a master's degree in public health. She lived in Rome and southern Italy for many years where she worked in occupational health nursing. She also was a clinical researcher in the Division of Gastroenterology at the Emory University School of Medicine. Miceli is a first-generation Italian American.

Karen Lucas Breda, PhD, RN, earned a doctorate in anthropology at the University of Connecticut, and a bachelor of science in nursing and master of science in nursing at Boston University. She is an associate professor at the University of Hartford. She conducted research on the Italian National Health Service with support from the Fulbright Association and the *Fondazione Giovanni Agnelli*. Breda is a third-generation Italian American.

Maria Esposito Frank, PhD, earned a doctorate in Italian studies at Harvard University. She also holds university degrees from the *Istituto Universitario Orientale* in Naples, Italy, and Moscow State University in the former Soviet Union. She is an associate professor at the University of Hartford. Frank is a first-generation Italian American.

CHAPTER 23

JAPANESE

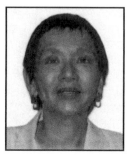
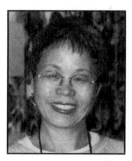
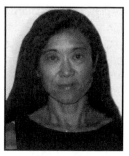

Gayle Shiba   *Yuko Matsumoto Leong*   *Roberta Oka*

CULTURAL/ETHNIC IDENTITY

- **Preferred term(s)**. Japanese American.
- **Census**. The 2000 U.S. Census reported 800,000 Japanese Americans, about 7% of the total Asian population of nearly 12 million. An estimated 274,000 were born in Japan. Census does not include the large number of Japanese who visit and/or temporarily reside in U.S. for school, work, or other purposes. About 5 million Japanese visited in 2000 and 312,936 Japanese were living in U.S. as of 2001 but did not intend to immigrate.
- **History of immigration**. Began immigrating in 1885, mainly to the West Coast and Hawaii. Immigration peaked in 1900–10. The 1924 National Origins Act barred Japanese and other Asians from entering U.S. until 1950, when immigration began again. In 1942, during World War II, an executive order required that all persons of Japanese ancestry living in California, Washington, and Oregon be forcibly relocated to camps because of their perceived threat to U.S. security. Japanese Americans acculturate on many levels yet maintain viable ethnic communities and identity. Theirs is the only ethnic group to identify itself formally according to birth generation, distinguishable by age, experience, language, and values. *Issei* means immigrants. Early *Issei* had a strong sense of national identity, which declines with each succeeding generation. Second-generation Japanese Americans (*Nisei*) were born and educated in U.S. While appearing acculturated, *Nisei*'s feelings and attitudes are rooted in Japanese culture. Third-generation (*Sansei*) and fourth-generation (*Yonsei*) Japanese Americans are more like people in the dominant culture; they are less connected to Japanese culture and many of them married persons of other ethnic backgrounds. *Shin* (new) *Issei* came from postwar Japan in the 1950s and 1960s. With economic growth in Japan,

the number of emigrants decreased, except for women who married American servicemen stationed in Japan. Small numbers of immigrants continue to be admitted each year. Recent immigrants tend to be well-educated and settle in large metropolitan areas with significant Japanese communities, such as San Francisco and Honolulu.

SPIRITUAL/RELIGIOUS ORIENTATION

- **Primary religious/spiritual affiliations**. Buddhism, Shintoism, and Christianity. Christianity accounts for largest group among Japanese Americans. Parents may have different religious affiliation than their children, especially in older-generation families (e.g., parents are Buddhist, children are Christian). Japanese immigrants most commonly practice Buddhism and Shintoism.
- **Usual religious/spiritual practices**. Depend on religious beliefs. In larger Japanese communities, people tend to join churches (of whatever religion) that have a number of Japanese American or Japanese immigrant members. Church has been, and continues to be, a means for socializing and acculturation.
- **Use of spiritual healing/healers**. Depends on religious beliefs. Prayer and offerings prevalent in Buddhism and Shintoism. In addition to such practices at a temple or church, Buddhist and Shinto families pray and make offerings in small shrines at home. Japanese usually combine prayer and offerings with traditional Western medicine.
- **Holidays**. Japanese New Year (January 1) is most important. Japanese associate New Year's with purification, renewal, and family gatherings. In Japan, New Year's celebration continues for at least three days; most businesses and schools are closed. Japanese Americans also celebrate Japanese New Year as an important holiday. New *Issei*, especially those in mixed marriages, may find it difficult to celebrate this holiday if they do not have extended family who can share traditional New Year's foods; may not have access to Japanese grocery stores. Women members of extended family usually prepare food together in a social gathering.

COMMUNICATION
ORAL COMMUNICATION

- **Major languages and dialects**. Japanese. *Nisei* are usually bilingual, but later generations speak English only. Newly immigrated Japanese usually can understand and speak some English. Most Japanese visitors have difficulty communicating in English.
- **Greetings**. Formal. Use surnames. Small bow more common among older generations, handshakes more common among younger generations. May acknowledge someone with a smile or small bow.
- **Tone of voice**. Among older generations and newer immigrants, soft tone is polite.

- **Direct or indirect style of speech**. Traditionally indirect. Careful about feelings of listener. Adjust speech according to other person's age, gender, and especially social status. Avoid direct expressions of disagreement or conflict. *Sansei* and *Yonsei* likely to be more assertive and outspoken. In general, Japanese Americans ask few questions about their treatment or care, deferring to clinician's authority. Their communication is influenced by three cultural concepts: *enryo*, *gaman*, and *haji*. *Enryo* is self-restraint in interactions with others; also described as polite refusal or polite hesitation, wherein patient refuses medication or assistance if it would be embarrassing or "inconvenient" for either the patient or clinician. *Gaman* is related to self-control and ability to endure. Stoic patients reflect this trait. Clinicians should phrase questions so that more than a "yes" or "no" answer is necessary, as patients may not question an explanation or ask for further explanation to avoid embarrassment. *Haji* is the concept of shame. It is to be avoided at almost any cost, as shame reflects poorly upon not only the individual but also the family and family name.
- **Use of interpreters**. Interpreters especially important for newly immigrated *Issei* and Japanese visitors. Japanese prefer that family members translate. To protect patient's privacy regarding sensitive issues, such as sex and diagnosis, interpreter should be a close family member or of same gender as patient.
- **Serious or terminal illness**. Clinician should first consult with family members—spouse and eldest son or daughter. Family may be reluctant to divulge terminal diagnosis and prognosis to patient. It may filter information for new immigrants and older patients who speak little or no English. Do not freely discuss illnesses, especially cancer, outside family as younger generations do.

WRITTEN COMMUNICATION

- **Literacy assessment**. Newly immigrated *Issei* tend to be well-educated, and read and understand English. Most *Nisei* are bilingual. Later generations—*Sansei* and *Yonsei*—predominantly speak English. Earlier generations may not speak English well (57.5% of Japanese Americans, according to a 2002 Census citation) but can usually read and understand it. *Sansei* and later generations have been educated in U.S.; most have graduated from high school and attended college.
- **Consents**. Clinician should explain procedures clearly and stop to elicit feedback and understanding of the information he/she is communicating. Should also emphasize important details; patients may be uncomfortable asking for clarification. *Nisei* more likely than *Sansei* and *Yonsei* to consent to procedure, based on a health care professional's recommendation, even though they may not fully understand. This may occur because *Nisei* believe that the doctor knows best.

NONVERBAL COMMUNICATION

In general, Japanese may value and trust nonverbal communication more highly than they do verbal communication. Are very aware of nonverbal cues that establish the meaning of a verbal message.

- **Eye contact**. Older Japanese may avoid direct eye contact with authority figures. *Sansei* and *Yonsei* are similar to dominant culture in this regard.
- **Personal space**. Immigrants may be more tolerant of crowding than dominant culture is. But they maintain social distance in new situations and may be uncomfortable with invasion of personal space. Varies by relationship, gender, and acculturation. Closeness among family members, but they have less physical contact in public than people in dominant culture do.
- **Use and meaning of silence**. Typically quiet and polite. Silence can mean that someone is disappointed or disagrees, depending on situation. This is related to generation; younger persons exhibit such behavior less commonly.
- **Gestures**. Not overly expressive with gestures. Tend toward self-restraint in interactions. Maintain self-control. Often interpret the "OK" sign as a symbol for money. Present and accept something, such as a business card, with both hands; this practice is more common in immigrant population.
- **Openness in expressing emotions**. More-traditional persons control their emotions in public or formal situations. "Face" or "saving face" an important concept. Do not condone expressions of anger or loss of temper, as it reflects negatively on family. Avoid overt conflict even within family. Younger persons, *Sansei*, and *Yonsei* are more open in expressing emotions with family, friends, and others.
- **Privacy**. Despite strong respect for authority, patient may self-disclose sensitive information only if trust has been established and, usually, only when clinician elicits it. Sensitive to shame and saving face; younger and acculturated persons are less sensitive in this regard.
- **Touch**. Japanese culture is relatively low-touch. Touching in public less common among older Japanese than among younger generations. Acceptable to touch most parts of the body when necessary for care. Older women less comfortable than younger women are when clinician examines them. If health care professional states that examination must be performed, older Japanese do not question authority and generally consent.
- **Orientation to time**. Promptness important, especially among older persons. Often early for appointments. Past orientation reflected in respect for elderly and maintaining family honor. Future orientation reflected in working hard, saving for success, and valuing education.

ACTIVITIES OF DAILY LIVING

- **Modesty**. Very modest, particularly women. Modest even with family members, especially older persons, and those of opposite gender. Clinician-patient gender matching ideal.

- **Skin care**. Cleanliness and hygiene very important. Linked to belief that one must purify the body to help restore health. Prefer daily tub baths or showers, preferably in evening before bedtime.
- **Hair care**. Prefer to wash hair daily or several times a week. Older women frequently have their hair professionally washed and styled weekly.
- **Nail care**. Short and clean. Younger generations more likely to mirror practices in dominant culture; they get manicures and pedicures.
- **Toileting**. Use bathroom, primarily for privacy. Wash after toileting.
- **Special clothing or amulets**. May use prayer beads, particularly if Buddhist.
- **Self-care**. If able, patient performs personal hygiene. Family member, particularly spouse or elder daughter, may be able to help; patient prefers this to help by health care provider. Older adults may be more dependent on family members when ill.

FOOD PRACTICES

- **Usual meal pattern**. Three meals a day. Snacks between meals, which may include ethnic foods, such as rice cakes. Rice with most meals, particularly dinner. Younger generation has adopted a more Western diet (e.g., eats less rice). Food should be visually appealing.
- **Special utensils**. Chopsticks, depending on setting.
- **Food beliefs and rituals**. Prepare special foods and dishes during New Year's holiday and at other times of year (e.g., *ozoni*, a soup containing *mochi* [pounded rice] that is thought to bring good luck/fortune and good health to family during the year).
- **Usual diet**. Usually lower in fat, animal protein, cholesterol, and sugar but higher in salt content than Western diet is. Traditional protein sources are fish and soybeans with vegetables. Rice at dinner. Younger generation has adopted more Western dietary habits.
- **Fluids**. Primarily green tea, without cream or sugar. Older persons in particular favor green tea. Many Japanese drink coffee. Also rice wine (*sake*), especially new *Issei* and visitors on different occasions and at social gatherings.
- **Food taboos and prescriptions**. Many are lactose- or alcohol-intolerant. Older Japanese, especially, believe that combining certain foods, such as eel and pickled plums, watermelon and crab, and cherries and milk, causes illness. Often eat rice gruel or porridge with pickled vegetables when ill. Drink hot tea when ill or for stomach ailments. Use pickled plums and hot tea to prevent constipation or maintain normal bowel function, but this practice is more common among older Japanese and new immigrants.
- **Hospitality**. Very important, especially among family members. Offer and often serve food and beverages to visitors even if they decline. Usually serve men first at meals, but this is influenced by generation. Not partaking of food often viewed as disrespectful or ungrateful. Parents give up their own bed to family members from out of town.

SYMPTOM MANAGEMENT

Patients generally do not complain about symptoms and may not freely ask for medications to alleviate them. May delay seeking help until symptoms are severe. When assessing older Japanese and immigrants for symptoms and symptom severity, clinician should use word descriptors instead of numerical scales, as these patients understand word descriptors better. Younger Japanese most likely understand both scales. Before they seek medical assistance, older-generation Japanese may use nonpharmacological methods that family members or friends have recommended for controlling symptoms.

- **Pain** (*itami* [e-ta-mee] means "to have pain"; *itai* [e-ta-ee] means "it hurts"). Can be stoic in expressing pain or discomfort. Clinician should offer pain medication. Some Japanese have a high pain threshold, while others may refrain from asking for medication. Older generation especially concerned about becoming addicted to medication and may refuse. Others take medication as prescribed, preferring oral type rather than injections. May refuse rectal medications.

- **Dyspnea** (*iki-gurushii* or *iki-ga-dekinai* means "cannot breathe"). Accept oxygen. Less likely to accept or use narcotic medication.

- **Nausea/vomiting** (*hakike/haku*). Embarrassed when lose control of bodily functions. Some patients or family members clean up vomitus. May consume home remedies, such as rice gruel (*okayu*), *miso* soup, or green tea, before using medications.

- **Constipation/diarrhea** (*benpi/geri*). Uncomfortable when bowel routine disrupted. May disclose if asked. May prefer trying own remedies before taking medication. May try dietary options when recommended, but if results are not immediate, they are likely to discontinue. Use enema as last resort.

- **Fatigue** (*tsukare-yasui* means "easily get tired"). Generally tolerate fatigue. If necessary, Japanese may resort to foods that they think relieve fatigue. For example, pickled plums (*umeboshi*) and *miso* are thought to promote overall well-being.

- **Depression** (*utsu, utsu-byo*). Patient may not express psychological state or mood due to fear of social stigma and shame. Physical symptoms may be an expression of emotional disturbance or distress. Japanese use mental health services less often than dominant population does and also quit treatment more often. Because of stigma, those who seek care for such disorders may initially present with more-severe symptoms. May follow treatment plan, as long as it is not disruptive or likely to draw attention to themselves. If in therapy, may prefer therapist of similar ethnicity. May respond better to a counseling style that is directive.

- **Self-care symptom management**. Older generation may not respond to illness until it is advanced. Younger generations acknowledge illness more readily and are receptive to self-care for symptom management. Japanese are more likely to listen to a health care professional's recommendation for self-care than to a family member's. Older generations, especially males, may rely on spouse or female family member, such as a daughter or daughter-in-law, to help manage their illness.

BIRTH RITUALS/CARE OF THE NEW MOTHER AND BABY

- **Pregnancy care**. Traditionally, Japanese value pregnancy as a woman's destiny. She is pampered. Encourage pregnant women to get plenty of rest and not "overdo it." Mothers-to-be very health-conscious; eat properly, avoiding foods and beverages that may harm baby. Prenatal care an expectation early in pregnancy. Pregnant women often work up until their due date. Some pregnant women born in Japan may go back to their parents' home for last months of pregnancy and birth (a practice called *sato-gaeri*).

- **Preferences for children**. Traditionally prefer male children, to inherit family assets and to take responsibility for parents and siblings. This is less true among younger generations. In Japan, families have fewer than two children on average. In U.S., number of children appears to mirror that in dominant population; two are desirable, but families may have more if first two children are girls, reflecting the cultural preference for boys.

- **Labor practices**. Consistent with those of dominant culture, unless recently immigrated. In Japan, expectant mother may eat a full meal during labor. Clinician should assess patient for pain and offer adequate pain relief. Some women may not request pain medication or may refuse it until pain becomes severe.

- **Role of the laboring woman during birth**. May be assertive during labor, expressing her wishes and needs. Most women attempt to control vocal expressions of pain or discomfort, such as screaming. Modesty important.

- **Role of the father and other family members during birth**. *Sansei* and *Yonsei* fathers usually are present during labor and delivery. Father assumes active role if he attended childbirth preparation classes. Expectant woman's mother also may be present. If father not present during labor and delivery, expectant woman wants mother, sister, or friend to be there.

- **Vaginal vs. cesarean section**. Highly prefer vaginal delivery.

- **Breastfeeding**. Expected, at least for some period of time. Mothers who breastfeed may also bottle-feed (1–2 bottles a day). While breastfeeding, mother tends to be very conscious of health and diet, as they benefit baby. Mothers returning to work often discontinue breastfeeding and start bottle-feeding.

- **Birth recuperation**. Expect new mother to rest and recuperate for several weeks after birth. Some women ask their mother or mother-in-law to come from Japan or from elsewhere in U.S. to provide postpartum and infant care. Or a member of the extended family may stay with family to help with household activities and child care. Other family members and close friends may assist (e.g., by providing meals). Personal hygiene important. Mothers bathe, shower, and perform peri-care frequently.

- **Baby care**. Mother primarily responsible. Men in younger generations more involved in child care.
- **Problems with baby**. If family is newly immigrated, best if clinician consults with father before informing mother. Should also make sure father or other family members are present for discussion with mother. Otherwise, clinician can consult with mother initially. However, decision-making requires consultation with both mother and father.
- **Male and female circumcision**. Male circumcision common before discharge from hospital. Female circumcision not performed.

DEVELOPMENTAL AND SEXUAL ISSUES

- **Celebration of menarche or becoming a man**. Because of privacy and embarrassment, Japanese women generally do not mention menstrual periods when male family members are present. Becoming a man not celebrated.
- **Attitudes about birth control**. Birth control most acceptable within marriage. Single women who are sexually active use contraceptives but usually do not tell family. Women may undergo tubal ligation when they no longer want to become pregnant. Men less likely to undergo vasectomy. New *Issei* and visitors from Japan most likely to use condoms. Abortion quite common for birth control.
- **Attitudes about sexually transmitted infection (STI) control, including condoms**. Young adults are more knowledgeable about STIs and likely to protect themselves with condoms. Older generation believes that only promiscuous persons are likely to acquire STIs. Newly immigrated persons and visitors from Japan may not be knowledgeable about safe sex.
- **Attitudes about abortion**. Unacceptable to older-generation Japanese; expect parents to marry if the woman is pregnant and couple is unwed. Abortion more acceptable in younger generation. Choice of abortion as birth control method more common among new *Issei* and Japanese visitors.
- **Attitudes about unwed sexual experimentation**. Older Japanese frown upon sexual activity outside of marriage. Younger persons accept it but keep it secret from family.
- **Sexual orientation**. Older generation does not acknowledge or openly accept gay and lesbian relationships; may view such relationships as shameful or as a disgrace to family. Close family members may be supportive of a gay or lesbian family member.
- **Gender identity**. Strong expectation that women and men assume their appropriate gender roles. Gender ambiguity unacceptable. Parents may pressure children to conform.
- **Attitudes about menopause**. Generally regard it as normal. However, women may not openly discuss symptoms with health care providers. If women have symptoms, more likely to try over-the-counter or home/folk remedies recommended by family members or friends before they seek med-

ical advice. Women whose diets are rich in soy products may have fewer symptoms than do those in dominant culture.

FAMILY RELATIONSHIPS

- **Composition/structure**. Japanese are family-oriented; subordinate self to family unit. In older families, members have well-defined roles. Family structure is hierarchical and patriarchal, with father being head of household and major authority; characterized by solidarity, mutual helpfulness, and interdependency (*amae*). Values include importance of family as unit, duty to family, responsibility, obligation, and maintaining harmony. Other strong influences are respect for age and authority, and filial piety (duty and obedience to parents, and duty of parents to children). Younger generations less likely to live close to parents.

- **Decision-making**. Women, especially those in younger-generation families, usually involved in decision-making. However, a male—usually the eldest male member present—tends to be family spokesperson.

- **Spokesperson**. Father, eldest son, or daughter. In younger-generation families, mother often serves as spokesperson before son or daughter does.

- **Gender issues**. More-traditional families consider women to be subordinate. In younger families, women have more equality with males.

- **Changing roles among generations in U.S.** *Nisei* elders are more closely linked to traditional Japanese values. Subsequent generations have become acculturated, typically have assumed American cultural values, and are more American than Japanese.

- **Caring roles**. Women—mother, wife, daughter, or daughter-in-law—are primary caregivers for family. Men are pampered. Even if women are sick, they tend to continue care-taking and household activities.

- **Expectations of and for children**. Revere children, who are taught to be polite, quiet, shy, humble, and deferent to elders. Emphasize conforming to expectations. Discourage emotional outbursts. Positive reinforcement and discussing one's personal achievements unusual. Expect grown children to care for parents if necessary. Family values emphasize and support education and educational achievement leading to valued or respected occupations, such as medicine, pharmacy, law, or teaching. Newer immigrant families more strongly emphasize this than do families that have lived in dominant culture for several generations, due to acculturation. In both cases, education is an important value.

- **Expectations of and for elders**. Respect elders. Healthy elders may help in household, including caring for children and grandchildren. Elders frequently maintain separate household from their children and grandchildren. When sick, eldest son's family traditionally cares for them at home. Though family is expected to care for elders at home, younger generations may place sick elder in nursing home, although choice is difficult and may cause much guilt.

- **Expectations of hospital visitors**. Family member, particularly spouse, may want to remain at patient's bedside. Older generations less likely to stay overnight; younger family members likely to do so. Entire family and close friends considered to be part of the family visit. Visitors likely to bring a gift, such as flowers, fruit, or Japanese food. Patient and family may give food to staff.

ILLNESS BELIEFS

- **Causes of/attitudes about physical illness**. Naturalistic causes include being out of balance from lack of sleep or poor diet. Holistic causes may include loss of spiritual, family, or environmental harmony. May attribute chronic illness, such as cancer, to karma (a result of bad behavior in this life or a past life) or to actions of another family member. May attribute disease or illness to contact with a contaminated source that disrupts the body's balance or harmony. Also may believe that spirits of deceased loved ones are watching over them. Younger generations have more Western beliefs about physical illness.
- **Causes of/attitudes about mental illness**. Attribute mental illness to evil spirits that cause a loss of mental self-control or believe that it is punishment for improper behavior or not living a good life. View loss of mental self-control as lack of will power, over which one is expected to have control. Families often view a mentally ill member as not trying hard enough to deal with the situation. Japanese frequently do not think of mental illness as a real illness. It is stigmatized and brings shame on one's family; thus, family may delay or avoid seeking professional help. Younger persons more likely to seek mental health services. Japanese may require lower doses of psychotropic medications than do Whites or Blacks.
- **Causes of genetic defects**. May interpret defects as punishment for parents' or family's bad behavior.
- **Attitudes about disabilities**. Attitudes of younger Japanese similar to those in dominant culture. Older generations and newly immigrated *Issei* tend to view disabilities as shameful or disgraceful. May believe that disability is punishment for something one has done in his/her life or for something a family member has done. If a disability is not overtly visible, Japanese attempt to conceal it from others.
- **Sick role**. Women primarily care for sick persons, who assume a passive role. In such cases, women caregivers are not expected to perform their usual duties. However, women who are sick may continue to fulfill household duties, although other family members may help.
- **Home and folk remedies**. Some Japanese, particularly those in older generation, may use herbal medicine to cure ailments (e.g., by applying a topical form of capsaicin to skin at site of pain for pain relief). They obtain these medicines through local herbalists in "Japantown," where Japanese stores and

businesses are located, or at stores catering to persons of Japanese descent. Immigrants may bring remedies from Japan or have family members there send them. Younger generation generally relies on Western biomedicine.

- **Medications**. Compliant with Western medications, which they may use in conjunction with folk remedies. Older generations are likely to try folk remedies before seeking Western medical attention.
- **Acceptance of procedures**. Blood transfusions and donations acceptable. Organ transplants are a recent phenomenon in Japan; new immigrants may not accept them, due to beliefs about maintaining body's integrity. Clinician should thoroughly explain procedures. Japanese generally accept Western biomedicine, unless it conflicts with cultural or religious beliefs.
- **Care-seeking**. Older generation may not respond to illness until it has advanced. May try home remedies before seeking medical attention. May use such complementary methods as acupressure (*shiatsu*), acupuncture, moxibustion (*okyu*), or massage in addition to biomedicine.

HEALTH ISSUES

- **Concept of health**. Associate good health with taking care of oneself, being able to maintain independence, and living free of disease. Balance and harmony among the individual, society, and universe are important.
- **Health promotion and prevention**. Western beliefs about health promotion becoming more accepted. Younger generations more readily adopt healthy lifestyles regarding diet, exercise, and smoking.
- **Screening**. Health maintenance important, particularly among younger generations. *Nisei* may have more difficulty providing information related to screening if issue is sensitive (e.g., regarding sex or something that may reflect negatively on family). However, most disclose information because they respect health care professionals. *Nisei* less likely to undergo screening. May avoid even a recommended procedure, such as a colonoscopy or mammogram, if they view it as invasive, embarrassing, or a threat to privacy.
- **Common health problems**. As generations have become more westernized and acculturated, health problems reflect those of general population. Common problems are hypertension, heart disease, stroke, arthritis, benign prostatic hypertrophy, and cancer, especially of the stomach, colon, rectum, and liver.

DEATH RITUALS

- **Beliefs and attitudes about death**. Traditionally in Japan, death not openly discussed. Varies depending on religious beliefs. For example, Buddhists believe that death is a natural progression and that the deceased will be reincarnated. Shinto believe that the soul has an eternal life.
- **Preparation**. Clinician should discuss imminent death with spouse or eldest son or daughter. Sometimes, both the family and patient know that patient

is seriously ill or dying but avoid talking about it with each other. Do-not-resuscitate is difficult choice for Japanese. Entire family decides.

- **Home vs. hospital**. Prefer hospital in cases of acute illness. When choosing between home and an intermediate care facility, prefer home if they have the resources and care can be provided there. In terminal cases, prefer to die at home. Family may not initially accept hospice care because it does not want to acknowledge to patient that family considers death inevitable.

- **Special needs**. Family member(s) may request to stay with patient if illness serious or terminal. Women openly grieve, while men remain stoic. Clinician must thoroughly assess whether family has special needs, as it may not request help and may even deny it needs assistance.

- **Care of the body**. Important that body is clean and that dignity and modesty of the deceased are preserved for viewing. Many Buddhists and Shinto have body cremated.

- **Attitudes about organ donation**. Older Japanese less likely to agree to organ donation. Strongly believe that when someone dies, body should be kept intact, as it was at birth. Younger generations more likely to agree to donation. However, clinician should respect elders' wishes. *Sansei* and *Yonsei* may consider organ donation.

- **Attitudes about autopsy**. Older Japanese less likely to agree to autopsy, unless there is a good justification for it. May view autopsy as a violation of the body. Younger generations more receptive.

SELECTED REFERENCES

Fujita, S. S., & O'Brien, D. J. (1991). *Japanese American ethnicity: The persistence of community.* Seattle: University of Washington Press.

Hosokawa, B. (1998). *Out of the frying pan: Reflections of a Japanese American.* Niwot, CO: University Press of Colorado.

Ishida, D., & Inouye, J. (2004). Japanese Americans. In J. Giger & R. Davidhizar (Eds.), *Transcultural nursing: Assessment and intervention* (4th ed.) (pp. 333–360). St. Louis, MO: Mosby.

Kitano, H., & Stotsky, S. (Ed.) (1995). *The Japanese Americans.* New York: Chelsea House Publishers.

Leininger, M. (2002). *Japanese Americans and culture care.* In M. Leininger & M. R. McFarland (Eds.), *Transcultural nursing: Concepts, theories, research and practice* (3rd ed.) (pp. 453–464). New York: McGraw-Hill/Appleton & Lange.

Leong, Y. M. (2003). Japanese. In P. St. Hill, J. G. Lipson, & A. I. Meleis (Eds.), *Caring for women cross-culturally* (pp. 188–201). Philadelphia: F. A. Davis.

AUTHORS

Gayle Shiba, RN, MS, DNSc, is an associate professor at the University of Memphis Loewenberg School of Nursing in Tennessee, where she teaches in the undergraduate and graduate nursing programs. Her research interests are symptom occurrence and symptom management of patients with head and neck cancer. She is a third-generation Japanese American whose grandparents emigrated to the U.S. in the early 1900s from Japan and whose parents were relocated during World War II.

Yuko Matsumoto Leong, RN, MS, is a public health nurse for the City of Berkeley, CA. She was a nurse-midwife and an instructor of maternal nursing in Japan. Her primary interests are the transitional experiences of immigrant women who married American men and the experience of their children in such households. She immigrated in 1980 and married a fourth-generation Chinese American.

Roberta Oka, RN, ANP, DNSc, is an assistant professor in the University of California-San Francisco School of Nursing. Her research interests are risk-factor modification and vascular biology in various populations. Born and raised in Hawaii, she is a third-generation (*Sansei*) Japanese American.

CHAPTER 24

KOREANS

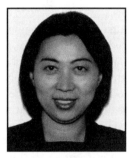

Eun-Ok Im

CULTURAL/ETHNIC IDENTITY

- **Preferred term(s)**. Korean (*Han-Kuk Yin* or *Han-Kuk Saram*) or Korean American (*Jae-Mi Kyo-Po*). Korean Americans maintain a strong ethnic identity.
- **Census**. The 2000 U.S. Census estimated a population of more than 1 million. Between 1990 and 2000, 60% were foreign-born. Koreans are dispersed throughout the U.S., but the largest Korean community (with more than 20% of the total) is in Los Angeles County. New York City also has a large population.
- **History of immigration**. Began in 1903. By 1905, when the Korean government prohibited further emigration, there were 10,000 Koreans in Hawaii and 1,000 on the mainland. The U.S. Immigration Act of 1924 halted further immigration until the law was amended in 1965, after which most immigration occurred. Between 1970–80, the number of Koreans in the U.S. increased to 354,529 from 70,000. Between 1990 and 2000, the population grew another 35%.

SPIRITUAL/RELIGIOUS ORIENTATION

- **Primary religious/spiritual affiliations**. Korean culture mingles Shamanism, Taoism, Confucianism, Buddhism, and Christianity. Shamanism (spirit worship) was practiced before the other religions and still influences some Koreans today. About 85% of Koreans in U.S. are Christian and regularly attend Protestant or Catholic churches.
- **Usual religious/spiritual practices**. Confucian and Buddhist traditions combined with Shamanism prevail, including a mixture of faiths within households. Buddhists may chant, Christians may pray, and Shamanists may

chant and place a talisman or amulet in a secret place around the patient (e.g., under the pillow or in his/her underwear).

- **Use of spiritual healing/healers**. Koreans may hire a *moodang* to discover the cause of an evil spirit and how to get rid of it. Christian prayer healing is prevalent among Koreans.
- **Holidays**. Traditional holidays that first-generation and older immigrants in U.S may celebrate include New Year's Eve, Lunar New Year's Day, Fifth Day of the Fifth Month, and Seventh Day of the Seventh Month. Traditionally, women went to the well at dawn on New Year's Eve day to be the first to draw "lucky water," then prepared the feast for the next day. The family settled outstanding debts by midnight and stayed awake after midnight to prevent their eyebrows from "turning white." On Lunar New Year's Day (*Seollal*), most families visit husband's family. Children perform the New Year's bow (*sebae*) in front of all the elders and wish them good fortune (*bok*) in the coming year; children are rewarded with good advice and money. Families play traditional Korean games, such as a four-stick board game (*yunnori*), and participate in tug-of-war, kite-flying, and see-sawing. They eat a soup containing slices of rice cake (*tteokguk*), which symbolizes getting one year older. Families offer food and drink to ancestors. Korean age is calculated based on *Seollal*, not on one's date of birth, although birth date is celebrated. The Fifth Day of the Month, or "Double Five" (*Dano*), welcomes the beginning of summer and involves memorial rites for ancestors. Traditionally, women gathered herbs and washed their hair in water in which iris roots had been boiled. *Dano* was the one day of the year that married women were free to visit their own families. Regarding the Seventh Day of the Seventh Month (*Chilseok*), legend holds that the Vega and Altair stars are the celestial reincarnations of two lovers, Herd Boy (*Gyeonu*) and Weaving Maiden (*Jiknyeo*), who meet only once a year. Koreans believe that it usually rains on this day because the two lovers cry when they meet. Foods included rice cakes, zucchini pancakes, noodles, and pickled cucumber (*kimchi*). On Korean Thanksgiving Day (*Chuseok*), families again visit the husband's family to celebrate a good harvest. In the past, families received new clothes, but today they dress up in Korean traditional clothes (*hanbok*). People pay respects to their ancestors with rice wine, half-moon-shaped rice cakes (*song-pyeon*), and newly harvested fruits and grains, such as persimmons, apples, Korean pears, and chestnuts.

COMMUNICATION
ORAL COMMUNICATION

- **Major languages and dialects**. The major language, Hangeul, is thought to be one of the most scientific and efficient in the world, with 14 consonants and 10 vowels. It contains some words of Chinese and Japanese origin.

Vocabulary and verb endings reflect the status relationship between speakers. There is one written language but several dialects as a result of geographical differences. Because North Korea has been separated from South Korea since 1950, the oral languages have developed differently.

- **Greetings**. Correct etiquette important. Persons address each other using "Mr.," "Mrs.," or "Ms." and last name unless they are relatives or close friends. Show respect for elders and authority figures by quarter-bowing quickly. Highly respect medical doctors but have mixed feelings about nurses because, in the old days, nurses were novice doctors' assistants and did not have a formal nursing education.
- **Tone of voice**. In standard Korean language, tone is very flat. But it varies among regional dialects. For example, in Kyung-sang-do province, people speak in a wide variety of pitches and use loudness to emphasize something important, while in Choong-chung-do province, they speak in a very slow and flat tone of voice. Korean Americans raise their voice when they want to emphasize something or are excited or upset.
- **Direct or indirect style of speech**. Prefer indirect style because they perceive direct indications of intention or opinions as rude. Agree with health care provider in order to avoid conflict or hurting someone's feelings even if request is impossible to comply with. Important for others to "read between the lines." Koreans growing up in U.S. may adopt the dominant American communication style.
- **Use of interpreters**. Patients frequently need an interpreter and help filling out forms. Family members often accompany children, women, and elderly persons to health care encounters to assist. Clinician should use family members as much as possible because it makes patient feel more comfortable. Gender of interpreter might affect answers to health/illness problems regarding sexual organs.
- **Serious or terminal illness**. Hesitant to talk about death. Clinician should inform family, preferably the head of the household, of the diagnosis or prognosis, and family will then inform patient.

WRITTEN COMMUNICATION

- **Literacy assessment**. Immigrants have acculturated slowly; very few use English at home. About half have difficulty with English and do not read American printed media. Language is a major barrier to health care access. Elderly immigrants may have very limited or no English skills. However, ability to speak English does not necessarily equate with Koreans' ability to read and write in English. Although direct communication is not usually appropriate, clinician must directly ask patients or family if they understand what he/she is telling them.
- **Consents**. Clinician should explain procedures in a clear and understandable manner, and give patient time to think or review. Because Koreans

respect and trust health care providers, they tend to give consent without an adequate understanding of procedures, side effects, and/or complications. Thus, it is important not to rush or pressure them.

NONVERBAL COMMUNICATION

- **Eye contact**. Avoid direct eye contact out of respect for older persons and authority figures, including health care providers. May avoid direct eye contact with strangers. Women may avoid direct eye contact with men out of modesty. Younger persons educated in U.S. may adopt the dominant-culture communication style of eye contact.
- **Personal space**. Share close personal space (less than 1 foot) with family members and close friends. Inappropriate for strangers to step into "intimate space" unless necessary for health care.
- **Use and meaning of silence**. Traditionally, Koreans emphasized silence as a virtue of educated persons. Even among Korean Americans, those who are silent (especially men) are viewed as humble and well-educated.
- **Gestures**. Rarely use gestures to communicate nonverbally. Using a finger or a foot to direct a person is rude.
- **Openness in expressing emotions**. Do not express emotions directly or in public. Especially among men, expressing emotions in front of others, including family members, causes shame. A common belief is that men should cry only three times in their lives: when they are born, when their parents die, and when their country perishes.
- **Privacy**. Pride and shame prevalent. Trust must be established for patients to reveal personal or pertinent information; are reluctant to disclose information if they feel embarrassed. Health care providers should be sensitive to their own and patient's words and facial expressions when explaining some aspect of care or diagnosis. Clinicians may consider an issue to be nonprivate, but Koreans may consider it to be very private.
- **Touch**. Touching, friendly pushing, and hugging acceptable among family members and close friends. Among strangers, however, touching is disrespectful unless necessary for care.
- **Orientation to time**. Generally clock-oriented, but conception of time depends on circumstances. Koreans recognize that punctuality is necessary for clinical appointments and work. They tend not to be punctual for informal gatherings, and joke about arriving at parties and visiting family or friends within 30 minutes of the agreed-upon time. Many are future-oriented, which is related to Koreans' belief in karma.

ACTIVITIES OF DAILY LIVING

- **Modesty**. Very modest, especially women. Many women do not participate in breast cancer screening because of modesty. Women are much more comfortable with female health care providers, particularly for ob/gyn problems.

Health care staff should provide robes and pajama pants for both men and women.

- **Skin care**. Tend to be very clean; do not like to feel dirty. A common practice is to rub skin with rough cloth while bathing to help exfoliate dead skin. Many women use lotions, moisturizers, and nourishing creams to protect their skin.
- **Hair care**. Many older women do not shampoo daily; they may wash hair only once or twice a week. Younger men and women shampoo daily and use hair gels or creams.
- **Nail care**. Prefer very clean and well-trimmed nails, especially first-generation Koreans. Frequently trim nails, even out nail breaks, and remove hangnails. Nail care among second generation and younger women similar to that in dominant culture. Men only trim nails.
- **Toileting**. Prefer bathroom for privacy. Clinician must ensure privacy for patients who use commode or bedpan, especially when clinician is of opposite gender.
- **Special clothing or amulets**. On traditional holidays and special occasions, wear traditional Korean clothes (*hanbok*). Normally, Koreans wear minimal jewelry, which signals wealth. Some Christians wear crucifix and some Buddhists wear prayer beads around their neck for use in chanting.
- **Self-care**. Younger patients perform their own hygiene. Family members care for older patients, a duty of children generally. Caregiving is a female responsibility.

FOOD PRACTICES

- **Usual meal pattern**. Three meals a day. Dinner is main meal, a time that most family members spend together.
- **Special utensils**. Chopsticks and spoons.
- **Food beliefs and rituals**. Do not usually welcome cold fluids, such as iced beverages. Associate cold with an imbalance of *um* (*yin*—related to cold) and *yang* (related to hot) that may result in illness.
- **Usual diet**. High in fiber and spicy, consisting primarily of rice, tofu (bean curd), vegetables, seafood, lean meats, and pickled vegetables (*kimchi*). Many meals consist of soups or broth prepared with lots of vegetables, noodles, and small portions of meat.
- **Fluids**. Older Koreans do not like water directly from tap, fearing contamination, so many boil dried corn in water to purify it, then store the water in refrigerator before drinking it. Many drink bottled water.
- **Food taboos and prescriptions**. Rarely consume dairy products; many Koreans are lactose intolerant. May treat someone who has a "hot" condition with "cold" foods, such as bean curd, cold noodles, or crab. A "cold" condition requires "hot" foods, such as ginger, peppers, or onions. Commonly use ginseng to increase vital energy (*ki*) and promote health. There

are specific instructions for food consumed during pregnancy (see below).
- **Hospitality**. Provide food and drink to guests. Even when guest is already full, he/she is expected to eat at least a small amount as gratitude for hospitality.

SYMPTOM MANAGEMENT

- **Pain** (*ah-poom nida*; *jook-get-so* or *jook-get-da* means "killing pain"). Tend to be stoic regarding pain. Perceive complaints about pain as a sign of impatience. Women tend to describe pain in detail. Men tend not to report pain and do not verbalize it. Koreans do not often take pain medications for fear of addiction or complications, or due to limited financial resources. Prefer oral and IV routes rather than intramuscular, which they view as invasive.
- **Dyspnea** (*soomi-chap-nida* means shortness of breath or dyspnea). Frightening for Koreans; perceive shortness of breath or dyspnea as a sign of serious disease. May not welcome oxygen, fearing that they have progressive disease or that their condition is worsening.
- **Nausea/vomiting** (*to-ha-gue-seub-nida* means nausea and feeling like one will vomit soon). Many do not tell health care providers before they vomit, due to embarrassment or desire to vomit in private.
- **Constipation/diarrhea** (*byun-bi/sul-sa*). Due to modesty, patients may not inform health care providers unless condition is severe. May take medications to assist with defecation. Prefer oral medications to enemas or suppositories.
- **Fatigue** (*pee-lo-hab-nida* and *pee-kon-hab-nida*). May not report fatigue, although may avoid daily activities and ambulation, and nap frequently. Do not want to take medication for fatigue.
- **Depression** (*chim-ool-hab-nida* and *woo-wool-hab-nida*). Because of stigma attached to mental illness and/or mental health problems in Korean culture, may not reveal depression unless asked. Even when Koreans acknowledge and report depression, they may be hesitant to use antidepressants.
- **Self-care symptom management**. May delay seeking health care until symptoms are severe. May choose herbal and/or folk remedies for symptom management first.

BIRTH RITUALS/CARE OF THE NEW MOTHER AND BABY

- **Pregnancy care**. Practice standard prenatal care in first trimester. However, pregnant women maintain their cultural values, attitudes, and practices in pregnancy. Many place great importance on following exactly what health care providers recommend. Pregnancy is an important and welcomed family event, accompanied by practices to ensure a healthy baby. Although pregnancy taboos protect the woman from danger, they may also keep her from getting essential nutrients or isolate and depress her. Folk beliefs prescribe or prohibit specific foods during pregnancy. Primigravidas may avoid eating as many as 20 different foods. Koreans may believe that duck, rabbit, eggs, and crab affect infant's appearance or character. Seaweed soup is good for anemia and bleeding. A pregnant woman's and/or relative's conception dream (*tae mong*) predetermines the baby's future.

- **Preferences for children**. Koreans in U.S. and South Korea openly acknowledge their preference for sons. Regard first son as a continuation of family lineage. Once the family has a son, it welcomes the first-born daughter as an important household resource. If a family has limited resources, it may provide health care for sons rather than daughters, and for husbands rather than wives.

- **Labor practices**. Any female family member can be a birth attendant. In recent years, husbands have been encouraged to participate, contrary to their minimal involvement in the past. With introduction of Western biomedicine in Korea, babies usually are delivered in hospitals by health care professionals. Koreans may view pain control during delivery as potentially harmful to baby.

- **Role of the laboring woman during birth**. In the past, women were expected to be strong and to tolerate labor passively under the worst circumstances. Today, they are encouraged to be more active. They often vocalize during contractions, although older in-laws or family members may discourage shouting or crying out, believing that it shows aggressiveness.

- **Role of the father and other family members during birth**. Traditionally, male family members were not involved. Today, fathers are as actively involved as their counterparts in dominant culture. Female family members usually help with preparations and postpartum care of mother and baby.

- **Vaginal vs. cesarean section**. Women prefer vaginal delivery but choose whichever method will reduce negative health outcomes for infant. Recently in South Korea, some women have been opting for cesareans so they can select the exact date and time of birth, based on the belief that the birth date, hour, and minute determine baby's destiny.

- **Breastfeeding**. At one time, Korean women breastfed exclusively. After Western medicine was introduced, they began to bottle-feed. In recent years, bottle-feeding has become the preferred practice, especially among working women. Most Korean American women are working mothers who do not favor breastfeeding. When they do choose to breastfeed, they must be taught ways to incorporate feedings into their everyday activities and/or how to keep pumped breast milk fresh and safe for baby.

- **Birth recuperation**. Traditionally, expected new mothers to stay in bed for 21 days, not bathe, and eat lots of seaweed soup. Postpartum women are protected from exposure to cold air, water, and foods; usually do not bathe for several weeks to prevent exposure. Female family members provide care. Typical postpartum recuperation is 6–8 weeks, but new mothers rarely stay in bed now because of economic pressures.

- **Baby care**. Family protects newborn by allowing only close relatives to visit. Mothers tend to view infants as passive and dependent, and do not encourage autonomy. Mothering is molded more by rituals and societal rules than by individual desire or choice. Women often seek family or folk information about infant care rather than professional advice.

- **Problems with baby**. Clinician should inform head of family first (e.g., father) as soon as diagnosis or illness is noted. Korean mothers may blame themselves, attributing the problem to improper behavior during pregnancy. Clinician should reassure her and family members that no one is to blame.
- **Male and female circumcision**. Traditionally, neither males nor females were circumcised. Modern Koreans and Korean Americans usually have male babies circumcised after weighing the pros and cons.

DEVELOPMENTAL AND SEXUAL ISSUES

- **Celebration of menarche or becoming a man**. No special rituals.
- **Attitudes about birth control**. Women responsible for contraception. When it fails, pregnancy is woman's responsibility. Most women use Western biomedical methods, including pills for convenience, intrauterine devices, or tubal ligation. Male partner plays an important role in deciding number and spacing of children, but he rarely determines type or use of contraception.
- **Attitudes about sexually transmitted infection (STI) control, including condoms**. STI stigmatizes a person and his/her family. Thus, STIs usually are kept secret even among family members, which makes it is difficult to determine STI prevalence. Despite the stigma, STIs in men are relatively acceptable because their extramarital sexual relationships are much more tolerated than women's are. Men usually do not use condoms. HIV/AIDS education programs have persuaded younger persons to start using condoms, but more education is necessary.
- **Attitudes about abortion**. Since 1973, when South Korea legalized abortion, it has become widespread and available for a moderate price at most private ob/gyn clinics. Korean American women tend to have a positive attitude about abortion; it is a procedure to be used when necessary. Women may perceive abortion as similar to menstrual periods; some immediately resume their usual activities after abortion without complaint, although they may feel guilty. Some upper-class or middle-class women believe that abortion affects the body in a manner similar to that of childbirth, so they may take postpartum measures, such as rest, eating seaweed soup, and covering their body for warmth.
- **Attitudes about unwed sexual experimentation**. Virginity important. Sexual activities and pregnancy at puberty stigmatize the family, regardless of social class. Some young persons experiment before marriage but never tell their parents. They might tell a close friend or sibling in secret, but in general, talking about sexuality, contraception, or pregnancy in public is taboo. Other young persons do not talk about sexuality because their parents strongly emphasized modesty in upbringing.

- **Sexual orientation**. Korean families do not accept sexual minorities. Gay men especially are a disappointment to their parents, who expect sons to continue the family lineage.
- **Gender identity**. Korean families typically do not accept a member whose gender identity is ambiguous or opposite to his/her birth gender. Most families are not pleased with very masculine girls or very feminine boys.
- **Attitudes about menopause**. Korean women tend to view menopause more positively than Western women do—as a normal developmental process that does not require special coping mechanisms. Korean women report lower levels of hot flashes, dizziness, and night sweats than Western women do.

FAMILY RELATIONSHIPS
- **Composition/structure**. Families are both nuclear and extended; three-generation households not uncommon. Filial piety and family loyalty very important. One gains self-esteem through family identification, family honors, and approval from other community members.
- **Decision-making**. In traditional patriarchal culture, the head of the household made decisions. Today, decision-making is more family-focused, although husband/father or eldest son may have more authority. Studies show that Korean patriarchal culture still is alive among first-generation families. Second-generation families may adopt American styles of decision-making.
- **Spokesperson**. Husband, father, or eldest son/daughter.
- **Gender issues**. Traditional patriarchal and Confucian norms subordinated women and wives, who were confined to home and bore major responsibility for household tasks. Husband was breadwinner and did not share in household tasks. Wives tended to be physically overloaded and psychologically distressed; exploitation was hidden under Confucian norms that praise women who sacrifice themselves for family and nation. This tradition persists among Korean Americans, despite women's financial contributions to family. Husbands still occupy center stage, exercise authority, and make major family decisions. They expect their wives to work full-time outside the home and also handle housekeeping and child-rearing. In recent years, some women have broken away from male domination by divorcing and marrying non-Koreans or by remaining single and pursuing a professional career. Most women, however, quietly endure without complaining, for the sake of family and the future of their children.
- **Changing roles among generations in U.S.** Women hold the family together and are dedicated to the welfare of their husbands and children. They may work 10–15 hours a day, seven days a week and play a vital role in family's and community's economic base. Second-generation Koreans born and raised in U.S. tend to adopt norms of dominant culture. For example, they may not respect the elderly as much as the older generation does, and some women refuse to sacrifice themselves for family.

- **Caring roles**. Women responsible for bedside care. Mothers responsible for care of their children, and daughters-in-law for care of mothers- and fathers-in-law.
- **Expectations of and for children**. Most families set extremely high standards for, and have high expectations of, children. "Giving a whip to a beloved child" is the philosophy behind discipline. Rear children to be obedient and orderly, especially outside the home. Do not promote early independence; family is most important. Primary goal is education; college education is a must.
- **Expectations of and for elders**. Confucianism emphasizes respect for the elderly and familial bonds. Caring for elderly kin is the family's customary duty. Koreans treat elders with utmost respect. Elders are welcome to live with family for duration of their lives. Grandparents frequently care for grandchildren while parents work. If family cannot care for elder at home, he/she may be placed in nursing home, which is less desirable.
- **Expectations of hospital visitors**. Nonfamily visitors frequently come to see patient out of respect, especially if he/she is older. When family members care for hospitalized patient, they want to stay with him/her. They bring in Korean foods and feed patient.

ILLNESS BELIEFS

- **Causes of/attitudes about physical illness**. Traditionally view physical illness as an imbalance between *yin* (*um*) and *yang*, and as an imbalanced state of *ki* (*ch'i*, or life energy). Shamanism and Buddhism may influence beliefs. For example, some Koreans believe that illness is a result of bad luck or misfortune, and others that it is a consequence of having done something wrong in the past (karma). Such patients may be resigned to physical illness and feel helpless or depressed, believing that they cannot change the course of luck. Others attribute illness to restless ancestors or ghosts.
- **Causes of/attitudes about mental illness**. View it as a disruption of the spiritual self. Mental illness stigmatized, such that when family members are asked about a relative's mental disorder, they may downplay the extent of the illness to save face. May use traditional healing modes, such as Shamanism.
- **Causes of genetic defects**. Traditionally viewed as payback for something ancestors did wrong. Today, many Koreans acknowledge familial genetic influence. Parents may feel responsible for their children's genetic defects. Some favor caring for child at home, others favor institutionalization.
- **Attitudes about disabilities**. Traditionally viewed birth disability as punishment for ancestors' sins, as shameful for family. Also viewed disability caused by accident as a family's misfortune; disabled persons were ridiculed in public. Negative attitudes have since moderated, but many Koreans still consider disability to be a family stigma.
- **Sick role**. Expect patients to be passive and "act like a patient." Family

members meet patient's basic needs and actively participate in his/her care.

- **Home and folk remedies**. Shamanistic approach is based on the belief that restless ancestors, ghosts, and angry household gods bring home afflictions, such as illness, financial loss, and domestic strife. It attempts to cure illness attributed to hovering ghosts with a simple exorcism to drive them away and clean the body of illness. Traditional Korean medicine (*hanbang*) includes four common treatments: acupuncture (*chi'm*), herbal medicine (*hanyak*), moxabustion (*d'um*), and "cupping" (*buhwang*). Some herbal remedies have toxic elements or interact with pharmaceuticals.

- **Medications**. Immigrants tend to self-treat as much as possible to save money. Older persons are likely to try folk remedies or Korean traditional medicine before seeking Western medical help. Often combine folk remedies with Western medications, which usually are acceptable, although compliance varies. Sharing medications acceptable and common. Some Koreans reduce dose or frequency, believing that American medications are too strong for them. Tend to stop medicating when immediate symptoms are alleviated. Some prefer imported Korean medications, claiming that they are made for Koreans and therefore best.

- **Acceptance of procedures**. Koreans respect health care providers and accept suggested procedures, even when they do not fully understand them or do not agree. Elderly may fear drawing of blood as removing life energy (*ki*). Clinician should double-check patient's understanding of procedure. Family members need to be involved in decision-making. There are no cultural objections to blood transfusions, but Korean Jehovah's Witnesses do not allow them.

- **Care-seeking**. Koreans take a pluralistic approach to health care. May use Western biomedicine, traditional medicine, and Shamanism. The combination of, and emphasis on, these approaches vary by age, gender, education, socioeconomic status, and acculturation.

HEALTH ISSUES

- **Concept of health**. Traditionally, good health is a result of harmonious relationships in the human and supernatural worlds, and in the universe at large. The key is maintaining vital energy (*ki*) and balance in all aspects of one's life. Balancing *yin* (*um*) and *yang* in diet and other areas of life is particularly important for avoiding illness. Koreans still view health holistically, as a balanced state in all aspects of life.

- **Health promotion and prevention**. Balancing all aspects of one's life promotes and maintains health. Korean diet includes rice, vegetables, fruit, lean meats, and bean curd, although there is a lot of sodium in foods such as pickled vegetables (*kimchi*), hot sauces, and soy sauce. Vigorous exercise popular among younger generation; older generation frequently walks to promote health.

- **Screening**. Accept screening if it is thoroughly explained. Women more likely to accept breast cancer screening and Pap smear if female clinician does the procedure.

- **Common health problems**. Stomach cancer, liver cancer, and stroke are most common, but there are also high rates of hypertension, lactose intolerance, dental problems, and stomach ulcers. Less heart disease and breast cancer than in larger U.S. population.

DEATH RITUALS

- **Beliefs and attitudes about death**. Although Koreans are hesitant to talk about death, they consider a peaceful death to be one of life's five blessings (the others are longevity, wealth, health, and virtue). Peaceful death places no undue emotional burden on children. Traditionally, the death of unwed men, women, or children is considered shameful; they are regarded as undutiful children because their death renders them unavailable to care for parents as they age. A mixture of Shamanism, Confucianism, Buddhism, and Christianity influences attitudes about death. Christians believe that the dead go to heaven or hell, and Buddhists that the dead will be reborn. According to Shamanism, and depending on the individual or circumstances of death, souls either wander the earth and possibly harm survivors, or settle down in heaven. Traditionally, bodies were buried intact so the dead would rest peacefully; if bodies of ancestors were damaged in any way, misfortune would befall descendants.
- **Preparation**. Clinician should tell head of family first about imminent death, who will then relay the information to family. Family unites and prepares for death by ordering a coffin and white clothes for the patient, preparing white clothes and pins for family members for the funeral and mourning, and arranging funeral services at a church and/or burial ground.
- **Home vs. hospital**. Family may prefer to move patient home before death due to traditional belief that when someone dies outside the home, his/her ghost will wander. Some choose to have patient remain in hospital if family members must work and cannot provide 24-hour care.
- **Special needs**. Some families chant, pray, burn incense, or observe other mourning traditions. Spouse and family members wear white clothes and white pins for 100 days after the death.
- **Care of the body**. Family may want to spend time with the deceased and may request that the body be cleansed. Some Koreans associate cremation with destroying the dead person's soul or spirit. However, cremation is increasing in South Korea because of limited land space. Cremation rare among Korean Americans, except for those who have no family or who die at a young age.
- **Attitudes about organ donation**. Typically negative; family may refuse. View organ donation as tampering with the body, soul, and spirit.
- **Attitudes about autopsy**. Family usually refuses. May consider autopsy in cases of sudden death.

SELECTED REFERENCES

Im, E. O. (2002). Korean culture. In P. St. Hill, J. Lipson, & A. Meleis (Eds.), *Caring for women cross-culturally: A portable guide*. Philadelphia: F. A. Davis.

Kim, Y., & Grant, D. (1997). Immigration patterns, social support, and adaptation among Korean immigrant women and Korean American women. *Cultural Diversity in Mental Health*, 3, 235–245.

Martinson, I. M. (1998). Funeral rituals in Taiwan and Korea. *Oncology Nursing Forum*, 25, 1756–1760.

AUTHOR

Eun-Ok Im, PhD, MPH, is an associate professor at the University of Texas at Austin. She was born and raised in South Korea, and moved to the U.S. to study. She received her PhD in nursing from the University of California-San Francisco in 1997 and did postdoctoral study there. Her primary research interests and expertise are feminist and international/cross-cultural approaches to women's health issues, including menopause, cancer pain, and breast cancer. She has developed a number of computer programs for the health care of culturally diverse groups of women.

CHAPTER 25

MEXICANS

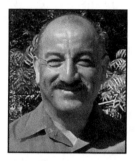

Peter Andrew Guarnero

CULTURAL/ETHNIC IDENTITY

- **Preferred term(s)**. Acculturated Mexican Americans may prefer American. Militant persons favor *Chicano(a)*, *Raza*, or *Mexicano(a)*. Recent arrivals prefer *Mexicano(a)*. Indigenous peoples may prefer their tribal name.
- **Census**. The 2000 U.S. Census estimates a Mexican population of more than 20.6 million. It does not distinguish between the foreign-born and those born in the U.S. People of Mexican origin account for 58.7% of the Hispanic/*Latino* population. These figures do not include undocumented persons, among whom Mexicans are the largest ethnic group. The largest numbers are in California, Texas, Illinois, and Arizona.
- **History of immigration**. The Spanish settled in the Southwest in 1598, but Mexico lost its land north of the Rio Grande River to the U.S. in the Mexican-American War (1846–48). Mexicans have a long history of migration; they crossed the border in both directions. The first documented influx of immigrants (1900–30)—the so-called Great Migration—was spurred by political upheaval in Mexico and economic opportunities in the southwestern U.S. The Depression created anti-immigration sentiment, increased racism and discrimination, and resulted in government-initiated massive deportations, which at times included U.S. citizens. The Bracero Program, which recruited Mexican workers to fill agricultural jobs, began during World War II when many American men enlisted. But lawmakers let the program expire because of growing anti-immigrant pressure. Despite poor working conditions, the influx of undocumented immigrants continued. More recently, there has been an increase in immigration of men, women, and children as a result of economic depression and upheaval in Mexico, especially the devaluation of the peso in the late 1970s.

SPIRITUAL/RELIGIOUS ORIENTATION

- **Primary religious/spiritual affiliations**. Most are Roman Catholic, but Protestant and Pentecostal missionaries have converted many Mexicans in recent years. Traditional men view religious practices as a preoccupation of women. More-acculturated persons tend not to attend church services regularly and may engage in New Age practices, such as channeling, yoga, or Eastern mysticism.

- **Usual religious/spiritual practices**. Traditional persons light candles; attend church; pray to God, Jesus, the Virgin Mary, and the saints; and hold baptisms and confirmations. Families may pray together. May visit shrines throughout Mexico dedicated to the Virgin Mary (e.g., *La Virgen de San Juan de los Lagos* in Guadalajara). May have home shrines. Protestant and Evangelical church services focus on Bible or sacred scriptures that may have special healing power.

- **Use of spiritual healing/healers**. Traditional persons may consult a folk healer (*curandero*) or spiritualist (*espirituista*). *Curanderos* usually are located in private homes. Mexicans consult them regarding a variety of ailments and life situations. Some Mexicans visit a health care provider and a *curandero* simultaneously. They may consult a *curandero* instead of a biomedical professional because they lack insurance or access to care. Some traditional faith healers are willing to work with health care professionals in treating patients.

- **Holidays**. Many celebrate *Cinco de Mayo* (May 5), although in Mexico, Independence Day (September 16) is more important. American entrepreneurs promote *Cinco de Mayo*. Mexicans also celebrate regional holidays. Catholics celebrate Ash Wednesday, Palm Sunday, Good Friday, Easter Sunday, and *Virgen de Guadalupe* (December 12). Holidays vary among Protestants and Pentecostals.

COMMUNICATION

ORAL COMMUNICATION

- **Major languages and dialects**. Acculturated persons often speak only English, but some speak Chicano Spanish. Recent arrivals prefer Spanish, although many attempt to learn English for occupational advancement. Recent immigrant children struggle to learn English in school, but once they master English, they prefer to speak it. Many are bilingual. Mexico has 62 living languages. Many recent arrivals are indigenous persons from central and southern Mexico who speak Spanish but cannot read or write it.

- **Greetings**. Traditional persons prefer the formal "you" (*usted*) rather than the informal *tu* when addressing an elder, professional, or senior family member. Clinician should politely ask patient how he/she prefers to be addressed. Handshake appropriate at first meeting. More intimate friends greet each other with an embrace/hug (*abrazo*). Many women greet each other with a light kiss on each cheek. As a gesture of respect, patient and his/her family may stand when clinician enters room.

- **Tone of voice**. Consider loudness to be rude and inappropriate when addressing someone. Shouting may cause patient to disengage and not follow through with treatment regimen. Commands and/or requests should be in a nonconfrontational tone of voice—for example, "I want to ask you a favor" or "It is necessary that you follow the prescription I am going to give you" (*Es necesario que sega usted la recita que le voy a dar*). Loud, friendly banter between family and friends common. Depending on circumstances, Mexicans address children in a loud, firm voice for discipline.
- **Direct or indirect style of speech**. May preface a conversation with a story or small talk to lessen the tension and get a sense of clinician's style of relating. Tend to be tactful and diplomatic, and indirect rather than blunt, with health care providers. May agree with a suggestion or prescription simply out of courtesy.
- **Use of interpreters**. Clinician should avoid using a relative as interpreter because it may put the relative in a compromising position of learning information the patient does not want to share. Interpreter should be someone who understands regional differences in Spanish language and who is of same gender as patient and also about the same age.
- **Serious or terminal illness**. Clinician should inform patient and family together and as soon as possible about serious or terminal illness. Should also ask patient who should be included in the discussion.

WRITTEN COMMUNICATION

- **Literacy assessment**. Recent arrivals may have only a fifth- or sixth-grade education. Some Mexican nationals cannot read or write in Spanish. Appropriate for clinician to ask patient directly if he/she can read and write in Spanish and/or English. Most Mexican Americans can read and write in English.
- **Consents**. Undocumented immigrants tend to be suspicious of any type of consent, especially written consent. May fear they are signing away their rights and will be deported. Consent forms should be written at a fifth-grade level in Spanish and procedures should be explained in simple Spanish. Hispanic/*Latino* health care provider may be helpful in obtaining consent. Many Mexicans unfamiliar with how research is conducted. A clear, concise explanation of a research project should accompany consent.

NONVERBAL COMMUNICATION

- **Eye contact**. May interpret staring as a challenge or intimidation. Gazing into another's eyes indicates a high degree of familiarity and is reserved for intimate relationships. Clinician might consider looking at something behind patient while conversing in a warm but respectful manner. Mexicans avoid sustained eye contact with authority figures and opposite gender.

- **Personal space**. Depends on context and relationship. Many value intimate space (up to 18 inches), but this varies by kinship and level of assimilation. May prefer to keep an appropriate social distance (9–12 feet), especially with strangers.
- **Use and meaning of silence**. May indicate disapproval, disappointment,
  or anger. Also may suggest politeness, deference, or not understanding.
- **Gestures**. Handshake appropriate, especially between strangers. Usually
  reserve hug (*abrazo*) for close relatives or friends. Clinician should avoid gestures that might be misinterpreted. Impolite to point finger or use index finger to signal "come here." Standing with hands on hips suggests hostility.
- **Openness in expressing emotions**. Varies by level of acculturation,
  assimilation, education, and social class. Persons who are more acculturated,
  have more education, and come from a higher social class are less expressive;
  they subdue their emotions and maintain control. Women tend to express
  emotion more than men do and may use dramatic body language.
- **Privacy**. Usually share information about illness with spouse, children, and
  selected members of extended family. Do not usually share family problems/
  conflicts with persons outside the family. Do not spontaneously reveal to
  health care providers their use of home remedies or folk healers/spiritualists.
- **Touch**. Generally enjoy touching family members and close friends but may
  find it uncomfortable to touch, or be touched by, strangers. Clinician should
  inform, and seek permission from, patient before touching any area of
  his/her body, especially an intimate area.
- **Orientation to time**. Usually focused on the here and now; leave the future
  in God's hands. Time is often flexible; may arrive late for an appointment
  because there was an important family matter. Acculturated and educated
  persons understand the need to be on time, especially for work and health
  care appointments.

ACTIVITIES OF DAILY LIVING
- **Modesty**. Greatly valued. Most Mexicans uncomfortable exposing their
  bodies to someone of opposite gender. Men and women may prefer clinician
  of same gender. Clinician should avoid unnecessary exposure or disrobing of
  patient. Should offer a blanket to cover his/her lower extremities.
- **Skin care**. Usually take daily baths or showers. Make every effort to remain
  very clean, especially when ill. May like soothing lotions on all extremities.
- **Hair care**. Customs vary. Some women prefer long hair so they can have
  braids (*trenzas*), while others prefer current hair styles. Wash hair daily with
  regular shampoo. Some men and women use brilliantine on their hair.
- **Nail care**. Varies as in dominant culture. More-affluent or acculturated persons may have regular manicures and pedicures. Many do not pay attention
  to foot care. Diabetics need thorough education on foot care.
- **Toileting**. Practices vary depending on level of affluence and acculturation.

Toileting is a private matter that Mexicans cannot easily discuss with persons they do not know well. Clinician should respect patient's modesty by providing privacy if bedpan or commode is necessary.

- **Special clothing or amulets**. Vary widely. Include crucifixes, scapulars, and religious medals. Clinician should handle amulet respectfully and, if removal is necessary, give it to family member for safe-keeping.
- **Self-care**. Generally expect hospital staff to help with self-care. May also wait for family members to arrive and help with care. At home, patient may try to be self-sufficient, especially if he/she perceives care as a burden on others.

FOOD PRACTICES

- **Usual meal pattern**. Varies depending on acculturation level. Most have a big meal at lunch and a lighter meal in the evening with nuclear family or extended family, including grandparents, uncles, aunts, and cousins. However, there is a growing tendency among Mexicans to eat fast food or meals on the go.
- **Special utensils**. None.
- **Food beliefs and rituals**. Traditional persons believe in "hot"/"cold" foods, preserving health through balancing "hot" and "cold," or treating a "cold" illness with "hot" foods. Examples of hot foods include chocolate, eggs, oil, red meat, chilies, and onions. Cold foods include fresh vegetables and tropical fruits, dairy products, and fish or chicken.
- **Usual diet**. Traditional foods include rice, beans, meat, chicken, and corn and flour tortillas. Prepare some traditional foods with lard, but this practice has decreased as Mexicans learn about the need to limit fat in food preparation. Snacks include Mexican sweet bread and pastries. Acculturated persons eat a wide range of foods.
- **Fluids**. Prefer cool drinks in summer, especially fruit juices. More-traditional persons like fresh-fruit coolers (*aguas frescas*), particularly cantaloupe (*agua de melon*), watermelon (*agua de sandia*), and tamarind (*agua de tamarindo*), available in many *taquerias* and restaurants. Like coffee with breakfast, hot chocolate on special occasions. Men, especially, consume lots of alcohol. Clinician must encourage patients to drink more water.
- **Food taboos and prescriptions**. Traditional persons may subscribe to "hot"/"cold" theory. May abstain from certain foods, such as dairy products, that can cause increased acidity and thus nausea. Acculturated persons may not believe in need to balance hot/cold. Some Roman Catholics abstain from meat during Lent, the 40 days before Easter. A grandmother or neighborhood pharmacy may recommend herbal teas, especially spearmint (*yerba buena*) or chamomile (*té de manzanilla*), for some conditions.
- **Hospitality**. An important aspect of home life among all social classes. Polite to offer coffee and pastry to visitors. Hospitality is a mark of being well-mannered (*bien educado*).

SYMPTOM MANAGEMENT

- **Pain** (*dolor*). May want pain relief as quickly as possible. Using words to describe pain may be easier than using numbers, but it depends on patient's level of comprehension. Accept narcotic analgesia (preferably oral) if it is explained appropriately.

- **Dyspnea** (*Me falta la respiracion* means "I lack breath"; *No puedo respirar* means "I cannot breathe"). May fear being short of breath, interpreting it as a sign of imminent death. Words may be easier than numbers to describe the degree and intensity of dyspnea, but this depends on patient's level of education and comprehension. May interpret use of oxygen as a bad sign. May readily accept oxygen and medications to calm or relieve dyspnea if these are explained. Reassurance and emotional support allay fears of suffocation and death.

- **Nausea/vomiting** (*náusea, vómito,* or *deponer*). May attribute nausea/vomiting to eating too much food or intoxication, or, in some instances, to the evil eye (*mal de ojo*), especially in children. This depends on acculturation, although many assimilated persons still hold traditional or folk beliefs. Words rather than numbers easier to describe amount, color, and frequency. May prefer oral rather than IV medication, depending on circumstances. Some prefer a home remedy (*remedio casero*). Sometimes drink chamomile tea (*té de manzanilla*) to relieve nausea.

- **Constipation/diarrhea** (*estreñimiento/diarrea*). May attribute constipation to eating food that "hardens the stomach." May express a high degree of discomfort and want relief. Many use purgatives, laxatives, and sometimes enemas. May attribute diarrhea to eating spoiled food. Treat diarrhea at home with foods such as jack cheese, which hardens the stomach. Beliefs of more-acculturated Mexicans similar to those in dominant culture.

- **Fatigue** (*fatiga, cansancio*). May attribute fatigue to illness or everyday stresses. May prefer words rather than numbers to describe fatigue. Home remedies, such as chamomile tea (*té de manzanilla*), may be appropriate.

- **Depression** (*depresión*). Usually under-diagnosed. There may be more somatic than emotional complaints, especially among women, but this varies. May accept medication if they receive clear and concise information about it. Clinician should emphasize need to continue taking antidepressant even if patient feels better. Should also carefully assess for use of nonpharmacological treatments; there is some anecdotal evidence that herbs in combination with psychotropic medications may trigger a manic episode.

- **Self-care symptom management**. May self-treat, especially if uninsured or of questionable legal status. May use folk remedies, such as herbal remedies that a relative suggests, before seeking medical care. Also may use spiritual healing or prayer, or seek healing by visiting shrines. Those who live along U.S.-Mexico border may travel to Mexico to seek health care and purchase affordable medications.

BIRTH RITUALS/CARE OF THE NEW MOTHER AND BABY

- **Pregnancy care**. Inadequate money or transportation problems may preclude standard prenatal care. Recent arrivals, especially those of unknown legal status, may fear that health care providers will report them, resulting in deportation. Some women see no need for prenatal care because childbirth is a natural part of life. Affluent and acculturated persons are more likely to seek prenatal care. Those from rural areas of Mexico may have had access to midwives (*parteras*) and may feel more comfortable with them. Mexicans discourage expectant mothers from doing heavy work, smoking, or drinking; encourage them to avoid stressful situations or strong emotional shocks, as these may negatively impact fetal development; and to rest, get adequate sleep, walk, and eat well for baby.

- **Preferences for children**. Generally protect and cherish children. Men may prefer boys to girls. Traditional persons favor large families, but Mexicans increasingly are using contraception to limit family size.

- **Labor practices**. Traditional persons view labor as a woman's task; few men get involved. Recommend walking for a quick birth. Fear of unnecessary medical interventions and separation from family members keeps some women laboring at home until they are in advanced labor. Acculturated women tend to come to the hospital earlier; they may not have female family members with childbirth experience who can provide support.

- **Role of the laboring woman during birth**. Traditional expectation was that she be passive and deliver a child to her husband. Feminism has empowered women to take control of labor. Family members, especially females, actively participate and encourage expectant mother during labor and birth. Acculturated couples take childbirth preparation classes and more actively participate in birth process.

- **Role of the father and other family members during birth**. Fathers traditionally have played a peripheral role. Today, however, more-affluent and acculturated persons expect father to be present. Mother, sisters, or aunts also may be present.

- **Vaginal vs. cesarean section**. Prefer spontaneous vaginal delivery. May view cesarean section as a drastic measure; clinician should carefully explain the need for, and the consequences of, having one.

- **Breastfeeding**. Traditional women opt for breastfeeding. However, the introduction and marketing of infant formula has reduced the prevalence of breastfeeding. Educational materials promoting breastfeeding should be made available in English and Spanish.

- **Birth recuperation**. A special time. Traditionally, women have 8–12 weeks to regain strength; family members help care for mother and child. May be different for women who must return to work.

- **Baby care**. In more-traditional families, members may help care for baby, and grandmothers, aunts, and close female relatives may babysit. Some affluent families hire a nanny to care for infant. Acculturated persons have live-in babysitters or use day care centers if available and economically feasible.

- **Problems with baby**. At hospital, clinician should discuss problems as soon as possible with parents. At home, new mothers discuss baby problems with female family members or friends, and some seek information on the Internet. May seek information from a health provider if one is readily available. Some use home remedies if nothing else is available. May need information on managing diarrhea and dehydration.
- **Male and female circumcision**. Traditional persons prefer not to circumcise infant boys. Acculturated persons tend to favor it, although not uniformly. Female circumcision not practiced.

DEVELOPMENTAL AND SEXUAL ISSUES

- **Celebration of menarche or becoming a man**. Many Mexicans and Mexican Americans mark a girl's transition to womanhood with a formal coming-of-age party (*quinceañera*) on her 15th birthday. No similar celebration for boys. Initiate some adolescent boys into sexual activity as part of their transition to manhood.
- **Attitudes about birth control**. Many married and single women use birth control. Acculturated women more likely to request information about it. Men may have a negative attitude about birth control, especially condoms; may interpret it as enabling women to have extramarital affairs. Women who use birth control may prefer pills or tubal ligation.
- **Attitudes about sexually transmitted infection (STI) control, including condoms**. Usually associate STIs with "bad" persons. Do not think married men are at risk for STIs, although some men engage in sex with other men. Men may be reluctant to use condoms, associating them with "bad" women or HIV transmission. Women who insist on use of condoms may be viewed with suspicion by their male partners because "good" women do not use condoms. Clinician should educate both men and women about using condoms to prevent STIs.
- **Attitudes about abortion**. Attitudes depend on acculturation and adherence to religious beliefs. Unacceptable among more-conservative persons. May consider abortion in cases of rape or incest.
- **Attitudes about unwed sexual experimentation**. Traditional or conservative families frown on unwed sexual experimentation and discourage it, especially among girls. However, this varies across acculturation and socioeconomic spectra, as evidenced by a high adolescent birth rate.
- **Sexual orientation**. No uniform family or community response, but many communities highly stigmatize homosexuality. Men tend to greet gay men with derision. Conservative families have negative attitudes about gay or lesbian members. Some organizations advocate for a better understanding of gay, lesbian, bisexual, and transgender persons. *Latina* lesbians have become a vis-

ible group in response to oppression and want to write about their experiences. HIV/AIDS pandemic has made gay and bisexual men more visible.

- **Gender identity**. Ambiguous genitalia or lack of differentiated genitalia not well-documented. Anecdotal evidence suggests that families perceive a child who has ambiguous genitalia to be a consequence of something mother did or something done to her. May choose not to discuss child's situation with others. Requires culturally sensitive and realistic interventions and treatment alternatives. Peers taunt effeminate boys and masculine girls; reactions to effeminate boys are more negative.

- **Attitudes about menopause**. View this change of life (*el cambio de vida*) as part of a natural progression. In the past, menopausal women received hormone replacement therapy, which is rare now. Attitudes and symptoms vary among women, who usually discuss menopause with other women and sometimes with their partners.

FAMILY RELATIONSHIPS

- **Composition/structure**. Traditional family consists of parents, children, grandparents, aunts, uncles, and cousins, and may include children's godfather and godmother (*padrino* and *madrina*). Social changes have dramatically altered family composition and structure. Economic necessity forces men and women to leave rural communities and go to large cities or U.S. for work. Parents sometimes leave children behind until parents have stable employment. Immigrants often settle in Mexican enclaves, especially if other relatives are living in same area; they move in with established family members and start working. Once settled into a community, many parents go to great pains to bring their children to U.S. Questionable legal status and possible deportation can disrupt family; children born in U.S. may remain behind in a relative's custody or foster care.

- **Decision-making**. Family unit traditionally makes decisions, but mobility or acculturation may alter this. Family members may consult with extended family in making decisions, but this varies. Some individuals make decision, then inform rest of family. Clinician should ask patient how decisions are made in his/her family, especially regarding treatment. End-of-life and other serious issues affect entire family.

- **Spokesperson**. Varies among families and by adherence to traditional family norms. May be a senior man or woman in family, a younger family member, or a family member who has the most education, money, or influence.

- **Gender issues**. Traditionally, man is head of the household and woman is subservient to him. Today, many women head households as single parents raising children and holding one or two jobs, attending school, and/or caring for a parent. More families are striving for egalitarian gender roles. Men are taking a more active role in child-rearing, especially as women move into job market.

- **Changing roles among generations in U.S.** Acculturation and assimilation have changed family roles and interactions. While family researchers and advocates idealize the notion of familism (*familiarlismo*), it exists in varying degrees. Because of socioeconomic needs, people move miles away from family; the interconnectedness that characterized previous generations is no longer as common.
- **Caring roles**. Women usually assume caring role, although some men may decide to take on that role.
- **Expectations of and for children**. Expect children to behave honorably toward elders and family. Many people place great value on family name; expect boys to carry it forward. Traditional families foster independence in boys and dependence in girls, but these expectations vary among communities and by acculturation level. Planning for a child's future depends on socioeconomic resources. While parents may encourage children to stay in school and earn a high school diploma and/or college degree, lack of academic preparation may preclude it. High school drop-out rate remains high. Those able to attend college may find it difficult, due to lack of academic skills, racism, discrimination, and poverty.
- **Expectations of and for elders**. Elderly may be revered, but acculturation reduces sense of obligation toward them. Mexicans often consult elders regarding important family decisions. Usually encourage elders to be as independent as possible; elders do not want to burden family. Families may feel obligated to care for an elder parent or relative, but this obligation does not preclude placement in a long-term-care facility. Many elders live on tight budgets and depend on family to supplement their fixed income.
- **Expectations of hospital visitors**. Family members constantly present. Some sleep at bedside, especially when patient is an elder or child. May view a limited-visiting policy as an attempt to hide something from family.

ILLNESS BELIEFS

- **Causes of/attitudes about physical illness**. May view physical illness as an act of God—therefore, as something to be endured—or the result of living a bad life or lifestyle. Persons who are more highly educated tend to perceive physical illness as a sign of an unhealthy lifestyle and within the individual's control. Cultural causes of illness include humoral imbalance and folk syndromes, such as the evil eye (*mal de ojo*), fright (*susto*), and intestinal blockage (*empacho*).
- **Causes of/attitudes about mental illness**. May view mental illness as God's punishment for living immorally. Some attribute mental illness to an enemy's hex or to witchcraft stemming from envy or vengeance. May be willing to undergo counseling or therapy if these are explained. Mental illness remains stigmatized; Mexicans do not discuss it with strangers.
- **Causes of genetic defects**. Usually attribute defects to God's will, mother's

failure to care for herself, or a hex placed on her. However, radio and television programs have somewhat altered these viewpoints; women have become more aware of the need for prenatal care to prevent or diagnose genetic defects.

- **Attitudes about disabilities**. More-traditional and religious persons view disability as a fate to be accepted. Acculturated persons may view it as a challenge to be overcome. Disabilities remain stigmatized; family may conceal a disabled member.
- **Sick role**. Illness affects entire family. Traditionally, families expect patient to be passive and allow family members to provide care. Migration and acculturation have affected perceptions of sick role and family members' ability to care for ill person, who may need to be less passive and attend to his/her own needs.
- **Home and folk remedies**. More-traditional persons use home and folk remedies (an art passed down from previous generations), possibly in conjunction with biomedical drugs. While more-acculturated persons may not use home and folk remedies, some may still believe in their efficacy. May not readily admit to using such remedies for fear of ridicule by health care provider.
- **Medications**. Most Mexicans are aware of and use Western medications. Patient may stop taking medication when he/she feels better or cannot afford it.
- **Acceptance of procedures**. Most accept blood transfusions; Jehovah's Witnesses refuse them, based on religious belief. Discussion of organ donation uncommon while patient is still alive; some Mexicans fear that speaking or thinking about death may hasten or cause death. Clinician should discuss transplant surgery in simple, nontechnical terms. Many Mexicans are aware of surgical advances and may welcome the possibility of better health. Some do not trust the health care system, fearing that, in the event of a transplant, they will receive the wrong organ.
- **Care-seeking**. More-affluent persons seek care from allopathic or osteopathic physicians. May be unaware of scope of practice of advanced practice nurses. May be wary of nurse practitioners or, under the care of nurse practitioners, think they are getting substandard care due to lack of resources. Many are aware of midwives, the only health care providers available in many poor, rural areas of Mexico.

HEALTH ISSUES

- **Concept of health**. Perceptions vary depending on income, acculturation, and education. Most believe that health is the ability to rise in the morning and work, and freedom from pain. More-affluent persons may think of health as going to the health club and eating nutritious foods; acculturated persons may think of it as engaging in vigorous exercise and eating low-fat foods. The primary concern of poor persons is survival; they view life as being in God's hands.

- **Health promotion and prevention**. Survival is the focus of many Mexicans. They may not place much stock in biomedical suggestions for health promotion and prevention, believing that life is in God's hands. Depending on level of acculturation and access to health care, may consider changing their eating, exercise, and smoking habits.
- **Screening**. May respond to health education about the importance of screening. Monolingual Spanish speakers need information about screening and tests that has been accurately translated into Spanish.
- **Common health problems**. Diabetes, with hypertension and obesity as comorbidities; lack of treatment results in higher prevalence of diabetic complications among Mexicans than among Whites. Also HIV/AIDS, childhood obesity, and trauma from gun violence.

DEATH RITUALS

- **Beliefs and attitudes about death**. Often view death from any cause as God's will. May view it as a release from the troubles of this life and passage to a better life. Many believe in an afterlife, going to heaven. Religious beliefs greatly influence perceptions of death and dying.
- **Preparation**. Clinician should inform family of impending death. Prudence and tact are crucial, especially when death is unexpected, sudden, or caused by violence. Family needs private space to deal with loss.
- **Home vs. hospital**. May prefer to die at home, although this varies depending on resources. May choose to die in hospital, as it will spare family from having to witness death. However, some Mexicans fear that spirit of deceased may get "lost" in hospital. Family wants supportive atmosphere. Depending on level of acculturation, education, and resources, may seek hospice care.
- **Special needs**. Keep rosary beads or religious medallions near patient. Roman Catholics request visit by priest to anoint the sick; if unavailable, clinician should summon hospital chaplain to administer this sacrament. If patient dies before priest arrives, the sacrament still should take place, before body is removed. Protestants and Evangelicals may request visit by their pastor. Many families become emotionally distraught, wailing and fainting. Clinician should give family members extra time to say good-bye to deceased.
- **Care of the body**. If patient dies in hospital, family members may ask to view body before it is moved to mortuary; some may want to help prepare it. Burial rather than cremation is most common. Catholics say a rosary the night before burial, a solemn mass of resurrection. More-traditional persons observe nine days of prayers. Acculturated persons may forego prolonged mourning. Protestants and Evangelicals request a minister or pastor to conduct a service for the deceased and family.
- **Attitudes about organ donation**. May be negative, based on belief that

the potential donor's body should be buried intact. Highly educated persons and those who value biomedicine may be receptive if clinician broaches the issue with a senior family member so family can discuss it.

- **Attitudes about autopsy**. Family may request autopsy. If autopsy necessary to confirm a diagnosis, clinician should approach senior family member so family can discuss it.

SELECTED REFERENCES

Browner, C. H., Preloran, H. M., Casado, M. C., Bass, H. N., & Walker, A. P. (2003). Genetic counseling gone awry: Miscommunication between prenatal genetic service providers and Mexican-origin clients. *Social Science and Medicine*, 56, 1933–1946.

Gonzales, M. G. (1999). *Mexicanos: A history of Mexicans in the United States.* Indianapolis: Indiana University Press.

Rehm, R. S. (2003). Cultural intersections in the care of Mexican American children with chronic conditions. *Pediatric Nursing*, 29, 434–439.

Williams, N. (1990). *The Mexican American family: Tradition and change.* Dix Hills, NY: General Hall.

AUTHOR

Peter Andrew Guarnero, BSN, MSN, PhD, received his bachelor's in nursing from Loyola University Chicago, a master's in nursing from the University of California-Los Angeles, and a PhD from the University of California-San Francisco. He completed postdoctoral study in health-related problems of vulnerable populations at the UCLA School of Nursing and is currently an assistant professor at the University of New Mexico College of Nursing. His clinical specialization is psychiatric mental health nursing. His research interests include health promotion among Hispanic men, and the impact of family and community on the social and sexual lives of Hispanic gay and bisexual men.

CHAPTER 26

NIGERIANS

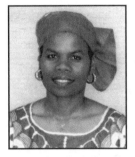

Marcellina Ada Ogbu

CULTURAL/ETHNIC IDENTITY

Nigeria, in West Africa, has more than 250 ethnic groups. The major groups include Hausa, Yoruba, Igbo, Kanuri, Fulani, Tiv, Ijaw, Ibibio, Bini, Nupe, Junku, Efik, and Itsekiri. Hausa, Yoruba, and Igbo make up 60% of the population. Hausa live predominantly in the North, Yoruba in the Southwest, and Igbo in the Southeast. Although these groups share some core cultural values and beliefs, there are considerable differences in religion, language, political history, and customs. This chapter focuses on shared beliefs and practices.

- **Preferred term(s)**. Nigerian.
- **Census**. According to the 2000 U.S. Census, 137,448 people report Nigerian ancestry and 112,877 indicate they were born in Nigeria. But nearly 1 million reported their ancestry as "African," of whom Nigerians are probably the largest group. Another estimate suggests that 3 million Nigerians reside in the U.S. Immigrants live in every part of the U.S. but are concentrated in urban centers, such as Los Angeles, the San Francisco Bay Area, Houston, New York City, Newark, and Atlanta. Ethnic groups tend to congregate in specific areas (e.g., Igbos in the San Francisco Bay Area and Houston).
- **History of immigration**. Began at the end of World War II. Nearly all immigrants before 1970 were male students who planned to return home at the end of their studies. Subsequent events changed this pattern. These included a 1986 congressional ruling that granted amnesty to undocumented aliens, permission by the Nigerian government to hold dual citizenship, continued economic stagnation in Nigeria, and the 1990 U.S. Immigration Act that expanded the number and diversity of countries from which people were granted permanent visas. Today, Nigerians are the largest group of African immigrants; one in four Africans is Nigerian. In contrast

to prior decades, many recent immigrants come for economic reasons rather than schooling and they include families, single women, and older persons. Most have jobs offering limited opportunity for advancement. For example, a Nigerian with a PhD may drive a taxi in New York City or work as a security guard. However, others are employed as professors, doctors, engineers, architects, lawyers, accountants, and civil servants in local, state, and federal governments. Many have become small business owners in fields such as accounting, real estate, and sales.

SPIRITUAL/RELIGIOUS ORIENTATION

- **Primary religious/spiritual affiliations**. Three formal religious traditions: Islam (50%), predominantly in the North and of the Sunni sect; Christianity (40%), mostly Catholic, Presbyterian, Episcopal/Anglican, Evangelical/Pentecostal, and African Christian (Aladura), and predominantly in the South; and indigenous religion (10%), which permeates all other religions. Persons hold traditional beliefs as well as other faiths (Islam or Christianity); they participate in two religions. Most immigrants are Christian. Indigenous beliefs include a supreme being, deities, and spirits, with ancestor worship an important component. Functionaries, who can be both benevolent and malevolent, serve as intermediaries between the faithful and their deities and ancestors. Such powers affect health, family, life, and death; humans must learn to live in balance with them.
- **Usual religious/spiritual practices**. Vary by ethnic group and beliefs. In general, most say prayers, read the Bible or Koran, and attend church or mosque. Aladura emphasizes divine healing, vision, prophecy, and the worship of God through a cultural medium, such as priests or objects. Nigerians wear religious objects—rosaries, crosses, amulets, Koranic verses, and charms—around their neck, ankle, waist, and wrist. Many homes have statues, posters, and pictures to ward off evil spirits, protect the household, and promote good luck, health, and fortune.
- **Use of spiritual healing/healers**. Traditional healers rare in U.S. Some immigrants return home to consult healers or they ask family members to do so on their behalf. Distinguish between what Western biomedicine and what traditional healers can cure. For example, some Nigerians consult healers regarding infertility, having only female children, or tragic or unexpected deaths. Use spiritual healing extensively, especially Evangelicals, born-again Christians, and followers of Aladura.
- **Holidays**. Traditional calendar year ranges from 10–13 months, depending on ethnic group; a week ranges from 4–8 days. Each ethnic group has its own indigenous holidays. Traditional New Year's (in southern Nigeria) falls in August/September and coincides with celebration of the New Yam harvest. Dates of Islamic New Year (*Muharram*) and Ramadan, the month of obligatory fasting, change yearly based on Islamic calendar. Other Muslim holidays

include end of Ramadan (*Eid el-Fitr*); end of *Hajj*, the time when Muslims should make their pilgrimage to Mecca (holy land) (*Eid el-Kabir*), and Mohammed's birthday (*Eid el-Maulud*) in September. Christians observe religious holidays similar to those in the West: Christmas, Lent, Palm Sunday, and Easter Sunday and Monday. Official secular holidays include Independence Day (October 1), the only one celebrated in U.S.; Boxing Day (December 26); Workers' Day (May 1); and Children's Day (May 25), which only children observe.

COMMUNICATION
ORAL COMMUNICATION

- **Major languages and dialects**. There are about 500 languages and 5,000 dialects in Nigeria, but most of the population speaks a language in one of these groups: Hausa, Yoruba, Igbo, Fulani, Edo, Adamawa/Fulfide, Efik, Ibibio, or Idoma. English is the official language of Nigeria and most immigrants speak it. Recent arrivals and elders with no schooling are likely to speak and understand Pidgin English (mixture of English and one or more other languages, using simple grammar) or minimal English. Many are multilingual; they speak English, two or more Nigerian languages, and other foreign languages. Muslims may also speak Arabic.
- **Greetings**. Highly valued. Consist of long, ritualized verbal exchanges, including asking about the other's and family's well-being. Nigerians do not rush greetings; they give others time to respond and expect them to be pleasant and cheerful. It is almost obligatory to greet someone, particularly in the morning. Usually expect younger person to initiate the exchange. Men shake hands and pat on the back; also shake hands with friends and strangers. Bowing and kneeling are formal, polite greetings in presence of elders and authority figures. In some ethnic groups, persons greet royalty, religious leaders, and chiefs by prostrating themselves. Some Igbo groups greet by placing an open right hand on the other's chest and returning the hand to their own chest. Nigerian Americans are beginning to incorporate hugging into their repertoire of greetings. Address most parents as father or mother of the first-born or surviving child, never by given name. Use "Uncle" or "Aunty" when addressing family members, friends, and sometimes other unrelated adults. Younger siblings address older ones as "Sister" or "Brother" followed by the sibling's first name (e.g., "Sister Ngozi"). Everyone, including nonrelatives, greets all older men and women as "Mother" (*Ma, Mama*) and "Father" (*Pa, Papa*) or the equivalent in their ethnic language. Educated persons tend to use "Sir" and "Madam" for other adults. Children may address their father as "Sir," but "Papa" or "Daddy" is becoming more common. Men, in particular, prefer to be addressed by their titles (e.g., "Dr.," "Chief," "Prince," "Barrister," "*Oba*"/"*Eze*" [chief/king], or "Professor").
- **Tone of voice**. Nigerians are soft-spoken, polite, cheerful, and noncon-

frontational. The nature of a conversation may influence intensity of the tone and sound.

- **Direct or indirect style of speech**. Varies by ethnic group, but all Nigerians view direct and abrupt styles of communication as impersonal and impolite. Traditionally important to exchange pleasantries, provide context, and establish social relations before addressing the main issue. Immigrant patients may give very short answers, believing that short answers are expected. Nigerian society is hierarchical; questioning authority is rare. Patients and family members do not complain or question medical treatment even if they have doubts, fearing that questioning the provider will cause alienation, conflict, or disappointment that might influence care. Women, in particular, may not mention their reservations about a treatment regimen, remaining silent, shrugging their shoulders, or rolling their eyes rather than questioning the provider. Men can be reserved but demanding, especially if they feel patronized and resentful about being treated as uneducated.

- **Use of interpreters**. Older and recently arrived immigrants may need interpreter for medical information. Family members usually escort them, but if none is available to interpret, patient or family must approve use of another interpreter. May be reluctant to do so; Nigerians still view many illnesses and misfortunes as punishment for personal misdeeds, which they fear an interpreter might expose. Nigerians may be residentially scattered, but because they are in constant contact through weddings, wakes, birthdays, baby showers, group meetings, and other community activities, there are numerous avenues for gossip. Out of fear of disclosure, may not report deeply personal matters, such as abortion, exposure to sexually transmitted infection, and mental health issues, to interpreter. Interpreters must navigate between what is professionally required and what is culturally acceptable.

- **Serious or terminal illness**. Traditionally, do not inform patient of poor diagnosis or prognosis; inform male family member instead. Because of immigration dynamics, another family member, close friend, or pastor might serve as initial recipient of bad news. Best if clinician asks patient initially who he/she would like to involve in communications. Family members decide what to tell a loved one, as the illness is a family crisis that requires a communal response. Patient must be protected from news that may aggravate his/her situation.

WRITTEN COMMUNICATION

- **Literacy assessment**. Many speak, read, and write in English, although about 10% in U.S. (including elderly) may have minimal education and need someone to translate and explain medical procedures. Clinician should ask patient if he/she can read and write in English.

- **Consents**. Patients generally believe in the healing power of healers, physicians, and other providers. Relationships are based on mutual trust. Uneasy

about signing consent forms, especially those that describe risks. May interpret such forms as meaning an illness is serious, that provider is absolving
him-/herself from responsibility, and that patient is accepting the risk.
Essentially, patients take consents literally. Some may refuse treatment even
when risk is low.

NONVERBAL COMMUNICATION

- **Eye contact**. Direct eye contact disrespectful, particularly with older persons and authority figures.
- **Personal space**. Do not value private space; wanting it is considered self-
  ish. In Nigeria, multiple family units live in large compounds. In U.S., not
  uncommon for many nuclear/extended family members, friends, and
  acquaintances to live together, sharing space, clothing, and other personal
  items. Nigerians tend to stand or sit very close to others when talking.
- **Use and meaning of silence**. Silence a very common form of communication. Use it in many ways. Silence can signal deference to authority figure or
  someone who is older. For example, Nigerians expect younger persons not to
  talk when authority figure or elder is speaking. Also use silence to avoid conflict and to express frustration or disagreement.
- **Gestures**. Express displeasure with children by pointing or waving finger, or
  using it to summon. Such gestures are insulting to adults. Say good-bye by
  waving hand right and left. Pushing the palm of the hand forward and
  spreading the fingers is considered vulgar. Nigerians frequently nod (yes) or
  shake their heads (no) in response to questions.
- **Openness in expressing emotions**. Usually reserved and stoic. Health
  care providers may have difficulty gauging severity of illness/pain because
  facial expressions often do not correspond to what the patient describes.
  Nigerians rarely express intimate behaviors—kissing, touching, caressing, or
  holding hands—in public. In some families, a hug is closest expression of
  love or caring, which are expressed instead through mutual respect and fulfilling responsibilities to family.
- **Privacy**. Families are very private. Individuals selectively share information
  about illness and misfortune. Patient may view these as punishment for personal failure; therefore, ill person may fear that clinician, friend, or community will perceive him/her negatively. Often, information that Nigerians
  share with outsiders is that which shows patient or family in a good light.
  Clinician should use open-ended questions, clearly explain need for honest
  communication, and assure patient of confidentiality.
- **Touch**. Touching, a gentle push on the shoulder, or patting someone's back are
  acceptable ways of communicating and are not an invasion of private space.
  Due to modesty, patients may be uncomfortable when health care providers
  touch genitalia/pubic area or breast. Nigerians widely use touch in traditional
  healing. Massaging a sick person's hands, feet, and back is common. Touching

the forehead with front or back of hand assesses fever. Clinician should explain why he/she wears gloves, as Nigerians view gloves as impersonal and may construe them as an expression of superiority, avoidance, or not caring.

- **Orientation to time**. Common to joke about Nigerian (African) time, the tendency to be late. Tardiness applies mostly to social situations; Nigerians value punctuality in work-related and formal situations. Most ethnic groups are relaxed about time, which they savor and do not rush. In health care settings where productivity is critical, Nigerians may perceive hurried providers as abrupt and/or perceive such behavior as rude, uncaring, or meaning that staff cannot provide adequate care. Traditionally, time and dates do not follow the Western calendar or clock. Nigerians view time as fluid; past, present, and future form a continuum. Traditional time, which Nigerians associate with landmarks, events, and activities, may be problematic when clinician tries to determine onset of disease, pregnancy due date, birth date, or medication schedule.

ACTIVITIES OF DAILY LIVING

- **Modesty**. Very modest and very private about their body. Disrobing for medical procedures or exposing oneself for pelvic exams may cause discomfort.
- **Skin care**. Depending on ethnic group and personal preference, Nigerians may shower once or twice daily. Generally apply lotion all over body. Muslims may ritually wash face, feet, and hands before prayers.
- **Hair care**. In Nigeria, women braid hair or cover it with a scarf. Many immigrant women process their hair. Individual preference dictates hair maintenance. Men have short or clean-shaven hair and may wash it daily.
- **Nail care**. Men generally keep nails short. Women's nail care based on personal preference, although Nigerians consider it improper for married women to have very long or painted nails.
- **Toileting**. Prefer bathroom out of modesty. Patients use bedpan or commode if necessary but prefer that there be no staff in room.
- **Special clothing or amulets**. Depends on religion or ethnic group. Muslims wear Koranic verses around their neck. Christians may wear crosses, rosaries, or other religious symbols. Members of all ethnic groups may wear amulets, such as cowry shells or beads. Some ethnic groups practice scarification of the face, body, and hands—sometimes for beauty but, in many cases, for protection from evil spirits.
- **Self-care**. Sick role is highly ritualized. Expect ill persons to rest; help them with most self-care. Patients are willing to ambulate or breathe deeply after surgery if necessary.

FOOD PRACTICES

- **Usual meal pattern**. Varies among ethnic groups, but breakfast, lunch, and dinner are common. Breakfast may be light or heavy, followed by a heavy lunch/supper and light dinner. Southerners eat very heavy meals compared to those from the North, where a meal may be a light porridge. Some families may eat leftover dinner for breakfast. Meal patterns are changing, with breakfast consisting of tea with milk, bread, pap custard (made of cornstarch, sugar, and milk), and bean cake (*akara*) or egg.

- **Special utensils**. Staple in southern Nigeria is *fufu* (made from cassava/ manioc or African yam), which usually is eaten with fingers. Many Nigerians prefer spoons to forks for foods such as rice. In Nigeria, persons eat from a common bowl.
- **Food beliefs and rituals**. Vary by ethnic group. Some throw a bit of food on floor before eating to invite ancestors to partake in meal. Initiate all major events and celebrations with libations. Adults, particularly father/husband, are fed before the children are.
- **Usual diet**. Traditional southern diet includes lots of starch and vegetables. Nigerians generally eat meat on ceremonial occasions. Southerners eat *fufu* almost daily; Nigerians in U.S. use wheat flour, cornmeal, or rice flour as a substitute. Eat *fufu* with a variety of stews or soups made with local vegetables, such as bitter leaf, okra, *utazi*, *ugu*, *okazi*, peanut, *egusi*, *ogbono*, and benniseed. In the North, particularly among the Hausa, the staple is *tuwo*, a thick porridge made from guinea corn and millet flour, and eaten with soup (*miya*). Both northerners and southerners eat legumes, particularly black-eyed peas and cowpeas. Usually prepare these as porridge, steamed (*moimoi*) or fried (*akara*). Other foods are jollof rice, plantain, and yams. Common meats include goat, chicken, guinea fowl, dried cod and other fish, and beef (*suya*). Guinea fowl rare in U.S., where Nigerians mostly use beef in stews. Dairy products generally not consumed in southern Nigeria, but they are important in Fulani diet and in diet of some ethnic groups in the North. Nigerian meals very spicy. Use generous amounts of palm oil in cooking. Prefer that meals be served hot.
- **Fluids**. Cocoa and tea with milk are the preferred morning beverages. Milk main beverage for northerners. Soda, hard liquor, and beer are common drinks. Palm wine common in the South and millet-based brews common in the North, but these are unavailable in U.S. Drink ice-cold water with every meal in the hot, humid weather of Nigeria. Immigrants may drink less fluid partly because of colder weather; many prefer water at room temperature.
- **Food taboos and prescriptions**. During pregnancy, prohibited foods that affect mother and fetus include rice (causes rash), spicy food (causes heartburn), certain vegetables, and various wild meats. Postpartum, encourage mother to eat spicy foods, lots of meat, fish, and rice. Some groups discourage consumption of vegetables, believing that they cause infant diarrhea. Religion and ethnic group dictate food taboos. For example, Islam forbids wild meats and pork, and food must be prepared in a religiously prescribed manner. Many Muslims fast during month of Ramadan, although children,

pregnant or lactating women, the sick, soldiers on duty, and travelers are exempt. Many Christians, particularly practicing Catholics, eat fish rather than meat on Friday. Some fast occasionally (e.g., on Friday and during Lent). Nigerians believe that warm, soothing foods, such as hot porridge and spicy soup, help the sick.

- **Hospitality**. Guests may drop by uninvited and unannounced, and provide food, regardless of time of day. If food has not already been prepared, host asks guest to wait. Depending on relationship, guest is expected to decline and take a rain check. Host offers visitor food or refreshment, which comprises kola nut and water. Nontraditional food and refreshments for visitors include biscuits, battered and fried dough (*chin-chin*), fruit, garden egg (a variety of eggplant eaten raw), and drinks (soft drinks, beer, or liquor). Host generally does not ask guest what he/she wants; automatically presents a tray with various refreshments. Inappropriate to refuse food/refreshment (i.e., host expects guest at least to taste food and sip drink). Also consider it impolite for guest to eat everything on plate. In some ethnic groups, guest should compliment the host rather than say "thank you." Throughout visit, guest receives special attention, which may include special meals, sitting in the best chair, and sleeping in someone's bed.

SYMPTOM MANAGEMENT

Varies by perception of illness cause or character. Anxiety, depression, and symptoms resulting from punishment for personal misdeeds are usually vague; may include generalized pain. Can use numerical scales, but words may be more accurate. Nigerians take medication for symptoms that are obvious or have a known etiology, such as those caused by malaria and diarrhea.

- **Pain**. Both genders have very high pain threshold. In some ethnic groups, acceptable for women and men to moan; in others, it is not. Ritualized moaning may be part of sick role and not necessarily reflect pain severity. Providers may have difficulty gauging pain by facial expression or description of symptoms. For example, patients commonly describe a painful condition with a smile. Clinicians should assess pain level by means other than numerical scale because of gender/cultural variation in pain tolerance or expression.
- **Dyspnea**. Sometimes families contribute to patient's hyperventilation and panic by hovering over him/her. Creating calm and providing assurance are key to reducing anxiety. May accept medications.
- **Nausea/vomiting**. Patients generally embarrassed. Women likely to clean up vomitus before health care provider can assess it. Some men, while embarrassed, may wait for provider. Traditionally use lemon to control nausea; sometimes take quinine diluted with water.
- **Constipation/diarrhea**. Traditional remedies for constipation include herbs, special foods, and laxatives. Modesty may inhibit acceptance of enema. Sometimes use fermented and dehydrated cassava in water (*garri*), pap

(*akamu*), or boiled ripe plantain to treat diarrhea. Use herbal concoctions, such as bitter-leaf water or salted water, for upset stomach.

- **Fatigue**. Until recently, Nigerians commonly napped after lunch. View fatigue as a normal part of illness. Often assume sick role based on fatigue as symptom.
- **Depression**. Recognize depression and consider it a normal response to loss, personal/group misfortune, or hardship. A prolonged state of sadness beyond the cultural norm is unacceptable. For example, Nigerians believe that grieving for too long after a death makes it difficult for the deceased to pass to the other world or that the depressed person may have contributed to the death in some way and feels guilty. Nigerians do not treat depression itself. They express depression through vague symptoms that apparently do not have an organic basis.
- **Self-care symptom management**. Over-the-counter medications prevalent among immigrants. They tend to self-diagnose and self-medicate, a carryover from Nigeria, where there are few health facilities and many prescription drugs are available over the counter. Patients likely do not understand when a clinician refuses to prescribe pain medications such as codeine. Self-care for chronic illness uncommon, except for illnesses such as arthritis and asthma that have symptoms.

BIRTH RITUALS/CARE OF THE NEW MOTHER AND BABY

- **Pregnancy care**. Traditionally, pregnancy evokes joy, anxiety, and secrecy. Nigerians neither publicize nor celebrate pregnancies out of fear that such display could engender the evil eye, causing miscarriage, premature delivery, or fetal malformation. Usually do not acknowledge or refer to pregnancy until the birth, although others chide the expectant mother for her size, appetite, and cravings. Women continue their regular activities throughout pregnancy, including sexual activity, which is believed to make the fetus stronger. Husbands may not accompany wives to prenatal visits, as pregnancy is considered a woman's domain. There is limited prenatal care in Nigeria, except in cities. In U.S., Nigerians begin prenatal care as soon as pregnancy is confirmed. Uncommon to attend childbirth preparation classes, as Nigerians view pregnancy and birth as natural events.
- **Preferences for children**. Although Nigerians welcome both boys and girls, how they receive a first-born depends on type of descent (matrilineal, patrilineal, and/or double descent), which varies among ethnic groups. In patrilineal groups, fathers prefer sons because of inheritance issues and the need to perpetuate lineage. Although some mothers prefer that first-born be a girl because she will help with babysitting, trading, and household chores, sons increase a woman's status in the husband's lineage. Daughters take care of their mothers long after they marry. Average number of children in Nigeria is six; in U.S., usually about four. Nigerians have one of the highest rates of twins in the world.

- **Labor practices**. Traditionally, a self-trained midwife, birth attendant, or older female family member assists with delivery. In urban Nigeria, most babies are delivered in hospital. Nigerians mostly consider labor pain to be normal and an obligatory part of motherhood. Women tend to tolerate pain well, but some moaning, grunting, and screaming are acceptable during contractions. Some women reject pain management strategies because of unfamiliarity or are hesitant to take medication for fear of harming baby. Female family members and friends comfort laboring woman by massaging her back and feet. Traditionally, women walk about during labor and squat during delivery; for many in U.S., lying down is very uncomfortable. Labor practices are changing; immigrants are adopting the usual birth-setting practices.
- **Role of the laboring woman during birth**. Takes active role. Efforts should be made to cover her, as modesty is still expected.
- **Role of the father and other family members during birth**. Traditionally, fathers and male family members not allowed to be with birthing woman. Babies born in all-female environments; unlike other health situations, Nigerians do not expect family members to participate. In U.S., father's participation varies. In some cases, he consoles and encourages (and limits intimate contact with) his wife during labor/delivery; in other cases, he waits outside. High percentage of fathers do not participate, many out of respect for modesty or because they cannot bear to see their wife in pain.
- **Vaginal vs. cesarean section**. Prefer vaginal delivery. Consider cesarean birth unnatural—almost equivalent to breech birth, which Nigerians view as an abomination. Also fear that a cesarean may interfere with future births.
- **Breastfeeding**. Traditionally, expect mothers to breastfeed for an average of two years, on demand. No taboo about breastfeeding in public. Growing number of immigrant mothers bottle-feed instead, some because they need to work and others out of ignorance (they associate bottle-feeding with high status). Nursing mothers eat special foods—essentially, a much more balanced diet than normally.
- **Birth recuperation**. Ethnic group, religious practice, family size, and wealth determine how long mother and baby are secluded; duration ranges from 1–6 months. Female family members help new mother bathe and care for baby. Nigerians consider both mother and baby to be delicate, making every effort to protect them from disease and harm. Mother is fed special foods, including chicken and other meat, delicious soups, and stews. Food and beverages must be warm. Childbirth is a joyous event for the family, neighbors, and community; friends and family bring food and gifts. Traditionally, parents do not name baby immediately; use generic name instead. Time between birth and naming ceremony ranges from four days to one year. Parents delay naming out of fear that child could be a target of the evil eye or because they believe that newborn needs time to decide whether to stay or return (die); delay protects them from emotional attachment if child chooses to return.

Naming follows established cultural rules. For example, child may be named after a parent or based on an event that took place around the time of birth.
- **Baby care**. Expect new mother to be with baby 24/7. Infant sleeps with mother so he/she can suckle through the night. Mother and female family members hold baby constantly and do not allow him/her to cry. Expect maternal and paternal grandmothers and female members of extended family to help with child care. Husbands and male family members not expected to care for infant, but they do provide some respite for new mother. Some fathers in U.S. are beginning to share infant care, but their involvement generally remains limited.
- **Problems with baby**. Ordinarily, father is informed. Acceptable in U.S. to inform father or mother. Although fathers may make final decision regarding problem with baby, most health-related responsibilities are the mother's.
- **Male and female circumcision**. In most ethnic groups, both males and females are circumcised. Two forms of female circumcision in Nigeria: clitoridectomy, or removing part or all of clitoris (more prevalent in the South); and excision, or removing part or all of clitoris and labia (practiced mostly among Muslims in the North). Infibulation (sewing up vulva) is not practiced in Nigeria. Age of child at circumcision varies. Boys' circumcision takes place 4–8 days after birth in some groups; in others, it is a rite of passage at puberty. Some communities perform female circumcision a few days after birth; others perform it at puberty. Female circumcision is declining, partly due to education and Christianity.

DEVELOPMENTAL AND SEXUAL ISSUES
- **Celebration of menarche or becoming a man**. Varies by ethnic group. Some groups merely acknowledge menarche with a special meal; others note it with elaborate celebrations. For example, Ibibio girls are circumcised at puberty and secluded for a period of time. In most ethnic groups, menstruation restricts female participation in social life. For example, a girl may not be allowed to leave the house or bathe, as she has special but harmful powers. Such beliefs are waning in U.S. and Nigeria. Afikpo-Ibo of eastern Nigeria consider boys' puberty a rite of passage and acknowledge it with an elaborate initiation into manhood.
- **Attitudes about birth control**. Modern contraceptives not widely available in Nigeria. Traditionally, women were expected to have as many children as "God gives." Even when contraceptives are available, Nigerians do not widely use them. Responsibility for birth control is almost solely the woman's. Traditional methods include abstinence while breastfeeding, douching after sex, inserting objects into vagina, and eating high concentrations of certain plants and seeds. Use of contraceptives has increased as a result of changes in Nigerian society and the realities of American life. Nigerians prefer methods that are not complicated or invasive.

- **Attitudes about sexually transmitted infection (STI) control, including condoms**. Knowledge about STIs is limited. Untreated STIs prevalent. Condom use is low and varies by education, age, and religious beliefs.
- **Attitudes about abortion**. Nigerians marry to have children, who are cherished. Abortion is illegal and stigmatized in Nigeria, and rare within marriage but frequent among unmarried high-school and college students. It is not uncommon for couples married in a civil ceremony to wait for the wife to become pregnant before having a church wedding. Some men fear that women may be infertile due partly to prior abortion. Douching with vinegar, lemon, salt, potassium, and traditional plants is a common abortion method.
- **Attitudes about unwed sexual experimentation**. Dating and sexual activity before marriage unacceptable. Out-of-wedlock pregnancy brings shame on family and girl, making it difficult for her to marry. Fear of being unmarriageable contributes to high abortion rates.
- **Sexual orientation**. Consider homosexuality very unnatural and therefore unacceptable, given the strict gender roles that characterize Nigerian society. Shun and ostracize gays and lesbians. Very limited information available about Nigerian gays and lesbians in U.S.
- **Gender identity**. Ambiguous gender identity strongly stigmatized and not discussed openly. A male child who clings to his mother is a source of worry for the community. Parents fear that he will grow up to be too effeminate.
- **Attitudes about menopause**. Traditionally, Nigerian women continue to have children until menopause, which tends to arrive quite early. For some, menopause is a welcome end to monthly periods and childbearing. It elevates their status and frees them to participate in religious activities, governance, and other social activities from which they previously were barred because they were menstruating. Nigerians do not generally discuss menopause, but women do not appear to be worried about it. Unclear if they experience typical symptoms; no information available on how women manage them.

FAMILY RELATIONSHIPS

- **Composition/structure**. Family structure tends to be hierarchical, with the elderly and males wielding a lot of power. Extended family most common, traditionally consisting of multiple households of related family members, such as grandparents, cousins, nephews, aunts, uncles, and in-laws. In U.S., households likely to include persons from outside the family.
- **Decision-making**. Family members work very closely together in discussing issues that require decisions. Traditionally, the father, eldest son, or other older adults, including women, play key roles in decision-making. In U.S., decision-making is somewhat diffuse. Although Nigerians seek input from older family members, family defers to member who is the most acculturated or has expertise or resources.
- **Spokesperson**. Father and uncles speak on family's behalf, followed by eld-

est son or daughter. In U.S., the most acculturated family member or a trusted friend assumes spokesperson role.

- **Gender issues**. Traditional system of polygamy still exists in Nigeria, but immigrants do not practice it. Husbands expect wives to be significant wage earners and to contribute financially to family's upkeep. Some families pool resources, others maintain separate finances. Some men cling to traditional gender roles and do not help with household tasks. Extended-family system creates conflicts in gender relations; often, the husband's relatives have greater influence on him than his wife does. Although some women have power and financial independence, power relations are not equitable. Women defer to men regarding major decisions (e.g., children's education, breaking bad news, and funeral arrangements).

- **Changing roles among generations in U.S.** Role reversal a major source of family conflict; youth are forced to be mediators in, and interpreters of, the new culture. Some families benefit in that mothers and children become closer as they learn together, producing greater levels of understanding rather than conflict. In many other families, particularly those that are less educated, role reversal puts children in difficult situations. They are exposed to adult experiences that children normally are shielded from, such as health problems, family finances, and frustrations in adjusting to a new country. Child-rearing practices in U.S. also are a source of conflict. Nigerian parents perceive American parenting as unacceptably permissive, while youths want to behave like Americans regarding style of dress, choice of music, recreational activities, dating, discipline, and parent-child relationships.

- **Caring roles**. Mothers, grandmothers, sisters, aunts, and other female family members are usually the main caregivers. Other family members, regardless of gender, may provide care when a parent is ill.

- **Expectations of and for children**. Child-rearing is informal and noncoercive. A young Nigerian child is indulged, never allowed to cry, constantly carried by mother or other family members, and fed on demand. Parents very protective. Although discipline begins by the third year, child's life is carefree. As child grows older, there is very limited formal teaching; he/she is expected to learn by observing adults or older siblings, with a focus on obedience, respect for elders, cooperation, and politeness. Immigrants strongly emphasize education, believing it is the only route to the American dream. The idea of children becoming independent at age 18 is alien. In most cases, young adults live with parents and grandparents until they marry (girls) or take a job elsewhere (particularly boys). Children maintain lifelong attachment to their families, attending to their needs, seeking their advice, and respecting their wishes.

- **Expectations of and for elders**. Family relationships are based on seniority. Nigerians respect elders, who expect their adult children to care for them once the children achieve success. There is no social security in Nigeria, so adult children are responsible for taking care of elderly parents in children's or parents' home. Do not generally consider nursing homes an option; institutionalizing a parent may be shameful.

- **Expectations of hospital visitors**. Family members and friends tend to hover over patient, never leaving him/her alone. Also may want to assist health care provider. Hospitalized patients expect visitors. Family members and friends visit constantly throughout the day.

ILLNESS BELIEFS

- **Causes of/attitudes about physical illness**. Naturalistic causes of illness include eating contaminated food, drinking polluted water, drinking or eating too much, and exposure to heat, cold, or wind. Supernatural causes are evil spirits, the gods, and the gods' functionaries. View illness—especially illness with no obvious symptoms or etiology—and misfortune as punishment for wrongdoing, ill will against others, failure to perform ritual obligations and offerings, and breach of social taboos.

- **Causes of/attitudes about mental illness**. Traditionally, attribute ailments—mental illness, epilepsy, and others with no known etiology—to evil spirits, personal failings, or group misdeeds. Families keep mental illness secret and generally do not tell clinician, as exposure may result in ostracism. Most families avoid marrying into families with mental illness. Such stigma discourages persons with symptoms from seeking treatment. Another barrier is the belief that diseases caused by evil spirits, including mental illness, must be treated differently than diseases that have naturalistic etiologies. For example, mentally ill persons in Nigeria may be beaten to exorcise the evil spirit, and those with epilepsy may be tied down to contain the spirit.

- **Causes of genetic defects**. Punishment by the gods. Consider genetic defects an abomination. Family members care for patient at home but conceal him/her. Families unwilling to institutionalize.

- **Attitudes about disabilities**. Strong stigma associated with disabilities, which Nigerians attribute to evil spirits or punishment by the gods. Generally, family members care for the disabled person, whom outsiders rarely see and whose involvement outside the family is limited.

- **Sick role**. Excuse sick persons from most activities and expect them to be passive and dependent. Expect family members and friends to attend to the sick, pamper them, bring soothing foods, take care of their obligations, and avoid anything that may cause them worry.

- **Home and folk remedies**. Use them extensively. Distinguish between diseases that can be treated with folk medicines and those that respond to Western medicine. Generally treat punishment illnesses with folk remedies; herbalists, native doctors, and spiritualists play major roles. All ethnic groups have large pharmacopoeias (e.g., palm-kernel oil for fever, bitter-leaf water for upset stomach, chewing stick for gum disease, lemon grass for malaria, shea butter for skin conditions, and other herbal preparations). The Hausa use up to 264 plants and roots as medicine.

- **Medications**. Nigerians do not seek care until they have pronounced symptoms; only then do they take medicine. Managing a chronic disease, such as hypertension, may be difficult because it has no obvious symptoms, so patients should be educated about the need to take medication consistently. Best to tell older patient to take medication after each meal rather than at a specific hour. Nigerians often combine folk or over-the-counter medications (even though they may be contraindicated) with prescription drugs, especially if patient fails to see immediate improvement.
- **Acceptance of procedures**. Patient and family members rarely disagree with clinician regarding suggested treatments. Patients generally fear all invasive procedures, including surgery; they need reassurance and education. Traditional and religious beliefs influence patient's willingness to donate or receive blood. Some Nigerians believe that blood carries the spirit or represents the soul. Nigerians are increasingly receptive to blood transfusion when they see it as a necessary adjunct to treatment.
- **Care-seeking**. Generally delay seeking medical attention. Often try home remedies first. Some consult family members and friends before seeking care. The perceived cause of illness influences when, where, and how Nigerians seek care.

HEALTH ISSUES

- **Concept of health**. View health from a holistic perspective, as a state of harmony with one's environment, including the supernatural world (gods, ancestors' spirits, and deities). Disease is the result of disharmony and conflict.
- **Health promotion and prevention**. Indigenous health system includes preventive measures such as massage, dietary restrictions, taboos, incantations, offerings to the gods, wearing special amulets, prayers, and ritual bathing. To promote health, one should eat and drink moderately, avoid emotional distress and exposure to atmospheric changes, be active, rest, and keep peace with the community. Nigerians make offerings to the gods for protection. Preventive strategies include taboo on sexual activity by lactating mothers. Do not commonly follow U.S. diet guidelines. Recreational activities and exercise are recent practices that Nigerian culture has yet to incorporate.
- **Screening**. A new concept for most Nigerians, as customary preventive measures do not include screening. Treat disease when someone becomes ill. Although some Nigerians are amenable to screening if educated about its value, a significant percentage do not use screening regardless of whether they have health insurance or access to care.
- **Common health problems**. Many are lactose intolerant. Other common problems include hypertension, malaria, obesity (traditionally perceived as a sign of good health), and diabetes. Sexually transmitted infections and cervi-

cal and prostate cancer are emerging problems. Some women have vaginal area tenderness and sensitivity, keloid scars, or irritation due in part to circumcision.

DEATH RITUALS

- **Beliefs and attitudes about death**. Death and afterlife are central to customs and traditions, particularly among those from southern Nigeria. Believe in reincarnation. Also believe that dead ancestors aid the living; Nigerians pray to them for well-being. Although Nigerians acknowledge that God ordains death, there is still an underlying belief that no death is natural—that jealousy, witchcraft, or a curse of the gods causes it. However, Muslims view and accept death as God's will. Many ethnic groups distinguish between good and bad deaths. Bad or shameful deaths include dying during childbirth; dying when young, before parents die; dying without offspring; and suicide. One who dies a shameful death does not receive traditional burial or funeral rites; the death is not celebrated for fear that reincarnation may cause families to go through the same pain again. This is a confusing period for the family; it acknowledges the loss, but coping rituals are absent. In southern Nigeria, death is a highly ritualized event with elaborate wake, burial, and funeral ceremonies. Although participants cry, the events are more celebratory, featuring dancing and feasting. In the North, particularly among Muslims, burial and funeral rites are less elaborate and follow religious custom.
- **Preparation**. Usually, Nigerians first inform friends of a death. These friends then assemble at the house before family is informed, to provide support. For weeks, there is a constant stream of visitors.
- **Home vs. hospital**. Traditionally, Nigerians die at home. In U.S., deaths often occur in hospital. Regardless of how sick a loved one is, there is always hope that he/she will get well. Therefore, Nigerians may not welcome hospice care at home, as it is acknowledgment the loved one will die. Hospice care outside the home may be acceptable if it is perceived as an extension of care. Families always want to be with the patient.
- **Special needs**. Emotional outbursts or public expressions of grief vary. Acceptable in some ethnic groups for men and women to cry out loud, fall to the ground, or beat their chests. Other groups frown upon such displays. In some groups, wailing is common or women cry and men shed silent tears. Mourning periods vary from one month to one year, with different rituals marking each phase. Widows wear a mourning dress and refrain from numerous activities. Family members generally shave their heads. Close family and friends bring food and drinks, and stay with the family for some time. Many of these customs continue among immigrants, although family members must return to work as soon as they can. They do not participate in social events until the end of the mourning period, during which they are excused from a number of obligations.
- **Care of the body**. In Nigeria and U.S., mortuary commonly prepares and

preserves body for burial. Most Nigerians want to be buried in homeland with ancestors. Cremation unacceptable.

- **Attitudes about organ donation**. Ancestral worship and belief in reincarnation discourage organ donation, as one is expected to return to ancestors whole. General reluctance to donate organ because that may mean the deceased cannot reincarnate or will return in another life with deformities. Attitudes about receiving organs vary depending on education and religious belief.
- **Attitudes about autopsy**. Presents same dilemmas as organ transplants do. But some Nigerian families are willing to accept autopsy, especially when they suspect that patient received inadequate care.

SELECTED REFERENCES

BBC News, UK Edition. (February 26, 2004). Nigeria leads in religious belief. Retrieved July 4, 2004, from http://news.bbc.co.uk/1/hi/programmes/wtwtgod

Embassy of the Federal Republic of Nigeria. (2004). Nigeria: History and people. Retrieved July 4, 2004, from http://www.nigeriaembassyusa.org/history.html

Etkin, N. L. (2002). Local knowledge of biotic diversity and its conservation in rural Hausaland, northern Nigeria. *Economic Botany*, 56, 73–88.

MoneyNett.com. (August 24, 2000). The comet: 3M Nigerians reside in U.S., says minister. Retrieved August 24, 2000, from http://www.moneynett.com/news/3m.html

Nnedu, C. C. (2004). Nigerian Americans. In J. Giger & R. Davidhizar (Eds.), *Transcultural nursing: Assessment and intervention* (4th ed.). St. Louis, MO: Mosby. Retrieved July 4, 2004, from http://evolveweb.elsevier.com/product Pages/s_0323022952.html

Ogbu, M. A. (1995). *Girl to woman in a changing African society: The impact of modernization and development on sexual socialization of adolescents*. Doctoral dissertation, University of California-Berkeley.

Olupona, J., & Falola, T. (1991). *Religion and society in Nigeria: Historical and sociological perspectives*. Ibadan, Nigeria: Spectrum.

Toubia, N. (1999). *Caring for women with circumcision: A technical manual for health care providers*. New York: RAINBO.

AUTHOR

Marcellina Ada Ogbu, DrPH, is chief operations officer for primary care services at the San Francisco Department of Public Health. She also teaches at City College of San Francisco and has taught at San Francisco State University. As a public health practitioner, she has worked as a community health education specialist, senior health planner, and health administrator. She received both her undergraduate and graduate degrees from the University of California-Berkeley. She was born and raised in Nigeria and has lived in the U.S. for more than two decades.

CHAPTER 27

PAKISTANIS

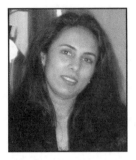

Saleema S. Hashwani

CULTURAL/ETHNIC IDENTITY

- **Preferred term(s)**. Pakistani American, South Asian, Pakistani Asian, or Pakistani. Within close communities, individuals sometimes identify themselves by social and ethnic class status (e.g., *Sheikh* or *Khan*).
- **Census**. A 2003 report by RAND cites 849,386 immigrants in U.S. According to the 2000 U.S. Census, 266,726 were born in Pakistan. Most immigrants are highly educated, earn a good income, and live in large metropolitan areas, such as New York, Washington, Los Angeles, San Francisco, Dallas, Chicago, Cleveland, and Detroit.
- **History of immigration**. Pakistan, formerly part of the British empire and India, became an independent Muslim state in 1947. People from the Indian Subcontinent first arrived in the U.S. in 1898. They were described as "Asian labor." In 1946, the U.S. first began allowing South Asians to immigrate and become citizens, but their numbers were limited to 100 per year. U.S. immigration law was revised in 1965, opening the doors to highly educated, technically trained persons from all countries, including Pakistan. Since 1990, 10,000–13,000 Pakistanis have legally immigrated annually. Though predominantly Muslim, their culture is strongly influenced by Hinduism. (This chapter emphasizes Islam; see the "East Indians" chapter for Hindu and Christian variations.) Immigrants vary socially and culturally according to their level of education, social class, religious affiliation, urban or rural background, and number of years they have resided in the U.S. Pakistanis also are divided along political, ethnic, and tribal lines. Their mixed culture comprises a number ethnic groups, the most predominant being Sindhi, Punjabi, Pathan, and Baluchi.

SPIRITUAL/RELIGIOUS ORIENTATION

- **Primary religious/spiritual affiliations**. Most are Muslim, but there are also many Hindus, Parsis, and Christians. Majority of Muslims belong to Sunni and Shi'ite (or Shi'ah) sects. Sunni Muslims adhere to the practices and teachings of Prophet Mohammed; there is no clear hierarchy of religious leaders. Shi'ite Muslims seek religious guidance from religious leaders (*imams*).

- **Usual religious/spiritual practices**. The five pillars of Islam are belief in one God (Allah) and his messenger, Prophet Mohammed (*Shahada*); prayer five times daily after ritual ablution, at home or in congregation at a mosque; fasting during the month of Ramadan (ninth month of the Muslim calendar); giving alms tax (*zakaat*); and pilgrimage to Mecca at least once in a lifetime. Sabbath prayers on Friday afternoon important. Islam influences all facets of life—birth, marriage, family, politics, economics, and social relationships. Muslims usually seek religious guidance through special prayers, visits to religious shrines, and consultations with religious scholars.

- **Use of spiritual healing/healers**. In Pakistan, may consult an herbalist (*hakim*), religious healer, or homeopathic physician while simultaneously using Western biomedicine. Many believe in spiritual healing. For example, reciting certain verses from the Koran eliminates illnesses or eases suffering. May also go to a spiritual leader (*pir*), who prays for sick person and may give him/her a packet containing Koranic verses (*taawiz*) to wear. Family members provide spiritual care, praying in groups or reading passages from Koran to patient.

- **Holidays**. Religious holidays include two yearly *Eid* festivals: *Eid ul Fitr*, at the end of the month of Ramadan, and *Eid ul Azha*, a festival after pilgrimage. Others are Prophet Mohammed's birthday (*Eid-e-Milad-un-Nabi*) and *Muharram*, a holy day commemorating the martyrdom of Prophet Mohammed's grandson, Hussain, in the battle of Karbala. Most religious holidays are based on lunar calendar. During religious celebrations, believers give charity to the poor, widows, and orphans to ensure spiritual and material prosperity. Typical practices include group prayer and visiting families, relatives, and neighbors. Secular holidays include Pakistan Independence Day (August 14). Some immigrant families also celebrate Easter, Thanksgiving, and Christmas.

COMMUNICATION

ORAL COMMUNICATION

- **Major languages and dialects**. English is official language of Pakistan. National language is Urdu. Pakistanis speak many other languages, including Punjabi, Sindhi, Pashto, Gujarati, Kashmiri, and Baluchi.
- **Greetings**. Express greetings verbally and with gestures. Muslims put palm of right hand to forehead, bow slightly, and utter, *Asallam Wallaiqum*, for

peace and prosperity. Men usually shake hands and hug each other, but women usually do not. Uncommon to use first or last name of older persons, although persons in same age group address each other or younger persons using first name. Address older persons using general terms (e.g., *Baji* for woman of older sister's age, *Bhaiya* for older brother, *Chachi* [aunt]/*Chacha* [uncle] for persons of parents' age, and *Ammah* [female]/*Baba* [male] for persons of grandparents' age).

- **Tone of voice**. Most Pakistani languages call for a soft tone of voice. Pakistanis may interpret loudness as disrespect, a command, an emotional outburst, anger, and/or violence. May give commands to younger persons, but older persons expect to be treated respectfully and politely. From childhood, emphasize and admire modesty, humility, shyness (*sharm*), tolerance, and silence.
- **Direct or indirect style of speech**. Politely acknowledge a message with a simple nod or smile usually. Sometimes silence indicates approval and acceptance; Pakistanis consider nonconfrontation a good quality. It may be rude or disrespectful to ask older persons direct questions. Usually direct with each other and health care providers but avoid topics related to genitals, breasts, or sex. Older persons tend to speak in stories rather than with brief answers.
- **Use of interpreters**. Prefer close family member who is older and of same gender to interpret in health care settings and offer advice. Regarding sensitive issues such as sex, may prefer to consult with older family members of same gender and age. Privacy important when discussing personal matters.
- **Serious or terminal illness**. Pakistanis prefer that physician first disclose diagnosis and prognosis to close family member; normally, husband or eldest male is appropriate. Then it is up to family's discretion whether to tell patient. Muslims believe that one should never give up hope; to do so would be to resist God's will.

WRITTEN COMMUNICATION

- **Literacy assessment**. Immigrants usually are well-educated professionals, although urbanites are more likely to be fluent and literate in English than are those from rural settings. Traditionally, Pakistani society emphasized education of males, but in recent years more women have obtained a university education. Expect young children to speak native language at home but also believe that learning English is important for career. Elderly immigrants may not understand English and may need interpretation to understand disease process. Before giving out forms or instructions, clinician should ask patient directly if and how well he/she understands and reads English or other languages.
- **Consents**. May prefer that a close family member be present for moral support and consultation. Some, especially young adults and women, feel uncomfortable with written consents. Clinician should explain procedure in simple

terms. Pakistanis tend to rely on health professionals to make treatment decisions. Sometimes husband, father, or older brother takes responsibility and
gives consent for care of a female patient.

NONVERBAL COMMUNICATION

- **Eye contact**. May view direct eye contact as rude or disrespectful, especially
  among elderly. From the age of puberty, Muslim men and women usually
  lower their gaze in presence of opposite gender, and avoid touching those of
  the opposite gender if they are not married or blood relatives.
- **Personal space**. Personal space varies by relationship, gender, and acculturation. Space between close friends and family is closer than in dominant
  culture. Traditionally, unrelated men and women maintain 2–3 feet distance
  from each other, often socializing in separate areas of a room.
- **Use and meaning of silence**. Mostly consider silence a good quality;
  emphasize and admire it beginning in childhood. Silence usually indicates
  acceptance, approval, and/or tolerance.
- **Gestures**. Inappropriate gestures include pointing a finger in conversation,
  which shows disrespect or dismissal. May make a point in discussion by holding index finger. Usually express themselves facially rather than with hands
  when talking to someone. Disrespectful for women to sit with legs apart.
  Consider it obscene to step on or touch someone with foot; offender should
  apologize immediately.
- **Openness in expressing emotions**. Repressing emotions may be a way of
  coping. Men usually mask their emotions; rarely cry in public because it is
  viewed as "unmanly." Women frequently express sadness, pain, and appre-
  hension to family, friends, and health care providers of same gender.
- **Privacy**. Most Pakistanis have strong sense of privacy. Are careful not to discuss family matters in public. Keep family secrets within the family; do not
  discuss them with strangers or unrelated outsiders.
- **Touch**. At and beyond puberty, Muslim men and women avoid touching
  those of the opposite gender if they are not married or blood relatives.
  Express love and caring through eyes and facial expressions rather than kissing or hugging.
- **Orientation to time**. May not be extremely time-conscious; dislike monitoring every minute of daily life. Tardiness acceptable for social gatherings,
  but it is important to be on time for medical appointments and work. Time
  orientation depends on situation. It includes focusing on past, present, and
  future (e.g., on the present in social interactions, on the future in terms of
  hard work and commitment to family prosperity).

ACTIVITIES OF DAILY LIVING

- **Modesty**. Patients usually prefer clinician of same gender, especially
  women, who require privacy to discuss health matters. Men comfortable

with loose pants (*shalwar*). Women prefer not to wear hospital gowns that reveal body parts; prefer *shalwar* and top (*kamiz*), below knee length. Many women prefer to cover head and chest with rectangular cloth (*chader*, about 3-by-6 feet). Health care providers should refrain from asking patient to remove any piece of clothing unless there is a clear need.

- **Skin care**. Most prefer a daily morning shower. Patients with respiratory tract infection or who have undergone surgery prefer bed bath. Use lots of running water while bathing, as running water is a symbol of purity and cleanliness. Important that menstruating women take full body bath, including hair wash, at end of period to purify self before praying.
- **Hair care**. Many women consider long hair a sign of beauty. Wash hair once or twice weekly. Women regularly massage scalp with coconut or mustard oil, and comb hair daily. Usually wear a head covering. No restrictions on cutting or shaving body hair.
- **Nail care**. Keep nails short and clean. Usually do not cut nails at night; doing so after sunset is believed to cause misfortune. All nail parings must be thrown in sink with running water.
- **Toileting**. Prefer private toilets for elimination but accept bedpans, urinals, or bedside commodes during hospitalization. Like thorough peri-wash with water after elimination; staff should provide pint-size, plastic water pitcher near toilet or commode. Must use left hand to wash and wipe perineal area. Avoid elimination at certain times of day (e.g., at time of prayer [*azan*] in mosque). Must purify themselves by washing hands, face, and feet before praying.
- **Special clothing or amulets**. Clothing related to age and acculturation. Immodest for women to bare skin. Women from very religious families may dress in a manner that reveals only face and hands. Women may wear gold or silver charm containing name of God (Allah) on neck chain as protection against illness or other bad fortune. Muslims sometimes wear Koranic verses folded in small cloth (*taawiz*) for protection; spiritual person usually provides these. Health care provider should remove *taawiz* only after patient or family member gives permission, or tie *taawiz* onto patient's gown.
- **Self-care**. Sick persons assume dependent role; expect caregiver or family member (usually a woman) to assist with personal hygiene and meals. In hospital, close family members prefer to stay with patient and help with activities of daily living.

FOOD PRACTICES

- **Usual meal pattern**. Typically eat 2–3 meals a day. Prefer big meal at lunch and small meal at supper. May prefer supper in late evening. Sometimes prefer snacks with evening tea or when guests arrive. Prepare elaborate and lavish meals for guests.
- **Special utensils**. None. May prefer clay cookware, which Pakistanis consider to be healthy.

- **Food beliefs and rituals**. Highly respect food. Encourage others to eat with love and compassion, and to be thankful to Allah for providing food that alleviates hunger and nourishes body and mind. Avoid distractions such as watching television, reading, or excessive talking while eating. Many wash hands before touching food. Islam discourages overeating, which is believed to reduce life span and lead to illness. Those who believe in Ayurvedic medicine classify foods as "hot"/"cold," which is related to content rather than temperature. Prescribe "hot" foods in winter for "cold" diseases or states, such as arthritis, respiratory tract infection, circulatory problems, fever, and after surgery. Hot foods include all kinds of meat and fish, eggs, honey, most oils, nuts and seeds, most herbs, and spices. One should eat "cold" foods in hot weather, including milk, butter, cheese, yogurt, most vegetables and fruits, and some grains and legumes, such as wheat, rice, barley, and lentils.
- **Usual diet**. Most common staples are rice or flat, baked bread made from whole wheat flour (*chapati*) eaten with meat, vegetable, or lentil curry. Sweet dishes are not part of regular meal. Breakfast typically comprises cereals, bread or eggs, tea, and milk. Lunch is rice or *chapati* with another dish. Dinner is similar. Teenagers and children eat fast food similar to those in dominant culture. Pakistanis usually entertain guests with cookies or salty snacks and beverage.
- **Fluids**. Beverages of choice are water, buttermilk (*lasi*), or mango shakes, which are believed to aid digestion. Tea with milk is a common hot beverage instead of coffee.
- **Food taboos and prescriptions**. Muslims fast during the month of Ramadan; no food or fluids allowed from sunrise to sunset. Young children, persons who are ill or traveling, and women who are menstruating, pregnant, or breastfeeding are exempt from fasting. Pork and alcoholic beverages strictly prohibited. Allowed to eat only fish with fins and scales. Permitted to eat most meat products from animals slaughtered in a particular manner (*halal*). Pakistanis believe certain foods are incompatible when eaten together. For example, eating fish and milk, red meat and milk, or sour fruit and milk can lead to production of toxins in body. Recommend fasting for fever, gastrointestinal problems, cold, or arthritic pain. During acute illness, may like bland, liquid, or easily digested foods.
- **Hospitality**. Most Pakistani cultures view guests as a blessing from Allah. Hosts ensure that guests are well-fed, offering a meal and drinks such as tea, juice, or other beverage. Host family expects guest to accept food or beverage; some families may consider it rude to refuse.

SYMPTOM MANAGEMENT

- **Pain** (*darad* in many South Asian languages). May understand numerical scale for quantifying pain. Muslim patients may refuse narcotics for mild to moderate pain, as Islam forbids narcotics. Some prefer intramuscular analgesics but not while fasting. Many prefer home remedies to manage acute muscle pain and joint inflammation secondary to trauma. Common reme-dies are mustard-paste poultice applied to painful muscle, and turmeric paste warmed and applied on gauze to painful joint and wrapped with bandage overnight. Accept analgesics for postsurgical pain or pain associated with chronic illnesses, such as cancer and arthritis.

- **Dyspnea** (*sans ukhrna*, or breathlessness). May get very anxious and hyper-ventilate. Accept oxygen if explained. Clinician should approach patient calmly. Some Pakistanis may use home remedies, such as ginger and herbal teas. Some patients prefer to keep themselves warm with extra clothing to avoid getting cold, as Pakistanis consider dyspnea to be a "cold" disease. For patient's comfort, family caregiver usually recites Koran or reads special prayers from it.

- **Nausea/vomiting** (*budhazmi/ulti*). Believe that nausea/vomiting is caused by toxins in stomach that body must eliminate. Typically, Pakistanis do not initially seek medical treatment for nausea/vomiting; they are encouraged instead to refrain from eating regular food and rest their gastrointestinal tract. May consume herbs and spices, such as black pepper and/or dill seeds. If severe, may go to hospital and may accept IV or rectal medication.

- **Constipation/diarrhea** (*kabz/dast*). Believe that constipation causes abdom-inal distention and discomfort, headache, and bad breath. Use herbal reme-dies (e.g., 1 teaspoon of *ghee* [clarified butter] mixed with hot milk, taken at bedtime). Usually encourage eating fiber to relieve constipation. Generally accept enemas. For diarrhea, consume a paste of fresh ginger mixed with but-termilk. Also believe that black coffee, cumin, or nutmeg cures diarrhea. Avoid regular meals; prefer soft or liquid diet and more fluids.

- **Fatigue** (*thakan lagna*). Elderly tend to complain that they are always tired due to aging, which makes it difficult to distinguish illness-related fatigue. Describe fatigue as "I do not feel like doing anything all day." Women more likely to report fatigue than men are; take multivitamins or iron tablets. Those who complain of fatigue are advised to get enough rest and eat a proper diet. Believe that taking a warm bath or shower and drinking a warm glass of milk with some sugar just before bedtime promote sleep and allevi-ate fatigue. Generally receptive to medications and other methods to reduce fatigue if these are explained clearly.

- **Depression** (*dil uddas hona* or *saya* in Urdu, Punjabi, and Gujarati lan-guages). May view depression as a sign of spiritual unhappiness. Associate it with mental illness, which is highly stigmatized. Depressed persons are encouraged to seek help from family and usually resist seeking, or following through with, psychiatric treatment. May seek help from psychiatrist or spir-itual healer in cases of extreme or psychotic depression. Many do not know what depression is and seek medical care for physical symptoms. Women usually somaticize depression. Clinician should be cautious about mention-ing diagnosis, as patient may think it implies that something is very wrong with him/her. Some pray and meditate. With more public awareness, Pakistanis generally are receptive to taking antidepressants and are becoming more receptive to nonpharmacological treatments, such as psychotherapy, group therapy, meditation, and exercise.

- **Self-care symptom management**. Usually prompt in responding to symptoms that cause discomfort. Tend to rely on Western medications along with home remedies to alleviate symptoms. Early ambulation and deep-breathing exercises acceptable in hospital; believe that these improve blood circulation. Chronically ill patients prefer to do their own self-care (e.g., diabetic blood testing, dietary control, and monitoring of blood pressure).

BIRTH RITUALS/CARE OF THE NEW MOTHER AND BABY

- **Pregnancy care**. View pregnancy as a healthy state. Pregnant woman's mother and mother-in-law or elder female family member offer advice. Allow expectant mother to perform usual tasks, except heavy lifting, and protect her from emotional stress and shock. Especially during first trimester, she must avoid "hot" foods, such as meat, eggs, nuts, herbs, and spices, as these are believed to cause miscarriage. Prenatal care becoming common, due to greater emphasis on preventive health practices and health education. In U.S., women receive regular prenatal care and younger adults attend childbirth preparation classes. Husbands sometimes attend classes; depends on level of education and acculturation.
- **Preferences for children**. Some families value sons more than daughters, as sons carry on the family name. Expect young girls to help mother with household chores. Sometimes punish girls more severely than boys for misbehaving. Recent Pakistani emphasis on family planning and birth control has resulted in smaller families in Pakistan. Families prefer two children; consider a son and daughter ideal.
- **Labor practices**. In Pakistan, most deliveries occur in hospital, but some families prefer home birth. In U.S., prefer hospital deliveries. Encourage women to walk during labor. Advise light meals. Usually do not encourage pain medications, as they may delay delivery.
- **Role of the laboring woman during birth**. Usually assumes passive role and follows instructions from health care providers or family members. Moaning, grunting, and screaming acceptable, but older female family members encourage her to suppress expression of pain if possible.
- **Role of the father and other family members during birth**. Female family member stays with mother for emotional support. Fathers usually not present at delivery but remain within reach in case of emergency. Better-educated and more-acculturated fathers prefer to stay with wife to provide emotional support. Do not reveal baby's sex to mother until placenta has been delivered. Show baby to mother first, then to father and other family members. In Muslim families, father or grandfather recites the Muslim calls

to prayer—*Azan* in newborn's right ear and *Iqama* in the left—to ensure infant hears these words first as an invitation to follow God.

- **Vaginal vs. cesarean section**. Usually prefer vaginal delivery. Accept cesarean if necessary.
- **Breastfeeding**. Encourage breastfeeding for at least six months and for as long as 2–3 years, mostly on demand. Working mothers may combine breastfeeding with bottled formula for convenience. Pakistanis encourage breastfeeding mothers to eat nutritious meals rich in carbohydrates and fats for sufficient lactation.
- **Birth recuperation**. In U.S., family or close relatives care for mother and baby for six weeks after delivery. Generally expect new mother and baby to remain at home for 40 days, during which time mother should get adequate rest. Offer her special foods along with regular meals to restore energy she lost during pregnancy and childbirth. Older woman gives new mother back massages with warm oil. Strongly emphasize that mother should stay warm. She may bathe only once a week but can take partial baths and wash perineal area with warm water every time she eliminates. During the 40 days, relatives and friends visit to congratulate family and bring gifts for newborn. Party may be held to celebrate birth. Muslim family may perform ceremony (*Aqiqah*) in which newborn's head is shaved and one or two goats are sacrificed.
- **Baby care**. Mother, maternal grandmother, or older women in family hold and comfort infant. Older women in family usually provide baby care for six weeks to three months after delivery. Common to give baby body massages with warm oil, followed by bath, and to wrap baby tightly to prevent cold from entering his/her body. Father may participate in baby care. Working mother may arrange infant care or have older, female family member provide such care.
- **Problems with baby**. Clinician should tell mother first, but if illness is serious, may approach father or mother-in-law first. Pakistanis expect physician, rather than nurse, to inform parents of diagnosis. Generally accept nurses' opinions about managing ongoing health problem.
- **Male and female circumcision**. Male circumcision is an Islamic ritual that should be performed before age 7, but there is no minimum or maximum age. Girls never circumcised.

DEVELOPMENTAL AND SEXUAL ISSUES

- **Celebration of menarche or becoming a man**. No specific celebration for either gender.
- **Attitudes about birth control**. Many Pakistani married couples accept birth control. Sometimes the decision is mutual, but it is more common for woman to use birth control after she obtains permission from husband. Single women who are sexually intimate secretly use birth control methods such as oral contraceptives. Birth control more common in younger generation.

- **Attitudes about sexually transmitted infection (STI) control, including condoms**. There has been more emphasis recently on discussing responsible sexual behaviors with adolescents, particularly girls. Families usually rely on health care providers to discuss importance of STI control. Information on women's risk of STIs tends to exacerbate stigma and confusion. Testing positive raises concerns about trust, fidelity, blame, and protection among women in long-term monogamous relationships. Older generation believes there is no risk of acquiring an STI in marriage. Young adults more knowledgeable about STIs and more likely to protect themselves, including using condoms.
- **Attitudes about abortion**. Therapeutic abortion acceptable if mother's life endangered. Islam forbids abortion by choice, as fetus is considered to be a person 120 days after conception. Family usually wants to be given fetus or stillborn baby for burial. If woman becomes pregnant outside of marriage, she might have an abortion; if she does, immediate family keeps it a secret, never revealing it to outsiders.
- **Attitudes about unwed sexual experimentation**. Consider it a sin that brings shame on family. Allow sexual relationships only after marriage. Forbid and discourage premarital sex among both genders, particularly girls. If parents learn that a young woman has been sexually active, they or other family members may punish or disown her. Acculturated young persons usually keep their sexual relationships secret.
- **Sexual orientation**. Parents and other close family members do not approve of same-sex relationships. Uncommon for individuals or families to disclose minority sexual orientation to family or community, as Pakistanis consider sex to be a private and personal matter.
- **Gender identity**. Strong traditional expectations of women to be lady-like and of men to be very masculine. Parents may pressure children who do not fit these ideals to change.
- **Attitudes about menopause**. View it as a normal physiological process. Older women may welcome it because they gain respect and decision-making power in family. Often seek and follow medical advice if symptoms persist.

FAMILY RELATIONSHIPS

- **Composition/structure**. Concept of family encompasses several households living in different locations but counted as one family. Typical household comprises parents, children, grandparents, and older relatives living together. Family members interdependent. They are more concerned about the unit than about themselves individually; family responsibilities normally come first. In U.S., some prefer to live as nuclear family. Extended family comprises grandparents, their sons and families, and unmarried daughters. Usually expect daughter to move in with husband's family after marriage. Same-gender couples/parents unacceptable.
- **Decision-making**. Oldest male family member, usually father or eldest son,

has decision-making power within and outside of the family. However, he rarely makes decisions in isolation; consults other family members and considers their opinions before making final decision.

- **Spokesperson**. Commonly the father, eldest son, or other male family member.
- **Gender issues**. Gender roles in Pakistan vary depending on social class and educational level; an additional factor in U.S. is level of acculturation. Men are primarily breadwinners and responsible for activities outside the home. Women are primarily responsible for taking care of and raising children, and for housekeeping. Working women also handle domestic responsibilities, with minimal support from their male counterparts. In some families, women still are subservient to husband's wishes and demands.
- **Changing roles among generations in U.S.** First-generation Pakistani Americans may reflect traditional hierarchical family structure in terms of gender and age; gender roles and relationships are clearly defined. Relationship between husband and wife, and between parents and children, is both close and formal. Most marriages are arranged and divorce rate is low. Young women in second generation prefer to select their own mates. Females experience more stress than males do regarding prohibitions on dating and/or any expression of sexuality. Women are becoming more active professionally and providing equal financial support for their family. Some Pakistani couples now have egalitarian relationships.
- **Caring roles**. Mother, wife, daughter, or other female relative usually cares for sick family members, including children and elders. Young male patients prefer to be cared for by their mother or wife rather than have another female caregiver touch them. Pakistanis hospitalize sick persons only if they are seriously ill or require medical intervention for complex illness.
- **Expectations of and for children**. Expect children to obey parents. Teach children to behave well and respect others, especially elders; to work hard; and to be religious. Treat children affectionately and pamper them but only up to a certain point. Acceptable to punish children for misbehavior. Children rarely make decisions independently; seek opinion of an elder or authority figure, which usually carries much weight. Children often rely on parents to choose their career. In Pakistan, there is a greater emphasis on vocational training than on formal education. Pakistanis often encourage children to take up the father's or family's occupation/business.
- **Expectations of and for elders**. Highly respect elders. Do not permit younger family members to boast around elderly or belittle them. Consider the mere presence of an elderly family member to be a blessing from Allah. Advise children and grandchildren to be grateful to elderly, as they are the reason one exists. Elders usually live with their children (preferably married sons) and grandchildren. They sometimes babysit and teach cultural values and religion to grandchildren.

- **Expectations of hospital visitors**. Close family member usually stays with sick person and wants to participate in care, even overnight. Other family members may bring in fruit or home-cooked food.

ILLNESS BELIEFS

- **Causes of/attitudes about physical illness**. Attribute illness to natural causes, such as "germs," dirt, cold or wind, seasonal changes, stress, or failure to take proper care of the body. Traditional humoral belief holds that "hot"/ "cold" imbalances cause sickness; hot/cold qualities describe food, drinks, medicinal herbs, individual human nature, and specific illnesses. Also believe that illness has supernatural causes, that it results from bad actions. Illness washes away a person's sins and engenders God's mercy; therefore, one should never complain to God about illness but rather recite prayers to alleviate suffering.

- **Causes of/attitudes about mental illness**. Often believe that psychosis is due either to spells cast by an enemy or to the body falling prey to an evil spirit. Cultural factors that inhibit Pakistanis from seeking counseling or psychotherapy include a prohibition on talking about personal matters with anyone other than family members; social denial of mental illness, which brings shame and stigma upon family; and little emphasis on self as opposed to family obligations. Often prefer to seek spiritual advice first for curing mental illness.

- **Causes of genetic defects**. Some families believe that genetic defects occur when pregnant woman picks up sharp objects, such as scissors, knives, and needles, during a lunar or solar eclipse. Some believe that persons with hereditary or congenital problems must have been exposed to toxins or chemicals during mother's pregnancy. (See "East Indians" for Hindu beliefs.)

- **Attitudes about disabilities**. Have limited understanding. Disabled family member often feels isolated and not respected, and is forced into a passive role and undervalued within family. Parents may regard disability as a tragedy, with implications not just for their own future but also for the child's development and family life. Consider persons with disabilities to be free of sin. Families sometimes believe that it is a blessing to care for a disabled member.

- **Sick role**. Sick persons usually assume passive role, are encouraged to rest, and are relieved of daily responsibilities. Pakistanis do not expect ill women to cook or do housework.

- **Home and folk remedies**. Folk remedies are passed down from generation to generation. Such remedies include honey in warm milk for cough and cold, turmeric paste as an antiseptic to heal wounds, and ginger and lime juice with sugar for stomach upset. To cure earache, boil fresh garlic in mustard oil, cool it to room temperature, and place concoction in affected ear overnight. Some use cloves for toothache.

- **Medications**. Most use home and folk remedies, such as certain leaves and herbs available at Pakistani or Indian stores, before consulting physician. Believe that natural substances cure many ailments. Usually take Western medications for a physical health problem, such as pain, fever, or cold. Sometimes take herbal medicine concurrently with other medication. Some families keep over-the-counter medications imported from Pakistan as first-aid remedies at home. Younger persons comply with medications, but the elderly stop medication, especially antibiotics, when symptoms decrease.

- **Acceptance of procedures**. Generally receptive to blood transfusions but may prefer to receive blood from persons of same religion. May fear giving blood, as blood donation can cause severe weakness. Organ transplants acceptable.
- **Care-seeking**. Usually prompt in responding to symptoms that cause discomfort. Typically accept Western biomedical practices. Some prefer to consult homeopaths or herbalists; others consult a spiritual healer in conjunction with biomedicine. Tend to rely on Western medications along with home remedies to alleviate symptoms.

HEALTH ISSUES

- **Concept of health**. Balance among body, mind, and spirit; senses that function normally; and body, mind, and consciousness harmoniously working as one.
- **Health promotion and prevention**. View health as a precious gift that one must enjoy. Observe practices that preserve, maintain, and protect health. To stay healthy, one should get adequate rest and sleep, rise before sunrise, and go to bed early; maintain personal hygiene; eat in moderation; exercise; and pray regularly. Too much sex is unhealthy. Negative emotions, such as hate, anger, greed, jealousy, fear, and worry, may negatively affect health and should be avoided. In U.S., young Pakistanis are becoming aware of healthy lifestyle, including stress management, exercise, and good nutrition.
- **Screening**. Usually accept all screening procedures. Exception is unmarried women who may not allow vaginal examination to preserve virginity. Younger, educated persons undergo screening more routinely.
- **Common health problems**. Coronary heart disease, hypertension, and diabetes. Incidence of hypertension and depression is higher in women than men.

DEATH RITUALS

- **Beliefs and attitudes about death**. Muslims believe that all people are born free of sin and that on judgment day everyone will be accountable for their deeds. Accept death, believing that people must go to the other world when their time comes, that their time in the mortal world is completed. Acceptable to express grief. Family may accept life support initially but not continue it for a long period, viewing it as playing with Allah or nature.
- **Preparation**. Pakistanis tell immediate family first and as soon as possible

so they can inform other relatives and family members. If death is imminent, family members and relatives must be called and allowed to stay at patient's bedside. Family decides whether to tell dying person; usually, it does not. Muslim family may offer special prayers for dying person to ease his/her suffering. Sometimes, when patient is near death, family summons religious leader (*imam*) to offer special prayers.

- **Home vs. hospital**. Usually prefer death at home in the presence of all family members. Family may wish to perform religious rituals at time of death. Many families do not accept hospice.
- **Special needs**. Some families may want to call spiritual leader, who prays for dying person and gives him/her holy water to drink to purify the body internally just before death. Surviving family members mourn openly by crying. Muslims mourn for three days and then hold periodic memorial gatherings (e.g., one week later, then one month later).
- **Care of the body**. After someone dies, body, arms, and legs are straightened, eyes are closed, toes are fastened together with bandage, and body is covered with a sheet. If the deceased was an adult, body is ritually washed by another Muslim of same gender just before burial, then wrapped in a white cotton shroud and placed in coffin. Body buried as soon as possible after death. Muslims do not believe in embalming.
- **Attitudes about organ donation**. Muslims usually resist organ donation because Islam forbids it.
- **Attitudes about autopsy**. Most Pakistanis do not accept autopsy unless absolutely necessary. Muslims request that, if autopsy performed, organs be returned to body afterward.

SELECTED REFERENCES

Ibrahim, F., Ohnishi, H., & Sandhu, D. S. (1997). Asian-American identity development: South Asian Americans. *Journal of Multicultural Counseling and Development, 25,* 34–50.

Immigration Statistics for U.S. States. (2003). *RAND California 2003.* Retrieved October 15, 2003, from http://www.ca.rand.org/cgi-bin/annual.cgi

Krikorian, M., Pipes, D., Skerry, P., & Camarota, S. (2002, August). Muslim Immigrants in the United States. Center for Immigration Studies Forum. Retrieved October 26, 2003, from http://www.danielpipes.org/article/453

McKennis, A. T. (1999). Caring for the Islamic patient. *AORN Journal, 69,* 1187–1202.

AUTHOR

Saleema S. Hashwani, RN, MSN, is a PhD candidate in the University of California-San Francisco School of Nursing and an immigrant from Pakistan who has five years of community health and teaching experience. She is using the grounded theory method to study the resettlement experiences of first-generation Pakistani immigrants in the U.S. Her studies focus on self- and ethnic-identity construction, and on the beliefs and attitudes immigrants have about physical and mental health, health care needs, and utilization of health care. She is a project manager at Lumetra, a quality improvement organization in San Francisco.

CHAPTER 28

POLISH

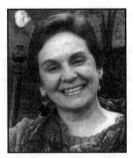

Eileen M. Carol

CULTURAL/ETHNIC IDENTITY

- **Preferred term(s)**. Polish or Pole, from the Polanes tribe, which established the state in the 10th century. "Polak" considered derogatory.
- **Census**. The 2000 U.S. Census estimates more than 9 million people of Polish ancestry, but of these, only 471,000 were born in Poland. Live predominantly in New York, Chicago, and Detroit areas, as well as in Pennsylvania, New Jersey, California, and Wisconsin. Historically and today, Chicago has the most well-developed Polish community.
- **History of immigration**. Poles came to America in the early 1600s as glassblowers. Society also valued their skills in manufacturing pitch, tar, and resins for the shipbuilding and lumber industries. Poland was partitioned among Prussia, Russia, and Austria between 1772–1919 but maintained its language and culture through a strong, Catholic, religious tradition. Political uprisings against partition resulted in emigration of Polish patriots, intellectuals, and poorer nobles to the U.S. The first communities were in Texas (1854) and Wisconsin (1855). A massive first wave of immigrants arrived between 1854–1924, especially after the 1870 Franco-Prussian War. They left Poland for economic, political, and religious reasons. Most were poor peasants who came first from the Prussian annex; others from the Russian and Austrian annexes followed. Many were illiterate and unskilled; they took low-paying jobs as laborers and lived in crowded conditions, establishing close-knit ethnic clusters in Buffalo, New York City, and Chicago. The second wave, after World War II, included émigrés escaping Soviet oppression, political prisoners, dissidents, and intellectuals from refugee camps. This educated group aligned itself with middle-class and professional groups in the U.S. A smaller third wave of immigrants arrived during the 1980s,

when martial law was imposed in Poland. Many were highly educated and have done well in business and academia.

SPIRITUAL/RELIGIOUS ORIENTATION

- **Primary religious/spiritual affiliations**. About 95% are Roman Catholic. Remainder are Orthodox, Protestant, or Jewish. Most Poles in U.S., especially younger persons living in Polish communities and the elderly, are deeply religious. More-assimilated Poles are less religiously observant.
- **Usual religious/spiritual practices**. In addition to the Catholic belief in a trinitarian God comprising the Father, Son, and Holy Spirit, Poles believe in, and are devoted to, many saints and angels (e.g., Satan is a fallen angel and source of all evil in an ongoing spiritual battle between good and evil). Catholics attend church at least weekly, pray daily and before meals, and plan activities around baptisms, name day, first communions, confirmations, weddings, and funerals. Strongly devoted to Blessed Virgin Mary, Mother of God (*Matka Boska*). A goal for many is to make a pilgrimage to Our Lady of Czestochowa in Poland. Believe in spiritual properties of prayer books, rosary beads, medals, and consecrated objects and relics of saints (bone or clothing). Openly express this belief in the home with crucifixes, pictures, statues, candles, and a devotional corner. Poles who practice other religions range from devout to less so.
- **Use of spiritual healing/healers**. Polish Catholics strongly believe in prayer and God's intervention in physical healing. Priest confers sacrament of healing (prayers and blessing with holy oil) on ill or dying persons. Prayers also invoke saints and family members who died previously. Family members may bring relics, such as bone or clothing, of saints and devotional items to bedside of ill or dying person, or pin them on him/her.
- **Holidays**. When Poland adopted Christianity in 10th century, Catholic Church incorporated native traditions and became the primary preserver of Polish folkways for 1,100 years. There are major Catholic feasts monthly, but main focus is on Christmas and Easter. Christmas season begins with four weeks of Advent and ends with Feast of the Epiphany on January 6. Easter season begins with Ash Wednesday, when priest traces a cross of ashes on forehead as a reminder of mortality and the need for penance. Forty-day fast of Lent follows, and the season ends with a Holy Week celebration on Easter Sunday. Easter meal, blessed by priest, includes bread, paschal lamb (made of cake, butter, or sugar), smoked meats, bitter herbs, greens, wine, salt, decorated eggs, and pussy willows (Polish palms). Catholic children named after saints celebrate the feast day of their particular saint as a birthday with gifts and other remembrances. Poles in U.S. celebrate two major secular holidays: Feast of St. Joseph the Worker (May 1), a national holiday in Poland, and Freedom of Constitution (July 22), commemorating the liberation of Poland after World War II. American sec-

ular holidays have little significance for most older Poles, but more-acculturated persons celebrate them.

COMMUNICATION
ORAL COMMUNICATION

- **Major languages and dialects**. Polish, with minor regional differences. Under communism (1945–89), Poles were not permitted to speak or read English; German and Russian supplemented Polish in schools. Since the fall of communism, the country has encouraged English; most younger Poles and university students realize its importance. Educated immigrants speak English on arrival, but older adults typically do not.
- **Greetings**. Very formal and polite. Commonly shake hands with strangers. Occasionally greet with a gentle kiss or touch on each cheek if they know the person. Gender, age, and title important in establishing social hierarchy. Persons of lower social status show deference to those of higher status. Use "Mr." (*Pan*) and "Mrs." (*Pani*). Never use first names, unless they receive permission to do so. Pleased if foreigner attempts to speak their language, even if pronunciation is incorrect. "Hello"/"Good morning" (*Dzien dobry*, pronounced zhen dough-brie) is a common greeting.
- **Tone of voice**. Very self-confident. Poles have strong opinions and may appear to be pushy, but a seemingly raised voice may just reflect assuredness. Enjoy a hearty, animated conversation. Facial expressions may indicate tone of conversation.
- **Direct or indirect style of speech**. Very direct. Poles look directly in another's face and say what is on their mind. Freely share thoughts and ideas, especially as a sign of hospitality. In general conversation, easily say "no" when they do not agree. Polite to authority figures, such as physicians; do not want to offend them by being disagreeable.
- **Use of interpreters**. Spouse may be able to interpret. If unavailable, best to match patient's and interpreter's gender. Inappropriate to use younger children to interpret for adults or elderly.
- **Serious or terminal illness**. Father or spouse should be informed first; he/she makes most decisions and then appropriately shares information with rest of family. If family member unavailable to make decision, patient defers to physician, who is highly respected.

WRITTEN COMMUNICATION

- **Literacy assessment**. American-born Poles literate in English; most not literate in Polish unless parents taught them. Most adult immigrants have at least a high school education and read, write, and speak Polish. Great variation in ability to read and write in English because of English-language ban in Poland until 1989. Acceptable for clinician to assess patient's literacy by asking him/her directly. Difficulties with English have hindered immigrants from working in their trained field and have lowered their social status.

- **Consents**. Should be formalized in writing for all patients. Clinician also should carefully discuss consents with older Poles, as they may not completely understand a procedure. Patients may be hesitant to sign written consents or participate in research.

NONVERBAL COMMUNICATION

- **Eye contact**. Look at others directly in the eye while talking, and prefer that others do the same. Direct eye contact indicates one is listening. No variation by age or social status.
- **Personal space**. Comfortable in close proximity with family members and friends, similar to other Northern European Americans. Keep greater distance from strangers, including health care providers.
- **Use and meaning of silence**. Means one is listening (acknowledgment). Poles also use silence with children to indicate disapproval.
- **Gestures**. Very expressive with hands. No specific cultural gestures.
- **Openness in expressing emotions**. Very expressive. Display emotions freely. Although very open with family and friends, they may restrict expression with strangers until a trusting relationship has been established. Praise the deeds and good works of others but are less apt to acknowledge how they feel about one another. Adults express love for other adults covertly; do so more freely for young children, with tenderness.
- **Privacy**. Do not share personal information with strangers until a trusting relationship has been established. Never share some personal information. Willing to share public information first (facts about themselves or their illness) as well as thoughts and ideas. Comfortable talking about job, family, spouse, and misfortunes.
- **Touch**. Common among family and friends as an expression of caring. Not overly demonstrative. Because Poles have profound trust in physicians, they allow any body part to be touched in an exam or during routine health care. Clinician should avoid casual body contact and ask permission before touching private body parts.
- **Orientation to time**. Punctuality very important. Poles are on time or early for appointments. In social situations, expect others to arrive on time and stay late. Maintaining family traditions (e.g., all older children go to mother's house) demonstrates strong orientation to past. Also future-oriented; strong work ethic pushes Poles to achieve.

ACTIVITIES OF DAILY LIVING

- **Modesty**. Personal modesty and privacy very important. Prefer health care providers of same gender. Women accept male clinicians for gynecological exams but prefer females. Men prefer male providers.

- **Skin care**. Bathe daily. No special soaps or lotions. Most use fragrances or perfumes.
- **Hair care**. No special customs regarding hair cutting or products. Shampoo hair daily if oily, otherwise more infrequently.
- **Nail care**. Older persons trim nails short. Younger females may leave fingernails long and paint them.
- **Toileting**. No restrictions or rituals. Always wash hands afterward. Expect privacy.
- **Special clothing or amulets**. Wear religious items, such as crucifixes, medals, or cloth scapular around neck. Prefer to keep these items on, especially while hospitalized, for spiritual support.
- **Self-care**. Women try to care for themselves as much as possible; if seriously ill, they expect help. Men may expect more assistance while hospitalized or at home.

FOOD PRACTICES

- **Usual meal pattern**. Usually a hearty breakfast of coffee, bread, sausage, and eggs, and a mid-morning snack. Main meal is in mid-afternoon—soup, meat, potatoes, hot vegetable, and dessert. May also have a light, cold snack in evening. In U.S., three-meal daily pattern, with main meal in evening.
- **Special utensils**. None.
- **Food beliefs and rituals**. Food is a very important symbol of hospitality and sustenance. No specific food-preparation or eating rituals. Many religious holidays involve special fasts or feasts with special foods.
- **Usual diet**. Before the end of communism, staple diet was chicken, pork, millet, barley, potatoes, cabbage, turnips, beets, beans, and onions. Eat hearty bread at every meal and a variety of dumplings, including *pierogi*. In cold weather, stews and soups common. Favorite desserts include coffee cake (*babka*), pastries, and poppyseed roll. Polish foods and cooking similar to German, Russian, and Jewish dishes. Diet usually high in saturated fat from fried food, sour cream and butter, and fatty meats (e.g., Polish sausage [*kielbasa*] is 40% fat). Processed ham and pickled foods increase sodium content. Polish diet often deficient in fresh fruit and vegetables; in Poland, these are limited to apples, cherries, and plums, and beans, beets, cabbage, carrots, and potatoes. Poles in U.S. eat a greater variety and have fewer deficiencies.
- **Fluids**. All drink water and milk. In Poland, prepare juices from fresh cherries and other locally available fruits. Adults drink tea, coffee, and alcohol (wine, beer, or hard liquor, such as vodka). Children also drink sodas. Excessive alcohol consumption a problem for many Poles, including those in U.S.
- **Food taboos and prescriptions**. Some Polish Jews keep kosher, eating only meat from which all blood has been drained, avoiding pork and shellfish, and keeping meat and milk products strictly separate. Some Catholic holidays restrict certain foods. During Lent, for example, these Catholics

may not consume meat; also fast, eating only small meals. For health promotion and illness, hot clear soups and herbal teas very important; also a diet balanced with fruit and vegetables. Special foods for ill persons include soups, especially chicken soup with parsley, carrots, and sometimes other vegetables.

- **Hospitality**. Food a very important symbol. Serve food to guests at home and expect them to eat. In lieu of main meal, offer snacks, desserts, or drinks. Visitors commonly bring a bouquet of fresh flowers or candy and should plan to stay late.

SYMPTOM MANAGEMENT

Generally stoic about all symptoms. Able to express symptom severity on numeric scale. Often seek care only when symptom is severe.

- **Pain** (*ból*). Meaning may be religious. Suffering atones for one's offenses against God and for personal salvation. Many immigrants have worked as laborers and are accustomed to tolerating bodily aches and pains. Tend to minimize pain or persevere. Avoid pain medication but follow physician's recommendations and use analgesics when necessary. Also use herbal remedies and folk treatments (e.g., heat and ice, rubbing compounds, and poultices for muscle and joint aches and pains).

- **Dyspnea** (*trudno oddychać*, pronounced trud-no o-de-hach). After immigrating, Poles often worked in large industrial settings. Air pollution and respiratory problems common, exacerbated by high incidence of cigarette smoking. Believe that respiratory problems are due to inadequate air or poor ventilation, and that breathing fresh air in the sun helps alleviate them. Older patients seek medical help only when other methods do not work. May seek care or express dyspnea only when severe. Accept oxygen and other physician-recommended remedies. Treatment in Poland often included visits to spas. For example, at Tezniowy Park in Ciechocinek, built in 1824, windmills pump mineral water into an extensive, elevated system of twigs that release a vapor believed to heal respiratory ailments. Poles also may breathe vapors prepared from steamed herbs, but this practice is less common in U.S.

- **Nausea/vomiting** (*mdłości*, pronounced dwos-chi)/*wymioty*, pronounced v-maoaw-te). Believe that infection or poisoning causes nausea/vomiting. Report nausea/vomiting only if asked or if it interferes with daily activities. Expect a care provider to clean up vomitus. Use a variety of teas, including chamomile, as well as soda and herbal remedies to treat gastrointestinal disorders. Poles hydrate with clear soups and broths, and herbal teas. If these do not work, they seek physician's help, especially if patient is a child. Accept all prescriptions for medications.

- **Constipation/diarrhea** (*zatwardzenie*, pronounced zot-far-zen-ya)/*biegunka*, pronounced be-ah-gun-ka). Try a variety of herbal treatments, vitamins, soups, and teas before seeking physician's help. Accept suggested medications, enemas, and dietary changes.

- **Fatigue** (*zmęczenie*, pronounced czem-chen-ya). Because Poles have a strong work ethic, they are always tired. Most tend to work through fatigue, a symptom clinicians do not typically see. If fatigue present, clinician should carefully evaluate it.
- **Depression** (*depresja*, pronounced de-pres-chia). Recognize depression. Even though Poles frequently talk about their difficult lives, especially during war and under the former communist regime, they tend to turn to mental health providers only as a last resort. For psychosocial problems, they seek help from family members or parish priest. Older immigrants may get depressed because they lack the language or coping skills to help them function in U.S., and are especially vulnerable when adult children leave to begin their own families. Visit physician and accept medication when they can no longer function.
- **Self-care symptom management**. Try various self-care treatments before seeking health care. Most Poles are expected to carry out their normal daily functions when sick, and will do so as long as possible, even if chronically ill. Often neglect self-care for sake of family. Once a physician identifies the problem, Poles do what is necessary for care.

BIRTH RITUALS/CARE OF THE NEW MOTHER AND BABY

- **Pregnancy care**. In the past, pregnant woman took precautions to ensure a strong and healthy baby. Many old wives' tales included avoiding looking at or into a fire, which might cause the baby to have a red birthmark; looking at a mouse, which might cause moles; looking through a keyhole, which might cause crossed eyes; and seeing a lame person, which might cause the baby to be lame. Poles also believed that crossing over a rope on the ground or under a clothesline resulted in problems with the umbilical cord during childbirth. They concealed a pregnancy as long as possible to protect mother and infant from jealousy, witchcraft, and the evil eye. Having a baby shower brought bad luck; even now, grandmothers may be reluctant to give gifts until after the birth. Not all of these traditional beliefs have been passed down to second- and third-generation Polish Americans. Poles respect pregnant women. They consider prenatal care important and expect women to seek preventive health care, eat well, and obtain adequate rest in order to ensure a healthy baby. Emphasis on eating well means making sure women do not gain excessive weight during pregnancy. Poles rarely take childbirth preparation classes.
- **Preferences for children**. Value both boys and girls. Greatly desire children. In Poland and among early immigrants to U.S., women tried to ensure fertility by eating herbs and meat from animals considered to be fertile, by praying, and by making pilgrimages to holy places. Children enhanced a family's status and were an economic necessity. During war and in times of poverty, Polish families spaced their children. Today in U.S., prefer smaller families (2–3 children).

- **Labor practices**. At one time, untrained midwives were common in rural Poland, but today hospital births are typical there. In U.S., Poles may use a midwife if they consider her to be as good as a physician. In the past, they removed or undid anything with knots (including plaited hair) to ease labor pains. Also used garlic and onions to chase away spirits that might interfere with delivery. Today, Poles more commonly invoke Virgin Mary's assistance through prayer and saying the rosary.
- **Role of the laboring woman during birth**. Goes to hospital while in labor. Cooperates with staff recommendations. Labor practices vary. For example, some women prefer to walk and others to lie in bed. Takes an active role in labor and birth. Women have a strong constitution and prefer not to be medicated for pain, but they request medication if pain is intolerable.
- **Role of the father and other family members during birth**. Consider labor to be a woman's domain. She usually needs help and special care from an older and respected woman, such as her mother, sister, or close female friend. Women born in Poland may feel uncomfortable with family-centered care or with men in the delivery room; instead, men stay in waiting room. Family members usually absent during delivery. American-born Polish men are more involved in labor and birth, and present in labor and delivery rooms.
- **Vaginal vs. cesarean section**. Prefer vaginal delivery but accept C-section if necessary. Defer to physician.
- **Breastfeeding**. Expect mother to breastfeed. Consider it beneficial and healthy for infant. According to an old belief, placing infant on left breast first makes the child left-handed. Most children weaned by two years; in the past, many superstitions determined when weaning should occur (e.g., on certain feast days, not on fasting days, during the full moon or harvest, or in the fall). In U.S., new mothers nurse as long as they can if they remain at home but bottle-feed if they must return to work. Rarely combine breast- and bottle-feeding.
- **Birth recuperation**. Expect women to rest for first few weeks after delivery. Infants generally sleep with mother or in same room until the christening, usually at age 4–6 weeks. In Poland, nurse comes to the home daily to help with baby until umbilical cord falls off. Most often, woman's mother cooks and helps care for the infant, household, and other children for at least one month. This practice is the same among new mothers in U.S.
- **Baby care**. Do not expect father to help care for infant. Grandparents have an important role; Poles often expect grandmother and older women in family to help with infant and provide instruction on care during first month.
- **Problems with baby**. Clinician should tell both parents as soon as possible. Should not tell friends or members of extended family; family will inform them at its discretion.
- **Male and female circumcision**. Neither practiced, unless male child is Jewish.

DEVELOPMENTAL AND SEXUAL ISSUES

- **Celebration of menarche or becoming a man**. No special celebrations. In the past, girls beginning their menses received little information; they were expected simply to know what was happening. American-born mothers prepare daughters for menarche. Girl tells only her mother that she has begun to menstruate. Periods never mentioned in presence of male family members.

- **Attitudes about birth control**. Although Catholic Church strongly opposes birth control, many second- and third-generation Polish Americans use various methods. Most common one is avoiding sexual intercourse during times of fertility. Poles highly value children. Also still value chastity until marriage (i.e., "no marriage, no children"). Third-generation Poles in U.S. do not share that attitude.

- **Attitudes about sexually transmitted infection (STI) control, including condoms**. Personal responsibility and monogamous relationships are a priority. Attitudes about sexuality are changing, especially among younger Poles. Young adults are more knowledgeable about STIs and protect themselves, including using condoms.

- **Attitudes about abortion**. Most follow Catholic teaching that opposes abortion, believing that everyone has a spiritual soul from the moment of conception. Abortion unacceptable even among young adults who are not staunch Catholics.

- **Attitudes about unwed sexual experimentation**. Frown upon sexual activity outside of marriage for both sexes but especially for women. Prefer that couples marry. Some acculturated young persons have sexual relationships but do not reveal them to family.

- **Sexual orientation**. Strong expectation to fulfill traditional roles and have heterosexual relationships. Families do not approve of gay or lesbian relationships. Gay or lesbian family member remains closeted. Polish community may ostracize same-gender couples.

- **Gender identity**. Strongly emphasize male and female gender identities, although parents do not pressure a masculine girl or feminine boy to change. Older Poles do not accept ambiguous gender identity. Younger American-born Poles may be more accepting.

- **Attitudes about menopause**. Accept it as part of life. Releases women from childbearing responsibilities. Poles treat older women with more respect. Women never discuss menopausal symptoms. If symptoms interfere with daily activities, women seek physician's help. Younger-generation women more willing to discuss symptoms with women their own age.

FAMILY RELATIONSHIPS

- **Composition/structure**. Family is the core of Polish life. Extended family is the norm, including aunts, uncles, and godparents. Long-time friends become aunts or uncles to Polish children. Patriarchal social structure, with father the head of the family. In the past, families were very large; today, parents have only a few children. Numerous family rituals and socializing around holidays and family gatherings, such as births, marriages, and name dates. Poles traditionally expect husbands to be faithful to their wives and provide financial support. Also expect wives to be faithful and obedient. Both parents work very hard for the family and children. Major priority is enhancing family's position in the community.

- **Decision-making**. While father is the head of the family, women express opinions and participate in decision-making. Nuclear family makes major health decisions, but it may seek help from an extended-family member, knowledgeable friend, or parish priest. Parental authority remains important even into old age. May ask more-educated children or friends to intervene and provide information for decision-making.
- **Spokesperson**. As head of the family, father speaks for it. Parents speak for children. Women often make decisions about matters within the home.
- **Gender issues**. Consider men and women to be equal. Men have more authority and are expected to provide financial support, but women have more control in the household. Women cook and tend the children and house. They often have jobs and provide additional income.
- **Changing roles among generations in U.S.** Older Poles, especially the foreign-born, have more-traditional beliefs and roles. Those born in U.S.—especially the third and succeeding generations—tend to be acculturated to American values and lifestyle. However, the Polish value of family solidarity remains very strong. View divorce as a last resort. Acculturated children remain loyal to their parents and do not neglect them. Given the emphasis on English language and American education, children tend not to continue speaking or learning Polish.
- **Caring roles**. Women are the caretakers in sickness and health. Poles expect women to continue their duties as wife and homemaker even when ill; other women fill caretaker role when a woman becomes sick. Men never assume caretaker role, but this may be changing among younger Poles.
- **Expectations of and for children**. Expect children to obey parents and older siblings. Any behavior that undermines parental authority is unacceptable. Parents may be demonstrative with young children (through toddler age) but do not show affection for older children by way of teaching them to be strong and resilient. Praise children for doing well and for self-control. Do not spank children. Parents make decisions for, and plan the futures of, children until they reach adulthood yet support the decisions their children make. Poles expect children to be educated, have a good job, and provide for their elderly parents. In the past, parents sought prospective marriage partners for their children, but American-born Poles do not. Parents tend to be vocal and influential regarding children's dating partners and activities.
- **Expectations of and for elders**. Greatly respect older persons, who con-

tribute to the family economically, help in the daily routine (including raising and assisting grandchildren), and maintain Polish customs and religious values. Families try to keep aged family members at home, but work schedules and demands of care may force them to consider placing elderly in extended-care facility or nursing home.

- **Expectations of hospital visitors**. Family present in hospital, though not continuously at bedside. Family members are willing to help with patient care (bathing or feeding) if allowed. Often summon priest to pray with family at bedside. Family also may hold a quiet prayer vigil at bedside. Close friends may visit. Family and friends stay overnight only if situation is critical. Do not expect food to be brought from home.

ILLNESS BELIEFS

- **Causes of/attitudes about physical illness**. Believe in biomedical causes of illness (e.g., that "germs" cause infections and that some diseases are inherited). Also believe in natural causes (e.g., wet hair in cold temperatures). Believe that excessive drinking/smoking or improper diet can cause some illnesses or make them worse. Older Catholics often believe that illness is God's will and that suffering has a purifying and redemptive purpose. Do not believe in other supernatural causes of illness.

- **Causes of/attitudes about mental illness**. Mental illness denotes a lack of personal strength. Poles often look for a physical cause. May initially present with somatic complaints. Usually some degree of shame is associated with mental illness, especially among older persons. Family accepts and supports mentally ill member. Seek care from physicians and accept their recommendations regarding medications, therapy, or hospitalization.

- **Causes of genetic defects**. Accept children with genetic, birth, or congenital defects as God's will. Because of intense family loyalty, such family members receive love and care at home.

- **Attitudes about disabilities**. Accept disabilities as God's will for that person and his/her family. Take disabled persons out into public along with family. Family loves and cares for disabled member at home as long as possible; accepts institutionalization only if it can no longer do so. Even after institutionalization, family continues providing support, given that Poles honor family loyalty.

- **Sick role**. Many do not accept sick role easily. May underplay symptoms. Focus on maintaining daily functioning. More readily accept acute episodic illnesses, such as cold or flu, than chronic illnesses. Expect ill women to continue performing their duties as mothers and wives.

- **Home and folk remedies**. Drink herbal teas with honey and spirits. Believe that one should "sweat" a cold. Take over-the-counter medications and vitamins; clinician must ask specific questions to obtain this information. Most Poles wear religious medals or cloth badges attached to undergarments.

- **Medications**. About 25% of medical prescriptions in Poland are for herbal remedies. In U.S., Poles still value herbs and vitamins; many have small herb gardens. May use herbal remedies in conjunction with medical treatments. Because they respect physicians, Poles use biomedical drugs and other modalities as ordered.
- **Acceptance of procedures**. Accept recommended procedures out of respect for physicians. Consult with family (especially the father) before making final decision. Uncommon for Poles to approve extraordinary efforts to keep patient alive. No taboos against blood transfusions or organ transplants, but the cost and impact on family play important roles in decision. Most Poles do not want to be a burden on their family. Do not practice euthanasia.
- **Care-seeking**. Most try home remedies first. If inadequate and symptoms interfere with functioning, Poles seek care from physician but often only if they truly suffer or have so much pain that family must care for them. Prefer physician who is warm and caring. Will switch physicians if they think they are receiving inadequate care. Willing to seek advice from chiropractor, pharmacist, and family members.

HEALTH ISSUES

- **Concept of health**. Equate health with performing normal daily routines and with lack of symptoms.
- **Health promotion and prevention**. In Poland, do not practice preventive care or have annual physical exams, but they advocate spas and mineral springs for rest and relaxation. In U.S., most undergo annual exam if they have health insurance; still, concept of preventive care is difficult for them. Most Poles value eating a balanced diet and doing what is necessary to maintain health, such as resting properly and exercising. However, older Polish Americans and newer immigrants do not value preventive practices. Many smoke and drink, get little regular exercise outside of work, and have poor dental care. More-educated persons tend to pay closer attention to preventive health behavior and exercise.
- **Screening**. Difficult concept for most Poles, as most visit a physician only when ill. Clinician needs to explain reasons for screening. Women more likely to see health care provider of same gender for routine female care. Younger or acculturated Poles more easily accept annual exams and screening, such as mammograms.
- **Common health problems**. Smoking-, obesity-, and alcohol-related problems are common. Others are cardiac disease, gastrointestinal disorders, thyroid disease, and dental problems. Respiratory disease and cancer common among miners and those exposed to industrial pollution in Poland and U.S.

DEATH RITUALS

- **Beliefs and attitudes about death**. Catholics believe that when someone dies, Jesus Christ judges the soul and rewards the good and punishes the evil; goal is to attain eternal bliss with God in heaven. Stoically accept death as a normal part of life. Religious Poles believe that soul leaves body upon death and lives eternally.

- **Preparation**. Best if physician informs spouse or children in private, away from bedside. Desirable to have another family member present for emotional support. Family then notifies other family members and friends. Important to have family members at bedside or in waiting room. If Catholic, family wants priest to pray and anoint patient with holy oil while he/she still is conscious; this is a highly valued ritual that protects the soul from spiritual harm and claims it for God.
- **Home vs. hospital**. Preference depends on nature of illness; if acute or more serious, hospital acceptable. After death, body is transferred to funeral home. For a more chronic problem, prefer home. Hospice care at home acceptable. Family and friends stay with dying person and women take care of him/her. Visitors show their concern by bringing food for family, caring for children, and helping with household chores. Grown children responsible for funeral arrangements.
- **Special needs**. Rosary, statues, candles at bedside, and other religious objects. Very important to have priest present as a personal and spiritual friend.
- **Care of the body**. Spouse or eldest child removes religious items. If body is at home, women prepare it. Even today in Poland, body is not embalmed, so immigrants in U.S. may not understand this practice. Dress body for burial in coffin. If death occurs at home, hold a three-day vigil, which includes prayer and visitation by family and friends. After vigil, hold a mass and religious burial. If death occurs in hospital, visitation held in funeral home. Often take photographs of attending family members and deceased in coffin as a memento for those who could not be present. Cremation acceptable. Families tend grave site for years and honor the dead by attending mass and making special offerings to the church on All Souls Day (November 1).
- **Attitudes about organ donation**. Unacceptable among older Poles. May be acceptable among younger generations.
- **Attitudes about autopsy**. Poles generally do not have autopsy performed, unless legally required.

SELECTED REFERENCES

Davies, N. (1982). *God's playground: A history of Poland*. New York: Columbia University Press.

From, M. A. (2003). People of Polish heritage. In L. D. Purnell & B. J. Paulanka (Eds.), *Transcultural health care: A culturally competent approach* (2nd ed.) (pp. 294–306). Philadelphia: F. A. Davis.

Knab, S. H. (1996). *Polish customs, traditions, and folklore*. New York: Hippocrene Books.

Paleczny, T. (1999). *A comparative study of emigration to the United States from Ireland and Poland.* Krakow, Poland: University of Jagiellonski.

AUTHOR

Eileen M. Carol, RNC, FNP, PhD, is a graduate of the University of California-San Francisco School of Nursing. For her dissertation, "Interpreting Information: Health Care Communication Among Family Nurse Practitioners, Interpreters, and Cambodian Refugee Patients," she developed a research model describing the variables that affect the outcome of using an interpreter. She also worked in Poland and the former Czechoslovakia with Project Hope, helping to improve the clinical expertise of Polish, Czech, and Slovak hospital nurses. Her grandparents immigrated from Prussia and the Austro-Hungarian Empire (now Poland and the Slovak Republic). She currently works as a family nurse practitioner in a medical office in Healdsburg, CA.

CHAPTER 29

PUERTO RICANS

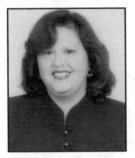

Tereza C. Juarbe

CULTURAL/ETHNIC IDENTITY

- **Preferred term(s)**. Puerto Rican, *Puertorriqueño(a)*. Also *Boricua*, a term used with great pride that originates from the name given to the island by its original inhabitants, the Taíno Indians. *Jíbaro* refers to rural persons with profound cultural roots.
- **Census**. There are an estimated 3.5 million Puerto Ricans in the U.S., representing 8.6% of the country's *Latino* population. Largest numbers reside in urban areas of New York, Connecticut, Illinois, and Florida. Families migrate state to state, East to West (including Hawaii), and between northern and southern states. Such migration has been especially typical in the last 10 years.
- **History of immigration**. Early immigrants came to the U.S. in search of economic opportunities and social mobility, and to join family members. Recent immigrants want better education and higher professional income. The first natives immigrated in the late 1400s. Starting in the 1830s, immigration increased under a Spanish merchant agreement that allowed Puerto Ricans to work in the U.S. The Jones Act of 1917 gave Puerto Ricans U.S. citizenship if they agreed to mandatory military service; it also made immigration easier. The largest wave came after World War II. In the 1950s, a yearly average of 41,000 Puerto Ricans immigrated. By 1970, at least 1.4 million were living in more than 30 U.S. cities. But economic decline in the U.S. between 1970 and the 1990s prompted thousands to return to Puerto Rico. Immigration has declined since 2000. Puerto Ricans are moving back and forth in a "boomerang" pattern.

SPIRITUAL/RELIGIOUS ORIENTATION

- **Primary religious/spiritual affiliations**. Eighty-five percent of Puerto

Ricans in U.S. practice Catholicism. The remainder practice Protestantism, especially Pentecostalism or other evangelical faiths. Simultaneously, many Puerto Ricans practice *espiritismo* (spiritualism), which is a blend of Indian, African, and Catholic beliefs that involves communicating with and using evil and good spirits, and *Santeria*, a tribal religion brought to the Caribbean by African slaves that involves worshipping African gods (*orishas*) and Catholic saints. *Espiritismo* practice has declined, but even those who do not practice *espiritismo* still respect it.

- **Usual religious/spiritual practices**. Religious days are very solemn; certain foods and daily activities prohibited. For example, some believers do not eat meat or do not shower. Clinician should ask patient about his/her dietary preferences on those days.
- **Use of spiritual healing/healers**. Want priest/clergy present to bless patient before surgery or special procedures, to welcome and bless new infant, to give sacrament of the sick, or to take confession. Most commonly used healers are *espiritistas* and *santeros*, who apply topical herbs, aromatic ointments or liquids, prayer, and biomedicine. Puerto Ricans may consult *santeros*, in particular, regarding mental problems. Clinician must be willing to share information with priest or traditional healers, who often are available to attend to spiritual needs of hospitalized patients. Clinician should provide time for healing practices without interruption.
- **Holidays**. Puerto Ricans celebrate many U.S. holidays, including Presidents' Day, Thanksgiving, and Christmas. Kings' Day (*Día de los Reyes*) (January 6), also known as Epiphany Day, has unique cultural and religious value. It is more meaningful than Christmas for some Puerto Ricans, who may keep their children out of school. Also celebrate Saint John's Day (*Día de San Juan*) (June 25) with parades, concerts, and other festivities in honor of this Catholic saint and patron.

COMMUNICATION
ORAL COMMUNICATION

- **Major languages and dialects**. Spanish and English have been the official languages for many years. Language is a sensitive issue because, in 1900, Puerto Rico was forced to adopt English as the official language of instruction, even though few people knew it. In the last three decades, official language has alternated between Spanish/English and Spanish with each government change. Puerto Ricans use Spanish in schools, mass media, and business, and at home. Those from metropolitan areas are more likely to read, understand, and speak some English. Puerto Ricans highly respect clinicians and may be embarrassed to ask them to speak slowly.
- **Greetings**. Women greet each other with a hug and kiss on cheek. Men greet with strong right handshake as left hand strokes greeter's shoulder; may greet godfather (*compadre*) or family members with a hug. Puerto Ricans

greet health care providers with friendly handshake; after trust is established, some greet with a hug. Clinician should show respect in addressing adults by using "Mr." (*Señor* or *Don*) or "Mrs./Ms." (*Señora/Doña*) and last name. Single women prefer to use mother's and father's surname. Married women drop mother's name and add husband's last name, preceded by *de* (of). Younger and more-acculturated women may take husband's name.

- **Tone of voice**. Non-Puerto Ricans often interpret loud pitch and inflections as confrontational rather than ordinary. Clinician should consider content and context of conversation before judging.

- **Direct or indirect style of speech**. Young and more-acculturated persons use direct style. Some use the word *unju* when indicating disagreement or a sense of mistrust. Some also respond with *¡Está chévere!* to convey understanding, to be courteous, or to avoid embarrassment. When in doubt, clinician should ask patient to repeat instructions to make sure patient understands. Tend to interrupt each other frequently.

- **Use of interpreters**. Most commonly use family members, neighbors, or *compadres/comadres* (godfathers/godmothers) as interpreters. Clinician must consider gender when discussing sensitive issues. Should discuss stigmatized health care issues, such as HIV/AIDS, sexual behaviors, and tuberculosis, with help of interpreter rather than family member. Puerto Ricans often communicate concerns to interpreter that they would not want disclosed to clinician. Before interpretation begins, clinician should ask interpreter to suggest to patient that patient not disclose any information he/she does not want revealed to clinician.

- **Serious or terminal illness**. Often do not tell patient, particularly if he/she is elderly, about terminal illness to protect him/her from more suffering (*más sufrimientos*) and to provide optimism and better quality of life for patient. On admission, clinician should ask patient (and document) the name of the family member ultimately responsible for patient's health decisions (self, eldest daughter/son, partner, or caregiver) to avoid conflict with family. Should also consider the literacy and educational background of decision-maker when providing information.

WRITTEN COMMUNICATION

- **Literacy assessment**. Greatly value education. Many Puerto Ricans immigrate for higher education. High incidence of school dropout; small percentage goes on to receive professional education. Puerto Ricans of urban origin are likely to understand English but may be unable to speak or write it; those from rural areas are more likely to be monolingual. Clinician should initially assess literacy level by asking patient about his/her proficiency in English and Spanish, and provide information and instructions slowly and clearly.

- **Consents**. Nodding affirmatively may not mean agreement or understanding. Acceptable for clinician to ask patient to repeat or clarify information.

Nipa indicates a strong "no." Clinician should provide verbal and/or written information in English and Spanish. Very important to give patient sufficient time to read information and consult with family members before patient makes a decision. Clinician should consider obtaining verbal approval from a woman's partner. Puerto Ricans prefer verbal consent to signed consent, if feasible.

NONVERBAL COMMUNICATION

- **Eye contact**. Among younger persons and those born in U.S., eye contact is direct. Those raised in rural areas may limit eye contact out of respect, especially with elderly persons, who command respect and are knowledgeable. Out of modesty, single women may avoid direct eye contact with men. Parents may ask children to look into their eyes when disciplining them as acknowledgment of parental authority and control.

- **Personal space**. Varies by age, generation, and gender. Compared to Northern European Americans, personal space among Puerto Ricans is closer between family members and friends.

- **Use and meaning of silence**. Puerto Ricans often are labeled as noisy and loud (*alborotosos*). Rarely observe silence, except during periods of grief, loss, or depression or in the absence of trust (*confianza*). Individuals or whole families may use the punishment of silence (*el castigo del silencio*) with a family member as a sign of anger, rejection, censure, or frustration.

- **Gestures**. Use numerous hand, face, and body gestures along with verbal communication to convey messages. Clinician may misinterpret loud voice and gestures as threatening, violent, antagonistic, or angry behavior. Not unusual for men to look at attractive women and wink an eye and/or whistle. This may be problematic if female clinician or staff interprets it as harassment; a warning is adequate to preclude further gestures.

- **Openness in expressing emotions**. Puerto Ricans are very loving and affectionate (*cariñosos*), want to be likable and warm (*simpáticos*), and desire smooth interpersonal relationships. Generally express emotions openly and easily, although some men suppress their emotions with male friends or family members to avoid being perceived as less masculine. Very likely to express emotions, physical ailments, and discomforts to health care professionals.

- **Privacy**. Prefer to discuss health matters in private. Patient expects clinician to be respectful and use soft tone of voice. Rooms without doors connote disrespect and are conspicuous, especially if patient must remove clothes or disclose information.

- **Touch**. May express themselves with an array of hand motions that include intermittent touching and taps or strokes to the upper bodies of those around them. Clinician should explain procedures step by step before and during exams that require touching breast or genitalia. Patients prefer health care provider of same gender for breast and prostate exams.

- **Orientation to time**. Flexible view of time. May be late for medical appointments. Puerto Ricans have difficulty staying within predetermined duration of appointment; may talk at length (*dar lata*), providing detailed and candid responses to straightforward questions, and thereby delaying subsequent appointments. For them, quality of the interaction is more important than time limit. Clinician should tell patient about time limit at beginning of visit.

ACTIVITIES OF DAILY LIVING

- **Modesty**. Most men and women greatly value modesty. Important to match patient's and caregiver's gender. Have difficulty disclosing sexuality issues, such as birth control, impotence, sexually transmitted infection, and infertility, especially older adults. Generally avoid the word "sex" (*sexo*); instead, use the expression *tener relaciones* ("to have intimate relations"). Some men cope with impotence through denial. Most women prefer to discuss health issues with clinician before they change their clothes for breast, vaginal, or complete physical exam. Hospitalized men and women prefer to wear underwear and pants under hospital gown.
- **Skin care**. Daily shower essential for promoting health and for personal appearance, except during illnesses such as cold, flu, or viral infection. Women may use rice or lemon water to wash face. Women use roots of a medicinal plant (*maguey*) with Epsom salt to prevent and treat acne.
- **Hair care**. Prefer to shampoo daily. Exception is menstruating women, who avoid shampooing. Some believe that washing hair during menstruation or after giving birth may cause bleeding, stroke, abdominal pain, or arthritis. In shampooing, not uncommon for women to use strong peroxide solutions with chamomile water, which are believed to brighten and strengthen hair.
- **Nail care**. Both men and women pay particular attention to maintaining clean and well-groomed nails. Men typically keep short nails, as longer nails are associated with being gay. Important for clinician to emphasize foot care among older women in rural settings, who are more likely to wear open sandals or walk without shoes.
- **Toileting** (*dal del cuerpo*). While hospitalized, some avoid having bowel movements rather than use a bedside commode or bedpan. Staff should provide privacy and ample toileting time. Patient may prefer wet, warm washcloth to clean hands.
- **Special clothing or amulets**. No longer wear traditional clothing. *Espiritistas* and some religious sects may dress in white outfits, hats, and handkerchiefs on Sundays and other special occasions. Amulets have lost popularity over the years, but Puerto Ricans from both urban and rural areas sometimes use a small black fist (*azabache*) or small black rabbit foot to protect children from evil. Believe that removing this object results in illness, misfortune, or even death; often request priest's benediction before doing so. Clinician should always ask permission before removing amulets. Family members like

to keep rosary beads on patient. If family members approve, clinician might remove rosary beads from patient's neck and wrap them loosely in his/her hand. Often bring candles, pictures of saints, and/or holy water to patient's bedside and place them as close as possible to him/her. Many like to rub patient's body with aromatic oils and lotions as protection from evil.

- **Self-care**. When sick, most Puerto Ricans prefer to perform self-care and personal hygiene as they normally would or with minimal help from a family member of the same gender. They accept help doing chores, such as housekeeping, cooking, and buying groceries, with the focus on loved ones' help rather than individual self-care. Family care may prevail over self-care in chronic-illness cases. Puerto Ricans expect a sick person to be passive, which may hinder recovery and contradict clinical notions about self-care. In hospital, by way of encouraging patient's cooperation with activities such as deep breathing and coughing, hygiene, and ambulation, clinician should explain importance of self-care for earlier discharge.

FOOD PRACTICES

- **Usual meal pattern**. Three full meals a day: breakfast (coffee with milk, eggs, bread, hot cereals, bacon/sausage or ham, potatoes), lunch, and dinner. Many still continue tradition of coffee time at 10 a.m. and 3 p.m. Boil fresh milk and add it to strong coffee with plenty of sugar. Some add canned condensed milk to freshly made cup of espresso.
- **Special utensils**. None.
- **Food beliefs and rituals**. From birth to death, arrange all events around food to honor guest and as a symbol of wealth. Many still adhere to the "hot"/"cold" classifications of foods to promote physical, emotional, and spiritual balance.
- **Usual diet**. Eat rice, beans, fried plantains (*plátanos*), and bread with practically all meals. Serve rice plain or cooked with beans, chicken, codfish, vegetables, sausage, corned beef, and other foods. Use a special blend of spices (*sofrito*) to season stews. Roots such as cassava, pumpkin, sweet potatoes, celery, and chayote squash are an essential part of Puerto Rican diet. Hospitalized patients may find North American meals to be flavorless and unappetizing.
- **Fluids**. Coffee, which Puerto Ricans even introduce to young children. Prefer ice in drinks, except when they have a cold or respiratory illness (cold drinks are believed to promote illness). Encourage menstruating women to drink hot herbal tea rather than cold drinks or sodas.
- **Food taboos and prescriptions**. Most prohibitions are related to spiritual beliefs, illness, pregnancy, and postpartum period. During special religious events, such as Holy Week, Puerto Ricans do not eat red meat or chicken; may eat fish. When afflicted with a cold, flu, or virus, use a mixture of honey, lemon, and rum as expectorant and antitussive. Consume a malt beverage

(*malta*), fruit juice, or egg yolk stirred with sugar and added to warm milk to increase hemoglobin and strength of chronically or terminally ill persons, persons who have a cold, women after they give birth, and thin children. Some believe that the elderly must take small, daily portions of brandy added to black coffee to increase blood pressure and enhance the functioning of their "old" heart.

- **Hospitality**. Puerto Ricans like homes filled with friends and family, whom they welcome with music and large quantities of food and alcoholic beverages. May express respect and gratitude to health care providers by offering gifts, such as homemade, traditional food. May interpret refusal of such gifts as an insult or rejection.

SYMPTOM MANAGEMENT

Educated Puerto Ricans can use numerical pain scale but may prefer words for other symptoms. Especially among Evangelical and Charismatic families, frequently use prayer as a nonpharmacological method of controlling all symptoms.

- **Pain** (*dolor*). Very loud and outspoken when expressing pain. Clinician should not censure pain expression or view it as exaggeration. ¡Ayyy! and ¡Ay bendito! are verbal moaning expressions of pain that accompany rubbing of painful area with hand (by oneself or a significant other). Numerical scale to express pain level might be difficult for low-literacy, rural, and elderly Puerto Ricans. Prefer oral or IV medications to intramuscular or rectal. Use herbal teas, heat (heating pads and hot water bags), and prayer to manage pain. Mix camphor (*cubitos de alcanfór*) and mint leaves in bottle of *alcoholado* (similar to isopropyl alcohol or witch hazel, and pronounced "alcolao") and rub solution on painful area.

- **Dyspnea** (*asfixiao*, or shortness of breath). Believe that fanning or blowing into a patient provides oxygen or relieves dyspnea. Also believe that tea made from alligator tail, snails, or a plant leaf (*savila*) improves or heals dyspnea-related illnesses such as asthma and congestive heart failure. Some apply hot wet compress and/or Mentholatum™ to reduce dyspnea.

- **Nausea/vomiting** (*asco/deponer* in rural areas, *nausea/vómitos* among the educated). An alarming and embarrassing symptom of illness. Many Puerto Ricans like to smell *alcoholado* or apply it to forehead to relieve nausea. Some put head between legs to stop vomiting. Boil mint, orange- or lemon-tree leaves, or star anise seeds to brew tea for relief of nausea/vomiting or stomach illness. Seldom use suppositories. Clinician should explain use of suppositories, as many Puerto Ricans believe that they induce diarrhea.

- **Constipation/diarrhea** (*estreñimiento* [*estar tapao* means "being clogged"]/ *diarrea* [*estar de carreritas* means "have the runs"]). Consider both conditions to be a result of harmful food. For constipation, use several natural and common laxatives (e.g., milk of magnesia or castor oil) or hot prunes. Many from rural areas frequently and inappropriately use enemas. Use clear chicken broth, rice water, and tea for diarrhea. In children, use water or natural teas with sugar (*sueritos*) to supply fluids.

- **Fatigue** (*fatiga*). A symptom of illness, anemia, malnutrition, or nervousness (*nervios*).

- **Depression** (*depresión*). Commonly use this term to convey sadness, grief, or anguish, not necessarily clinical depression. Rather, Puerto Ricans typically use nervousness (*nervios*) or attack of nerves (*ataque de nervios*) to describe depression symptoms. Clinician should not mistake *ataque de nervios*—a culturally learned expression to denote that an anxiety, fear, or tension climax has been reached—for panic attacks. Thorough mental health assessment is critical. Puerto Ricans might not disclose clinical depression and other mental illnesses that carry stigma or shame. Widely prefer medications and other treatments to psychotherapy. Clinician should acknowledge confidentiality of any information the patient provides.

- **Self-care symptom management**. Drink natural herbal teas for signs or symptoms of illness. Many consult family and friends before consulting health care provider. Often consider pharmacists to be close community members who play a vital role in symptom management.

BIRTH RITUALS/CARE OF THE NEW MOTHER AND BABY

- **Pregnancy care**. In many families, pregnant woman is indulged; she is granted all of her wishes by way of promoting her and the baby's well-being. Pregnant women carefully follow guidelines for good hygiene and diet (e.g., avoid hot sauces, chocolate, beans, oily foods, and citrus; consume milk, beef, chicken, vegetables, and fruit). Exercise deemed inappropriate. Pregnant women prohibited from lifting heavy objects. Recommend rest and plenty of sleep. Clinician should encourage regular exercise and good nutrition. Also should assess for "pregnancy wantedness," a cultural and migration construct associated with a desire to continue or not continue with pregnancy. Puerto Ricans encourage prenatal care, which usually begins in first trimester among more-acculturated adult women, who are more likely to attend childbirth preparation classes with spouse/partner. Clinician should discuss birth options early in pregnancy and educate patient about them. Many women refrain from sexual intercourse (*tener relaciones*) during and after second trimester. Men may use this opportunity for extramarital sexual activities. With sensitivity, clinician may ask men, and educate them about, the risk of sexually transmitted infection and HIV/AIDS.

- **Preferences for children**. Men more likely to prefer male first-born to ensure that family name continues. In some traditional families, boys have greater symbolic value (e.g., they may demonstrate father's virility and strength). Some families continue to reproduce until a boy is born. Younger generation prefers smaller families. Family size a common point of disagreement between younger and older generations.

- **Labor practices**. Highly value hygiene and modesty during labor. Women prefer to have their body covered and not to be examined frequently. Prefer bed position in hospital. Also want spouse, mother, or sister present during labor. Expect close family members and members of extended family to remain in waiting room as a sign of *familismo* (the central importance of family as the social unit), which may create disruption and overcrowding.
- **Role of the laboring woman during birth**. Active and assertive. Loud or noisy expressions of pain acceptable and encouraged as a means of coping with pain and discomfort. Medications acceptable. Clinician should discuss pain-management choices, risks and benefits, and birth alternatives with couple.
- **Role of the father and other family members during birth**. Fathers assume passive, supportive role during labor. Young fathers who attended birth preparation classes help during labor. Others prefer not to be present during labor but want to be updated frequently.
- **Vaginal vs. cesarean section**. Prefer vaginal delivery. For some Puerto Ricans, cesarean carries a "weak woman" stigma, which clinician should discourage among patients and their partners.
- **Breastfeeding**. Women of rural origin may prefer breastfeeding in first year. Those who work outside the home may use formula, breastfeeding, or both. Women avoid beans, starch products, and eggs during breastfeeding; believe that such foods make infant colicky.
- **Birth recuperation**. Clinician should assess support systems available to the new mother and help her use them. First meal after delivery should be fresh, homemade chicken soup. Puerto Ricans encourage new mothers to avoid wind, cold temperatures, lifting heavy objects, and doing housework during first 40 days after birth (*cuarentena*). Some women who work outside the home experience great distress when they cannot follow such cultural values/norms. Some do not wash their hair during *cuarentena*. Good hygiene encouraged; use plenty of soap, body lotions, and light fragrances.
- **Baby care**. Caregiving roles vary. Puerto Ricans expect most new mothers to care for baby with support from spouse/partner and family members. Commonly, woman's mother or mother-in-law visits for first three months to help care for new mother and baby.
- **Problems with baby**. Mother wants to be informed first, preferably directly by pediatrician, and to tell others herself. She consults close family members and friends first about common pediatric issues, such as rash, colic, crying, fever, and colds.
- **Male and female circumcision**. Male circumcision traditionally performed at birth. Some rural or traditional families prefer not to circumcise child for fear of causing pain, bleeding, or harm. Female circumcision never performed.

DEVELOPMENTAL AND SEXUAL ISSUES
- **Celebration of menarche or becoming a man**. No specific events. While

Puerto Ricans welcome this transition in young men, menarche (*hacerse señoritas*) signals risk of pregnancy. Parents may become overprotective. A young woman's 15th birthday (*quinceañero*) represents both a social and religious transition to womanhood; it is similar to a wedding, involving a religious ceremony and festivity.

- **Attitudes about birth control**. Most are receptive to education about, and discussion of, birth control. Catholics are encouraged to practice sexual abstinence or rhythm method (*el ritmo*). Due to public health pressure in Puerto Rico and U.S., tubal ligation is the most common form of birth control in U.S. (23%), followed by oral contraceptives (8.7%). Some women opt for tubal ligation/sterilization at a younger age as permanent protection from pregnancy.
- **Attitudes about sexually transmitted infection (STI) control, including condoms**. Many consider STIs and condom use taboo topics. Some men believe that using condoms may lead to perception of them as being less *macho* or infected with STI. Negative attitudes of male sex partners, lack of education, gender power issues, and cultural acceptance of male extramarital sex interfere with condom use. Clinician must explore possibility that recommending condoms for preventing pregnancy and STI will place woman at risk for partner violence.
- **Attitudes about abortion**. Many perceive it as immoral and disgraceful but acceptable if mother's life is in danger. Being a single mother may be more acceptable than undergoing abortion.
- **Attitudes about unwed sexual experimentation**. Traditional and religious families discourage it among women. Expect women to remain virgins until marriage. *Machismo* fosters pre- and extramarital sexual practices among men, but they are encouraged to marry a virgin. Pregnancy rates among Puerto Rican teenagers and single women higher than in other Hispanic groups, but single women do not disclose that they are sexually active.
- **Sexual orientation**. Same-sex orientation usually not disclosed to avoid rejection by family. For some, sex between men is a sign of virility and power rather than sexual orientation. Have difficulty disclosing same-gender partner; often do so only in extreme situations, such as illness. Partners might not be accepted at family gatherings or in illness situations. Special accommodations for timing of hospital visits may be necessary.
- **Gender identity**. Family may suspect ambiguous gender identity but not disclose or talk about it. May punish open verbal and nonverbal expressions of gender uncertainty among children and adolescents. Such expressions might lead to social, spiritual, and emotional rejection.
- **Attitudes about menopause**. View *el cambio de vida* either as a normal process leading to the prime of life and/or as a shortfall of sexual value. Acceptable for women to become depressed. May use alternative treatments to relieve symptoms, such as relaxation, massage, acupuncture, chelation, or herbs (e.g., black cohosh, evening primrose, St. John's wort, and sarsapa-

rilla). Often consult with folk healers. Acculturated women and/or those with health insurance more likely to use hormone replacement therapy.

FAMILY RELATIONSHIPS

- **Composition/structure**. Family is nucleus of community (*familismo*), the locus of all activities, decisions, and social and cultural standards. Value family solidarity over individual interests and rights. Nuclear and extended-family structure. Traditionally patriarchal; man demands respect and expects obedience from wife and children. Expect children to live at home until they marry or leave for college.
- **Decision-making**. Many consult elderly persons regarding decisions, as a sign of respect and to tap their wisdom. In some families, may consult several family members, such as godfather or godmother (*compadre* or *comadre*). In many families, eldest son or daughter has power to make final decision concerning health matters. Clinician must consult husband to obtain verbal consent for woman's treatment to prevent physical or emotional harm; should ask patient if her husband's authorization is necessary before she consents to surgical or nonsurgical procedures. Acceptable for clinician to ask family about decision-making process.
- **Spokesperson**. Eldest son or daughter, or older woman in family. Husband is spokesperson in cases involving young children or women.
- **Gender issues**. Traditionally expect men to be *macho*, powerful, and strong; dominant over women; and financial provider. Women are socialized to focus on family, motherhood, and home care, and to discipline and guide children. Older women may have a powerful and respected role in family. In younger families, expect men to take responsibility for decision-making.
- **Changing roles among generations in U.S.** In Puerto Rico and U.S., women increasingly are working outside the home and participating in politics and traditional, male-oriented roles. Younger and more-acculturated couples share family roles, caregiving, providing for family financially, and decision-making. Traditional gender roles may cause conflict, but many women are gaining equality in sexual relationships.
- **Caring roles**. Emphasize family care over self-care. Expect close family members and those in extended family to help care for children. Eldest son or daughter may assume care for elderly. In caring for ill persons, women assume an active role and men a passive role, but men are expected to finance health care.
- **Expectations of and for children**. Children are the center of family life. Puerto Ricans strongly emphasize respect, education, and religion among children and expect them to follow family roles and traditions. In many homes, male children are socialized to play a more independent, *macho* role, while girls are taught about home economics and family dynamics. Parents use both positive and negative inducements to encourage discipline, respect, and sub-

mission among children; use belts on children's legs or buttocks for physical discipline, which mother usually delivers.

- **Expectations of and for elders**. Grandparent or elderly figure (*abuelo[a]*) commands respect, admiration, and wisdom. Many children are taught to address grandparent as *Mama* or *Papa*, which denotes respect for elders as parents. Both men and women care for elderly; distribute and share such responsibilities with family members and close network members. Families make noble financial and manpower efforts to keep elderly at home. Puerto Ricans view nursing homes and extended care facilities as inappropriate and inconsiderate; institutionalization can lead to depression and distress among family members.
- **Expectations of hospital visitors**. Expect close and distant members of family, neighbors, and friends to visit. Clinician can ask family spokesperson to communicate information and visitation rules to visitors.

ILLNESS BELIEFS

- **Causes of/attitudes about physical illness**. Hereditary factors, lack of personal attention to health, humoral imbalance, or negative environmental forces, such as toxins, cause illness. Supernatural causes include punishment for sins, evil spirits, or the evil eye. Some believe that destiny or God's will (*si Dios quiere* means "if God wants") controls life, health, and death, which helps Puerto Ricans cope with crisis, death, or grief. This belief may influence perception of future disease risks and whether one can control them. Most Puerto Ricans are receptive to such a discussion, so clinician must assess patient's perceptions of forces that determine health and illness.
- **Causes of/attitudes about mental illness**. Greatly stigmatized. Many do not disclose any past or present mental illness in family. Some believe that mental illness is hereditary, others believe that suffering (*sufrimientos*) is a precursor. Many camouflage mental illness by calling it nervousness (*nerviosismo*) or an attack of nerves (*ataque de nervios*). May seek help from friends, family, or folk healers before seeking biomedical treatment.
- **Causes of genetic defects**. Genetic defects create great family stress. Puerto Ricans blame women for any defect; many argue that a woman who has a child with a genetic defect did not take care of herself during pregnancy. Keep such a child at home rather than institutionalize him/her.
- **Attitudes about disabilities**. May blame a baby's disabling condition on mother's lack of self-care, working during pregnancy, or personal suffering. Puerto Ricans are caring and helpful regarding disabled persons. Some families initially hide children who are physically disabled; less likely to hide disabled adults, especially if they are older family members or parents. Prefer to care for disabled family members at home. Rear disabled children so they can still attend school and outdoor programs. Religion plays critical, supportive role in lives of families with disabled children. Support groups for such families are helpful.

- **Sick role**. Sick person usually assumes passive role. Family members must provide all care, including preparation of soups (*caldos*) and special or favorite foods. Expect family members to take active role in providing resources and care for someone who is chronically or terminally ill.
- **Home and folk remedies**. Often use home and folk remedies before, or in combination with, biomedicine. Most do not interfere with biomedical treatments but rather enhance adherence to them. Folk healers (*santeros* or *espiritistas*) may suggest herbs for patient to drink or bathe in, incense, prayers, and illness-related figurines that promote health. Drink a variety of herbal teas to treat illness and promote health. Examples are mint, orange- and lemon-tree leaves, camphor, eucalyptus oil, and menthol for body aches, colds, pneumonia, and other flu-like symptoms. For eye illnesses or insect stings, mix a small amount of fresh urine (from anyone around) with mud and apply compound to affected area. Use baking soda for diarrhea, stomach illnesses, and heartburn. Drink warm milk with sugar to treat ulcers and reduce gastric secretions. Treat parasites with laxatives and, when available, gentian violet. Use olive oil for ear ache or disorders. *Maravilla* water, a liquid astringent, is available in most homes for treating bruises, contusions, sprains, slight cuts, scrapes, and muscular pain. Most Puerto Ricans openly display their home remedies; clinician should ask family about patient's current or concomitant use of them.
- **Medications**. Family and friends commonly share prescribed medications. Older and rural adults may stop treatment when symptoms subside.
- **Acceptance of procedures**. Fear blood transfusions and donations, worrying that shared blood will transmit HIV. Accept surgery if clearly explained. Some families need reassurance about spiritual issues related to organ transplants, such as the meaning of another person's organ in one's body and its lack of influence on the recipient, particularly the transcendence of his/her soul, memories, and life.
- **Care-seeking**. Pharmacist plays significant role in care-seeking. In health matters, most Puerto Ricans consult family members and friends before consulting physician or nurse. May consult folk healers (*espiritistas*) for mental illness or other conditions that do not respond to home remedy or biomedical treatment.

HEALTH ISSUES

- **Concept of health**. Perceive health as not being too thin and being clean (*llenitos y limpios*) and as an absence of mental, spiritual, or physical discomfort. Underweight or thinness also a symbol of economic disadvantage. Consider someone who is worried or *nervioso(a)* to be ill.
- **Health promotion and prevention**. Eating well and drinking fruit beverages are common health promotion practices. Commonly take multivitamins. Clinician should emphasize regular exercise, as Puerto Ricans do not perceive it as a health promotion practice and they discourage exercise dur-

ing illness. Clinician also should encourage and reinforce a low-fat, low-cholesterol diet and teach about body weight and its influence on the development of heart disease and other illnesses.

- **Screening**. Older men often resist it. Wives and sisters very influential in men's screening decisions. Women view screening for breast and pelvic cancer as intrusive and embarrassing; thus, they delay or avoid it. Clinician should inform women about their options for annual exams. Younger women more likely to use screening. Son or daughter may be able to convince elderly person of need for screening and follow-up care. Puerto Ricans follow screening recommendations for children. Prefer clinician of same gender.
- **Common health problems**. Major causes of death are heart and cardiovascular disease, cancer, and diabetes. Hypertension, smoking, and physical inactivity put Puerto Ricans at risk. High rates of alcoholism, illicit drug use, and sex-related illnesses. Substance abuse in Puerto Rican families can lead to unintentional injuries and violence between intimate partners. Disproportionately high rate of asthma among children. Visual impairment often not diagnosed. Early health-promotion interventions to reduce risk factors are effective.

DEATH RITUALS

- **Beliefs and attitudes about death**. Even when a death is expected, Puerto Ricans view it as a calamity. Religious values mostly shape beliefs. Important to involve as many family members as possible in death decisions to avoid delays. Puerto Ricans often view hospital's time constraints as insensitive to family death rituals and expectations.
- **Preparation**. In a private room or environment, clinician should notify family spokesperson when death is imminent. Customary to have priest/clergy present when such news is disclosed to other family members. At hospital or home, family members usually are present around the clock; if death imminent, many family members stay in waiting area day and night. Some believe that daughters, sons, sisters, and brothers must be physically present at time of death and burial. Expect family spokesperson to notify family members elsewhere, even in other countries, so they can be present before and at death. This requires emotional and spiritual energy and may delay burial, creating anxiety and frustration among family members. Do-not-resuscitate decision difficult to accept, even in the worst scenario; important for clinician to emphasize quality of life and suffering (*sufrimientos*) when family is making this decision.
- **Home vs. hospital**. If diagnosed with chronic or long-term illness, some Puerto Ricans prefer a skilled nursing facility or tertiary, palliative-care unit to reduce burden on family. If spouse is healthy or if an older daughter is available, many families prefer to provide care at home and have the sick member die there. Hospice an option if financial resources are available and geographical location allows it.

- **Special needs**. Catholics place candles, rosary beads, and figurines of special or patron saint near patient. Protestant or Evangelical families may hold worship services with music, Bible readings, and prayer at bedside. Expect spiritual leaders to be with patient at moment of death. Family members want to touch and kiss body before removal. Loud and unmanageable crying or thunderous talking to God or other deities very common. Some faint, feel nauseated, vomit, or experience physical illness as a result of an attack of nerves (*ataque de nervios*) or nervousness (*nerviosismo*). Clinician should minimize interruptions and promote privacy to facilitate supportive atmosphere.
- **Care of the body**. In U.S., for financial or cultural reasons, some families keep body at home rather than at a funeral parlor. Some prefer to bury body within 24 hours but may delay burial until all family members are present. Clinician should explain U.S. customs and legal practices regarding funeral homes and care of body.
- **Attitudes about organ donation**. Often practiced. Puerto Ricans view organ donation as an act of goodwill if it benefits another human being, especially a child. Might need authorization from several family members. Meeting and knowing organ recipient very important.
- **Attitudes about autopsy**. Consider the body sacred; regard it with great respect. Usually view autopsy as a violation of the body. Clinician must obtain verbal authorization from family.

SELECTED REFERENCES

Juarbe, T. C. (2003). People of Puerto Rican heritage. In L. D. Purnell & B. J. Paulanka (Eds.), *Transcultural health care: A culturally competent approach* (2nd ed.) (pp. 307–326). Philadelphia: F. A. Davis.

Ramírez de Orellano, A. B. (1999). Death as a sentinel event: The mortality experience of Puerto Ricans in the United States. *Puerto Rican Medical Association Bulletin, 91*, 81–84.

Therrien, M., & Ramirez, R. R. (2001). *The Hispanic population in the United States: Population characteristics* (U.S. Census Bureau, Current Population Reports for March 2000, P20-535). Washington, DC: U.S. Government Printing Office.

AUTHOR

Tereza C. Juarbe, RN, PhD, is an assistant professor in the Department of Family Health Care at the University of California-San Francisco. Her research focuses on health promotion behaviors among *Latina* women regarding cardiovascular disease and breast cancer. She is a first-generation Puerto Rican who emigrated to the U.S. in 1983.

CHAPTER 30

ROMA (GYPSIES)

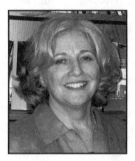

Anne H. Sutherland

CULTURAL/ETHNIC IDENTITY

- **Preferred term(s)**. *Rom* is the Gypsy word for man and *Roma* is the plural, meaning people. In the U.S. and elsewhere, Roma are the largest group of Gypsies, subdivided into several "nations." Other groups of Gypsies include the Romanies (English origin), Travelers (English and Irish origin), Gitanos (Spanish origin), and other subgroups. The groups all recognize each other but do not necessarily mingle. The term "Gypsy" often is not appropriate for non-Gypsies to use.
- **Census**. There are no reliable census figures for Roma. Most are born in the U.S., but a small number still immigrate. Because Roma are relatively few (probably numbering about 250,000), they are very noticeable in the health care setting.
- **History of immigration**. The largest immigration from Europe (mainly of Roma) was during the late 19th century. In the 1920s and 1930s, large numbers of Roma migrated from the East Coast to the West Coast.

SPIRITUAL/RELIGIOUS ORIENTATION

- **Primary religious/spiritual affiliations**. Nominally Christian (Roman Catholic or Orthodox). Some have recently converted to Pentecostalism. Traditional belief system is related to spirits, saints, and other supernatural beings, but new converts reject much of that system.
- **Usual religious/spiritual practices**. Family may bring in figures of saints and other objects of spiritual importance or that promote good luck. Home often has a shrine where family members pray.
- **Use of spiritual healing/healers**. Family may ask for priest or chaplain to be present. An older female relative who is also a spiritual healer (*drabarni*)

may bring in certain plants and medicines for patient. Healer works in conjunction with Western medicine and respects medical specialists.

- **Holidays**. Thanksgiving, Christmas, and some religious holidays, such as those honoring saints. For example, the Machwaya and Kalderasha (Roma groups) celebrate St. Mary's Day and St. Anne's Day.

COMMUNICATION
ORAL COMMUNICATION

- **Major languages and dialects**. "Roma" refers to those who speak inflected Romany (or Romanes), the language they have used for hundreds of years and that derives from Sanskrit. The Gitanos of Spain speak creolized Romany, which has Spanish grammar and structure rather than the original Sanskrit structure. All Roma in U.S. speak English as well as other languages.
- **Greetings**. Raise palm of hand up and call out, *Baxt hai sastimos* ("luck and health"). Prefer that others use the title "Mr." or "Mrs." in English with last name, especially for older adults. Acceptable to use first name after short acquaintance, especially with younger Roma. Handshake not necessary.
- **Tone of voice**. Can be loud or argumentative, even threatening. But this style is best handled by ignoring it, as it often indicates anxiety or fear of illness and death.
- **Direct or indirect style of speech**. Generally very direct. Often use repetition to ensure understanding and to communicate to other Roma in the room.
- **Use of interpreters**. The best interpreters are young adult relatives, male or female.
- **Serious or terminal illness**. In private, physician with senior ranking should first tell the oldest relative who appears to be the leader (male or female). Then physician should tell patient in presence of leader and/or other relatives. Traditional expressions of mourning include outrage and extreme behavior (wailing loudly, showing anger, pulling hair), which need not concern medical personnel. News of illness and death travels rapidly through Roma community, whose members gather in times of crisis. Best if clinician provides space (e.g., a garden area) for large numbers to gather and grieve rather than try to keep them out.

WRITTEN COMMUNICATION

- **Literacy assessment**. Older and some younger Roma have no formal education and cannot read or write, other than sign their name. Clinician must read important documents to them rather than ask if they can read, as Roma are sensitive about illiteracy. Or clinician should ask if there is a family member who can read aloud to patient. Roma may appear to understand medical terminology when in fact they do not; clinician needs to confirm their understanding.
- **Consents**. Clinician should explain procedures clearly and ask for feedback. Should not underestimate patient's intelligence and ability to grasp complex

procedures but also should make sure that one or two unfamiliar words have not led to misunderstanding. Roma associate cancer with certain death; clinician must explain risk immediately. Patient can sign written consent after verbal explanation.

NONVERBAL COMMUNICATION

- **Eye contact**. Sustained and penetrating.
- **Personal space**. Closer than in dominant culture.
- **Use and meaning of silence**. Indicates extreme discomfort. In large groups, everyone tends to talk at once.
- **Gestures**. Hand gestures very common and recognizable to any American.
- **Openness in expressing emotions**. Very open to medical personnel and each other. Very demonstrative. Often gregarious and assertive. Mood can shift quickly from aggressive to begging for help. Facial expressions may reflect suspicion. First reaction often is mistrust.
- **Privacy**. Clinician should ask for personal information only in presence of family member of same gender, never in mixed company. Roma are reluctant to discuss personal body issues with health care providers or family members of opposite gender. Men and women extremely modest regarding procedures dealing with lower body, women more so than men. Very sensitive to lower-body exams and discussion of body fluids (e.g., menstrual blood, urine, or feces); ashamed of, and embarrassed by, these topics but not topics related to upper body and upper-body fluids (e.g., vomit or spittle). Women sometimes pinch each other's breasts to show affection.
- **Touch**. Taboo to touch body parts below waist, but Roma allow doctor of same gender to do so when absolutely necessary. Avoid close contact with non-Roma and impure surfaces (e.g., toilet, floor, or areas the lower body has touched).
- **Orientation to time**. Generally not clock-oriented, as Roma do not hold jobs or attend school. Understand appointment times but may not show up unless aware of importance. Understand past, present, and future.

ACTIVITIES OF DAILY LIVING

- **Modesty**. Very modest regarding lower body. Staff should offer clean robe plus gown and pants for men. For exams, clinician should be of same gender as patient. Gender separation very important.
- **Skin care**. Prefer to keep skin moist; staff should offer cream. Roma view hygiene (i.e., keeping lower body separate from upper body) as essential to moral character. Staff should offer separate towels and soap for each half of body, and allow frequent hand washing.
- **Hair care**. Symbolically important to keep head clean. Men in particular must keep their heads "pure." Staff should provide clean pillowcase when possible and not touch it or patient's head.
- **Nail care**. Wash hands frequently. Separate nail care of hands and feet; nail

cutter must be sterilized after use on feet for use on hands.

- **Toileting**. Prefer privacy. If bedpan necessary, someone of same gender should help patient and keep bedpan away from patient's upper body.
- **Special clothing or amulets**. Most Roma (especially children) wear an amulet around their neck. Staff should allow patient to place amulet under pillow or on bedside table; should never put amulet at foot of bed. Man's hat and woman's scarf also must be kept by patient's head and not at foot of bed.
- **Self-care**. Clinician should allow patient and his/her family to provide care when possible. Family members very attentive. Long-term self-care is problematic, as Roma often stop medication when they feel better.

FOOD PRACTICES

- **Usual meal pattern**. Three meals a day. Larger meals at lunch and dinner. Light breakfast or just coffee.
- **Special utensils**. No metal silverware; only disposable plastic utensils. Roma prefer to use their hands if they can wash before eating.
- **Food beliefs and rituals**. Food must be prepared in "clean" manner (wrapped in plastic or put on paper plates or in/on anything disposable). Avoid eating anything on plates that have been used and washed.
- **Usual diet**. Heavy and greasy, high in salt and cholesterol. Eat white bread with every meal. Prefer barbecued meat and salad with lots of dressing. Usual diet related to many illnesses that are common among Roma, including diabetes, hemorrhoids, hypertension, and heart disease.
- **Fluids**. Drink lots of coffee, sweet tea, beer, and colas.
- **Food taboos and prescriptions**. Some Roma prefer fish on Friday. Some fast on Friday or avoid animal products. Relatives of sick person sometimes fast and/or avoid animal products to help him/her recover. Do not eat food that non-Roma have handled too much. If food comes with a cover, staff should allow patient to remove cover. Generally believe that eating impure food causes illness. Breastfeeding mothers avoid greens (e.g., cabbage), pickled foods, and tomatoes. Shun sour foods (e.g., sour cream, lemon, and vinegar) when someone dies. Certain foods promote luck and good health. View garlic, black pepper, red pepper, salt, vinegar, onions, and pickled foods as especially healthy; use these as cures and often in amulets worn around the neck or sewn into clothes.
- **Hospitality**. When visiting or receiving visitors, customary to offer a drink of some kind, such as coffee or cola. Do not give food gifts.

SYMPTOM MANAGEMENT

- **Pain**. Describe pain willingly. But Roma lack accurate knowledge of anatomy, so they use nonspecific terms to describe pain location. Avoid rectal pain medications; prefer oral or IV route. Adults are not stoic and may moan loudly; children are more stoic. Understand numerical pain scale.

- **Dyspnea**. Prone to excitement and hyperventilation. Usually accept oxygen but generally fear anesthesia, which Roma refer to as "little death." May mistake oxygen mask for administration of anesthesia.
- **Nausea/vomiting**. Readily report nausea/vomiting. No prohibitions on vomiting. One of Romas' most powerful medicines is "ghost's vomit," a slime mold (*Fuligo septica*) found in wood piles and garbage dumps.
- **Constipation/diarrhea**. Avoid discussing diarrhea. Constipation and hemorrhoids very common because of diet; may need help with constipation. Use enemas as a last resort.
- **Fatigue**. Very often report fatigue. Effectively use number scale to describe fatigue. Take medications for fatigue or to sleep.
- **Depression**. Generally uncommon. May not recognize or report depression.
- **Self-care symptom management**. Avoid hospitals and doctors until illness is advanced. Do a poor job of long-term self-care or medication. Roma tend to stop self-care unless they fear death or are in great pain.

BIRTH RITUALS/CARE OF THE NEW MOTHER AND BABY

- **Pregnancy care**. Generally avoid prenatal care, although more and more young Roma are beginning to use it. Prefer not to have internal exam and will avoid prenatal care to avert such exams. Need advice on healthy diet.
- **Preferences for children**. Value boys and girls.
- **Labor practices**. Roma midwives perform many deliveries. However, Roma increasingly accept hospital deliveries, usually on emergency basis when labor has begun. Clinician should offer pain relief, although some may refuse it. Father usually not in room. Woman's mother or other older female relative is the usual birth attendant.
- **Role of the laboring woman during birth**. Mother-to-be relies on assistance from older women relatives (mother, aunt, or midwife). They tell her what is happening only during labor, not before. Increasingly accept modern birth practices.
- **Role of the father and other family members during birth**. Preferred coach is mother or aunt. Father stays outside birthing room with other relatives. Father may absent himself altogether—not for lack of concern but out of modesty.
- **Vaginal vs. cesarean section**. Prefer vaginal delivery. If cesarean section necessary, mother prefers to be conscious.
- **Breastfeeding**. Many young mothers do not breastfeed, although breastfeeding was the norm in the past. Breastfeeding mothers avoid cabbage and other green vegetables and tomatoes, believing they give baby colic. Drink beer or whiskey to calm baby.
- **Birth recuperation**. Women who have given birth are "polluted" (*mahrime*) for nine days because of birth fluids. Must not touch men or cook food. Hospital births popular because hospital disposes of birth fluids, thereby reducing

new mother's time in ritual isolation. Allow older female relatives to be near new mother and baby but keep visiting family members to a minimum out of fear they will bring in spirit of the night (*Martiya*), who may harm baby.

- **Baby care**. Mother cares for baby, which often is tightly swaddled. Roma believe that baby is very vulnerable to the evil eye; carefully observe visitors lest they give baby the evil eye. Baby's fussing and/or colic viewed as evidence of the evil eye. Giver of evil eye may make a cross with spittle on baby's forehead. Not shameful if someone possesses the evil eye, as he/she cannot do anything about it. Believe that evil eye is more common in persons with bushy or heavy eyebrows or lots of body hair.
- **Problems with baby**. If baby dies, parents try to avoid its death and burial; they may depart hospital suddenly to avoid the association between death and bad luck/impurity (*mahrime*). Grandparents responsible for burying baby, but they, too, may leave everything to hospital.
- **Male and female circumcision**. Male circumcision not traditionally done but may be more acceptable due to higher incidence of hospital births. Female circumcision not practiced.

DEVELOPMENTAL AND SEXUAL ISSUES

- **Celebration of menarche or becoming a man**. A girl's life changes dramatically at menarche. She must adopt not only a new set of rules about washing, eating, and cleanliness but also must avoid contact with male relatives during menarche, adopt a new body language (downcast eyes and being quiet and modest), and abandon her childhood. Boys become men when they are able to have sex.
- **Attitudes about birth control**. Practice it but not openly.
- **Attitudes about sexually transmitted infection (STI) control, including condoms**. Very sensitive subject. STI extremely shameful. Men are reluctant to use condoms, but some do. Because Roma consider all lower-body fluids to be impure (*mahrime*), connecting lack of condom use with disease fits well into their beliefs about causes of illness.
- **Attitudes about abortion**. Generally unacceptable. However, pregnancy before marriage is very shameful, so some younger women may consider abortion to spare their parents the shame.
- **Attitudes about unwed sexual experimentation**. Not acceptable ideally, but adults are realistic about its occurrence.
- **Sexual orientation**. Unacceptable to remain unmarried or to be gay or lesbian. Often leads to complete rejection by community.
- **Gender identity**. Unacceptable to have ambiguous gender identity or gender that is opposite of one's birth gender.
- **Attitudes about menopause**. Gives women greater power, as they become "clean." Postmenopausal women are respected leaders in the family (especially if widowed) and have a great deal of clout in decision-making.

FAMILY RELATIONSHIPS

- **Composition/structure**. Large extended families comprising at least three generations, sometimes 4–5 generations. Nuclear family also large. Relatives on both mother's and father's sides of family important, but young persons usually reside and identify with one family line (*vitsa*). Households encompass 3–4 generations and have fluid composition. All close relatives in town stay and eat at each other's house. Gather daily. Relatives from out of town visit constantly. Family members fiercely loyal to each other; therefore, when feuds break out (usually between brothers vying for authority), they cause irreparable splits in family. Family takes strong interest in arranging marriages of next generation.

- **Decision-making**. Individuals make their own decisions but prefer to consult entire family first. Persons 35 years old and younger often prefer to leave decisions to older relatives. Eldest person usually the one in authority, unless he/she is senile. Men present themselves as spokesperson for whole family, but older women, such as spokesperson's wife, play critical role in decisions; she may in fact have the final word, as she is the one who knows "medicine." Clinician should always consult with husband and wife together regarding a permanent decision. Very old grandmother who is frail may be past her time as authority figure, but if relatives defer to her, she must be consulted, too. Decisions involving avoidance of moral impurity (*mahrime*) may be out of the hands of the immediate extended family and up to all elders in the area.

- **Spokesperson**. Parents speak for children but also listen to their wishes, often to the detriment of a child's long-term health. Mother- and father-in-law may make decisions for a daughter-in-law, but it is best if clinician contacts her parents.

- **Gender issues**. Men are ostensible leaders in political decision-making matters concerning the group. Women play a less obvious but crucial role. Women often are principal money earners; Roma view men's work as extra help. Men invest in women's careers. Women cook and care for children, and are responsible for providing household income (e.g., through fortune-telling). Men organize large festivities, such as a saint's day feast (*slava*), death ritual feast (*pomana*), or baptism. Women generally are keepers and communicators of medical and spiritual knowledge; thus, their role is very important in times of illness. In hospital, older female medical practitioner (*drabarni*) may administer her own medicine in addition to medications ordered by doctor.

- **Changing roles among generations in U.S.** Adults are more familiar with modern American life than grandparents are, and are beginning to take the lead on some issues. Influence of elders has become more fragmented. There is a tendency toward smaller families.

- **Caring roles**. Women take primary role in caring for sick but often do not follow clinician's instructions, instead providing their own notion of appropriate care. Women caregivers have strong feelings about what patient needs; patient accepts decision, sometimes to his/her detriment.

- **Expectations of and for children**. Indulge children and allow them free expression. Tolerate noisy, turbulent behavior, though parents recognize that non-Roma have lower tolerance level. Expect children to learn how to make a living the Roma way, marry someone their parents approve of or select, bear many children, and stay very close to family. Schooling is not an expectation, but some children like to attend school for a few years. However, family activities take priority over schooling. Expect children to learn how to be savvy and street smart, how to talk their way out of situations, and never to accept anything at face value but rather always to check something out with other sources. Children learn at an early age to fend for themselves, to handle money correctly, and not to get cheated. Children very close to parents, siblings, and members of extended family. Rebellion unusual, but it does occur.
- **Expectations of and for elders**. Highly respect elders for their superior knowledge of Roma culture and history, for their long experience in dealing with non-Roma, and for their ability to survive hardship. Also fear elders for their power to decide on membership in a group or expulsion from it, the worst punishment the group metes out. Elders decide questions of moral purity and make all political decisions for group. Head of household is elderly. Adult children care for their elders. Roma do not put elders in assisted living facilities or nursing homes.
- **Expectations of hospital visitors**. Expect large numbers of constant visitors. If this presents difficulties, clinician should ask eldest authority figure to organize a system (e.g., five visitors in patient's room at any given time) and to choose which close family members may stay at all times (should consult both male and female elders). Staff can manage hospital visitors by enlisting help of all elders. One option that often works is to designate a room or garden area where all Roma can gather; outside is best if weather permits. Roma prefer to segregate themselves from non-Roma; prefer to be outside where chances of coming into contact with a source of spiritual and moral impurity (*mahrime*) are less. Clinician should designate an older person on hospital staff to manage many visitors, answer their questions, and appeal to authority figure(s) to control the situation and be effective liaison(s) to hospital personnel.

ILLNESS BELIEFS

- **Causes of/attitudes about physical illness**. Traditionally, health, good luck, and prosperity are all a result of spiritual and moral cleanliness (*wuzho*). Lack of spiritual and moral cleanliness (*mahrime*) not only results in disease and bad luck but attracts certain spirits (*Mamioro, Martiya*) or the devil (*o beng*), harbingers of illness. Roma also accept and readily adopt Western medicine as powerful and effective. Are willing to try anything that cures.

- **Causes of/attitudes about mental illness**. Someone is deemed "crazy" or mentally ill primarily when he/she does not conform to Roma cultural rules of behavior. The cure is to get the person to conform. For example, someone who does not want to marry (a sign of mental illness) is cured by arranging a marriage. Also attribute mental illness (e.g., wild behavior or seizures) to possession by the devil.
- **Causes of genetic defects**. Roma accept genetic, birth, and congenital defects, do not understand or distinguish significantly among them, and care for afflicted persons at home. Generally refuse institutionalization.
- **Attitudes about disabilities**. Generally tolerant. Accept disability as bad luck.
- **Sick role**. Sick persons expect family to attend to their needs and care for them. Illness is a group as well as an individual crisis; patient must deal with both aspects.
- **Home and folk remedies**. Devil causes convulsions. Roma cure these by giving the afflicted person a spice (*asafetida*), which they call devil's dung. Spirit named Little Grandmother (*Mamioro*) brings a number of serious illnesses, such as flu, pneumonia, tuberculosis, cholera, and plague, which are cured by giving the sick person *Mamioro's* vomit, or slime mold (*Fuligo septica*). Regardless of these beliefs, Roma are very practical; they recognize that American doctors are also powerful healers and have very effective medicine. Roma frequently use both folk remedies and Western biomedicine just to make sure patient recovers.
- **Medications**. Use folk remedies and take Western medications concurrently. Compliance is good, but if patient feels better, he/she may stop medication. Clinician should explain importance of taking full course of medications.
- **Acceptance of procedures**. Greatly fear invasive procedures and operations ("going under the knife"). Also fear anesthesia ("little death"). Clinician should explain these very carefully to minimize fear and should emphasize the benefits. Roma refuse an operation they do not perceive as a matter of life or death. Gynecologic and proctologic exams highly embarrassing and shocking due to *mahrime* beliefs. Clinician should perform such exams only when absolutely necessary and after he/she has fully explained the necessity.
- **Care-seeking**. Roma use their own medicines (based on their own theories of illness causes) concurrently with "American medicine" (based, e.g., on "germ" theory).

HEALTH ISSUES

- **Concept of health**. Associate good health with moral purity, keeping upper and lower halves of body separate, and good behavior. Good health, prosperity, large families, and good luck inextricably intertwined. Romas' knowledge of anatomy is extremely weak.

- **Health promotion and prevention**. Promoting good health means staying clean (*wuzho*) and avoiding uncleanliness (*mahrime*). Roma know very little about preventive medicine, healthy eating practices, or exercise. Often smoke and drink heavily.
- **Screening**. Important for clinician to explain reasons for screening as it relates to health in general. Roma likely to resist screening for sexually transmitted infections.
- **Common health problems**. Obesity-related problems very common. Type 2 diabetes, hypertension, high cholesterol, and hemorrhoids common among both young and old Roma.

DEATH RITUALS

- **Beliefs and attitudes about death**. Consider death a tragedy when the deceased is young. Relatives express extreme grief. An old person who prepares for death has a "good" death that relatives can celebrate. Death of a relative causes the living to fear that the dead person's spirit may haunt them.
- **Preparation**. Clinician should inform eldest authority figure first and ask for help with informing other relatives and managing their grief. Family may want priest present for purification of body. Family wants window left open, preferably before death but also afterward, to allow spirit to leave. Grown children responsible for funeral arrangements for their parents. Roma do not avoid subject of death; may discuss it heatedly long before someone dies. Dying person is eager to have everything arranged for his/her death.
- **Home vs. hospital**. Preference varies by family, depending on illness and nature of death. For acute illness and illness requiring extensive treatment, may prefer hospital. Critical issue is presence of family. Likely to prefer home during terminal stages of chronic illness.
- **Special needs**. May ask for religious object or for dying person's favorite foods and a personal belonging, such as his fishing pole. May even set up a small home shrine. Want to have older female relative at window at all times to keep out night spirits and chase them away, and to allow dying person's spirit to leave. Moment of death highly significant: Feelings of dying person give relatives a sense of what will happen in the year after death, and close relatives want to hear his/her last words, which are very important.
- **Care of the body**. Body may be a source of spiritual danger for relatives. Usually want it embalmed immediately to remove blood, which Roma view as a source of the polluting effect of death. Want to sit with body day and night after death, and be able to eat and drink; funeral parlor usually is the most appropriate place. Except in cases of sudden death, Roma will have made all necessary arrangements.
- **Attitudes about organ donation**. In the past, organ donation was unacceptable. Today, however, Roma may donate/receive organs to/from a family member.

- **Attitudes about autopsy**. Very unlikely that family will agree to autopsy. If medically necessary, eldest authority figure decides.

SELECTED REFERENCES

Sutherland, A. (1992). Gypsies and health care. *Western Journal of Medicine*, 157, 276–280.

Sutherland, A. (1992). Health and illness among the Roma of California. *Journal of the Gypsy Lore Society*, 5, 19–59.

Thomas, J. D., Doucette, M. M., Thomas, D. C., & Stoeckle, J. D. (1987). Disease, lifestyle, and consanguinity in 58 American Gypsies. *Lancet*, 2, 377–379.

Vivian, C., & Dundes, L. (2004). The crossroads of culture and health among the Roma (Gypsies). *Journal of Nursing Scholarship*, 36, 86–91.

AUTHOR

Anne H. Sutherland, PhD (Oxon), is a professor of cultural and social anthropology at the University of California-Riverside. She received her PhD from Oxford University in 1972 and taught at Durham University in England for four years, at Macalester College in St. Paul, MN, for 19 years, and at Georgia State University for four years. She has conducted research on American Roma since 1968, on ethnic groups in Belize, and on identity and culture in Texas. The author of *Gypsies, the Hidden Americans* (1986) and numerous articles on American Roma, she has appeared in public television documentaries on the Roma, including "A Curse on the Gypsies" and "The Genocide Factor."

CHAPTER 31

RUSSIANS

AND OTHERS FROM THE FORMER SOVIET UNION

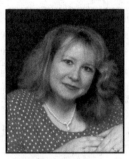
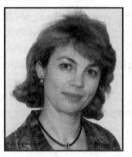

Luba Evanikoff del Puerto   *Ella Sigal*

CULTURAL/ETHNIC IDENTITY

- **Preferred term(s)**. Russian. In this chapter, the term includes other immigrants and refugees who have come from the former Soviet Union, most of them from the western (European) part of the country.
- **Census**. Between 1985–98, about 500,000 immigrants arrived. The 2000 U.S. Census estimates nearly 3 million people of Russian ancestry and 373,462 who are foreign-born. More than 900,000 people are of Ukrainian ancestry.
- **History of immigration**. Russia's 19th-century history of anti-Semitism included prohibiting Jews from owning property and requiring them to live within segregated, "Pale of Settlement" communities (*shtetls*). In the 20th and 21st centuries, most Russian immigrants and refugees have been Jewish. Those in the first immigration wave (1900–14) left Russia because of poor economic conditions and religious and political persecution. In addition to Jews, they included Orthodox Christians, Molokans (Christians who separated from the Russian Orthodox Church in the 18th century), and Catholics, mostly from Latvia, Lithuania, and Estonia. The second wave (1918–40) comprised primarily upper- and middle-class persons, army officers, and professionals who feared for their lives after the 1917 Bolshevik Revolution. There were about 20,000 immigrants in the third wave (1947–52), mostly war prisoners, slave laborers, and refugees who had fled to Germany during World War II and refused to return to Russia. The fourth wave (1971–91) comprised 181,000 Russian Jews who entered the U.S. for religious and political reasons. About 20% were older than 65, making this one

of the oldest immigrant populations. The fifth wave (1988–present) occurred after the rise of Mikhail Gorbachev and the break-up of the Soviet Union. The U.S. accepted 378,000 refugees, most of them Jewish and mainly from Russia and the western (European) part of the country.

SPIRITUAL/RELIGIOUS ORIENTATION

- **Primary religious/spiritual affiliations**. Predominantly Jewish and Eastern Orthodox. Others are Molokans, Baptists, Seventh Day Adventists, Pentecostals, Old Believers, Catholics, Buddhists, and Muslims.
- **Usual religious/spiritual practices**. Because of religious prohibitions in the former Soviet Union, most immigrants did not formally practice their religion there. Today, some pray privately rather than attend formal services.
- **Use of spiritual healing/healers**. Clinician should allow or summon a rabbi, priest, or minister only after consulting with patient and his/her family.
- **Holidays**. Immigrants celebrate most U.S. national holidays but still observe some of their own. Non-Jewish religious holidays include *Maslenitsa*, a week-long Christian Orthodox celebration that falls one week before the six-week Lenten fast. A special food during *Maslenitsa* is bliny. These round cakes, similar to crepes and containing various fillings, represent the sun's return after winter darkness and are an ancient tradition from the Spring Festival that later became Easter. Molokans, Orthodox Christians, and other Christians celebrate Easter. They fast for different periods of time, then pray and have a day of feasting. On Clean Thursday, before Easter, the faithful clean, wash, bake a special bread (*kulitch*) and other pastries, and color Easter eggs in the traditional way—by boiling them with onion skins. Some may observe Clean Thursday on Friday and request the day off. The ninth day after Easter is Parents' Day, when Russians bring flowers to the graves of their deceased parents. Jewish holidays are observed according to the Jewish lunar calendar (5765 corresponds with the Gregorian calendar year of 2005). Jewish New Year (*Rosh Hashanah*, which, translated from Hebrew, means "head of the year") is on the first and second day of the seventh month (*Tishri*), usually in September. The Day of Atonement (*Yom Kippur*) is the most important Jewish holiday; it falls on the 10th day of the seventh month. Even though many do not observe other Jewish traditions, on *Yom Kippur* they may refrain from work, fast for 24 hours, and/or attend synagogue services. Children and the severely ill are allowed to eat. A joyful holiday that some Orthodox Jewish families still observe is the Festival of Booths (*Sukkot*), which begins on the fifth day after *Yom Kippur*. The Festival of Lights (*Chanukah*) is the best-known Jewish holiday in the U.S. because it falls close to Christmas; families celebrate with elaborate gift-giving and decoration. *Purim*, which usually takes place in March, commemorates when Jews living in Persia were saved from extermination. Passover (*Pesach*) is an eight-day observance, usually in April, celebrating Jewish slaves'

freedom from Egypt. Families and friends gather for a lavish meal (*seder*) during which the story of Passover is retold. Some Jewish families observe Sabbath (*Shabbat*), which begins at twilight on Friday and continues until sundown on Saturday. During *Shabbat*, working, cooking, and driving are prohibited. Among secular holidays that Russians celebrate is New Year's, the most popular one. Many celebrate New Year's twice: on January 1 and, in accordance with the Julian calendar used in Russia before 1918, on January 14. On Women's Day (March 8), all women and girls—including female neighbors, co-workers, and friends—receive flowers, presents, and toasts from men. Another secular holiday is Victory Day (May 9), commemorating the millions of Russians who fell in World War II. People lay flowers and wreaths on graves, and veterans gather wearing their military uniforms and medals.

COMMUNICATION
ORAL COMMUNICATION

- **Major languages and dialects**. Russian, a Slavic language that uses the Cyrillic alphabet, is very rich, expressive, and difficult to learn. About 98% of Russians speak it as their native language. Three main dialects: One is spoken by the Nordic group of Russians (from Saint Petersburg to Siberia), another by the southern group (in most of central and southern Russia), and a third by the central group (in the area between the other two). Differences are minor; persons who speak the northern or southern dialect understand each other. Standard Russian is based on Moscow dialect (spoken primarily in the central part of the country) and includes characteristics of both the southern and northern dialects. Some Russians learned English as part of their education in Russia. Most also speak the language of the republic where they once lived, such as Ukrainian, Belarusian, or Latvian. Many elderly Jewish refugees speak Yiddish.
- **Greetings**. Take greetings very seriously. May shake hands or kiss one another on each cheek, depending on their relationship and place of origin. Kissing a woman on her forehead is reserved for funerals. Inappropriate to shake hands with an unfamiliar woman, except upon introduction. Some older men may kiss a woman's hand. In some Orthodox Jewish families, physical contact between men and women is inappropriate and prohibited by religious law. Expect to be addressed by "Mr." (*Gospodin*) or "Mrs." (*Gospodja*) and last name. Highly respect elders; address them as "Uncle" or "Aunt" even when there is no blood relationship. Socially unacceptable for health care provider to address patient by any term of endearment. However, family members and friends may show affection by using diminutives (e.g., Tania is Tanichka), cute animal nicknames (e.g., Bunny [*Zaichik*] instead of first name), or body parts (e.g., finger [*pal'chik*]).
- **Tone of voice**. Depending on family upbringing, some speak softly and oth-

ers loudly when trying to be understood, even in pleasant conversation.

- **Direct or indirect style of speech**. Russians are very straightforward and usually do not hesitate to say what they think in a way that leaves no room for misunderstanding. When persons meet or phone each other, they do not spend time on small talk but rather get straight to the point. However, if an elderly person is asked, "How are you?" he/she takes the question literally and answers with a sometimes lengthy explanation of his/her health problems.
- **Use of interpreters**. Clinician should use trained interpreters whenever possible. Family and friends become anxious when they do not have much information about a diagnosis or do not understand medical terminology. Uncommon for grandchildren to interpret.
- **Serious or terminal illness**. Prefer that spouse or eldest child be notified first about terminal illness; he/she will decide whether to inform patient. Usually, family members do not want patient to worry and be anxious about illness but rather to be at peace so his/her physical and emotional condition does not worsen.

WRITTEN COMMUNICATION

Russian is grammatically difficult; it has three genders and many rules. Words may be written differently than they are pronounced. Most parts of speech, such as verbs, adverbs, nouns, pronouns, and adjectives, change according to gender, tense, number, person, or mood. Even a last name might end differently, depending on sentence structure.

- **Literacy assessment**. Russians are highly educated and have a strong cultural history. Russia has the world's highest educational level; more than 40% of adults have a college/university degree. Many immigrants are highly educated professionals—doctors, nurses, engineers, musicians, and teachers. Both men and women are literate in Russian. Most immigrant children, adolescents, and young adults quickly become fluent in English soon after arriving. English can be a problem for older immigrants and those recently arrived. Some elderly are hesitant to admit that their understanding of English is limited. Clinician should assess patients' ability to read and write in English by asking them directly and giving them appropriate forms to fill out. Should always help elderly patients complete forms.
- **Consents**. Clinician should explain procedures, tests, and possible complications to patient and family together. Often a relative is or has been a health care provider and may serve as spokesperson or expert. In some cases, agreement by handshake may be more valid than signing a form, although patients realize that in the health care setting a signature is necessary. Russians do not usually consent to participate in research trials or experimental procedures.

NONVERBAL COMMUNICATION

- **Eye contact**. Direct eye contact is a sign of respect and trust. Russians use direct eye contact with everyone, even in public and among strangers. Socially appropriate to maintain eye contact throughout a conversation.

- **Personal space**. Depends on degree of friendship and familiarity. May prefer to maintain a social distance with health care providers (about 3–5 feet). Patients allow assessment and interventions in intimate space if they are informed first.
- **Use and meaning of silence**. Silence uncommon but can be appropriate in some situations (e.g., acceptable for health care provider to be silent after patient receives bad news about diagnosis).
- **Gestures**. Nodding is appropriate when agreeing, listening attentively, or answering a question. To show disapproval (seriously or jokingly), may raise a fist and shake it. To show approval, give the "thumbs up" sign.
- **Openness in expressing emotions**. Openly express emotions with family members through body language and facial expressions. May be more cautious about laughing, crying, joking, or arguing—emotions that may be inappropriate in some public settings. Russians become more open when trust is established.
- **Privacy**. Patients and parents may be reluctant to discuss emotional suffering with outsiders. Speak freely about physical problems. When hospitalized, patients tend to tolerate loss of privacy but still maintain privacy when a family member or friend of the opposite gender is present.
- **Touch**. Freely touch family members, intimates, and close friends. Touching acceptable in health care setting if clinician first explains the need for it. Acceptability of touching private body parts varies widely among individuals, depending on their place of origin and religion.
- **Orientation to time**. Value punctuality. Based on previous health care experiences, patients may try to make the most of their clinical time; often, they either arrive early for an appointment, in hopes of being the first to be seen, or late, so as not to waste time waiting. To others, Russians may seem demanding or difficult if their impatience grows in the waiting room. Mostly oriented to the future but also to the past and present.

ACTIVITIES OF DAILY LIVING

- **Modesty**. Value modesty. Gender of health care provider not an issue, but patient may prefer that a visitor of opposite gender leave the room for some procedures, such as peri-care or assessment of urinary catheter.
- **Skin care**. When sick, some avoid a daily shower, preferring sponge baths instead. Patient who showers may insist on being kept warm to avoid "catching cold."
- **Hair care**. No special preferences for hair cutting or products. Wash hair less frequently when sick, especially in hospital, for fear of "catching cold" or headache. If patient's hair must be washed, staff should shut windows and keep room warm, turning on heater if possible.

- **Nail care**. Both genders prefer neatly trimmed nails. Some women may request manicures and pedicures in hospital.
- **Toileting**. Urinals and bedpans acceptable to bedridden patients. Because of modesty, may avoid bedside commodes and may not save urine for measuring intake and output.
- **Special clothing or amulets**. Some elderly women wear warm clothing over hospital gown for fear of "catching cold" or pneumonia. Most patients wear handmade wool socks and sweaters. Some wear religious medallions and may want pictures of saints near bedside.
- **Self-care**. Patient, family member, or patient with help of nursing staff may perform hygiene. Staff should respect patient's modesty and ensure his/her privacy when family member of opposite gender is present. Patients generally like to have family members care for them while recovering at home.

FOOD PRACTICES

- **Usual meal pattern**. Three meals a day. Like many Europeans, Russians prefer largest meal at lunchtime. Enjoy hot tea between meals.
- **Special utensils**. Jewish families that keep kosher use separate sets of dishes and cookware for meals that include meat and milk.
- **Food beliefs and rituals**. Food is a universally binding element. Family dinners a tradition; encourage children and grandchildren to attend. Traditional recipes and preparation methods are related to folklore and holidays. Bread has a special meaning; in some religions, it is a holy food symbolizing abundance, future life, and happiness. Bread often described in folklore as promoting happiness. Use bread in certain rituals, such as weddings and remembrances of the deceased. Some Jewish families keep kosher, eating only meat from which all blood has been drained and not combining meat and milk products.
- **Usual diet**. Often high in fat, carbohydrates, and sodium. In the past, Russians had to preserve food without refrigeration, so they dried sausage and pickled meat, fish, and vegetables—popular foods that have a high salt content. Meals always include bread, which should be removed last and never thrown away. Consider potatoes to be the "second bread" and use them in a variety of dishes at every meal. Some eat too much red meat because it was scarce in Russia. But many take advantage of low-cost and available fresh fruit and vegetables in U.S.
- **Fluids**. Hot tea (chai) with lemon and honey or raspberry, strawberry, or lemon jam. Drink alcoholic beverages on social occasions and at home. Most Russians do not drink enough water due to the old belief that consuming too much water dilutes gastric juices, spoils the appetite, and causes bloating. Ill elders prefer tepid beverages; water pitcher should be labeled "no ice."
- **Food taboos and prescriptions**. Observant Jews avoid pork and shellfish; those who keep kosher do not combine milk and meat products. Some Jews

request kosher food only. Clinician should ask patient about dietary restrictions. Russian Molokans and Muslims forbid pork, and Molokans do not eat shellfish. When ill, prefer hot soups, such as vegetable, beet, and cabbage soup (*borscht*); various light-broth soups, such as chicken and rice soup; and soft and bland foods, such as oatmeal, ground-meat patties, boiled chicken, baked and mashed potatoes, fresh fruit, vegetables, and plain yogurt.

- **Hospitality**. Food symbolizes hospitality. Bread symbolizes abundance and future life; it is always served. Typical dinner for guests includes an abundant variety of appetizers, salads, and cold cuts along with the main course and dessert. Guests who do not eat heartily might offend the host, who may conclude they do not like the food. Host always offers hot tea, even during a short visit. Depending on religion, drinking alcohol may be an acceptable social tradition (e.g., dropping by a friend's house and having a drink). Men favor chilled Russian vodka; women favor Soviet champagne or dessert wine.

SYMPTOM MANAGEMENT

- **Pain** (*bohlyeet*). Russians tend to be very stoic. Because they fear that morphine will lead to addiction and pneumonia, clinician may need to encourage them to accept pain medication. Those acculturated to U.S. biomedical system are more receptive to such medication; prefer oral route. Accept any nonpharmacological methods first, such as ointments. Most Russians understand numerical pain scale.

- **Dyspnea** (*odish'ka*). Non-English speakers grasp chest and moan to express dyspnea. Most use words instead of numbers to describe level. Prefer pharmacological methods to relaxation techniques. May get more anxious because of language barrier. Accept oxygen.

- **Nausea/vomiting** (*toshnata'*). Some report nausea and describe the vomitus. Out of modesty, clean up vomitus. Accept nonpharmacological treatments first, such as lemon slices, ginger ale, mineral water, plain yogurt, and tea with lemon. May refuse medications and procedures when nauseated. Some believe that ingesting too many medications poisons the body or that taking medications on an empty stomach causes nausea. Clinician should offer snacks such as crackers.

- **Constipation/diarrhea** (*zapor'/ponos'*). Regular bowel movements a priority. Accept nonpharmacological treatments first. For constipation, clinician should offer prune juice, beets, and fruit, then a laxative such as milk of magnesia or one the patient chooses. He/she may refuse various procedures if constipated. For diarrhea in young children, Russians first try rice or rice broth, then accept medications.

- **Fatigue** (*ysta'lost'*). Prescribe rest and sleep as best treatment. Describe fatigue in words rather than numbers. Some accept sleeping pills for insomnia. Russians consider a good night's sleep essential; some become upset if interventions (vital signs, blood-sugar check, fluid input and output) require disturbing their sleep. Before patient's bedtime, clinician should explain need for interventions and, if possible, arrange for them to take place concurrently.

- **Depression** (*depresia*). Most do not directly acknowledge depression but are able to describe their symptoms in detail if asked. Russians, particularly the elderly, tend to describe depression in terms of multiple somatic symptoms because they have trouble labeling the problem "depression." Most elderly who have been placed in a skilled nursing facility exhibit symptoms of depression. Some young, educated persons or those previously treated in U.S. have no difficulty saying they are depressed. Most do not like to take excessive medication; prefer nonpharmacological treatments first, such as herbal supplements. Accept support and counseling. Clinician should discuss depression with patient and family.
- **Self-care symptom management**. Usually rely on self-care first before seeking medical attention. Commonly self-monitor blood pressure and blood glucose at home.

BIRTH RITUALS/CARE OF THE NEW MOTHER AND BABY

- **Pregnancy care**. Some pregnant women do not use prenatal care unless they are concerned something is wrong. More-acculturated women may begin prenatal care in first trimester. Couple may avoid announcing pregnancy during first trimester because of the belief that early news may harm fetus. Russians shield pregnant women from bad news, believing that it might harm fetus. Also discourage pregnant women from lifting heavy objects, skipping any steps on staircases, and performing heavy exercise, fearing that, as a result of such activities, umbilical cord will choke baby, baby may move to breech position, or baby will become past due.
- **Preferences for children**. Gender not an issue. Highly value children; most families welcome them. Normally have only 1–2 children.
- **Labor practices**. When a woman senses delivery is near, others encourage her to drink castor oil (although this practice is slowly fading) or give her an enema for easier birth. Physician or midwife assists with delivery. She is highly encouraged to walk when contractions begin to promote dilatation. Traditionally, Russians discouraged the expectant mother from taking any pain medication (e.g., epidural) during labor for fear of harming her or baby, but some women may want it. Lighting in birthing room should be minimal because Russians believe that newborn's eyes are not yet strong or mature enough and that too much light will cause baby to develop poor eyesight.
- **Role of the laboring woman during birth**. Generally assumes passive role and follows physician's or midwife's commands. Depending on the individual, Russian mothers are generally stoic and not very loud when giving birth.
- **Role of the father and other family members during birth**. Traditionally, father not allowed in birthing room; only closest female family member allowed, such as woman's mother, sister, or mother-in-law, depending on who

is available. Varies depending on acculturation level and is more acceptable among younger generation.

- **Vaginal vs. cesarean section**. Prefer vaginal delivery.
- **Breastfeeding**. Expect new mother to breastfeed until milk "runs out." May breastfeed into toddler years. Women value the health and immunological benefits of breastfeeding, and partners support and encourage it. In Russia, child care at work sites and an average maternity leave of 25 months foster breastfeeding. Believe that, during breastfeeding, too much noise or stimulation, or mother's nervousness, might make baby "hyper" later in life. Also believe that if mother is suddenly shocked or scared, breast milk should first be expelled rather than given to baby. Mothers breastfeed in dim light to preserve baby's eyesight. Believe that breasts should be kept warm at all times to prevent mother from developing breast cancer later in life. Mothers tend to avoid foods that cause gas, such as cabbage, cucumbers, garlic, broccoli, and turnips, to prevent indigestion in baby. Believe that maternal consumption of eggs, chocolate, citrus, corn, or nuts causes allergies in baby.
- **Birth recuperation**. Traditionally, 15 days of bed rest. New mother's mother or someone else cooks and does other household chores for up to 40 days, during which time the new mother should not go outside the home. Russians believe that new mother's internal organs should heal and return to the position they were in before pregnancy in order to prevent future physical problems. Traditionally, new mother wears pelvic binder to regain her figure. Pericare with warm water important.
- **Baby care**. Common for grandparents to raise grandchildren until age 4 or 5, especially if both parents work. If resources available, may also enroll toddler in a Russian day care center. Believe that it is important to keep baby warm at all times so bones develop normally and to prevent illness. Baby's head and feet should always be covered when exposed to cold, wind, or very hot sun.
- **Problems with baby**. Clinician should notify new mother first. She decides who else to tell but may not want anyone to know.
- **Male and female circumcision**. Clinician should discuss circumcision with parents. Most Christian parents do not believe in male circumcision. Most Jewish boys are circumcised on eighth day in a home ceremony (*brit milah*) conducted by someone (*mohel*) who has been trained to do circumcisions. Baby receives his Hebrew name at that time. Girls are not circumcised. Traditionally, a girl's birth was followed by prayers for her and her mother's health, and the birth was recognized by announcing baby's name publicly.

DEVELOPMENTAL AND SEXUAL ISSUES

- **Celebration of menarche or becoming a man**. Non-Jews do not celebrate either with any special ritual. After intensive study, Jewish boys are eligible for *bar mitzvah* at age 13 years and one day, which allows their full incorporation into religious life, including participation in a prayer quorum (*min-*

yan). After study, girls at age 12 years and one day can participate in *bat mitz-vah*. *Bar mitzvah* and *bat mitzvah* are religious ceremonies that take place in a synagogue, followed by celebration with food and dancing.

- **Attitudes about birth control**. Generally acceptable, but clinician should discuss it with each woman. Adolescents prefer pills, condoms, and patches, while women who have previously given birth prefer intrauterine devices and condoms. Adolescents seeking birth control and pregnancy testing tend to come in groups, having been referred by another Russian. Many come with their mothers, who speak on their behalf.

- **Attitudes about sexually transmitted infection (STI) control, including condoms**. When visiting health care providers, prefer to be screened for all possible STIs. Have positive attitude about condoms and use them very often.

- **Attitudes about abortion**. Medical abortions acceptable. Less commonly performed among unmarried women and teens. But in pregnancy, Russians take all measures to encourage mother to keep baby. Most parents offer support.

- **Attitudes about unwed sexual experimentation**. Generally frown upon it before age 16–17. Parents highly discourage it. Not uncommon to preserve virginity until marriage.

- **Sexual orientation**. In the past, homosexuals were persecuted in the homeland. Families and community may not approve of same-sex relationships or marriages, which are uncommon. Very few lesbians publicly reveal their orientation. Gay men are more public in the homeland but less obviously so than in U.S.

- **Gender identity**. Typically, family and community do not accept someone whose gender identity is ambiguous or opposite of his/her birth gender.

- **Attitudes about menopause**. Women easily accept it as a normal life transition. Russian women do not discuss menopause as openly as women in dominant U.S. culture do. Accept nonpharmacological remedies first. Some accept hormone replacement therapy.

FAMILY RELATIONSHIPS

- **Composition/structure**. Typical family is very close. Revere mother and elderly. Extended-family structure very strong. Contributing to this closeness was necessity in the past that several generations live under the same roof, depending on one another for child care and management of household. Divorce rate unusually low. Domestic violence uncommon, even though families may vigorously express their disagreement. Russian immigrants tend to have fewer children than other immigrants do.

- **Decision-making**. Father, mother, eldest son, and eldest daughter have the most say in making decisions about health care. Although husband and wife consult each other, some wives eventually give way to husband's opinion.

The more dominant personality probably prevails inside and outside the home. However, choice of, and decisions about, health care are novel to many immigrants; difficult for them to transition from a system in which all is predetermined to one that provides multiple options, especially when clear information is lacking.

- **Spokesperson**. Same as for decision-making or it is the family member who has a better grasp of English. In some cultures, such as Georgian, men are always head of the family.
- **Gender issues**. In Russia, women have had equal employment opportunities for decades. For example, most physicians and teachers are women, though their salaries and authority lag behind men's. Working women are nevertheless responsible for all household tasks and child care. Men still prefer to be family breadwinner.
- **Changing roles among generations in U.S.** Family roles have adapted to life in U.S. In some families, men help with household tasks. If a man loses his job, he becomes a "house husband." Because of their English skills, children have more family responsibilities, such as babysitting and interpreting when parents need help with certain tasks (e.g., paying bills, reading mail, or making appointments).
- **Caring roles**. Whole family pulls together during major crises for support and strength. All family members, including children, take turns caring for an ill family member.
- **Expectations of and for children**. Teach children to behave well in public, be obedient, be very respectful to elders, help rear younger children, and to study hard. Russians have strongly valued education for centuries. By the 1970s, those 25–34 years old had 16 years of education on average. Also expect children to broaden their knowledge in other areas, such as music, fine arts, and sports. Parents expect them to become independent and professionals while remaining involved with family, especially with ill family members. Some children prefer to stay near family rather than attend a distant college/university.
- **Expectations of and for elders**. Highly respect elderly, who remain very close to their children. Even if elders do not live with their children, they still are expected to help raise grandchildren and participate in decision-making. Some elders in U.S. take advantage of economic and other resources to lead a full and independent life; they volunteer, learn English, and participate in field trips and a variety of cultural activities. Russians generally do not favor nursing homes and other such facilities for elderly who need care. If an elder is placed in a facility, it should be near a family member's home.
- **Expectations of hospital visitors**. Expect family members and friends to visit; their strong bonds provide strength and support for patient. Happy to participate in care-giving. Most visitors stay overnight, alternating shifts if patient is seriously ill. Clinician should give them instructions on what they

can do to help and a quick orientation of hospital unit, such as location of pantry (if appropriate) and linen closet. Russians view the health care setting as serious and subdued; they expect staff and others to be serious, such that outbursts of laughter or loud expression of emotions may disturb them.

ILLNESS BELIEFS

- **Causes of/attitudes about physical illness**. Attribute illness to poor nutrition, not dressing warmly, exposure to draft, family history, stress, and mother not taking care of herself during pregnancy or ingesting too many medications. Some Christians believe that illness is God's will, a test of one's faith in God, or punishment. Some elderly Jews view sickness as inevitable and health as the exception. Accept, and privately deal with, pain and misfortune.

- **Causes of/attitudes about mental illness**. Believe that suffering, stress, and genetics cause mental illness. Historically, Russians did not discuss emotional and mental health problems, even among family members. Hesitant to seek appropriate psychiatric care because they remember the widespread use of psychiatric treatment as an instrument of political repression in the former Soviet Union. Instead, Russians used individual outpatient services or relied mostly on themselves, family members, or friends. However, depression is common among recent, elderly immigrants who feel displaced; in U.S., they are encouraged to seek medical attention.

- **Causes of genetic defects**. Similar to causes of physical illness. Clinician should screen Jews for Tay-Sachs disease and Gaucher disease.

- **Attitudes about disabilities**. Accept disabled family member without stigma or shame. Some families who are highly supportive take disabled member out in public. Clinician should offer resources available in hospital and clinic settings.

- **Sick role**. Family always cares for ill member. It may bring nutritious and appropriate food from home for hospitalized patient. If patient has fever and/or is diaphoretic, Russians believe it is very important that he/she stay covered and to shut window because patient is most prone to catching pneumonia at this time. Ill patients generally place themselves on bed rest. Clinician should explain importance of ambulation and other self-care measures, such as using an incentive spirometer.

- **Home and folk remedies**. Russians diagnose and treat themselves first before seeking medical attention. Many Russian households have numerous books and magazines on various medical and nonpharmacological diagnoses and treatments. They believe that excessive drug use can be harmful and that all medications are somewhat poisonous. Home and folk remedies include rubbing camphor and other ointments/oils on the skin, cupping (*banki*, or pressing small, hot glass on skin of back and shoulders) for cold and flu, enemas, light exercise in fresh air and sunlight, mud baths, steam baths for respiratory infections, hot soups, sweet liquor, mineral water, herbal teas, and tea with lemon, honey, and jam. May treat back pain with dry heat and a raw dough plaster on the back or with a pad of coarse wool or animal hair on skin of lower back. Treat headache with strong ointment applied behind ears, on temples, and on back of neck. Treat rhinitis with drops of raw onion juice in the nostrils. Gargle with salt and baking soda for sore throat. Commonly use a mercurochrome-based green liquid (*zelenka*) to treat skin problems. Popular herbal remedies in U.S. include valerian root; motherwort; hawthorn berries for nervous conditions such as insomnia, headache, and regulation of blood pressure and cardiac conditions; and coltsfoot for cough, cold, and bronchitis. Use daisies (*romashka*) and *chistotel*, a member of the poppy family, for any skin condition. Patients may use herbal remedies and Western medications concurrently but do not mention such use unless asked.

- **Medications**. Due to shortages of imported drugs in the former Soviet Union and the low quality of Soviet-made substitutes dispensed by pharmacists, many immigrants refuse generic drugs; they insist instead on certain brand names. Some patients prefer Soviet medications they or friends have imported, claiming that American medications are too strong. Some "adjust" the dose or frequency on their own without telling health care providers. Compliance with hypertension medications may be problematic. For example, patient may discontinue such medications so doctor can see what his/her "true" blood pressure is, or take medication sporadically in the belief that medicating regularly reduces efficacy or causes low blood pressure. Others believe that hypertension is symptomatic; thus, the absence of headache or an inability to "feel" blood pressure means medication is unnecessary.

- **Acceptance of procedures**. Appreciate technologically advanced surgery that can result in better quality of life. Newer immigrants may not consent to blood transfusion for fear of contracting HIV/AIDS or other blood-borne conditions. Educating the patient helps. May accept organ transplant, depending on patient's religious beliefs.

- **Care-seeking**. Russians respect physicians. Disclose pertinent information. Often mistake American nurses for physicians because of nurses' professional role. Russians expect formality in health care settings and tend not to appreciate a light, chatty approach. Because the salaries of all health care professionals in Russia are low and tips are expected, newer immigrants may give caregivers in U.S. a tip or gift. Longer hospital stays customary in the former Soviet Union, so new immigrants in U.S. may insist on longer hospitalization. Some patients might seem demanding because they seek special attention and request extra procedures and tests, based on their homeland experience.

HEALTH ISSUES

- **Concept of health**. View health as regular bowel movements, absence of symptoms such as colds, and less exposure to stress.

- **Health promotion and prevention**. One maintains good health by dressing warmly, eating nutritious foods, having regular bowel movements, exercising (e.g., walking in open air and sunshine, and in good climate), and enjoying pleasant entertainment. When ill, emphasize staying warm, dressing warmly, and avoiding ice-cold drinks. Because of shortage of fruit and vegetables in the former Soviet Union, many immigrants may never have had a balanced diet there.
- **Screening**. Understand and may request additional diagnostic services. Although Russians appreciate advanced technology, elderly women in particular often do not undergo mammograms or Pap smears, but this depends on their education level. If offered diagnostic screening, Russians take advantage of it. Depending on their risk factors and education level, some patients demand diagnostic tests.
- **Common health problems**. High incidence of hypertension, heart problems, breast cancer, and diabetes. Very high rate of somatization, especially among recent immigrants, possibly because of their somatic rather than psychological orientation. Some studies show that a high rate of somatization is an expression of depression, perhaps caused by the enormous stress of immigration and acculturation. Very important for clinician to recognize symptoms of depression. Many Russians are heavy smokers. Those from large industrial cities often present with respiratory problems caused by air pollution and chemicals in large factories. Chest pain or pressure is a common complaint among those older than 40. Patients from the Chernobyl area should be screened regularly for illnesses related to radiation exposure. Although alcoholism is rare among Jews, Molokans, and Pentecostal Christians, it may be a problem among other Russian immigrants. Dental problems are frequent; immigrants are unfamiliar with regular dental checks, dental cleaning, or flossing.

DEATH RITUALS

- **Beliefs and attitudes about death**. If religious, Russians' beliefs about death are in accordance with their religion (e.g., Christians may believe that the deceased will go to heaven). Jews believe that death is a natural part of the life cycle and that the body is returned to the earth whence it came. Jewish law strictly forbids euthanasia, suicide, and assisted suicide.
- **Preparation**. Clinician should inform head of family first. To ensure a more peaceful death, family may not want patient to know. Clinician should ask family about notifying rabbi, priest, or minister. Some family members may choose not to resuscitate an elderly patient so he/she can die in comfort rather than on life support.
- **Home vs. hospital**. In cases of terminal illness, some families prefer that all family members care for patient at home rather than place him/her in a skilled nursing facility. If patient is acutely ill, family prefers hospitalization. Accept hospice care.

- **Special needs**. Many need a rabbi, priest, minister, or others to pray for patient. Clinician should consult family. Jewish practices have two purposes: to comfort the living and show respect for the dead. Moment of death and patient's last words are highly significant. Feelings of dying person at that moment give relatives a sense of what will happen in the year after death. Close relatives want to hear patient's last words.
- **Care of the body**. After a person dies, the eyes are closed, the body is laid on the floor and covered, and candles are lit next to it. Depending on religion, family members may want to wash body and dress it with special clothes. Jewish families never leave body alone until after burial, as a sign of respect. Some Jews believe that body should remain intact; thus, severed limbs should be returned to body if possible. Everything buried with body is that which will decompose with it, facilitating "from ashes to ashes, dust to dust." Embalming violates tradition because it impedes natural decomposition. Tradition encourages simplicity: burial in a plain wooden coffin with no metal hardware (because it will not decompose), no cut flowers (because they will wither in a few days, a painful symbol of family's loss), and a modest funeral service focusing on prayer, song, and ministry. In the Molokan tradition, the deceased and funeral attendees wear white. Depending on religion, most Russians (especially Molokans and Jews) do not believe in cremation.
- **Attitudes about organ donation**. Both Christians and Jews believe that the body is sacred, so organ donation uncommon. Jewish law requires that all parts be buried with body, unless a transplant will save someone's life.
- **Attitudes about autopsy**. Respect body and consider it sacred. Unless absolutely necessary, most Russians refuse autopsy.

SELECTED REFERENCES

Aroian, K. J. (1990). A model of psychological adaptation to migration and resettlement. *Nursing Research, 39*, 5–10.

Aroian, K. J., Norris, A. E., Patsdaughter, C. A., & Tran, T. V. (1998). Predicting psychological distress among former Soviet immigrants. *International Journal of Social Psychiatry, 44*, 284–294.

Brod, M., & Heutin-Roberts, S. (1992). Older Russian emigrès and medical care. *Western Journal of Medicine, 157*, 333–336.

Miner, J., Witte, D. J., & Nordstrom, D. L. (1994). Infant feeding practices in a Russian and a United States city: Patterns and comparisons. *Journal of Human Lactation, 10*, 95–97.

Salimbene, S. (2000). *What language does your patient hurt in? A practical guide to caring for patients from other cultures.* Rockford, IL: Inter-Face International. Retrieved May 28, 2004, from http://www.inter-faceinter.com

Werstman, V. (1977). *The Russians in America: A chronology & fact book.* New York: Oceana Publications.

Wheat, M. E., Brownstein, H., & Kvitash, V. (1983). Aspects of medical care of Soviet Jewish emigrès. *Western Journal of Medicine*, 139, 900–904.

AUTHORS

Luba Evanikoff del Puerto, RN, BSHS, BSN, is a clinical nurse at the University of California-San Francisco Medical Center in the Cardiology, Telemetry, and Cardiothoracic and Vascular Surgery Unit. She obtained her nursing degree from the University of San Francisco. Her parents emigrated from Russia in 1947 and 1949; they met, married, and raised Luba in the U.S.

Ella Sigal, RN, MS, NP, works in the Chemical Dependency Recovery Program in Santa Clara, CA. She received her education in Gorky, Russia. After emigrating with her family from Russia in 1995, she graduated from the University of California-San Francisco with an MS in nursing. Her family values their culture, language, and traditions, which she hopes her daughter will pass on.

ACKNOWLEDGMENT

Luba Evanikoff del Puerto is very grateful to her parents for encouraging and guiding her in preserving the Russian culture and language, which have enriched her life. In addition, she thanks her husband, who also supported her in preserving her cultural roots.

CHAPTER 32

SAMOANS

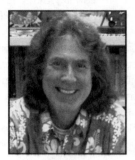

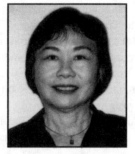

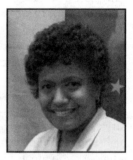

John F.
Mayer

Dianne N.
Ishida

Tusitala Feagaiga
Toomata-Mayer

CULTURAL/ETHNIC IDENTITY

- **Preferred term(s)**. Samoan. Politically, there are two Samoas: Samoa (formerly Western Samoa, *Samoa i Sisifo*), an independent nation with historically strong British ties, and American Samoa (*Amerika Samoa*), a U.S. territory. They share a common language and culture.
- **Census**. The 2000 U.S. Census reports 91,376 Samoans. They reside in every state, with the largest communities in California (37,498), Hawaii (16,166), Washington (8,049), and Utah (4,523). There are no data on the percentage of foreign-born Samoans for the U.S. as a whole, but census data for Hawaii indicate that about one-third were born in Samoa, one-third were born in American Samoa, and one-third are U.S.-born.
- **History of immigration**. In the 1920s, there was limited immigration to the U.S. Most of it was related to religious affiliation (e.g., the La'ie Samoan community in Hawaii, oriented to the Church of Latter Day Saints). In 1951, the U.S. Naval Base in American Samoa closed when administration of the territory was transferred to the U.S. Department of the Interior. About 2,000 American Samoan government workers and their dependents had immigrated to Hawaii and California by 1952. In the 1970s, a downturn in New Zealand's economy prompted many Western Samoans to immigrate to American Samoa and then to the U.S. In the 1980s, airport improvements in Western Samoa and increased airline services to both Samoas facilitated travel. Unlike previous waves, many later immigrants had less education and fewer marketable job skills. The immigration rate has remained steady since the 1980s.

SPIRITUAL/RELIGIOUS ORIENTATION

- **Primary religious/spiritual affiliations**. Since the introduction of Christianity in 1830, both Samoa and American Samoa have been virtually 100% Christian. The most common denominations are Congregational, Methodist, Catholic, Latter Day Saints, Seventh Day Adventist, and Assembly of God. Baha'i faith also has a following.
- **Usual religious/spiritual practices**. Christianity is the major foundation of Samoan social interactions. Therefore, some form of group prayer precedes and concludes all social events and family gatherings. Minister occupies highest rung of Samoan social ladder. Communal nature of Samoan society requires visits to hospitalized patient by church or religious-community subgroups (e.g., church choir, women's group, church youth group, or high-ranking officials in church community). Specific practices depend on religious denomination.
- **Use of spiritual healing/healers**. Traditional Samoan medicine is based on herbal lore, physical manipulation and massage, and spiritual harmony. Traditional medicine usually is confined to indigenous maladies and illnesses caused by social or spiritual imbalance. Traditional healers work in cooperation with Western health care providers and may come to the hospital to provide treatment.
- **Holidays**. Flag Day (*Aso o le Fu'a*) (April 17) commemorates the raising of the American flag in American Samoa in 1900; U.S. Samoan communities celebrate it. White Sunday (*Aso Sa Pa'epa'e/Lotu a Tamaiti*), on the second Sunday in October, is a religious and social holiday established by the early missionaries to honor children. Both Samoas and U.S. Samoan communities celebrate White Sunday. They also observe Christmas, New Year's, and Easter. American Samoa celebrates Thanksgiving and other U.S. cultural traditions, such as Halloween and Fourth of July.

COMMUNICATION
ORAL COMMUNICATION

- **Major languages and dialects**. Samoan is the official language of both Samoas. English is the language of instruction in schools after early grades. Government, business, and mass media use both Samoan and English, although Samoan preferred.
- **Greetings**. Prefer first names. Exposure to U.S. culture has created understanding and acceptance of use of last names. Many adults also have an honorific title—family chief (*matai*)—that greeters should use. Both men and women can serve as *matai*, but men normally assume the role of public representative in traditional family and cultural affairs. Handshake customary among both genders. Also shake hands when saying good-bye. Restrict kissing to instances of extreme emotion, although there is a greater tendency for Samoans living in Hawaii to greet members of opposite gender with a kiss (a

Hawaiian custom). Elderly may greet by touching noses, a practice that is becoming obsolete. Culturally appropriate to remain seated when shaking hands, although Samoans living in U.S. may stand in accordance with American custom.

- **Tone of voice**. Loud or disruptive levels of sound inappropriate. Restrict family conversation to levels within hearing of family members only. Because of high value Samoans place on politeness and formality, commands or requests are more acceptable when accompanied by a word or phrase (e.g., "please") indicating voluntary compliance. General rule: The less direct and sharp a statement is, the less chance there will be of giving personal offense.

- **Direct or indirect style of speech**. In Samoa, question-and-answer format of conversation among adults more appropriate for intimate conversation. In formal situations (e.g., conference involving clinician and patient's family), Samoans customarily expect to respond to a presentation by health care provider with a similar presentation by family spokesperson. Emphasize politeness and deference to authority figures, such as clergy, family chief (*matai*), elderly, and professionals; often express this by agreement or attempted compliance with requests or orders, whether or not they in fact agree or fully understand.

- **Use of interpreters**. Younger family members who are more proficient in English may serve as interpreters, as may nonfamily members, especially ministers of any denomination and professionals (e.g., social workers, police, and teachers). Male and female blood relatives in family avoid talking about sexual issues, a deep feature of Samoan culture that is fading among Samoans who live abroad.

- **Serious or terminal illness**. Clinician should convey information to family and patient as soon as possible. Samoan culture dictates that all family members be present for major life events, such as births, marriages, and deaths. Samoan families may extend from New Zealand to continental U.S. and beyond. Decisions concerning treatment, disposition of family resources, and postmortem issues require participation of all family members regardless of domicile. Clinician should pay special attention to linguistic considerations, such as availability of interpreter and the patient's and family's complete understanding of options.

WRITTEN COMMUNICATION

- **Literacy assessment**. Until recently, there was virtually universal and secular literacy instruction throughout both Samoas. Thus, most adults are literate in Samoan and speak English to some degree. Because of increasing levels of educational attainment, young adults have greater proficiency in English than their parents or grandparents do. Appropriate for clinician to question patient to determine his/her level of oral or written proficiency. Young Samoans often interpret for older family members. Because of New

Zealand English in Samoa vs. American English in American Samoa, immigrants from the former may not be familiar with American terminology or local idioms. Clinician should use simple medical terms.

- **Consents**. Caution: Minors may be under the care of adults who do not have legal guardianship. Although a parent or legal guardian must grant consent, the importance of other adult family members—especially a family leader, who is usually the family chief (*matai*)—cannot be overestimated. Traditionally, decisions require input from all adult family members. Clinician should consider using an interpreter early on and continuously to ensure complete understanding of medical condition and treatment options. Adult patient signs consent after family makes decision. Samoans resist written consent but not verbal consent.

NONVERBAL COMMUNICATION

- **Eye contact**. Generally avoid eye contact when speaking to a group. In personal conversation, eye contact may vary, depending on circumstances. Eye contact appropriate in casual or informal exchanges, except in situations where there is wide social disparity, as may be the case between patient and clinician.
- **Personal space**. Physical space important, especially among adults. Area in front of person is most important. Customary to say, "Excuse me" (*tulou*, pronounced two-LOW) and bow head slightly when walking in front of someone. Social distance among intimates is closer than American norm. With unfamiliar clinicians and in formal situations, social distance is much greater than American norm; persons may sit at opposite ends of table or room.
- **Use and meaning of silence**. Silence may indicate contemplation, lack of understanding, disapproval, disappointment, or anger. Smile may indicate happiness and contentment but could also be a defensive expression of unease or uncertainty. Samoan society stresses politeness and deference to authority figures (e.g., clergy, family chief [*matai*], elderly, and professionals), which often take the form of silence. Clinician should avoid rushing discussions or decisions as much as possible.
- **Gestures**. May informally raise eyebrows or move head upward to indicate affirmative response. Beckon someone by moving the hand, palm down, toward chest or by single nod of the head. Customary for inferiors to maintain a lower posture (e.g., seated) than superiors, although due to prolonged exposure to New Zealand and American customs, some Samoans may reverse this custom. Samoans understand most of the common, nonverbal gestures Americans use.
- **Openness in expressing emotions**. In normal situations, do not express emotions in public. In times of highly emotional experiences, express grief, anger, joy, and other emotions freely, intensely, and publicly; may direct such feelings to family members or health care providers.
- **Privacy**. During patient/family conference, clinician can elicit personal

patient information that does not threaten integrity of larger family unit. Patient's reluctance to continue discussion may indicate need for privacy. Information that might bring shame to family may not require family members' participation; thus, a confidante outside the family or a pastor may be able to help at this point, translating or rephrasing questions so they are more culturally appropriate, and explaining why the information is necessary. Highly respect Samoan ministers and, because of ministers' religious, educational, and social roles, accord them special privileges in such situations. Others who possibly can help include family chief (*matai*), elders, and recognized professionals in the community.

- **Touch**. Touching another person's arm or shoulder, or giving him/her a hug, is an acceptable sign of sincerity or intimacy. Touch is inappropriate in formal, public interactions. Samoans expect touching in clinical situations, but clinician should first explain why it is necessary.
- **Orientation to time**. Traditionally mark time by recognizing important personal or family occasions rather than referring to other time markers. For example, patient may set an important medical appointment but later give higher priority to a family event that takes place. Lack of transportation also may affect patient's ability to meet time commitments. Mainly present-oriented regarding health; little emphasis on past health conditions or events, or on maintaining health and preventing disease.

ACTIVITIES OF DAILY LIVING

- **Modesty**. Very modest in clinical situations. Prefer to wear own clothing. Women may be more concerned about exposing themselves below the waist (e.g., their thighs) than exposing breasts. Both men and women prefer health care provider of same gender; may have difficulty undressing for caregiver of opposite gender.
- **Skin care**. Daily showers very common; often shower twice. No preference for soap or special lotions. May apply Samoan coconut oil either as body lotion or as an ingredient in topical treatment, such as massage.
- **Hair care**. Frequent washing or shampooing common. No special lotions, soaps, or shampoos. Some women prefer not to wash their hair late at night or during menstruation.
- **Nail care**. Keep fingernails short. No special nail or toenail care. Pregnant women may not cut their nails.
- **Toileting**. No special rituals, but toileting is very private. Samoans may prefer to use bathroom with door closed rather than a bedside commode. May be offended when bedpan is offered or if they cannot use bathroom on their own. Wash hands after toileting.
- **Special clothing or amulets**. Men prefer a sarong or skirt (*lavalava*, pronounced lah-vah-LAH-vah) rather than hospital gown. Women also prefer to wear a *lavalava* over their clothing or hospital gown.

- **Self-care**. Perform activities of daily living if able, including ambulation and deep breathing after surgery. Otherwise, family member assists with overall care of patient. Samoans expect a family member to remain with patient throughout entire hospital stay.

FOOD PRACTICES

- **Usual meal pattern**. Traditionally, two main meals a day. Increasingly common for modern Samoans to consume three meals a day. Eat fairly large portions, which consist of starch (taro, bananas, rice, or breadfruit) and meat protein.
- **Special utensils**. May prefer to eat with fingers. Wash hands before and after meal.
- **Food beliefs and rituals**. May say prayer before every meal, especially dinner. Traditional custom requires adults to eat before older children do. In more-acculturated families, all family members may eat together, although adults might eat first when guests are present.
- **Usual diet**. Prefer hot prepared meals. Also prefer starch, such as taro, bananas, and breadfruit, but may substitute rice and potatoes. Eat these starches with beef, fish, pork, chicken, or canned meat. Sometimes combine two or three meats in one meal. May eat green salad but not frequently. Although they highly favor fish as a protein source, the modern Samoan diet leans heavily toward foods high in cholesterol and saturated fat. If there are no dietary restrictions, clinician can suggest that family bring in food prepared to patient's liking.
- **Fluids**. Prefer cool water or sweet drinks if available. Often consume tea or coffee with evening meals. Highly favor carbonated drinks.
- **Food taboos and prescriptions**. Pregnant and postpartum women may have food restrictions (see pregnancy care). Prefer warm soups and starches made with coconut cream. Generally give sick person fish soup or soup made with very basic ingredients, such as rice, onion, a few vegetables, and meats seasoned with salt and pepper or curry. Generally give sweet soup made with papaya or young coconut meat to children and postpartum women. Fish soup is the preferred meal for sick persons. OK to serve soup with or without coconut cream.
- **Hospitality**. There are formal rituals and daily practices for receiving guests in Samoan society. Visitors can expect a high degree of formality, especially during initial visits. Visitor should first approach eldest adult out of respect. A formal verbal welcome is required, especially if guest is unfamiliar. Host normally provides food and drink without asking; if host asks, acceptable for guest to refuse. Guest should at least sample food or drink, but he/she is not expected to finish all food served. Host expects a word of thanks (*fa'afetai lava*, pronounced fah-ah-fay-tie LAH-vah).

SYMPTOM MANAGEMENT

Numerical quantification difficult; prefer words.

- **Pain** (*tiga*, pronounced tee-NGAH). May be stoic and not complain. Often accept pain as God's will. Degree and type of pain may be difficult for some patients to verbalize or quantify. May use numerical pain scales. Pictures showing facial expressions of degrees of pain also helpful. Health care provider may need to offer pain medications. Narcotic pain medications of any kind are acceptable, but Samoans may be sensitive to medication effects. Prefer oral medication. Clinician should consider beginning with a lower dose and explain side effects. Traditionally, Samoans often use massage to treat pain.

- **Dyspnea** (*faigata le manava*, pronounced faye-gah-TAH leh mah-NAH-vah, means trouble with breathing; *sela*, pronounced SAY-lah, means shortness of breath). OK to administer oxygen after explaining procedure. Shortness of breath may cause anxiety. If clinician knows primary cause of dyspnea, he/she should explain it and treatment to patient. Prayer, massage, or presence of intimates may help reduce patient's anxiety.

- **Nausea/vomiting** (*fa'afaufau*, pronounced fah-ah-fow-FOW/*fa'asuati*, pronounced fah-ah-soo-AH-tee). During periods of nausea, patient may want to rest. Attribute nausea in pregnancy to food reaction. Traditional herbal medicine (both internal and external) addresses nausea. May attempt to clean up vomitus, but embarrassment is not a major concern.

- **Constipation/diarrhea** (*manava mamau*, pronounced mah-nah-vah mah-MAH-oo/*manava tata*, pronounced mah-nah-vah tah-TAAHH). Sometimes attribute constipation/diarrhea to food that one should not have eaten. Categorize gastrointestinal ailments based on those that cause constipation, diarrhea, or pain. Patients embarrassed to talk about feces. Nutritional controls acceptable. Traditionally treat diarrhea with guava juice/fruit. Use enemas as a last resort.

- **Fatigue** (*vaivai*, pronounced vie-VIE, means weak). Believe that overexertion, heat, or illness causes fatigue. May not attribute fatigue to underlying illness. Because Samoans traditionally tend to be early risers, afternoon nap is common.

- **Depression** (*fa'anoanoa*, pronounced fah-ah-no-ah-NO-ah, means sadness). Commonly associate depression with sadness or withdrawal from family participation. No stigma attached. If someone (especially a relative) is depressed, it is a signal for greater interpersonal interaction within the family to demonstrate that family values and loves the depressed member, who becomes the focus of physical, emotional, and psychological interaction. Samoans may tend to somaticize general complaints.

- **Self-care symptom management**. Samoans tend to avoid self-treatment even if a condition is minor. Other family members become involved. Family may consult traditional healer, who assesses the sick person and treats him/her with Samoan medicine. Family as a whole provides continuous care; in cases of chronic illness, this includes diabetes blood testing and injections.

BIRTH RITUALS/CARE OF THE NEW MOTHER AND BABY

- **Pregnancy care**. Consider pregnancy (*ma'itaga* or *ma'ito*) an illness. Prenatal care may vary tremendously and may involve early traditional practices or Western-oriented care. Samoans traditionally exclude men from participating, while U.S.-born men are more likely to become involved, including taking childbirth preparation classes. Many Samoans may not be familiar with the availability and scope of biomedical prenatal care. Pregnant women should not eat certain foods, such as octopus or raw fish, and should not eat alone or be left unattended, especially at night. Pregnancy prohibitions extend to garlands, jewelry, and garments fastened under the arms.
- **Preferences for children**. Prefer large families; average number of children in U.S. is 4–5. Consider children to be a gift from God and a sign that the marriage is blessed. Value boys and girls equally. Because descent lines are patrilineal, parents may be disappointed if there are no male children.
- **Labor practices**. Traditionally, midwife participates in birth process. Treatment includes gentle massage of abdomen and lower back to relieve discomfort and determine position of fetus. Readily accept giving birth in hospital. Birth is a family affair; adult female members may be present and assist. May use both Western and traditional treatments; latter include massage and herbal teas and ointments.
- **Role of the laboring woman during birth**. May choose comfortable position during labor. May be active (if able) or passive. May be stoic and refrain from loudly expressing pain. Traditionally, prefers not to take medication; if U.S.-born, more likely to request it.
- **Role of the father and other family members during birth**. Adult female relatives most important; they provide spiritual and emotional support as well as massage if permitted. Father may be present but traditionally not in birthing area. U.S.-born males may take a more active role.
- **Vaginal vs. cesarean section**. Prefer vaginal delivery.
- **Breastfeeding**. Expect mother to breastfeed if she can. Mothers working outside the home may resort to a combination of bottle- and breastfeeding. Sexual abstinence customary while breastfeeding. In the 1970s, popularity of baby formula prompted women in Samoa to switch to bottle-feeding; that attitude may persist today among some. There may be dietary restrictions for breastfeeding women, such as not eating certain kinds of seafood (e.g., octopus and raw fish).
- **Birth recuperation**. Traditionally after birth, midwife may give new mother an abdominal massage, focusing on uterus. Abdominal area also may be bound. Give new mother coconut porridge (*vaisalo*). Convalescent period may vary from two weeks to more than a month. Expect new mother to care

only for her baby, although family assists. At night, postpartum women do not carry baby about or stand in front of windows for fear of spiritual sicknesses that are believed to be prevalent at that time.

- **Baby care**. Generally expect mother to provide primary care for infant with help from other experienced female relatives, including grandparents, aunts, and older children. Father traditionally has minor role in baby care. Parents indulge very young children.
- **Problems with baby**. Clinician should discuss—with adult female relatives, especially baby's grandmother—any unusual problems. Family assists during convalescence of mother and baby, particularly with first-born child.
- **Male and female circumcision**. Generally, male circumcision is in accordance with usual Christian expectations. No female circumcision.

DEVELOPMENTAL AND SEXUAL ISSUES

- **Celebration of menarche or becoming a man**. Do not publicly celebrate menarche (*ma'i masina*). No modern male rite of passage.
- **Attitudes about birth control**. Large families culturally appropriate. Samoans are aware of birth control methods and understand the need to space children but may not follow through on contraception because of daily routine or sexual needs of mates. May use breastfeeding as a form of birth control. Those from American Samoa and those born in U.S. often are more aware of birth control methods and procedures. Traditionally, birth control among singles in Samoa is uncommon due to inaccessibility of methods and fear of family finding out. But birth control is becoming more common, especially among U.S.-born Samoans.
- **Attitudes about sexually transmitted infection (STI) control, including condoms**. Do not openly discuss sex and sexuality concerns, especially not with opposite gender. That may preclude awareness of, and knowledge about, STIs and stifle preventive measures. STIs highly stigmatized in traditional society; such stigma often hinders treatment. U.S.-born Samoans more likely to seek treatment for STIs because of patient privacy and confidentiality practices in U.S. Males do not like condoms (*pa'u fai*); often avoid using them.
- **Attitudes about abortion**. Do not discuss or publicly promote abortion (*fa'apa'u le pepe*). Individuals may consider a traditional or Western abortion as an option for keeping knowledge of an unwanted pregnancy from others. Abortions often performed in secret. If family already knows about an unwanted pregnancy, likelihood of abortion decreases. Abortion not congruent with Samoan Christian beliefs.
- **Attitudes about unwed sexual experimentation**. Samoans view it as a natural result of male-female interaction; therefore, gender separation in family and public activities starts from puberty. Family closely guards female virtue; view female experimentation negatively. More tolerant of male exper-

imentation. High teen-pregnancy rate among Samoans indicates active experimentation despite cultural and religious prohibitions.

- **Sexual orientation**. Tolerate sexual orientations other than heterosexual ones, which are the norm. However, public displays of sexuality, including kissing and holding hands, are inappropriate regardless of orientation. Homosexuality not congruent with Samoan Christian beliefs.
- **Gender identity**. Traditional society tolerant of transgender family members. Reluctant to discuss gender identity publicly. No overt social pressure to change behavior of feminine boys or masculine girls.
- **Attitudes about menopause**. Consider it a natural stage in female development. Do not generally discuss menopause. Look forward to menopause as a cessation of menstrual cycle. No traditional treatment for symptoms.

FAMILY RELATIONSHIPS

- **Composition/structure**. Large extended family (*aiga*, pronounced ah-ING-ah) common. May include those related by blood, marriage, or adoption, and those who serve family. Samoan family composition is fluid due to high mobility of family members. Authority vested in elders, adults, and traditional family chief (*matai*). Strong commitment to mutual aid and support within family and church.
- **Decision-making**. Involves all adults in family or extended family (*aiga*); therefore, families may want to include more than immediate family members in conferences. Before making a decision, they may need to consult other family members who are not present. Family chief (*matai*) and elders make decisions by consensus after seeking opinions of all adult family members. Value minister's opinion, but minister may not play active role in decision-making.
- **Spokesperson**. Customary for one spokesperson to represent family and voice its decisions. In interactions with non-Samoans, usually the family chief (*matai*), an elder, or, if English is a problem, the most educated family member serves as spokesperson. Man or woman may fill this role.
- **Gender issues**. Family members have gender-specific roles that often are adaptable, depending on circumstances. Men perform heavier outdoor activities, such as fishing, building, and preparing the earth oven, and take part in village council. Women and children perform tasks necessary to maintain household, such as caring for children and weaving. Both genders take part in agricultural activities and some food preparation.
- **Changing roles among generations in U.S.** Because Samoans travel frequently between family branches in Samoa and abroad, most families maintain a high degree of traditional social values and cultural practices. However, the English language and American cultural values and practices are dominant in the lives of an increasing percentage of U.S.-born Samoans, often enabling them to serve as interpreters. Younger generations participate in family affairs but have very limited understanding of their native culture or

language. Nevertheless, there has been little change in gender roles, even among U.S.-born Samoans.

- **Caring roles**. Women are primary bedside caregivers, but children may assist. Women and men who are blood relatives have a gender-avoidance taboo that may affect selection of caregiver. For example, a male may feel uneasy if his female relative is tended by a male caregiver.
- **Expectations of and for children**. Samoans value children, including those born out of wedlock. They expect children to be obedient, serve older family members, and avoid direct confrontation with authority figures. Parents indulge very young children. Older children are generally responsible for care of younger siblings and are expected to be highly autonomous at an early age. Peers play major role in socialization. Samoans traditionally encourage females to marry after high school, and males to seek employment and help with family finances. Younger generations of Samoans are more likely to attend college or join U.S. military. Samoans may continue to live at home even after marriage.
- **Expectations of and for elders**. Traditionally revere elders as sources of wisdom and knowledge of the Samoan way (*fa'asamoa*, pronounced fah-ah-sah-MOH-ah). Elders remain active members of family; they often assist in child care and decision-making, and oversee family activities. Elderly live with adult children. Samoans in U.S. may institutionalize elderly as a last resort if they cannot provide home care.
- **Expectations of hospital visitors**. Generally welcome visitors. In hospital, family member may intercede with visitors on patient's behalf.

ILLNESS BELIEFS

- **Causes of/attitudes about physical illness**. Attribute illness to apparent causes (such as trauma), effects of internal/external ecosystem (such as parasites, "germs," diabetes, or climate), or supernatural causes (illness as a consequence of past misdeeds or misconduct). Also may view illness as a consequence of one's actions toward the living or the dead, or one's violation of social or religious principles. The need for openness, trust, and harmony in healing process may require group confessions of misdeeds. Generally, illness disrupts normal family life; for this reason, Samoans tend to put off treatment until advanced illness requires hospitalization. Health beliefs and practices have expanded to incorporate Western beliefs and practices. Samoans believe that illnesses may be of European origin (*ma'i palagi*) or Samoan origin (*ma'i Samoa*). Imbalances in physical, spiritual, and mental harmony require a holistic approach to healing. Treatment for illnesses may involve both Samoan and non-Samoan cures; do not perceive conflict between the two. Samoan cures include massage, prayer, and herbal medicine.
- **Causes of/attitudes about mental illness**. Causes include spirit possession; stress from interpersonal relationships, family obligations, and social

constraints; and pressure from peer groups. Also may attribute mental illness to guilt resulting from misdeeds. Society is tolerant of mentally ill persons. Traditional treatment combines herbal medicine, massage, and family support. Hospitalization or Western medication or therapy is rare, but Samoans may consider these as a last resort.

- **Causes of genetic defects**. Often view defects as punishment for husband's bad behavior during pregnancy, pregnant mother's or family member's deviant or unacceptable behavior toward others, or violation of dietary taboos.
- **Attitudes about disabilities**. Generally accepting of disabled family member and willing to care for him/her at home, unless care becomes unmanageable. Generally accept disabilities as part of life. No stigma attached to disability, although joking about it is not uncommon. Family members may help disabled person, but Samoan culture encourages him/her to be independent and freely participate in daily activities.
- **Sick role**. Family members care for the sick and treat them well. Sick person may actively participate in his/her care and normal family activities.
- **Home and folk remedies**. Folk remedies such as massage (*fofo*) and herbs are prevalent, especially for illnesses attributed to Samoan causes. For example, Samoans may attribute general malaise to displaced life force (*to'ala*), which a healer, using therapeutic massage, can return to its proper location in the abdomen. Patients may not readily admit to using folk remedies. Traditional healers recognized by the family prescribe folk remedies, including massage with cordyline (*ti*) leaves for fever or body aches, and guava juice for diarrhea.
- **Medications**. Generally accept traditional herbal and Western medications. Often discontinue Western medications after symptoms abate because patient can participate in social and family activities again, and because dwelling any longer on illness might distract patient from such participation. More likely to continue taking traditional medication after symptoms abate because family is involved in administering it.
- **Acceptance of procedures**. Samoans accept surgery. May also accept blood transfusion or organ transplant if necessary for patient's survival. Do not commonly understand or practice organ donation.
- **Care-seeking**. Except in cases of severe trauma or diseases clearly of Western origin, Samoans usually consult traditional healer before seeking care from Western clinicians. Vagueness of Samoan or Western illness classifications may result in overlapping treatment approaches. Clinician should be aware of family members' tendency to rely on Samoan medicine if prognosis is uncertain or if treatment with Western medicine has been ineffective. Samoans often use massage (*fofo*) to treat a variety of conditions or symptoms. May use Western and traditional medicine concurrently, viewing them as complementary.

HEALTH ISSUES

- **Concept of health**. To live, rest, and be free of sickness (*soifua maloloina*). Traditional holistic view of health includes body, mind, and spirit. One should be attuned not only to obvious physical ailments but also to relationships with others (especially family), the environment, and the spiritual world (especially recently deceased ancestors).
- **Health promotion and prevention**. View ill health as a problem when it begins interfering with one's participation in day-to-day family and social activities; do not view it as something that needs to be prevented. Preventive health is not a well-established concept in Samoa. Samoans do not closely associate diet and physical activity with health. If they have limited English language competency, there is limited access to health education resources and programs. Younger generations in Samoa and U.S. tend to be more aware of preventive health care and programs.
- **Screening**. Because Samoans have great respect for authority figures, they accept screening if an elder, pastor, or other authority figure suggests it. May perceive questions about sexually transmitted infection, sexual relations, menstrual cycle, feces, genitalia, or mental aberrations as shameful and private. Clinician must clearly explain why such questions are relevant. Samoans may be reluctant to accept invasive screening procedures (e.g., Pap smear or colonoscopy) unless the need for them is clearly explained.
- **Common health problems**. In U.S., cardiovascular disease, diabetes, and hypertension. Obesity is particularly prevalent as Samoans adopt Western diets and lifestyles. View large body size as a sign of good health, unless it interferes with functional mobility and meaningful contributions to family and social activities. Tobacco use very high among adults. In Samoan communities abroad, teen pregnancy also is a concern.

DEATH RITUALS

- **Beliefs and attitudes about death**. Integrate traditional cultural beliefs with Christian tenets. Believe that the spirit inherits the Christian afterlife while still maintaining a close connection with the living. Samoans bury deceased relatives beside family residence. Integrity of the body (especially the head) after death is important. Believe that the spirits of the deceased return to cause illness and misfortune among the living if they were mistreated or abused when ill or after death. Must follow elaborate and strictly mandated cultural rituals before and after death. These include preparation of the body, ceremonial visitations and speeches, ritual exchanges (of fine mats, money, and food), and Christian hymns and prayers.
- **Preparation**. Patient and family members prefer to be informed of prognosis early. Interpreter is crucial if there are any language barriers. Family spokesperson is main communicator between family and health care provider.
- **Home vs. hospital**. Family almost always prefers home care rather than hos-

pitalizing patient or placing him/her in hospice facility. Hospice services at home acceptable.

■ **Special needs**. Family members, ministers, and church members provide major support for patient during his/her final days.

■ **Care of the body**. Under normal conditions, family prefers to prepare body. Preparations include washing body, applying traditional Samoan coconut oil, dressing body, and anointing it with perfume. Cremation very rare.

■ **Attitudes about organ donation**. Traditionally, Samoans do not consider donating organs; any such suggestion could offend family. Believe that body should be buried intact, as integrity of remains is culturally important. Acculturation may alter such views.

■ **Attitudes about autopsy**. Family generally does not consider autopsy, unless physician suggests it for medical reasons. Clinician should consult family spokesperson if autopsy is necessary.

SELECTED REFERENCES

King, A. P. (1990). A Samoan perspective: Funeral practices, death, and dying. In J. K. Parry (Ed.), *Social work practice with the terminally ill: A transcultural perspective* (pp. 175–189). Springfield, IL: Charles C. Thomas.

Kinloch, P. (1985). *Talking health but doing sickness: Studies in Samoan health.* Wellington, New Zealand: Victoria University Press.

Macpherson, C., & Macpherson, L. (1990). *Samoan medical belief and practice.* Auckland, New Zealand: Auckland University Press.

Mayer, J. F. (1992). *Samoan language for health care providers.* Honolulu: University of Hawaii Second Language Teaching and Curriculum Center.

Mishra, S. I., Hubbell, F. A., & Luce-Aoelua, P. H. (1997). *Cancer control needs among native American Samoans: Results from American Samoa, Hawaii, and Los Angeles.* Los Angeles: University of California-Irvine Center for Health Policy and Research.

Whistler, A. W. (1996). *Samoan herbal medicine.* Honolulu: Isle Botanica.

AUTHORS

John F. Mayer, PhD, is an assistant professor of Samoan language and culture at the University of Hawaii at Manoa. He has directed the Samoan Language and Culture Program since 1976. Before joining the university, he worked in the Peace Corps for six years in Western Samoa.

Dianne N. Ishida, PhD, APRN, is an associate professor in the University of Hawaii School of Nursing at Manoa. She is a nurse anthropologist whose focus is learning and culture in Pacific/Asian cultures, particularly Samoa. She is a co-director of dissemination at the school's Center for Health Disparities Research.

Tusitala Feagaiga Toomata-Mayer, BSN, RN, is a registered nurse of Samoan background. She is coordinator of the Breast and Cervical Cancer Control Program at St. Francis Medical Center in Honolulu. She lectures frequently on health care issues facing Samoans and other Pacific Islanders. She also is an international flight attendant with United Airlines.

CHAPTER 33

VIETNAMESE

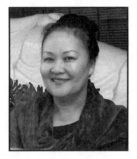

Thu T. Nowak

CULTURAL/ETHNIC IDENTITY

- **Preferred term(s)**. Refer to themselves as *người Viet Nam*. English speakers use the term Vietnamese. Many born in Vietnam are not ethnically Vietnamese but rather Chinese, Hmong, or minorities who have their own language, culture, and special needs.
- **Census**. The 2000 U.S. Census estimates more than 1.1 million residents of Vietnamese origin. The largest numbers are in California, Texas, and Washington, DC.
- **History of immigration**. At the end of the Vietnam War in 1975, the U.S. admitted many well-educated and professional refugees who supported the pro-Western government of South Vietnam. The next wave of refugees, whose 1978–79 exodus often was very dangerous, included those who were disenchanted with communism and their poor living standards. The third wave began in 1979 with the Orderly Departure Program, which provided safe, legal exit for those joining their family in the U.S. In 1987, a fourth wave began with the Amerasian Homecoming Act, which brought children of American servicemen and their Vietnamese mothers and close relatives to the U.S. It also provided for entry of former South Vietnamese military officers and other political detainees.

SPIRITUAL/RELIGIOUS ORIENTATION

- **Primary religious/spiritual affiliations**. In U.S., nearly 30% are Catholic and the rest Buddhist. Vietnamese are influenced by Confucianism, which stresses harmony through social order and worship of ancestors, and Taoism, which emphasizes allowing events to follow a natural course that one should not try to change.

- **Usual religious/spiritual practices**. Buddhists rarely visit temples or perform rituals but may pray silently or meditate while alone. Both Buddhists and Christians may maintain an altar at home for regular religious observances. In cases of severe illness, they may say prayers and make offerings at a temple.
- **Use of spiritual healing/healers**. A priest or monk commonly visits the seriously ill but should be called only at the patient's or family's request. Vietnamese may seek care from practitioners of traditional Oriental medicine or spiritual healers before seeking care from biomedical health care providers.
- **Holidays**. *Tet*, a three-day celebration corresponding to the Chinese Lunar New Year, takes place in late January or February. *Tet Trung Thu* celebrates the end of harvest in late August or September; families gather and there are parties, gifts, or excursions for children. Less popular are National Day (September 2), which celebrates independence from France in 1945, and Liberation Day (April 30), which celebrates the fall of South Vietnam in 1975.

COMMUNICATION
ORAL COMMUNICATION

- **Major languages and dialects**. Vietnamese is a single, polytonal language with mutually understood northern, central, and southern dialects. Each vowel can be spoken in five or six tones that may completely change the meaning of a word. Vietnamese is written in the Roman alphabet. Most Vietnamese who came to U.S. in 1975 or earlier either knew English or learned it soon after arriving, and many are studying it today. Most of those in subsequent immigration waves, who generally came from lower socioeconomic groups, did not know English; some still have not learned it. Nearly all American-born Vietnamese speak Vietnamese fluently, though many have some difficulty reading and writing it.
- **Greetings**. Unacquainted persons exchange formal names, a smile, and sometimes a gentle bow, especially if one of them is elderly. Men shake hands with other men but should not offer their hand to a woman, unless she extends hers first. Women usually do not shake hands with each other. Hugging and kissing rare in public, except among close relatives. Names consist of a family name, a middle name, and a given name, in that order. *Nguyen* (pronounced nwin) and *Tràn* are the family names of more than half of all Vietnamese. Terms of address are *Ong* ("Mr."), *Bà* (for older and/or married women), and *Co* (for young women).
- **Tone of voice**. Vietnamese language usually spoken softly by both genders, especially women. Monosyllabic structure of the language lends itself to rapidity; however, spoken pace varies according to the situation.
- **Direct or indirect style of speech**. Avoid expressions of disagreement that may irritate or offend another person. When asked a direct but delicate ques-

tion, many cannot easily answer with a blunt "no" because it may create disharmony. Unlikely to openly volunteer significant medical information. Women reluctant to discuss sex, childbearing, or contraception, demonstrated by giggling, shrugging, or averting their eyes. Traditionally stoic. Consider complaining a sign of weakness.

- **Use of interpreters**. Best not to use child interpreter. If qualified interpreter unavailable, an adult female relative fluent in English is best for asking about female health issues and filling out forms. Clinician should ensure that woman receives correct information on female health issues through female relative. Teenage girl may be more comfortable having an unrelated friend interpret. Men usually are comfortable with interpreters of either gender.
- **Serious or terminal illness**. Clinician should not tell patient without first consulting the head of the family. Many Vietnamese do not wish to add to a close relative's stress by informing him/her that he/she is dying.

WRITTEN COMMUNICATION

- **Literacy assessment**. Fewer than 10% of the elderly can read and write in English. About 50% of middle-age persons, especially those from socioeconomically deprived groups, read and write in English. Percentage is higher for early refugees and persons from higher socioeconomic levels. Nearly all young and U.S.-born Vietnamese are literate in English. To assess patient's literacy, best if clinician asks a relative or trusted friend. Otherwise, clinician should ask patient politely using helpful tone of voice, expression, and body language.
- **Consents**. Vietnamese word for "yes" does not necessarily express a positive answer or agreement; rather, it may show respect or a desire to avoid confrontation or to please. Some nod affirmatively to acknowledge that they heard, but in fact they may not understand or approve. Clinician should ask patient to verbalize what was explained to verify his/her understanding. Some hesitate to ask questions in a group; therefore, they should be permitted to ask individually. A common suspicion among Vietnamese is that divulging personal information could jeopardize their legal rights. Clinician should allow patient to discuss forms with spouse or trusted friend before signing.

NONVERBAL COMMUNICATION

- **Eye contact**. Should avoid direct eye contact with someone of unequal status or age, or someone of opposite gender. Direct eye contact could be offensive and may signal a challenge or intimacy. Vietnamese show respect (especially for nurses and doctors) by avoiding eye contact and slightly bowing head.
- **Personal space**. Vietnamese prefer more distance from nonfamily members than most Americans do. Large extended families live comfortably together in close quarters.
- **Use and meaning of silence**. Convey negative emotions and expressions, even pain, by silence or a reluctant smile. Use silence instead of verbal dis-

agreement. Clinician should interpret silence as a need to develop a context in which the problem can be discussed. A smile may be an appropriate response to criticism or when age or status differences preclude saying "I'm sorry" or "thank you."

- **Gestures**. Tend to be relatively unexpressive physically. Beckoning someone with an upturned finger is a provocation; waving the hand is more appropriate. Consider the feet to be profane; placing them on desk is offensive. Show respect by bowing and using both hands when giving something to someone. Gentle touch may be appropriate in conversation between persons of same gender. Younger Vietnamese more likely to use gestures that are the American norm.
- **Openness in expressing emotions**. Except with family, unaccustomed to expressing personal feelings openly. In times of distress or loss, often complain of physical discomforts, such as headache, backache, or insomnia. Consider loud expressions of emotion to be a weakness that interferes with self-control and to be in bad taste.
- **Privacy**. Vietnamese, especially women, unlikely to readily volunteer significant medical information. Woman may smile and say she is fine even if she is in pain. Family members who accompany patient can provide information. Clinician should not launch immediately into personal issues without taking time to establish trust. Should also be cautious when asking about sexual matters or women's health care issues, using a quiet, unhurried manner and watching for behavioral cues. Once a woman opens up, she may voice elaborate explanations and tell lengthy stories to explain her illness.
- **Touch**. Traditional Asian male practitioners avoided touching the bodies of female patients, sometimes using a doll to demonstrate a problem. Because of modesty, male clinicians should avoid touching females except when absolutely necessary and then only in the presence of a female friend or relative. Accept touching or exposure of young girl's or woman's body only with great reluctance and embarrassment, especially during breast and gynecological exams and even if clinician is female. Vietnamese consider the head to be a sacred body part that should not be touched.
- **Orientation to time**. Generally have a more fluid concept of time than Westerners do. May be less concerned about precise schedules and planning ahead. Frequently late for appointments, although acculturated persons are aware of the importance of punctuality. Persistent reminders, in the context of an overall effort to improve communication and dissemination of information, help encourage screening and follow-up treatment.

ACTIVITIES OF DAILY LIVING

- **Modesty**. Both Catholics and Buddhists favor modest behavior, although traditional social standards probably have a more dominant influence. The term *nam nu tho tho bát than* refers to the need to restrict contact between genders, thereby preventing problems and maintaining harmony in the community. Traditionally, a young girl is expected to be modest in behavior and conservative in dress, and to make sure most of her body is covered. Contact with boys is greatly limited, although an annual village celebration (*cúng dình*) allows formal interaction between genders. Such traditions are changing in America; extent of change depends largely on parents' will. Clinician should conduct exams in a private room and provide hospital gown and robe.

- **Skin care**. Vietnamese commonly bathe or shower daily. Good personal hygiene very important, especially peri-care. Some women accustomed to using a solution of warm salt water for peri-care, especially postpartum; less-acculturated women may use an herb (turmeric).
- **Hair care**. Cutting and styling are by individual choice, though some young women wear their hair very long and straight. Wash hair daily, except after giving birth. Never leave hair wet at night, as it is believed to cause headache.
- **Nail care**. Keep nails clean. Many women favor long, well-manicured nails.
- **Toileting**. Preferences are similar to those in dominant culture, but some insist on using bathroom instead of bedpan or urinal. Women peri-wash, especially before bedtime, and some prefer soap and water after urination.
- **Special clothing or amulets**. In Vietnam, the standard girl's garment (*áo dài*) exposes only the head, hands, and feet, although most Vietnamese wear Western clothing. Women favor jewelry, some of which has religious significance (e.g., a Buddhist amulet or Christian cross).
- **Self-care**. In Vietnam, family provides care even in hospital. Patients prefer to handle personal hygiene themselves or, if unable, to be assisted by a family member of same gender.

FOOD PRACTICES

- **Usual meal pattern**. Typically a light breakfast, large lunch and dinner, and sometimes snacks.
- **Special utensils**. Chopsticks and sometimes spoons. Knives seldom necessary, as meat and vegetables usually are cut into small pieces before serving.
- **Food beliefs and rituals**. Traditionally, dietary balance is based on the opposing forces of "cold" (*am*) and "hot" (*duong*), which correspond to Chinese *yin* and *yang*. These terms are unrelated to temperature and only partly associated with seasoning. Rice, flour, potatoes, most fruits and vegetables, fish, duck, and plants that grow in water are cold. Most other meats, fish sauce, eggs, spices, peppers, onions, and sweets are hot. Tea and water are cold, coffee and ice are hot. Vietnamese prefer hot foods and beverages after surgery or childbirth to replace and strengthen the blood.
- **Usual diet**. White or polished rice provides up to 80% of daily calories. Vietnamese serve rice with a salty, marinated fish sauce (*nuóc mam*). Typical meal includes green vegetables and pork, chicken, or tofu cut into slivers. A favorite is *pho*, a soup containing rice noodles, thinly sliced beef or

chicken, and scallions. Dessert includes fruit. Diet is basically nutritious but may be deficient in iron and calcium, and excessively high in sodium. Vietnamese Americans tend to use lots of sugar, even in traditional dishes.

- **Fluids**. Traditionally serve hot tea with meals. Iced tea also common. Sick persons drink warm tea or water at room temperature; juices and cold drinks are restricted. Most adults and many children are lactose intolerant.

- **Food taboos and prescriptions**. Few foods prohibited, except among Buddhists who are strict vegetarians. Many Vietnamese avoid cold drinks, especially with ice. Shellfish restricted for 3–6 months after surgery. Among foods that sick persons consume are light rice gruel (*cháo*) mixed with sugar or sweetened, condensed milk, and a few pieces of salty pork cooked with fish sauce; usually avoid fresh fruit and vegetables, which are too "cold."

- **Hospitality**. Meals are a means of honoring visitors. May set a lavish table, serving guests first. Special treats may require many hours of preparation. Hosts traditionally give up their bedroom to older family members or other honored visitors, and children sleep on floor so parents or guests can use their beds.

SYMPTOM MANAGEMENT

- **Pain** (*dau*). Because Vietnamese are influenced by the Confucian code of ethics, they maintain self-control and do not complain. Fatalistic attitudes and the belief that pain is punishment may reduce their expression of pain. Endurance of pain indicates strong character. Vietnamese' limited use of pain medication is due to deep cultural restraint against showing weakness, and to fear of addiction and side effects. Once they establish a relationship with clinician, older patients may report pain and want relief. Prefer oral or IV medications. Some can use numerical pain scale; if not, clinician should assess pain intensity by inquiring about it.

- **Dyspnea** (*khó tho* means difficulty breathing). Family more likely than patient to report dyspnea. May understand numerical scale but using it might be difficult as patient becomes anxious and begins hyperventilating. Accept oxygen. Reassuring words are helpful.

- **Nausea/vomiting** (*mua* or *ói*). Patients may be embarrassed and hesitant to report. Some may try to clean up and dispose of vomitus. Before reporting nausea/vomiting, may try a home remedy, such as Tiger Balm®, an analgesic ointment applied beneath the nose. More acceptance of medications (including IV meds) after many episodes of vomiting. Relaxation exercises may help control nausea/vomiting, especially during pregnancy.

- **Constipation/diarrhea** (*bón/ia chay*). Embarrassing. Patient unlikely to report constipation/diarrhea until it becomes serious or practitioner asks about it. Accept dietary measures to correct alteration in bowel function. Home remedies include increased consumption of fluids or green, leafy vegetables. Use enema for constipation only as a last resort.

- **Fatigue** (*met*). Generally do not report fatigue or take medication for it.

Respond to questions and may understand numerical scale. Consider sleep a part of healing process.

- **Depression** (*buon ba*). Refugees have high rates of depression, generalized anxiety disorders, and post-traumatic stress associated with military combat, political imprisonment, family separation, deaths of relatives and friends, harrowing escapes, and brutal attacks by pirates at sea. Few understand clinical depression and mental problems, which they consider shameful and seldom report. Social support from an established ethnic community and an intact marriage moderate the risk of depression. Family members or friends may try to cheer up patient by telling funny stories. Seek help from mental health professionals only when problems become very acute or obvious.
- **Self-care symptom management**. Many immigrants accustomed to depending on family and meeting health needs through traditional means. Family may try various home remedies, such as bed rest and medicinal herbs, or seek spiritual consultation. May let a condition become serious before requesting professional aid. Once they consult a Western clinician, Vietnamese usually are quite cooperative and respectful. View hospitalization as a last resort, when all else has failed.

BIRTH RITUALS/CARE OF THE NEW MOTHER AND BABY

- **Pregnancy care**. Traditionally few restrictions until late in pregnancy. Do not seek professional advice unless a severe problem develops, but this has changed recently with better education and clinic availability. Women believe that encounters with certain people and animals may adversely affect fetus. Conversely, a pregnant woman may frequently look at pictures of happy families, healthy children, or religious figures to ensure a successful birth. Vietnamese respect and assist pregnant women, but such women are considered bad luck at weddings, funerals, and New Year's celebrations. Home-based prenatal care includes ritual praying, commonly at a home altar. Prescribe foods in accordance with "cold" (*am*) and "hot" (*duong*) balance and those classified as "tonic" and "wind." During first trimester, women in a weak, cold, and antitonic state should eat hot foods, such as soup with chili peppers, salty meat and fish, and wine steeped with herbs. To provide energy to the fetus, pregnant woman also should follow a basic diet of tonic foods, such as steamed rice and pork. Women who are in a neutral state during second trimester continue tonic diet and add cold foods. Women in third trimester eat cold foods and avoid hot and tonic foods, which are believed to increase fetal weight and make birthing difficult. They avoid wind foods, including leafy vegetables, beef, mutton, and glutinous rice, throughout pregnancy. In practice, most women use this regimen as a general guide.
- **Preferences for children**. If a woman has only daughters, she may consider herself a failure and others view the family as less meritorious. Father is unlikely to totally abandon family, but he may seek another woman with

whom he can have sons. Vietnamese families in U.S. want at least one son. Traditional desire for large family is decreasing.

- **Labor practices**. Most women in U.S. deliver in hospital. Believe that birth is a critical time when the "hot"/"cold" balance is precarious. Mother sometimes prefers walking around during labor and squatting during birth. In Vietnam, pain medication is not usually prescribed, but in U.S. some women request it.

- **Role of the laboring woman during birth**. Tries to stay in control and may even smile continuously while suffering in silence. May moan or grunt; screaming unusual. Reassurance and comfort are helpful. Personal hygiene important (i.e., changing vaginal pads and keeping peri-anal area clean and dry).

- **Role of the father and other family members during birth**. Pregnant woman's mother and sisters are continuously present to provide comfort and advice. Traditionally keep father out and may chase him away if he persists, but he is expected to remain accessible. If couple attended childbirth preparation classes, appropriate for father to be in labor/birthing room.

- **Vaginal vs. cesarean section**. Prefer natural childbirth. Cesarean acceptable in a life-threatening situation.

- **Breastfeeding**. Traditional in Vietnam during the first year, although there is a trend toward formula or bottled milk in the mistaken belief that it is better for the child. Carefully educating women about the natural benefits of breastfeeding persuades them to return to it. Immigrant women who work might not realize that in some workplaces, they can breastfeed. After six months, new mother introduces infant to thin rice gruel, followed by thicker porridges.

- **Birth recuperation**. Because of loss of body heat during delivery, women avoid "cold" foods and cold or iced beverages, and consume more "hot" foods to replace and strengthen their blood. They eat most raw vegetables, fruits, and sour items in lesser amounts. Because water is "cold," traditionally do not fully bathe, shower, or wash their hair for 1–3 months after delivery. Practitioner should not urge bathing but should make sure that hot (or at least room-temperature) fluids are provided at bedside. Also should ask new mother what she prefers in terms of traditional recuperation practices, which include sleeping on a bed raised above hot coals and applying a hot, salty towel to vaginal area. Acculturated women rarely adhere to the old traditions, although some use the hot, salty towel. Some women welcome the opportunity to shower or bathe and they avoid other traditional practices, but many are reluctant to do so. Postpartum women avoid drafts and strenuous activity, wear warm clothing, and stay in bed or indoors for about one month.

- **Baby care**. Although mother is primary care-giver, her aunts and grandmother take much responsibility and extended-family members commonly are available. Mother is typically inactive and depends on other women for the first few months. Males traditionally do not get involved in baby care, but as both spouses increasingly work outside the home, fathers are starting to participate in basic care of young children.

- **Problems with baby**. Best to consult the father or other family support person. That person then decides who will tell new mother. Best to have physician present when mother hears the news.
- **Male and female circumcision**. Traditionally, neither sex is circumcised. However, males may be circumcised if clinician recommends it.

DEVELOPMENTAL AND SEXUAL ISSUES

- **Celebration of menarche or becoming a man**. No traditional rituals. Menstruation is a private matter; it may begin at age 13–14.
- **Attitudes about birth control**. Traditionally dislike contraception. Parents generally oppose it and young persons conceal their use of it. Buddhists accept contraception, but Catholicism officially opposes all unnatural forms of birth control. It is becoming acceptable among Vietnamese Americans, who commonly use oral contraceptives and intrauterine devices. Some women reluctant to use oral contraceptives because of fear of cancer. Men may not want their wives to use intrauterine device, though women often do so surreptitiously.
- **Attitudes about sexually transmitted infection (STI) control, including condoms**. Traditional restraints and dominance of family relationships tend to minimize concern about STIs among married persons. Young Asians are less sexually active than those in most other groups are; also at lower risk of HIV/AIDS. Vietnamese may have insufficient understanding of potential dangers. Males reluctant to use condoms because of allegedly reduced sensation. There is a tragically high rate of cervical cancer among Vietnamese women.
- **Attitudes about abortion**. Traditionally abhor abortion. Catholicism and Buddhism strongly oppose it because of the belief that the soul enters a being at time of conception. Teen abortions are performed to protect family reputation, more often in higher social classes; finances, religious proscriptions, and feelings of guilt constrain lower-class women. In U.S., abortion is becoming a more acceptable form of birth control.
- **Attitudes about unwed sexual experimentation**. Traditionally opposed to teenage dating, any display of sexuality, and contraception. Loathe pregnancy in unmarried teenagers. Strongly pressure young women to marry formally by age 21, fearing they might lose their virginity and thus be unable to enter a good marriage. Young men have fewer constraints. In U.S., it has become normal, if not fully acceptable, for teenage girls to date and to wear clothing that exposes much of the body.
- **Sexual orientation**. In Vietnam, knowledge and understanding of homosexuality are minimal. Among Vietnamese Americans, homosexuality is substantially less overt than it is among other groups. Gays and lesbians like-

ly hide their orientation for fear of being stigmatized by family and ethnic community.

- **Gender identity**. Families would deny or try to conceal matters such as masculine girls, feminine boys, or persons with ambiguous gender or persons who feel they were born with the wrong gender.
- **Attitudes about menopause**. Vietnamese term for menopause is *tát kinh*, which specifically means completion of a woman's job. Women favor a relatively early onset; late onset indicates bad karma reflecting misdeeds in an earlier life. Hot flashes, emotional changes, and becoming easily angered are common. Many try herbal teas and other traditional remedies. Some women terminate sexual relations at menopause because of cultural and religious influences rather than physical inclination. Many welcome menopause with relief; viewed as "too old," they no longer must be sexually active. Husband may seek another sexual partner. Women in U.S. more likely to want to extend their sex lives, sometimes with hormone replacement therapy or various stimuli.

FAMILY RELATIONSHIPS

- **Composition/structure**. Traditional family protects and guides the individual for life. Extended family is customarily large and patriarchal; it includes minor children, married sons, daughters-in-law, unmarried grown daughters, and grandchildren living under the same roof. A son's obligations to his parents may be more important than obligations to his wife, children, or siblings. Vietnamese define self more along the lines of family roles and responsibilities and less along the lines of the individual. Families in U.S. tend to be more nuclear, with more spousal interaction and interdependence, more egalitarian spousal relations, and shared decision-making.
- **Decision-making**. Male traditionally makes decisions. However, many women have used education to attain equal rights and a major role in controlling family decisions. Wives who do not earn a wage are more subordinate in decision-making. To maintain harmony, women sometimes defer to husband's final decisions. Traditionally consult elders regarding important decisions.
- **Spokesperson**. Usually the father/husband, but eldest son may fill that role if he is more proficient in English and more familiar with the context.
- **Gender issues**. Traditionally, women live with husband's family but retain their own identity. Husband is breadwinner and deals with matters outside the home, while wife is responsible for household. Although her role expands with age, wife is expected to be dutiful toward her husband and his parents. Vietnamese women often make family health-care decisions.
- **Changing roles among generations in U.S.** Vietnamese Americans in all subgroups experience some degree of role reversal in family. Father may no longer be the undisputed head of the household, which undermines parental authority. Women and children acculturate more quickly than men do. Wife and teenager/adult child may become wage earners because jobs traditionally

held by women, such as hotel maid, seamstress, and food service worker, are more readily available than male-oriented, unskilled jobs are. Children, who learn English and American customs more rapidly than their parents do, may become interpreters and family spokespersons. Older persons, accustomed to respect and esteem in Vietnam, may feel increasingly alienated and alone as younger generations adopt new values and ignore the counsel of elders.

- **Caring roles**. Family is primarily responsible for health care. Women attend to needs of sick persons, regardless of gender.
- **Expectations of and for children**. Value children because they carry on the family lineage. Expect children to avoid behavior that might dishonor family. Children are obliged to do everything possible to please their living parents and to worship parents' memory after death. Eldest son usually responsible for rituals honoring the departed. For boys, emphasis is on success in education and career. For girls, traditional emphasis is on avoiding pre-marital sex and pregnancy, and learning to serve family. These gender distinctions are blurring with acculturation, but a good education always has been important; parents pressure children of both genders to achieve it.
- **Expectations of and for elders**. Highly respect elderly. The expression *kính lao dác tho* means that the more one respects the elderly, the greater one's chances of reaching old age. Older family members transmit guidelines regarding social behavior, prepare younger persons for handling stressful life events, and provide support in coping with crises. Younger family members show deference by using a subdued tone of voice and standing when an older person enters room. Living in family unit helps elders adjust socially, but due to economic necessity and with younger women working, family may expect elders to prepare meals and care for grandchildren. Elders may experience conflict, homesickness, and despair about the future. Vietnamese expect younger adults to assume full responsibility for taking care of elders at home. Do not favor placing elders in nursing home.
- **Expectations of hospital visitors**. Expect family members to attend to needs of a hospitalized relative day and night. Some sleep at the bedside. Because of the constant flow of family and friends, private room is advisable.

ILLNESS BELIEFS

- **Causes of/attitudes about physical illness**. Many believe that poor health results from yin-yang (*am-duong*) imbalance. Some attribute illness to naturalistic causes, such as spoiled food or inclement weather. Belief in spiritual causes is common (e.g., *mác dàng duói* refers to a spirit taking over the body). Other supernatural causes include gods or demons, punishment for offending a deity, or violating a religious or moral code. Vietnamese do not reveal such beliefs to Western health care professionals.
- **Causes of/attitudes about mental illness**. Commonly attribute emotional disturbance to possession by malicious spirits, to bad luck in familial

inheritance, or, for Buddhists, to bad karma accumulated as a result of misdeeds in past lives. Many believe that mental illness results from offending a deity and must be concealed because it brings disgrace to family. Depression and anxiety, related to war trauma and separation, are common and sometimes severe. Vietnamese may enlist a shaman to help. Reluctantly seek psychotherapy and only with utmost discretion. Family usually cares for chronically mentally ill person, unless he/she becomes destructive and family seeks institutionalization.

- **Causes of genetic defects**. Punishment for wrong behavior in the present or past lives of family members. Affected child may be a source of shame, but family accepts him/her unconditionally and protectively provides care at home.
- **Attitudes about disabilities**. There are many physically disabled Vietnamese in Vietnam and U.S. Families and the government treat and care for them well, resources permitting. In contrast, family and society may stigmatize mentally disabled persons, who can jeopardize relatives' ability to find marriage partners.
- **Sick role**. Patient assumes passive role. Family members solicitously care for him/her.
- **Home and folk remedies**. Common treatments in Vietnam—and, to some extent, in U.S—include "rubbing out the wind" (*cao gió*) for cold, sore throat, influenza, or sinusitis. This involves spreading an ointment or hot balm oil across back, chest, or shoulders and rubbing with edge of a silver coin, which results in dark, striped bruises that allow offending wind to escape. Skin pinching (*be bao*) treats headache or sore throat. Repeatedly squeeze skin of affected area between thumbs and forefingers to produce bruises. Cupping (*giác*), for stress, headache, and joint and muscle pain, involves placing a small heated cup upside down on the skin, which creates a vacuum upon cooling to draw unwanted "hot" energy into the cup. *Xong* is a vaporized herbal preparation for relieving motion sickness or cold-related problems. Moxibustion (heated, pulverized wormwood or incense placed on skin at certain meridians) counters excess cold conditions. Acupuncture, acupressure, and acumassage relieve symptomatic stress and pain. Vietnamese consume herbal teas, soups, and other concoctions as "cold" measures to treat "hot" illnesses.
- **Medications**. Commonly share prescribed medications and combine them with traditional treatments without telling health care provider. Immigrants tend to stop medication when immediate symptoms are alleviated. Clinician should check patient's medication regimen repeatedly, obtain trusted relatives' observations, repeat instructions, and educate patient to ensure compliance.
- **Acceptance of procedures**. Invasive procedures may be frightening, the prospect of surgery terrifying. Believe that souls attached to different parts of the body can leave, causing illness or death. Fear loss of blood from any route. Patients may refuse to have blood drawn for laboratory tests; if blood is drawn, may complain of feeling weak for months, believing that tissue or

fluid removed cannot be replaced and that the body will suffer the loss in this life and the next. If a relative needs blood, family member may be willing to donate, but clinician must carefully explain the procedure and its necessity.

- **Care-seeking**. Typically treat illness with self-care, self-medication, and herbal medicines. Try traditional and natural remedies before consulting bio-medical practitioners.

HEALTH ISSUES

- **Concept of health**. Traditionally believe that good health is harmony and balance of the two basic, opposing forces: *am* (cold, dark, female, empty) and *duong* (hot, light, male, full). An excess of either force may lead to discomfort or illness. This holistic concept encompasses physical, spiritual, emotional, and social factors.

- **Health promotion and prevention**. One promotes health through *am-duong* balance by properly combining foods, medications, rest, cleanliness, and warmth or air. In the past, the typical Vietnamese was highly active and rarely overweight. Many Vietnamese Americans now are fully aware of the benefits of modern medicine and of promoting health through regular exams, exercise, and proper diet. Most are familiar with immunizations and diagnostic tests. Economically deprived persons and recent arrivals usually are too concerned with their immediate needs to worry about long-term prevention. They may require very basic instruction on matters such as careful hand washing to avoid communicable disease.

- **Screening**. Although many Vietnamese distrust Western methods, they generally respect professional authority and increasingly understand and accept screening if it is carefully explained. Follow-up and compliance are major problems. Tuberculosis screening is critical for Vietnamese; especially important for clinician to explain that the screening itself is not diagnostic but merely indicates a need for further testing. Most women with abnormal Pap smear results fail to return for follow-up care. To increase adherence to follow-up visits and care, clinician should carefully explain the consequence of inaction.

- **Common health problems**. Especially susceptible to tuberculosis, hepatitis B, diabetes, hypertension, lung cancer, and depression and other psychiatric conditions related to war trauma and social disruption. Lung cancer is associated with a high rate of smoking among men. Women have a very high rate of cervical cancer. Yeast infection is another persistent urogenital problem among women. Immigrants commonly return to Vietnam for visits, so they should be immunized against hepatitis A and B, typhoid, Japanese encephalitis, and rabies, and receive an antimalarial prescription.

DEATH RITUALS

- **Beliefs and attitudes about death**. Accept death as a normal part of life cycle. Beliefs are influenced by traditional stoicism, Buddhism's emphasis on cyclic continuity and reincarnation, and association of current activity with ancestral spirits. Give death more attention than they do marriage. There is considerable preparation for the time that one will become a venerated ancestor. Premature death (e.g., dying in childbirth) is traumatic for family. A dying person is encouraged to release life easily, without fear or anger. Vietnamese tend to avoid artificially prolonging life and suffering, though it may be difficult for relatives to consent to terminating active intervention.

- **Preparation**. If death is imminent, clinician should privately inform the head of the family, allowing time for notification of distant relatives and appropriate clergymen. If consent to remove life support is necessary, appropriate relative may wish to consult a religious adviser.

- **Home vs. hospital**. Most have an aversion to hospitals and prefer to die at home. Some believe that a person who dies outside the home becomes a wandering soul with no place to rest.

- **Special needs**. Families gather around body of recently deceased relative and sometimes express loud and uncontrolled emotion. Use various traditional prayers and rituals to help them accept the situation. Catholic families may place a religious medallion, rosary beads, or figure of a saint nearby. Family may pray with a priest in room. Buddhist families may light incense and have a monk lead a religious ritual. It is important to give families extra time with the deceased.

- **Care of the body**. Highly respect the body. Some families want to wash it themselves; others prefer to leave body as is or have funeral home handle it. Men traditionally wash and dress deceased males, and women deceased females. Dress body in good clothing, usually red if deceased was old. Do not use buttons or metal objects. Sometimes place rice in mouth of deceased. To prevent shifting of body in coffin, may fill coffin with tea leaves, if family can afford it, or crumpled paper, if family cannot. Although custom prescribes proper burial and maintenance of ancestral tombs, cremation is common among Buddhists. Traditional mourning practices include wearing white clothes for 14 days.

- **Attitudes about organ donation**. Because many Buddhists and some Catholics believe that the body must be kept intact even after death, they are averse to organ donation. Some who prefer cremation will donate body parts under certain circumstances.

- **Attitudes about autopsy**. Few Vietnamese families consent to autopsy unless they know and agree with the reasons for it.

SELECTED REFERENCES

Bong-Wright, J. (2000, July 16). Cervical cancer among Vietnamese-American women. Health awareness program for immigrants and National Asian Women's Health Organization. Annandale, VA.

Nowak, T. T. (1998). Vietnamese-Americans. In L. D. Purnell & B. J.

Paulanka (Eds.), *Transcultural health care: A culturally competent approach* (pp. 449–477). Philadelphia: F. A. Davis.

Shanahan, M., and Brayshaw, D. L. (1995). Are nurses aware of the differing health care needs of Vietnamese patients? *Journal of Advanced Nursing, 22,* 456–464.

Stauffer, R. (1995). Vietnamese Americans. In J. Giger & R. Davidhizar (Eds.), *Transcultural nursing: Assessment and intervention* (pp. 441–472). St. Louis, MO: Mosby.

AUTHOR

Thu T. Nowak, BSN, RN, is a public health nurse with the Fairfax County Health Department in Virginia. She was born and raised in South Vietnam and emigrated to the U.S. in 1970. Her work involves extensive contact with diverse ethnic groups, including the Vietnamese community in northern Virginia. She also teaches meditation therapy and relaxation exercises in the U.S. and Vietnam.

CHAPTER 34

WEST INDIANS/CARIBBEANS

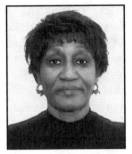

Patricia F. St. Hill

CULTURAL/ETHNIC IDENTITY

- **Preferred term(s)**. West Indian or Caribbean. Preferably Trinidadian, Jamaican, Barbadian, etc., depending on island of origin. Highly ethnically diverse population, consisting of individuals of East Indian, Chinese, Caucasian, and Black/African ancestry. While most see themselves as a single people, they are an ethnic melting pot. Focus of this chapter is on English speakers from countries that were former British colonies, including Anguilla, Antilles, Bahama Islands, Barbuda, Barbados, Caicos Islands, Cayman Islands, Dominica, Grenada, Jamaica, Montserrat, Nevis, Saint Kitts, Saint Lucia, Saint Vincent, Virgin Islands, Trinidad, Tobago, and Turk Islands.
- **Census**. Nearly 3.9 million Caribbeans live in U.S. In fiscal year 2002, an estimated 96,489 were admitted. Majority live in New York, Boston, and Miami.
- **History of immigration**. Documented immigration began in 1820 when 164 Caribbean nationals came to U.S. to help build railroads. Significant increases have occurred only since the 1970s, enabled by passage of the Immigration Act of 1965. It dispensed with the old quota system and permitted entry for relatives of U.S. citizens and permanent residents as well as those possessing skills needed in U.S.

SPIRITUAL/RELIGIOUS ORIENTATION

- **Primary religious/spiritual affiliations**. As a multiethnic/multicultural people, West Indians practice many different religions, depending on ancestral heritage, the former colonizer of their particular island, and the island's history. Trinidadians, for example, are predominantly Roman Catholics but include substantial numbers of Hindus, Anglicans, and Muslims. People from

Barbados are primarily Anglicans, as are Jamaicans. Jamaica also has sub-stantial numbers of Roman Catholics, Jews, Hindus, Muslims, Baha'is, and Rastafarians. The Baha'is, a worldwide religious community, believe in one God, one human race, and one evolving religion, based on new books of divine scripture revealed by Baha'u'llah, believed to be the modern messen-ger of God. Adherents follow spiritual teachings and apply logical and rea-sonable solutions to modern issues facing humanity. Rastafarians, who belong to a Jamaican messianic movement, worship the late Ethiopian Emperor Haile Selassie, who they believe is the only true God. Practices include using marijuana and chanting revivalist hymns.

- **Usual religious/spiritual practices**. Most families go to church on Sunday morning. In addition to Sunday morning mass, many Roman Catholics also go to confession on Saturday evening. At home, prayer is customary at bed-time and upon rising in the morning. Some families also have an altar in their home where they pray to their selected saints and burn candles. West Indians of other religions practice accordingly.

- **Use of spiritual healing/healers**. Not widely used; if they are, not openly acknowledged—done secretly to keep health care providers from knowing. Culturally, stigma and shame attached to such practices, which are equated with the supernatural, devil worship, or *obeah/voodoo*.

- **Holidays**. Most religious holidays appearing on the Christian calendar are observed in the Caribbean and by immigrants to the U.S. Include Christmas Day, Good Friday, and Easter (Gloria Saturday, Easter Sunday, and Easter Monday). The primary Muslim holiday is *Eid al-Fitr* that ends the Ramadan month of fasting, celebrated with food and prayers. The major Hindu holiday is *Divali* (in October), which is celebrated with decorations and lights in homes that signify the triumph of light over darkness. Secular holidays include New Year's Eve (or "Old Year's"); parties, family gatherings, and church attendance "bring in the New Year." Also observe New Year's Day. Boxing Day (December 26) often celebrated by horse racing and going to the race track. The date for celebrating Independence Day varies among islands, depending on date colonization ended. Carnival Monday and Tuesday (typi-cally in February, preceding Ash Wednesday and the beginning of the 40-day Lenten season) is equivalent to Mardi Gras; originated with African slaves brought to the islands to work on plantations. Celebrated on several islands and by émigrés residing in New York and Toronto.

COMMUNICATION
ORAL COMMUNICATION

- **Major languages and dialects**. Immigrants from the former British West Indies speak English mixed with a Creole dialect stemming from African ancestry. To the unaccustomed ear, the spoken word may not be readily rec-ognized as English. Clinician may need to ask patient to repeat or explain what he/she means by certain phrases and to speak more slowly. In Jamaica, it is called "Jamaican talk." Many, but not all, residents of the Dutch and French West Indies are also proficient in English.

- **Greetings**. Showing respect extremely important. Strangers and little-known acquaintances—especially if older—are typically greeted with a hand-shake and addressed by last name, unless greeter is told otherwise. Acceptable to greet relatives and close friends with an embrace or kiss on cheek.
- **Tone of voice**. A soft, nonassertive, and somewhat shy tone of voice is typical among females, especially when speaking with strangers and authority figures. Loud voice reflects hostility and an assertion of dominance or anger, and is likely to evoke an angry response.
- **Direct or indirect style of speech**. Direct and blunt speech is valued, but it may unintentionally hurt or offend persons unfamiliar with Caribbean culture. In contrast, when conversing with authority figures, recent arrivals and older persons may appear somewhat shy. May verbally agree with, and nod in response to, instructions and health information even though they might not fully understand. Asking questions of a health professional typically viewed as not having confidence in the provider or as questioning his/her ability.
- **Use of interpreters**. Unnecessary. Elderly may need an information interpreter, preferably a family member of same gender, to further explain or clarify information.
- **Serious or terminal illness**. Common and acceptable for patient to be told about a serious or terminal diagnosis/illness. Expect health care providers to tell them the truth. Emotional impact of bad news may be less taxing if a family member or trusted friend is present to provide support.

WRITTEN COMMUNICATION

- **Literacy assessment**. Literacy rate very high. A thick Caribbean accent and colloquial speech, especially when communicating with familiar persons, may lead health care providers to question patients' literacy. Quickest way to assess literacy is to provide written instructional materials and allow patients to ask questions after reading them.
- **Consents**. Written consents may be obtained directly from adult patients regardless of gender. Although patient may consult with close friends and/or family members, ultimate decision is his/hers. Patient may be reluctant to sign consent if explanation of the procedure, risks, and associated pain is insufficient.

NONVERBAL COMMUNICATION

- **Eye contact**. Maintain direct eye contact with peers or familiar persons. With authority figures, possible that recent arrivals and older persons will avoid sustained or direct eye contact in conversation and they likely will be shy.
- **Personal space**. Less well-defined than among Northern European Ameri-

cans. Accustomed to close proximity with strangers or in crowds (e.g., in outdoor markets or on public transportation). However, hugging and other close physical contact of a personal nature are typically reserved for family members and close friends.

- **Use and meaning of silence**. Often a sign of disapproval, anger, or disappointment.
- **Gestures**. Sucking one's teeth is a sign of disapproval or annoyance. Other gestures are same as those in dominant U.S. culture.
- **Openness in expressing emotions**. Generally not very expressive with authority figures, which is especially true among recent arrivals and seniors. Vocalize feelings with family members and acquaintances. May agree with authority figure out of respect, even if instructions are not clear.
- **Privacy**. "Not telling people your business" very important. Very reluctant to share personal information (especially regarding sex or abortion) with health care providers. Clinician should stress accuracy and importance of patient information. If a family member is present, patient may be even less inclined to provide such information.
- **Touch**. Typically not very physical. Touching, hugging, and kissing are greetings generally reserved for family members or very close friends. Casual acquaintances, including health care providers who attempt to comfort the patient with a gentle touch or hug, risk being perceived as disrespectful or "getting too familiar."
- **Orientation to time**. Consistent with the slower pace of Caribbean life, tend to be present-oriented and more casual about time and punctuality. Patients are likely to keep appointments but may not arrive on time.

ACTIVITIES OF DAILY LIVING

- **Modesty**. Extremely modest about private body parts. Embarrassed when they must expose their body to a clinician/stranger. If clinician is of the opposite gender or, worse, if clinician is younger than the patient, this "shame," as West Indians say, is even greater. Clinician should take extra measures to minimize exposure of patient's body and to create a safe, trusting environment.
- **Skin care**. Observe good personal hygiene. Shower daily. May shower again at night or do peri-care, referred to as "washing off." An ill patient, particularly one who has a fever or serious cold, refrains from showering out of fear that the body will be exposed to a "chill" or "draft."
- **Hair care**. Black females wash hair about once a week to preserve the natural oils in their naturally dry hair. Persons of Chinese, East Indian, or Spanish ancestry wash hair more frequently, given its different texture.
- **Nail care**. Preferred nail lengths vary. Maintaining clean nails is important.
- **Toileting**. Observe good hygiene. Very strict about hand washing after toileting and before preparing or touching foods. Do not object to urinal or bedpan but require privacy.

- **Special clothing or amulets**. May wear a cross on a chain around the neck or attach a pin of a saint to clothing. Clinician should leave such items in place if possible, as they afford the patient an extra sense of protection.
- **Self-care**. Typically do self-care, if able. If unable, a family member (usually the mother or grandmother) stays at the bedside to assist or provide personal care. If staff person provides care, patients prefer someone of same gender.

FOOD PRACTICES

- **Usual meal pattern**. Three meals a day with snacks between. In West Indies, lunch is biggest meal of the day.
- **Special utensils**. Some, especially those of East Indian descent, eat with their fingers rather than utensils.
- **Food beliefs and rituals**. Hot foods are served hot and cold foods cold. Consume primarily hot soups, hot tea, and broth when ill, when there are menstrual cramps, and after childbirth. Avoid ice and foods considered to be "cold," such as cucumbers, during these times.
- **Usual diet**. Rice a staple. Typical lunch is rice served with various stewed meats and gravies. On Sunday, lunch is a special and much larger meal typically consisting of more expensive foods not normally served during the week. Dinner is light—typically bread or homemade biscuits ("bakes") and a hot beverage (tea or chocolate). Minimal concerns about limiting fatty or high-cholesterol foods, or red meat. Food often cooked with coconut oil (extremely high in cholesterol) to enhance flavor. Because West Indian cooking is typically very spicy, patient may keep a bottle of hot sauce and/or other Caribbean spices at the bedside to add to hospital meals. Clinician should advise patient and visitors about dietary restrictions.
- **Fluids**. In their warm, dry climate, West Indians drink a significant amount of water and homemade fruit juices served with ice. However, they drink only warm liquids when ill.
- **Food taboos and prescriptions**. Muslims avoid pork. Food important in celebrating important occasions and for health promotion and protection. For example, West Indians drink stout mixed with milk and the white of a raw egg to restore energy or strength after an illness, or to "build up" if the person is considered to be anemic or weak. Soups and broths believed to be nutritious are routinely fed to the sick to rebuild strength. Balancing "hot"/ "cold" foods common. After birth and during menses, a woman's system is deemed "open" and susceptible to "lining cold" (a perceived disorder or cold affecting the uterus), so she avoids "cold" foods such as cucumbers. Also avoids acidic fruits at those times.
- **Hospitality**. Offer guests or those who drop in something to drink or eat; failing to do so is considered rude. Guest who refuses to eat may offend host. Certain special foods typify, and are prepared in accordance with, holidays or the season.

SYMPTOM MANAGEMENT

Patients are able to use numerical scales to describe symptom level if scale and ranking are explained to them.

- **Pain**. Signals onset of illness. Before seeking medical attention, most West Indians try home remedies, such as herbal or "bush" teas and ointments and balms (which may vary from one island to another) applied to pain site. Many fear that prescription pain medications can cause harm or addiction; may discontinue medications as soon as symptoms decrease. Given a choice, more likely to choose oral medications than intramuscular, IV, or rectal modalities. Greater likelihood of compliance with oral medications. May have reservations about and/or refuse acupuncture/acupressure, touch therapy, massage therapy, and the like for pain relief.

- **Dyspnea**. Viewed as a serious medical condition, generally associated with asthma. Seek conventional medical help. Accept oxygen and opioids to control dyspnea and, if asked, will express their breathing discomfort, using words to describe discomfort level.

- **Nausea/vomiting**. Generally associated with having eaten something disagreeable. Customary to drink hot tea and avoid solid foods for as long as the episode of nausea/vomiting lasts. Attempt to clean up vomitus quickly or seek help in getting it cleaned up. Accept medication for nausea/vomiting if offered. Hospitalized patients may believe that vomiting is a sign their condition is worsening.

- **Constipation/diarrhea**. Generally attribute change in bowel function to one or more particular foods. Some foods are thought to cause constipation. Do not recognize insufficient fluid intake or lack of exercise as a cause of constipation. If uncomfortable, patient will report constipation to clinician, although this topic is not generally discussed. Accept medication but may be reluctant to receive enema; will comply if its importance is explained. At home, treat constipation with a "purge or wash out" using harsh laxatives, such as Epsom salt or castor oil. Treat diarrhea with hot tea and avoid eating for a couple of hours to "rest the stomach."

- **Fatigue**. Means the person is "run down" or anemic and needs nourishing foods to "build him up." Report fatigue symptoms to clinician in very expressive terms. Willing to accept medications, preferably tonics.

- **Depression**. May hesitate to report because of stigma; depression viewed as a sign of personal weakness. If asked, patient likely to admit "feeling under the weather" and to describe signs and symptoms, but not very likely to use the word "depression." May resist therapy and medications. Unwilling to admit that a psychological disorder is causing symptoms.

- **Self-care symptom management**. Patient drinks appropriate herbal tea, based on symptoms. Also takes to bed or simply decreases household duties until condition improves. In cases of chronic illness, such as diabetes, patient performs self-care (e.g., monitors blood sugar) if properly instructed and if he/she understands what is required and why it is important.

BIRTH RITUALS/CARE OF THE NEW MOTHER AND BABY

- **Pregnancy care**. Regular prenatal care increasingly the norm on the larger Caribbean islands and in U.S. Women pay close attention to diet, avoiding foods they think are bad for baby and eating those that will nourish and fatten it. They do not believe it is important to monitor weight gain during pregnancy; the more weight gained, the healthier the mother and baby will be. Better-educated women and those of higher socioeconomic status may participate in childbirth preparation classes in their country of origin and U.S.

- **Preferences for children**. Prefer males, especially the first-born, although to a lesser extent than in the past. Those of East Indian descent still value male children most, but most couples prefer to have a family of boys and girls.

- **Labor practices**. In the Caribbean and U.S., midwives commonly attend births. Women are encouraged to keep walking during labor; many continue doing housework in the early stages. When contractions are closer together and pains intensify, a midwife is called and she begins monitoring and coaching the woman through delivery. Close female friend or relative is present to support her during labor.

- **Role of the laboring woman during birth**. Somewhat passive and follows clinician's instructions. To maintain dignity, "suffers in silence," stoically enduring labor pains and too ashamed to cry out as labor pains become more severe. This is especially true among women of higher socioeconomic status. Those of lower socioeconomic status tend to be more vocal/loud and even aggressive when staff attempts to instruct them on appropriate breathing. Accept medication (except epidural) for pain management.

- **Role of the father and other family members during birth**. Traditionally, baby's father not present nor involved in birth. May go out with friends, eagerly awaiting news of the birth, or remain at home to care for his other children. Men in U.S. likely to be more actively involved, coaching and supporting wife/partner during labor and birth.

- **Vaginal vs. cesarean section**. Prefer vaginal delivery but accept cesarean if medically necessary.

- **Breastfeeding**. Customary until child is about 9 months old. In the past, women used prolonged breastfeeding as a form of birth control. Today, working women often combine breastfeeding and bottle-feeding.

- **Birth recuperation**. New mothers stay in bed for about one week and are expected to refrain from heavy lifting and strenuous work. Observe same bathing and food restrictions as during menses, believing that the female system is "open" at these times and that exposure to cold showers and "cold" foods will cause "lining cold," a complication involving the uterus. Often a female relative, generally the woman's mother, stays with her to assist with housework and infant care.

- **Baby care**. Baby's mother is primary caregiver typically. Her mother and aunts may help with babysitting. Paternal relatives involved to a lesser degree.

- **Problems with baby**. Best to inform child's father or grandparents before telling the mother. It allows time to prepare her for bad news and for others to be there to provide support.
- **Male and female circumcision**. Male circumcision not customary, but if asked, most parents agree to have it done before discharge. Female circumcision not practiced.

DEVELOPMENTAL AND SEXUAL ISSUES

- **Celebration of menarche or becoming a man**. No formal recognition of puberty or transition to adulthood for either gender. Onset of menses is a private issue shrouded in secrecy and often embarrassing to the girl.
- **Attitudes about birth control**. Acceptance and use of birth control common among both married and unmarried women. Men much more resistant to condom use, partly due to cultural beliefs, the need to demonstrate one's manhood/fertility, and concerns about less sexual pleasure. Catholics may resist birth control. Family and community may frown upon teenage girls using it because such girls are considered too young to be sexually active.
- **Attitudes about sexually transmitted infection (STI) control, including condoms**. Reluctant to disclose private information about sexual activity or history of STIs. Men resist using condoms, believing they reduce sexual sensation. Some equate such use with prostitution. Expectations that a man will wear a condom even though he feels "clean" can result in hurt feelings or conflict. The high incidence of HIV/AIDS in Caribbean region—an estimated 500,000 cases in 2003, making it the leading cause of death among people 13–44 years old—is attributed to male resistance to condom use.
- **Attitudes about abortion**. Practiced but never openly discussed or acknowledged. Clinicians who need to discuss abortion with a patient must be particularly careful and sensitive, and may meet resistance. Women may hide the truth unless they have a trusting relationship with the clinician.
- **Attitudes about unwed sexual experimentation**. Although not condoned and people often do not admit to it, sexual activity outside of marriage is fairly common. Historically, common-law unions, visiting relationships, and having "outside" children were frequent occurrences. In visiting relationships, the man maintains, and lives with, a primary household/family and simultaneously establishes and helps maintain, financially, a second household/family with an "outside woman," whom he visits for sex.
- **Sexual orientation**. Homosexuality generally not accepted. Considerable shame associated with sex among lesbians and gay men. Most homosexuals are reluctant to reveal their sexual orientation to friends and family, fearing harassment, persecution, and unkind words.
- **Gender identity**. Little community and family tolerance for transgender identity or persons with ambiguous gender identity. Often a source of shame for families and likely to result in strained family relations. Members of same

gender feel extremely uncomfortable with such persons and tend to ridicule or harass them publicly.

- **Attitudes about menopause**. Menopause not openly discussed. "The change" is typically viewed as a natural phenomenon, part of the aging process. Women are more inclined to seek natural remedies and herbs than hormone replacement therapy to cope with discomforts such as hot flashes and mood swings.

FAMILY RELATIONSHIPS

- **Composition/structure**. Nuclear family, often including a widowed elderly parent, is customary. Very close ties maintained with members of extended family. The disapproved activities of individual family members generally bring shame to entire family.
- **Decision-making**. Men traditionally are the head of household and the source of power and decision-making. Increasingly, women (especially those employed outside the home) are sharing such power and participating in decision-making.
- **Spokesperson**. As head of the household, the man generally speaks for family. If a person is elderly and incapable of self-representation, an adult child generally takes over.
- **Gender issues**. Traditional male role in the family is that of provider, leader, and decision-maker. Traditional female role involves nurturing and caring for the family. These rigid roles are increasingly changing.
- **Changing roles among generations in U.S.** Roles tend to be less rigid today, as both partners work and bring money into household. In first-generation immigrant families, women still assume responsibility for most domestic chores and men help only if absolutely necessary. By the second generation, roles tend to parallel those in dominant American culture.
- **Caring roles**. Adult female—mother, daughter, or granddaughter—typically assumes the caring role in times of family illness. Sometimes, if no relatives are near or they cannot be there, a close family friend assumes caring role and comes to the house.
- **Expectations of and for children**. Good manners and respect for one's elders expected. Culturally, children are discouraged from expressing their views or speaking out; that is rude. "Children are to be seen and not heard" remains the primary motto for child-rearing. A good education and later a good job are very important and emphasized to children; they are expected to compete in school successfully. Poor families sacrifice their limited resources to pay for private lessons for their children.
- **Expectations of and for elders**. Expected to remain independent for as long as possible. Then they generally move in with an adult child and his/her family. Although treated with great respect, the elderly often are expected to help care for grandchildren. Placing elders in nursing homes not

widely practiced or accepted. Deeply ingrained in Caribbean culture is the belief that children are obliged to reciprocate their parents' and grandparents' kindness by caring for them when they no longer can safely care for themselves.

- **Expectations of hospital visitors**. Family and friends typically visit frequently. Those closest to the patient may take turns sleeping over to provide care during the night. If patient is not supposed to consume anything by mouth, family should be reminded not to bring meals from home, a common practice.

ILLNESS BELIEFS

- **Causes of/attitudes about physical illness**. Physical illness often attributed to the person's failure to properly care for him-/herself—e.g., not eating sufficiently nutritious foods, too much stress, insufficient sleep. Naturalistic explanations may include exposure to "germs" or cold air, causing one to "catch a draft." Supernatural explanations for illness, such as evil spirits or spells, are less prevalent today but still occur among less-educated and rural residents, both in Caribbean and U.S.
- **Causes of/attitudes about mental illness**. Mental illness still is highly stigmatized, almost never acknowledged or discussed, and is a source of shame for the entire family. Viewed as a weakness or inability to cope with worry and stress; less frequently, attributed to evil spirits or spell cast by someone. Denial often results in an unwillingness to accept psychotherapy and/or medications. Health care providers must strongly assure patients and families of confidentiality.
- **Causes of genetic defects**. Genetic defects in a child frequently perceived and explained as the work of God or as God's will for that family. Sometimes may be explained as an affliction from, or punishment by, God for parental sins.
- **Attitudes about disabilities**. Disability often viewed as a "defect," something to be ashamed of. Disabled persons less inclined to engage in social events, outings, etc. Nevertheless, families feel a responsibility "to care for their own" and are disinclined to institutionalize a disabled member. In U.S., employment outside the home may preclude this option.
- **Sick role**. Sick persons are expected to stay in bed and be cared for by relatives. Also expected to be fed nutritious foods to build up their resistance and body again.
- **Home and folk remedies**. Remain a significant and integral part of health care in West Indies. West Indians drink herbal teas, known locally as "bush tea," to prevent, control, and cure almost all "minor" ailments. Each ailment is assigned a plant, bush, leaf, flower, root, or bark. Choice and use of herbal teas, a form of folk medicine, is passed down from generation to generation by word of mouth. These choices vary among islands. West Indians also use

them when they think prescribed biomedical medication is not working, so there is a potential for drug interaction. If asked about their use of home remedies, patients generally disclose information to health professionals.

- **Medications**. When West Indians do take prescription medications, they tend to discontinue them as soon as symptoms disappear. Clinician should emphasize the importance of completing a course of medication and ask directly about herbal medications the patient is taking.

- **Acceptance of procedures**. In accordance with their respect for authority, most West Indians accept surgery, blood transfusions, organ transplants, and other suggested procedures deemed medically necessary.

- **Care-seeking**. Most Caribbeans begin with home remedies and herbal medications, and only seek medical attention when unable to perform daily tasks. Reliance on home remedies is largely responsible for advanced stages of disease when patients check into the health care system.

HEALTH ISSUES

- **Concept of health**. Define good health as absence of physical pain, ability to perform one's daily activities, and adequate weight, even if a person is overweight. In the West Indies, being thin is a negative condition often associated with disease. Very thin persons likely to be viewed as sick or even suspected of having tuberculosis or some other contagious disease, and are shunned.

- **Health promotion and prevention**. Promoting and maintaining good health associated with routinely eating well—large servings of heavy foods rich in carbohydrates. To prevent disease, few believe in or practice regular exercise, lowering sugar and salt content in foods, and lowering cholesterol level by eating fewer fatty foods.

- **Screening**. Annual physicals, Pap smears, mammograms, etc. not customary but accepted if suggested, especially in U.S. and if covered by health insurance. As very private people, West Indians are easily embarrassed and believe in keeping private matters strictly within the family. Do not readily disclose information about their sexual activity, history of STIs or any other contagious diseases, abortions, use of alternative medical treatments, or faith healing. In screening patients, clinician must discreetly ask about such matters.

- **Common health problems**. Incidence of hypertension, stroke, heart disease, and diabetes is relatively high among Caribbeans, similar to that among African Americans. HIV/AIDS has taken a stunning toll on this community in recent years.

DEATH RITUALS

- **Beliefs and attitudes about death**. This largely Christian society views death as the end of earthly life and strongly believes in the resurrection of the departed soul and an afterlife. For many others, the concept of death, what happens to people after death, and the power of the dead are veiled in superstition and mystery.

- **Preparation**. If a patient's prognosis is poor, he/she wants to be told the truth as soon as possible. When death is imminent, close friends and family want to gather at patient's bedside to pray and witness his/her passing. If there is little warning, surviving partner should be informed of the death as soon as possible, preferably in the presence of adult children/relatives.

- **Home vs. hospital**. Most families choose to care for the chronically ill/ dying person at home out of a sense of family obligation, loyalty, and respect. Because of work obligations, many immigrants cannot observe this cultural tradition and thus feel guilty. Hospice is an acceptable option but not perceived as a substitute for care provided by family.

- **Special needs**. Family members often request to view the body of the deceased in the hospital bed, as it was when the individual died. Clinician may offer to call a chaplain to meet with family, but most choose to be left alone with the deceased.

- **Care of the body**. Not customary for family to care for the body or prepare it for the mortuary. After death, hospital staff may take over.

- **Attitudes about organ donation**. Family members not likely to agree to donation. Maintaining integrity of the body is an important consideration in this culture, given the many myths surrounding death and the presumed afterlife. Clinician should approach family members discreetly regarding organ donation and make an extra effort not to pressure them.

- **Attitudes about autopsy**. Refuse autopsy, if not medically necessary, in order to maintain integrity of the body.

SELECTED REFERENCES

Bryce-Laporte, R. (1979). New York City and the new Caribbean immigration: A contextual statement. *International Migration Review, 13,* 214–233.

Garcia, J. (1986). Caribbean migration to the mainland: A review of adaptive experiences. *Annals of the American Academy of Political and Social Science, 487,* 114–125.

St. Hill, P. (2002). West Indians. In P. St. Hill, J. Lipson, & A. Meleis (Eds.), *Caring for women cross-culturally: A portable guide.* Philadelphia: F. A. Davis.

AUTHOR

Patricia F. St. Hill, RN, PhD, is an associate professor in the Hunter-Bellevue School of Nursing at the City University of New York. She was born in Trinidad but emigrated to the U.S. with her family in her early teens. She received her doctorate in nursing (community and cross-cultural health) from the University of California-San Francisco and a postdoctoral fellowship to study at the University of Washington-Seattle.

ACKNOWLEDGMENT

I wish to thank and acknowledge Hazel Holder, an undergraduate nursing student at the Hunter-Bellevue School of Nursing, who was born and raised in Trinidad, for corroborating the cultural material contained in this chapter.

CHAPTER 35

(FORMER) YUGOSLAVIANS

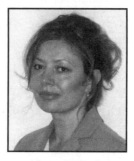

Alma Alikadic

CULTURAL/ETHNIC IDENTITY

- **Preferred term(s)**. A substantial number still call themselves Yugoslavs. Most refer to themselves by geographical origin, others by national identity (e.g., Albanian or Romanian). Very diverse—more than 25 nationalities and ethnic groups. Largest groups are Bosnians, Serbs, and Croats. Smaller groups include Slovenians, Macedonians, and Montenegrins.
- **Census**. The 2000 U.S. Census reports 545,000 former Yugoslavians, 234,000 of whom are foreign-born. Unofficial total is 1–3 million. Many did not specify their ancestry. Census does not include most recent refugees from Bosnia, Croatia, and Kosovo.
- **History of immigration**. Serbs and Croats have been coming to the U.S. since the 1820s. Accurate numbers are not available because the first arrivals often were mistakenly identified as Hungarians, Romanians, or Bulgarians. Slovenians and Macedonians immigrated throughout the 19th and 20th centuries for both economic and political reasons. Since 1993, more than 135,000 have arrived, including Macedonians, Montenegrins, Slovenians, Serbs, and Croats. Most were Bosnian refugees fleeing war; they typically spent 2–5 years in Croatia, Austria, or Germany before arriving in the U.S.

SPIRITUAL/RELIGIOUS ORIENTATION

- **Primary religious/spiritual affiliations**. Great religious diversity, but most Yugoslavs observe one of three religions. Orthodox Christians (49%) are dispersed throughout Serbia, Croatia, Montenegro, Bosnia-Herzegovina, and Macedonia. Roman Catholics (30%) live mainly in Croatia, Slovenia, Bosnia-Herzegovina, and Serbia; some reside in Montenegro. Muslims (10–12%) live mainly in Bosnia-Herzegovina, Kosovo, Macedonia, and Montenegro. The remaining 10% say they are "Yugoslavs," but most are Muslims. There are also Jews, Protestants, Methodists, Calvinists, and newer religious and spiritual orientations of Eastern origin.

- **Usual religious/spiritual practices**. Catholics pray, attend Sunday mass, take Holy Communion, and observe Christmas, Easter, and birthdays of major saints. Orthodox Christians celebrate the family patron saint, Orthodox Christmas, and Easter. Muslims observe the holy month of Ramadan and men say Friday's prayers in the mosque, but other Islamic practices vary among families. A significant number of Yugoslavs described themselves as "atheists" when communists were in power. Before the most recent war, people of different nationalities and religious backgrounds lived peacefully together, appreciating diversity and respecting one another. The war put an end to peaceful religious co-existence; instead, religious identity was used to politicize the population and turn people against each other. Bosnian communities in the U.S. organize large picnics that emphasize common (rather than religious) values and traditions, and that attract and reflect the diverse population of the former Yugoslavia.

- **Use of spiritual healing/healers**. Yugoslavs believe that faith and regular prayers help with illness and bring good health and good luck, but their priority is scientific biomedical treatment. They may call upon a priest to serve as spiritual healer when patient is receiving biomedical treatment or such treatment fails, although this is the exception rather than the rule.

- **Holidays**. Catholics and Orthodox Christians celebrate Christmas at different times, according to the Gregorian or Julian calendar. Families and friends visit and give gifts regardless of religious background. Orthodox families celebrate the family patron saint (*slava*). Muslims observe the month of Ramadan, which includes ritual fasting associated with the lunar calendar; it ends with three days of celebration (*Bajram*) during which families exchange visits and gifts. Almost every ethnic group celebrates New Year's. Another secular holiday is International Women's Day (March 8), marked by gifts and dinners for women, as was the practice in the former Yugoslavia.

COMMUNICATION
ORAL COMMUNICATION

- **Major languages and dialects**. Most spoke Serbo-Croatian in pre-war Yugoslavia; it was mandatory in all schools. After the republics gained independence, each named their language differently (e.g., Bosnian, Croatian, or Serbian). Nevertheless, Serbo-Croatian is mutually intelligible. Other languages include Slovenian, Macedonian, Albanian, Hungarian, Italian, and Slovakian. Most newer immigrants speak some English; many educated persons are fluent in English and also speak other languages.

- **Greetings**. Prefer title and last name. Common to use title such as "Dr." even in informal communication to show respect for someone's professional background. Firm and friendly handshake. Family members and friends prefer first name. They greet each other with affection—women with a hearty hug and kiss on cheek. Greet elderly person using a term of respect, such as "Aunt" (*Teta*) or "Uncle" (*Čika*).

- **Tone of voice**. Yugoslavs are open and friendly, prone to making jokes, and quick to laugh. Tone of voice among both men and women generally is loud. Clinician must assess emotional status by observing facial expressions and gestures rather than tone of voice.
- **Direct or indirect style of speech**. Direct, open, and sincere. Answers may be brief or expansive. Rarely tell stories in response to questions.
- **Use of interpreters**. Highly prefer a professional interpreter. No specific requirements regarding gender or age. If interpreter unavailable, prefer a family member or close friend to interpret in person rather than through a telephone translation service. However, interpretation by family member or friend often is unreliable due to patient's reluctance to talk about sensitive topics. Misinterpretations and mistakes also possible if patient does not understand medical terminology, has little medical knowledge, or speaks limited English.
- **Serious or terminal illness**. Clinician should tell spouse or eldest child first as soon as prognosis is confirmed. Depending on education level and family dynamics, common for Yugoslavs to hide prognosis from patient as long as possible; they may ask clinician not to inform patient. Prognosis should never be discussed in patient's presence or at home. Close family members tend to keep diagnosis secret from members of extended family because they do not want to spread bad news. If patient learns first about terminal diagnosis, he/she may hide it from family as long as possible or tell only his/her spouse or eldest child.

WRITTEN COMMUNICATION

- **Literacy assessment**. Clinician should use interpreter. Printed forms and instructions must be translated for, and carefully explained to, patients who know little or no English. Some elderly immigrants are not completely literate in their mother tongue; interpreter may need to explain the printed and translated consent form.
- **Consents**. Reluctant to sign consents because consents were neither common nor legally required in the former Yugoslavia. If a family member translates consent, he/she may purposely fail to translate or explain possible risks and complications in order to shield patient from fear or anxiety. Reluctant to fill out advance directives; believe that thinking or talking about end of life invites disaster or that physician is concealing important, unpleasant information about patient's health.

NONVERBAL COMMUNICATION

- **Eye contact**. Direct. While discussing sexual, mental-health, or other sensitive topics, eye contact may be fleeting or patient may totally avoid it. Health care professionals should not wink at patient of opposite gender; it is perceived as flirting.

- **Personal space**. Close between family members and friends. Keep strangers at a distance—about 3 feet or more—as Northern European Americans do.
- **Use and meaning of silence**. Varies among individuals and depends on the situation and the issue being discussed. Could mean embarrassment, approval, disagreement, disappointment, or protest. But Yugoslavs usually verbalize their thoughts; silence is of secondary importance in communication.
- **Gestures**. Common, as in most European cultures. Both men and women use hand gestures when speaking. Women are less expressive and open than men are. Rolling the eyes is a sign of disapproval and inappropriate. Inappropriate for women to sit with legs apart.
- **Openness in expressing emotions**. Though emotional, Yugoslavs are reluctant to express emotions; prefer to "keep it inside." Yugoslavian society is patriarchal: Men should not cry and women should not show anger or be overly talkative. With health care professionals, may be shy or embarrassed about expressing emotions.
- **Privacy**. Regardless of age, social status, or religious background, generally willing to share personal information with health care provider. Women are more cooperative than men are, but, because of embarrassment, they very rarely admit to domestic violence. Younger, acculturated generation similar to dominant U.S. culture.
- **Touch**. Most common form of touch is patting shoulder or lightly touching upper arm. In health care setting, best if clinician first announces and explains examination of private body parts.
- **Orientation to time**. More flexible about time than North Americans are. Usually not very late for appointments and expect tolerance if they are a few minutes late. Social time also is more flexible. May be oriented to the past, remembering "old times" (a favorite topic of conversation at social gatherings). Orientation to future reflected in Yugoslavs' emphasis on a good education and hopes of an easier life for their children. Many immigrants have incorporated American orientation to time.

ACTIVITIES OF DAILY LIVING

- **Modesty**. Most hospitalized patients bring their own robe and personal hygiene kit. Staff should ensure privacy during bathing. Women, especially those from rural areas, prefer female health care provider for gynecological exams.
- **Skin care**. Bathe daily if hospitalized. Some elderly patients use baby soap, lotion, and facial cream on the assumption they are mild and good for the skin. Otherwise, hygiene and use of beauty products vary among individuals. Men prefer to shave daily. Women of rural origin may shave pubic area before pelvic exam.

- **Hair care**. Cutting, styling, shampoos, and conditioners vary among individuals. Prefer neat hairdo. Younger persons wash hair daily. Some elderly wash hair once or twice weekly, believing that wet hair in windy or breezy weather can cause illness.
- **Nail care**. Men prefer short nails. Length and manicure vary among women. Some men keep the pinky nail longer as an expression of style. Toenails clean and short for men, sometimes longer and stylish for women.
- **Toileting**. Many prefer to wash genital area after toileting, especially after bowel movement. Wash hands frequently, especially after using toilet and before and after meals. Use bedside commode or bedpan if necessary; want privacy. May feel embarrassed but adjust to circumstances.
- **Special clothing or amulets**. In winter, some elderly patients wear thermal underwear. Some (but not many) wear religious amulets around their neck. Best if clinician asks permission to remove amulets. Some elderly women cover their hair with a scarf, especially if they lost a close family member in recent war. Occasionally tie red thread around baby's or toddler's wrist as protection from evil spells.
- **Self-care**. Close family members are caregivers. Yugoslavs believe that, by caring for ill family member, "God will bless and reward me for my good deeds." Expect and allow sick person to take sufficient time at home to recover completely, although patient may resist family care based on the attitude that "I've always been able to take care of myself." Hospitalized patients generally comply with all requests and actively perform self-care that may hasten recovery.

FOOD PRACTICES

- **Usual meal pattern**. Three meals a day. Late breakfast and dinner. Lunch is biggest meal, but many immigrants adjust to American lifestyle and work hours; for them, largest meal is at night, often as late as 9 or 10 o'clock. Serve coffee before breakfast and at around 5 p.m. Eat fruit, sweets, or simple sandwich as snacks, usually between lunch and dinner.
- **Special utensils**. None.
- **Food beliefs and rituals**. Prefer warm/hot cooked foods to cold or raw foods. Sometimes add spices. Believe that warm food tastes better and is healthier. To avoid getting sick, do not drink beverages from refrigerator after physical exertion or when body temperature is high. Never prepare meat with sweet dressing or gravy.
- **Usual diet**. Reflects a mixture of influences from Central Europe, the Balkans, the Mediterranean, and the Middle East. Immigrants tend to continue the eating habits they had back home. Biggest meal usually includes meat (any kind, including fish) with a starchy side dish and vegetables. Alternatives are filled pastries and salads or stuffed peppers, pasta, or roasted chicken with baked potato and vegetables. Want to consume soup daily, believing that "eating some-

thing with a spoon" each day is good for digestion. For breakfast and as a light dinner, elderly persons may prefer cheese, sour cream with bread or pastry, and fresh vegetables. Barbecued meat or fish, vegetables, and mushrooms popular for dinner, especially at social gatherings. Many Yugoslavs bake their own bread; the sugar in bread they purchase is odd to them.

- **Fluids**. Many do not drink enough water. Soft drinks and juices are favorites. Only adults drink coffee, at almost any time of day. Elderly persons like yogurt or a kind of buttermilk (*kefir*) served from the refrigerator. Children drink milk or cocoa in the morning and evening.

- **Food taboos and prescriptions**. Muslim and Jewish immigrants avoid eating pork and lard. Adults also avoid salami or hot dogs containing pork, but younger generation eats pepperoni pizza and hot dogs at school. Avoiding pork is a cross-cultural practice; many Yugoslavs of other religious beliefs also do not eat it for health reasons. Consume hot chicken soup and hot tea with honey and lemon to treat flu or cold. Believe that caramel milk eases the pain of sore throat and enables swallowing, and that lightly sweetened chamomile tea helps relieve stomach ache. Reduce cholesterol and blood pressure by consuming, on an empty stomach, fresh garlic or remedies made with garlic or other herbs soaked in alcohol.

- **Hospitality**. Extremely value hospitality. Having guests is a special occasion. Host always offers food, coffee, and choice of beverages and juices. Advanced meal preparation includes a variety of delicacies. Host serves guest first, often giving him/her the best piece of meat and a bigger/better piece of cake.

SYMPTOM MANAGEMENT

Comfortable with 0–10 scale but prefer to use words to describe pain or other symptom. Patient's numerical estimation often unreliable; needs a frame of reference and clarification. Clinician should ask patient to compare severity of his/her symptom with past severity.

- **Pain** (*bol*). Quite intolerant of pain. Few elderly persons accept pain as an inevitable consequence of aging. Younger persons impatient about learning cause of pain before taking medication. Hospitalized patients accept all types of analgesics or narcotics—via oral, IV, or rectal route—for intense or disabling pain. Communicate pain intensity mostly through facial expressions and/or in a qualitative rather than quantitative manner (e.g., by describing it as "throbbing pain" or "needle pain"). Fear sharp, sudden, intense pain the most; almost always go to emergency room. Dull, aching pain is less urgent, but they eventually report it. May not believe that pain is of musculoskeletal origin; think it comes from an internal organ "not working well." Women may be more willing to describe pain intensity, which may be their way of expressing depression and/or other emotional problems. Nonpharmacological remedies include hot compresses, a very warm shower, and cold compresses for headache.

- **Dyspnea** (*otežano disanje*). Consider dyspnea a very serious condition that requires immediate reporting, especially in a child. Describe it as "I cannot breathe" or "I'm going to die." Seek immediate medical attention on the assumption that it is a heart attack. Accept oxygen and any medication. Need strong assurance that dyspnea can be controlled to a certain degree.
- **Nausea/vomiting** (*mučnina/povraćanje*). Many attribute nausea/vomiting to excessive stomach acid. Report it and usually describe content of vomitus. Especially concerned if child vomits many times. Try to control nausea/vomiting with chamomile or other herbal tea before seeking help from health care provider. Accept rectal or IV medications.
- **Constipation/diarrhea** (*zatvor/proljev*). Try to control constipation with prune juice or yogurt. Accept laxatives. Report diarrhea, but elderly are embarrassed to mention it. Treat diarrhea with toast and unsweetened chamomile tea or rice cooked in water. Must be reminded to drink lots of fluids to avoid dehydration.
- **Fatigue** (*malaksalost*). Many say, "I feel tired all the time." Difficult to tell sometimes if fatigue is illness-related. Like to nap after lunch if circumstances allow. Generally reluctant to take pharmacologicals out of fear of addiction. Since the war, they are more willing to take medications.
- **Depression** (*depresija*). Very rarely recognize depression. Younger persons reluctantly admit "being depressed"; instead, they are more likely to complain about a physical symptom or be totally unaware of depression. Depression is somewhat taboo because Yugoslavs associate it with mental illness.
- **Self-care symptom management**. Tend to try herbal remedies, such as mint, chamomile tea, or chamomile tea warm compresses, and then herbs, such as *Althaea radix*, before seeking medical help. May delay seeking help out of fear the doctor might find "something wrong." Nevertheless, seek medical help when in pain. Hospitalized patients comply with any recommended activity for recovery, such as ambulation after surgery. Involvement of family members in activities of daily living varies. They may bring homemade food or help with bathing, based on the cultural importance of unconditional caring for sick family member. Chronically ill patients prefer self-care rather than dependence on family member. For example, most diabetic patients do their own blood testing or keep a blood-pressure diary. However, patients may need to be encouraged to manage their diet or to exercise.

BIRTH RITUALS/CARE OF THE NEW MOTHER AND BABY

- **Pregnancy care**. Pregnant women receive special attention. They are discouraged from carrying heavy loads and encouraged to get lots of sleep, eat well, and consume plenty of milk and yogurt for calcium. They satisfy food cravings. Moderate activity encouraged as due date approaches. Sexual intercourse inappropriate in late pregnancy. Childbirth preparation classes available in the former Yugoslavia; in U.S., younger, less-traditional couples attend them.

- **Preferences for children**. Families strongly desire a male child if they have more than one girl. Strongly believe that it is good to have at least one girl because she will care for elderly parents. Typical number of children is two, but the preferred number and gender vary. Avoid baby showers, believing that it is not wise to push one's luck by giving gifts before baby is born.

- **Labor practices**. Overall, laboring women are prepared for and tolerate pain but are expected to voice their suffering. In the former Yugoslavia, women in larger cities and better hospitals received epidural. In U.S., accept and appreciate epidural. Many women express their desire to have only medical staff present in labor room, fearing that husband might faint. Younger generation accepts father's presence.

- **Role of the laboring woman during birth**. Active. In home country, two trained midwives and an obstetrician guide laboring woman through birth.

- **Role of the father and other family members during birth**. Father usually waits in hospital to hear the happy news. Until recently in the former Yugoslavia, father was not allowed in labor room. Other family members wait at home. After baby is born, close family members and relatives have a small celebration.

- **Vaginal vs. cesarean section**. Prefer vaginal delivery. Accept C-section if medically indicated. In U.S., most Yugoslavs think that one day of postpartum care in hospital is much too short after vaginal birth. Women are accustomed to staying in hospital for 7–10 days in case baby develops jaundice.

- **Breastfeeding**. Popular and advocated. Advise new mothers to breastfeed as long as possible—even after baby begins eating solid food. Uncommon to breastfeed in public. If new mother must return to work, she is likely to pump breast milk.

- **Birth recuperation**. Usually 40 days to six weeks, during which time others help care for new mother and baby. They usually give her soup containing meat and other foods "stronger" in calories, such as cow's milk and yogurt, so she will have enough breast milk to feed baby. New mother avoids gas-producing vegetables, such as cabbage or beans, believing that they give baby abdominal cramps. Mother and baby usually stay indoors for the first 40 days; visitors other than family members discouraged. Younger generation has adopted U.S. practices of taking newborn outside on the second or third day and completely caring for baby beginning at birth.

- **Baby care**. Traditionally, grandmother on either side takes care of baby for 4–6 weeks, after which help is provided as needed.

- **Problems with baby**. Clinician should carefully give bad news to parents first, then to grandparents on both sides. Most common reaction is silent resignation and withdrawal for a period of time. Yugoslavs usually do not discuss problems with members of extended family.

- **Male and female circumcision**. Typically, Muslim and Jewish boys are circumcised five days to one month after birth. Sometimes older boys are circumcised. Circumcision performed in hospital on parents' request. Female circumcision never practiced.

DEVELOPMENTAL AND SEXUAL ISSUES

- **Celebration of menarche or becoming a man**. No particular celebrations. Daughter usually tells mother she has begun menstruating; unnecessary to tell father or others. Male adolescent may discuss puberty with father.
- **Attitudes about birth control**. Acceptable among married and unmarried couples in the former Yugoslavia. However, rural persons rarely use birth control, except early withdrawal (the "natural" way). Most sexually active persons in U.S. use some kind of birth control. Most common is condom, while married couples prefer intrauterine device or birth control pills. Some use interrupted intercourse or calendar method.
- **Attitudes about sexually transmitted infection (STI) control, including condoms**. Sexually active singles are cautious; most know about HIV and other diseases. Younger persons protect themselves against STIs, most commonly with condoms. Married couples are unconcerned about acquiring STI from partner and almost totally indifferent if partner has hepatitis B or C.
- **Attitudes about abortion**. Receptive to it. View abortion as a way to control family size. Religious beliefs prevent some women from having abortion. Rural women usually keep baby.
- **Attitudes about unwed sexual experimentation**. Practice and accept it. Somewhat taboo to discuss women's sexual activity. Men discuss their unwed sexual activity with their closest friends. Yugoslavs believe that men should not marry without previous sexual experience.
- **Sexual orientation**. Strongly averse to homosexuality. Consider traditional family sacred. Gays and lesbians typically conceal their sexual orientation; if it becomes public, others avoid or dislike them, and family members and friends may disown them. Within the last decade in the former Yugoslavia, gays and lesbians have begun to organize and express their orientation openly, especially after some public figures disclosed their sexual orientation.
- **Gender identity**. Expect gender norms. Reserved toward persons with ambiguous gender identity, who rarely are seen in public. Parents strongly disapprove if child's behavior is not in accordance with his/her birth gender.
- **Attitudes about menopause**. Accept it as part of life and aging. No special preparations or treatments. Women talk with health care provider about relief for hot flashes and insomnia. Female family members and friends discuss symptoms and problems. In the former Yugoslavia, women reluctant to take hormonal therapy, fearing excessive weight gain.

FAMILY RELATIONSHIPS

- **Composition/structure**. Consider family the core of life stability, happiness, and caring. Spend much time with members of nuclear and extended families. Extended-family members important, but they do not receive unconditional attention and help. Husband and wife share income and usually hold a joint bank account.

- **Decision-making**. In this patriarchal society, father/husband makes decisions, but decision-making varies by urban or rural origin. Urban couples may make mutual decisions, yet husband's influence is undeniable and he has the last word. Immigrants from the former Yugoslavia wary of involvement by social service agency in family matters, believing that parents (particularly father) are best suited to deal with family problems and circumstances.

- **Spokesperson**. Father is spokesperson regarding matters outside the home. Mother is in charge inside the home and, in husband's absence, outside.

- **Gender issues**. Since the 1970s, women have taken an active role in financially supporting the family, in contrast to earlier years when they were totally submissive to husband. Yugoslavs still expect women to keep house neat and clean, prepare fresh meals almost daily, and care for children. Middle-age and older immigrant couples maintain traditional gender roles, except that women work outside the home for economic survival, sometimes taking two jobs. Men may hold two jobs in order to provide for the family. Role changes forced by acculturation have caused some couples to separate, divorce, or face interventions by child-protection or domestic-violence agencies.

- **Changing roles among generations in U.S.** Older immigrants have same living habits they had in the former Yugoslavia. The middle generation (those in their 30s or 40s) are caught between adopting the American way of thinking and preserving the traditional way. Intergenerational struggles frequent.

- **Caring roles**. Women generally care for children and sick family members. If elderly sick person lives with son and needs care, daughter-in-law assumes care-giving responsibilities.

- **Expectations of and for children**. Expect children to avoid extremes of behavior. Value and advocate modesty and good behavior among children. Expect children to work hard at school, and to commit to and complete school assignments promptly. Generally encourage sports and other after-school activities. Newer immigrant parents strongly push their children to complete higher education to compensate for what the parents and children lost during war in the former Yugoslavia.

- **Expectations of and for elders**. Respect elderly persons and often seek their advice. Elderly usually live with their children, especially if widowed. Yugoslavs expect the elderly to help with household chores or babysit if adult children work. Shameful to place elderly person in nursing home, which demonstrates a lack of love and caring. However, that attitude has changed recently in the former Yugoslavia, where people take advantage of nursing homes when necessary. The elderly, particularly the most recent immigrants who came to U.S. in old age, usually tell their children where they want to be buried. Most want their body returned to country of birth for funeral and burial.

- **Expectations of hospital visitors**. Expect family members (spouse and/or children) to visit daily; they do not stay overnight unless patient asks them to. Family members usually bring homemade food and help patient shave or bathe.

ILLNESS BELIEFS

- **Causes of/attitudes about physical illness**. Natural causes include imbalances in daily living, such as poor eating habits, cold weather and wind, dirty or contaminated environment, too much stress, trying too hard to make a decent living, and, recently, war-related circumstances. Supernatural causes include God's punishment for not living a decent and moral life. Older persons may believe that illness is an inevitable consequence of aging and that, in any case, everyone leaves the world eventually.
- **Causes of/attitudes about mental illness**. Mental illness highly stigmatized. Mentally ill persons deemed less worthy than physically ill persons. Clinicians should exercise caution regarding diagnoses, including post-traumatic stress disorder. Yugoslavs may believe that mental illness is a special kind of punishment for improper lifestyle, as if one deserves it. Some think that mental illness runs in the family. In the last 5–10 years, Yugoslavs have realized the devastating impact that persecution, witnessing atrocities, and other events related to war in the former Yugoslavia (particularly Bosnia) had on mental health. They accept and explain post-traumatic stress and other acquired disorders in that context. Immigrants/refugees acknowledge that many among them have mental or emotional disorders as a consequence of war. Many Bosnians have sought professional help. Very few immigrants are diagnosed with serious mental illness. Families that have a seriously mentally ill member may feel shame and may fear the reactions of others.
- **Causes of genetic defects**. Fatalistically view them as God's will. Also attribute defects to extreme shock or stress during mother's pregnancy. Some families that have a disabled child live normally, providing undivided love and attention. Other families may feel shame and guilt, and live in isolation.
- **Attitudes about disabilities**. Do not discriminate against disabled persons. Some pity them. View disability as God's will. In most cases, families that have a disabled member take good care of him/her. Some families feel shame and guilt, and tend to isolate themselves.
- **Sick role**. Spouse or other close family member cares for sick person, providing much attention and caring. Usually expect patient to be passive, rest a lot, and eat appropriate food. Patients usually are not demanding. Yugoslavs generally do not expect women who are sick to do usual housework.
- **Home and folk remedies**. Use herbal remedies for illness or regularly for health maintenance. Drink chamomile tea for cold and flu symptoms, and often for stomach problem and indigestion. Also take baking powder mixed with lemon juice and water for indigestion and excessive stomach acid.

Believe that other herbal remedies "purify the blood" and lower cholesterol and blood pressure. Garlic, onion, and beet juice are thought to have great healing power; drink beet juice to treat cancer. For sore throat, use honey or apply compresses made with special brandy (*slivovitz*). Olive oil relieves sunburn and improves hair quality. Apply yogurt to burns to ease pain. Put sliced potato on forehead for headache. Soak socks in vinegar to reduce fever. Yugoslavs commonly use, share, and recommend these home remedies and many other special recipes.

- **Medications**. Former Yugoslavians use Western biomedical standards of compliance. Some persons do not understand the nature of illness and skip a treatment or take medicine only when they think they need to. Some use home remedies and receive biomedical treatment simultaneously.
- **Acceptance of procedures**. Accept procedures such as IVs, drawing of blood, transfusions, and surgery. Accept organ transplants without prejudice for donor's gender, age, or religion. Some elderly persons refuse surgery that could save their life because they think they have lived long enough, fear surgery risks, or place their destiny in God's hands.
- **Care-seeking**. If symptoms not too severe, Yugoslavs (especially elders) likely to try home remedies first. Prefer biomedical care to spiritual healers, whom they might consult regarding terminal disease or mental illness.

HEALTH ISSUES

- **Concept of health**. Good health is the most valuable treasure one can have. It is practically a synonym for happiness and joy in life, a relaxed state of mind, and endless possibilities for life achievement. Yugoslavs value and appreciate good health more when they begin to lose it or observe someone's struggle with illness. Older or chronically ill persons often tell others who face a dramatic life change after diagnosis, "Everything is good as long as you are healthy."
- **Health promotion and prevention**. Middle-age and older persons unenthusiastic about health promotion and prevention, which, until recently, were mostly neglected by the former Yugoslavia's highly sophisticated biomedical system. Yugoslavs commonly take action after illness has appeared; may seek medical care only when very sick. Promote health by eating lots of fruit and vegetables, and lean cuts of meat. May quit smoking after multiple counseling sessions or after clinician informs patient he/she has lung disease. May monitor diet if blood cholesterol is very high. For Yugoslavs, exercise is a half-hour walk or brief gardening. Younger persons have better understanding of, and are more likely to practice, prevention.
- **Screening**. Screening nonexistent in the former Yugoslavia. Common attitude is that one is better off not knowing too much about his/her health, so Yugoslavs generally avoid routine medical exams. Generally keep appointments for blood-pressure or diabetes check-up. Women do not undergo regu-

lar breast exams. Depending on age and education level, women may be under-educated about importance of annual Pap smear. Attitude regarding referrals for Pap smear, mammogram, or prostate screening is, "I do not have any problems with that." Need to be aggressively educated about the importance of dental checks and oral hygiene. Depending on education level, younger generation is more compliant with, and has some knowledge of, screening.

- **Common health problems**. Elevated blood pressure, hypercholesterolemia, diabetes, obstructive lung disease, arthritis, and rheumatic pain. Numerous Yugoslavs suffer from post-traumatic stress disorder, uncontrolled anxiety, or other mental health problems, mostly as a consequence of war. High percentage of immigrants are heavy smokers. Alcohol abuse not uncommon among males.

DEATH RITUALS

- **Beliefs and attitudes about death**. View it as an inevitable but frightening event. Grieve for a long time after someone dies. Some families are inconsolable; do not even seek spiritual comfort. Others accept the death of a loved one and live a quiet life with the stamp of grief on their face. Almost fatalistic, which makes death somewhat easier to accept. Yugoslavs accept life support; decision about whether to halt it depends on factors such as patient's situation, prognosis, and spiritual beliefs.
- **Preparation**. When it becomes obvious patient is dying, clinician should inform spouse and children before notifying anyone else. Sometimes adult children prefer to be notified first; then they very cautiously inform patient's spouse. Some families bring priest into hospital room for patient's last confession or comfort. Clinician should never summon priest without first consulting family.
- **Home vs. hospital**. In recent years in the former Yugoslavia, the most seriously or critically ill or dying persons have been taken to hospital for help or pain relief; thus, many die there. Some older persons prefer to die at home and therefore refuse hospitalization. Immigrants may prefer to take terminally ill person to hospital.
- **Special needs**. Entire nuclear and extended families present. Summon priest as soon as death occurs or when death obviously is imminent. Priest also gives a spiritual and comforting speech at funeral and attends family gathering and common meal afterward. Close friends and neighbors included; sometimes a close friend of deceased gives speech. Immigrants also observe these customs, depending on their finances and family dynamics.
- **Care of the body**. Family members, priest, or sometimes a specially designated person washes body. Muslims wash body and wrap it in a white cotton sheet. Christians dress the deceased. Show body before funeral so everyone can pay their last respects.
- **Attitudes about organ donation**. Reluctant to donate organs. Donation

ruins the body's integrity, a view probably related to the spiritual and religious belief in "life after life." Clinician should ask immediate family members about donating organs, waiting until after family deals with the initial shock. Recently, educated Yugoslavs have become more receptive to organ donation. They view it from the perspective of not knowing what life may bring, recognizing that they themselves or a family member may need a transplant someday.

- **Attitudes about autopsy**. Acceptable if fully explained to members of immediate family and there is a reasonable necessity. Family may request autopsy to resolve legal disputes between family members.

SELECTED REFERENCES

Bigby, J. (Ed.). (2003). *Cross-cultural medicine*. Philadelphia: American College of Physicians and American Society of Internal Medicine.

Kemp, C., & Rasbridge, L. (2003). Refugee health ~ immigrant health: Bosnians. Retrieved June 1, 2004, from http://www3.baylor.edu/~Charles_Kemp/bosnian_refugees.htm

Lipson, J., Weinstein, H., Gladstone, E., & Sarnoff, R. (2003). Bosnian and Soviet refugees' experiences with health care. *Western Journal of Nursing Research, 25,* 854–871.

Weinstein, H., Lipson, J., Sarnoff, R., & Gladstone, E. (1999). Rethinking displacement: Bosnians uprooted in Bosnia and California. In J. Lipson & L. A. McSpadden (Eds.), *Negotiating power and place at the margins: Selected papers on refugees and immigrants* (vol. 7, pp. 53–74). Arlington, VA: American Anthropological Association.

AUTHOR

Alma Alikadic holds a degree in teaching English and German, and also has completed two years of university-level law school in Croatia, where she was born. In 1996, she came to the U.S. as a refugee with her husband and two children. The Santa Clara Valley Medical Center in San Jose, CA, immediately hired her as a Bosnian language translator/interpreter. When Santa Clara County's Refugee Clinic opened in 1998, she became a full-time community worker. She translates written health-education materials and clinic brochures, and interprets for patients during medical appointments, including taking medical histories and providing health education. Alikadic also does community outreach and she interviews refugees and asylees. She just became a U.S. citizen.

OTHER UCSF NURSING PRESS TITLES

WOMEN'S PRIMARY HEALTH CARE: PROTOCOLS FOR PRACTICE, 2ND EDITION
STAR, LOMMEL, SHANNON
ISBN 0-943671-21-3

AMBULATORY OBSTETRICS, 3RD EDITION
STAR, SHANNON, LOMMEL, GUTIERREZ
ISBN 0-943671-18-3

SURGERY: A PATIENT'S GUIDE FROM DIAGNOSIS TO RECOVERY
MAILHOT, BRUBAKER, SLEZAK
ISBN 0-943671-19-1

MANAGING THE SIDE EFFECTS OF CHEMOTHERAPY AND RADIATION THERAPY
DODD
ISBN 0-943671-20-5

NURSE PRACTITIONER/PHYSICIAN COLLABORATIVE PRACTICE: CLINICAL GUIDELINES FOR AMBULATORY CARE
COLLINS-BRIDE, SAXE
ISBN 0-943671-17-5

ASSESSING & MANAGING COMMON SIGNS & SYMPTOMS: A DECISION-MAKING APPROACH FOR HEALTH CARE PROVIDERS
LOMMEL, JACKSON
ISBN 0-943671-16-1

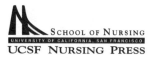

SCHOOL OF NURSING
UNIVERSITY OF CALIFORNIA, SAN FRANCISCO
UCSF NURSING PRESS

For order inquiries, contact:
UCSF NURSING PRESS
521 Parnassus Avenue, Room N535C
San Francisco, CA 94143-0608
Phone: (415) 476-4992 – Fax: (415) 476-6042
http://nurseweb.ucsf.edu/www/books.htm